CRITICAL CARE
NURSING

A
Physiologic
Approach

LINDA ABELS, R.N., M.S.N.

Adjunct Assistant Professor, School of Nursing,
Indiana University, Indianapolis, Indiana

with 156 illustrations

THE C. V. MOSBY COMPANY

ST. LOUIS · TORONTO · PRINCETON · 1986

MOSBY

A TRADITION OF PUBLISHING EXCELLENCE

Editor: Barbara Ellen Norwitz
Developmental editor: Sally Adkisson
Project editor: Suzanne Seeley
Manuscript editor: Kathy Corbett Hickman
Book design: Kay M. Kramer
Production: Kathy Burmann

Printed in the United States of America

The C.V. Mosby Company
11830 Westline Industrial Drive, St. Louis, Missouri 63146

Library of Congress Cataloging-in-Publication Data

Critical care nursing.

  Includes bibliographies and index.
   1. Intensive care nursing. 2. Human physiology.
I. Abels, Linda Feiwell, 1946-   . [DNLM: 1. Critical
Care—nurses' instruction. WY 154 C9329]
RT120.I5C745   1986   616'.028   86-5156
ISBN 0-8016-0083-9

A/VH/VH   9   8   7   6   5   4   3   2   1   01/D/005

Contributors

ANN BELCHER, R.N., M.N.
Assistant Professor, School of Nursing, Indiana University,
Indianapolis, Indiana

JOANN BROOKS-BRUNN, R.N., M.S.N., CCRN
Department of Medical Research, Methodist Hospital,
Indianapolis, Indiana

DEBRA GREENSPAN, R.N., M.S.N.
Clinical Nurse Specialist, Critical Care Units, Touro Infirmary,
New Orleans, Louisiana

ROSEMARY HUME, R.N., M.S.N.
Manager, Human Resource Development,
St. Vincent's Hospital and Health Care Center, Indianapolis, Indiana

MARY ROPKA, R.N., M.S.
Formerly Instructor of Nursing, School of Nursing,
University of Virginia, Charlottesville, Virginia

BARBARA RUSSO, R.N., M.S.N.
Director of Surgical Nursing and Former Coordinator of Critical Care Units,
St. Vincent's Hospital, Indianapolis, Indiana

JAMES SZWED, M.D.
Community Hospital of Indianapolis,
Indianapolis, Indiana

CHERYLL WODNIAK, R.N., M.S.N.
Indiana University, Indianapolis, Indiana

To my husband, Jon,
who has been supportive throughout my professional career;

To my children, Michelle, Benji, Matthew, and Bethie,
who patiently put up with a part-time mother on many occasions;

To my mother and father,
who gave me the courage to tackle the unattainable.

Preface

This comprehensive text utilizes a physiologic approach to review multisystem problems commonly seen in critical care. It serves as a reference for the critical care practitioner and other members of the acute-care health team. The text will also be of value in baccalaureate and graduate nursing programs, as well as in critical care orientation and continuing education courses.

The book is comprised of eight major units: Psychophysiology, Circulation, Respiration, the Nervous System, Fluid and Electrolytes, Alimentation, Coagulation, and Thermoregulation.

Each unit is organized systematically and includes a description of the following:

Developmental anatomy (embryology)
Physiologic review
Complete physical assessment
Synopsis of pathophysiology
Summary of current therapeutic modalities

The discussion of *developmental anatomy* is limited to information that will facilitate an understanding of the beginnings of life and the changes that occur during development. Such knowledge is essential to recognize the relationship between body structure and function.

The *physiologic review* is a study of mammalian functional systems. It describes anatomic, physiologic, and biochemical principles that are integral to the regulation of body activities.

Throughout the text, emphasis has been placed on those homeostatic mechanisms essential to the functional operation of each system. An exception is Unit 4, in which the nervous system is approached regionally.

Physical assessment is also described systematically. It consists of pertinent historical, physical, and laboratory data. Particular attention is directed to those concepts most applicable to critical care.

A *pathophysiologic analysis* is made of each symptom presented in the history. A concerted effort has been made to describe symptomatic rather than specific disease pathology.

In regard to the *therapeutic modalities* presented, both independent and dependent interventions are reviewed. Treatment protocols include pharmacologic, nutritional, and rehabilitative regimens. Current research is cited where applicable.

Acknowledgments

Many people have assisted in the preparation of this text. I am deeply grateful to all the nurses, professors, and physicians who have critiqued the manuscript and offered numerous suggestions. My illustrator, Karen Chevalier Smith, deserves a special thank-you for her creative artwork. In addition, this book would never have been completed without my babysitter, Carolyn Robertson, who has been loyal and reliable in rain, sleet, or snow, and without my typist, Joyce Lovelady, who typed, retyped, and retyped again and became as good a medical secretary as a legal secretary.

Linda Abels

Contents

CRITICAL CARE
NURSING

A
Physiologic
Approach

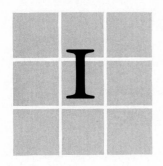

I Psychophysiology

DEBRA GREENSPAN

The evolution of critical care units has occurred rapidly over the past 29 years in response to the dramatic increase in available medical technology and subsequent role change among nurses. These factors have resulted in constantly improving critical patient care for urban and rural people regardless of socioeconomic conditions.

Florence Nightingale recognized that the critically ill patient needed to have more hours of direct nursing intervention. She recommended that patients be assigned beds according to the severity of their illness, with the most ill patients located closest to the nursing station. This method of bed allocation persisted for nearly 85 years with rare exception. In the ward environment, nurses and physicians experienced gross limitations in their ability to provide critically ill patients with lifesaving emergency measures, including readily available oxygen, suction, treatment room facilities, and specialized physician and nursing staff care. In 1923 a few farsighted thinkers at Johns Hopkins University Hospital realized the inadequacies of this system and developed a three-bed special care unit for the neurosurgical patient.

This unit was designed to provide round-the-clock qualified patient care using house staff and "specially trained" nurses. It must be realized that at this time in history, the role of the nurse was extremely limited, which can be attributed to the role of women in American and

European societies of that era. Women were to be protected from the horrors of death and destruction. They were perceived as feeble-minded, nymphlike beings incapable of handling the challenge of providing rational and scientifically based patient care to the critically ill. Consequently, the role of the specially trained nurse working in a special care area did not flourish until the onset of World War II.

Historically, war has brought technologic advances to civilization. World War II was no exception. Modern medicine boomed, rising to meet the challenge of saving war casualties wounded no longer by swords but by technologically advanced explosive weaponry. There was a new demand to refine surgical techniques and to develop anesthetics (needed for longer and more complicated surgical procedures) and antiinfective agents. Medical practitioners soon realized that they were too busy to provide bedside patient care and medical-surgical interventions simultaneously. Immediate postoperative patients required intensive monitoring and observation for at least 24 hours. Here was nursing's opportunity to demonstrate the valuable and necessary role of the specially trained nurse: a nurse who used her eyes, ears, and hands, as well as a highly trained intellect, to provide scientifically based nursing care to the recovering surgical patient. This need to care for postsurgical patients brought forth the concept of a recovery room—a special care unit designed to

Table 1-1. Potential stressors affecting the human organism

Intrapersonal	Body image
	Environment
	Control/power
	Awareness
	Perception/feelings
Interpersonal	Interactional patterns
	Culture
	Socioeconomic patterns
Biologic	Physical disruption of body processes
	Pain
	Decreased mental functioning (such as hypoperfusion)

provide immediate postoperative care, using the latest technology and a well-educated nursing staff. A recovery room made it unnecessary for operating rooms to hold unstable patients, which had been the practice in years past, and made maximum use of available medical, nursing, and auxiliary personnel in short supply.

With the 1950s came new bridges to be crossed by medicine and nursing. Poliomyelitis had reached worldwide epidemic proportions, with thousands of adults and children requiring respiratory-assist devices and intensive nursing care. Concurrently, cardiothoracic surgery had entered a new era, with refinement of intraoperative membrane oxygenation techniques. Children and adults with acquired and congenital heart defects, often living in faraway countries, were seizing the opportunity to live a more normal life by traveling to medical centers that performed the surgeries they needed. Therefore the need for critical care units became obvious in the medical center environment during the early 1950s. Out of this need arose the concepts of intensive and progressive patient care units as we know them today.

Oddly enough, however, it was the community hospital that became the pioneer in designing and implementing special care facilities. In the autumn of 1953 Manchester Memorial Hospital in Manchester, Connecticut opened a four-bed progressive care unit. This was followed by the establishment of an eight-bed critical care unit at North Carolina Memorial Hospital, in Chapel Hill, North Carolina, in January of 1954 and a six-bed critical care unit at Chestnut Hill Hospital in Philadelphia in May, 1954. By February of 1957 there were 20 hospitals in the United States with critical care units, and by May, 1958, there were nearly 150 such units. The concept of intensive care units with specially trained nurses and physicians had come to fruition.

During the 1970s, the term *ICU,* or *intensive care unit,* was gradually replaced with the term *critical care unit,* an umbrella phrase that includes all types of special care units, not just the postsurgical ICU. By 1979, virtually all hospitals had at least one critical care unit.

The challenge of the 1960s and 1970s was represented by an increasing degree of specialization within the medical community. With the accelerated development of new technologies, it was soon necessary to subspecialize ICUs; cardiovascular, renal, coronary, and respiratory ICUs were therefore created, matching nursing expertise with patient needs.

Beginning in the early 1970s, however, nurses became acutely aware that the recovery room design for critical care units was not conducive to the psychologic well-being of patients, their families, or staff members. The recovery room design allocated bedspace in an open ward environment, providing a small number of nurses with a great deal of visibility and ready access to patients. This concept did not consider the impact on patients of noise, lack of privacy, limited personal space, observing other patients during emergency situations, and other environmental stressors on psychologic health. In addition, the role that psychologic health plays in promoting the physical recovery of the patient was not considered. Concomitantly, the effect of this environment on critical care unit staff was not recognized. Indeed, nurses had now been given an opportunity to use their intellect and assessment skills in providing special care to the critically ill, but what would be the cost? Research now points to factors such as noise, high nurse/patient ratios, lack of personal space (such as break areas), and chronic patients or patients who have extended hospitalizations in critical care units as factors that promote "burnout"—the end result of prolonged stress without adequate coping reserves.

An increasing number of institutions have recognized this problem and have designed their new critical care units with private or semiprivate rooms, each with an outside window and other features of normalcy such as clocks, private or semiprivate bathrooms, and wall calendars. This environment appears to foster a higher level of patient and staff morale by limiting the impact of the previously mentioned stress-producing factors.

In a short 30 years, the critical care unit has gone from taking its first "baby steps" to running a multibillion dollar race between technology and disease. There have been many transformations in the environmental design of the critical care unit, as well as in nurse-patient and nurse-physician relationships, that bring form to the concept of the critical care unit. Prolonged patient hospitalizations have been shown to have a profound effect on nurses and on the depth and intensity of their relationships with patients and family members. The challenge that confronts the critical care nurse of the 1980s does not require monetary investments or budget juggling in these troubled economic times; it does require a personal investment in patients, their families, and fellow staff members. The critical care nurse of the '80s must begin to look beyond the patient's infected abdominal wound or acute myocardial infarction and attempt to examine the longstanding conflicts, character traits, and social factors of patients and families.

Within the critical care environment, a dynamic relationship exists among the patient, family, and health care team. Each system is composed of three subsystems: (1) intrapersonal (feelings), (2) interpersonal (communication),

and (3) biologic (Table 1-1). Each system has its own sphere of influence with an inherent capacity to affect and be affected by other systems. Within the critical care unit, the patient *(A)*, family *(B)*, and health care team *(C)* function as three interdependent systems (Fig. 1-1).

This relationship can be affected by stress-producing factors within the environment, as well as by intrapersonal, interpersonal, and biologic factors. Unchecked, these factors can and do significantly alter normal physiologic processes. Environmental stressors are easier to identify and augment than intrapersonal and interpersonal stressors. Therefore the remainder of this chapter will concentrate on using the nursing process to support the mental health of critically ill patients and their families without depleting the coping reserves of the nurse.

PSYCHOPHYSIOLOGY
Stress theory: a biopsychosocial perspective

Humans have always been very curious about determining cause and effect relationships. However, the connection between the mind and the body has remained somewhat elusive in spite of enormous research efforts over the past 60 years. From experience, we all know this body-mind connection is real. When we perceive the feeling of fear or anger, our palms

---

Fig. 1-1. This model demonstrates the interrelatedness of the systems found in the critical care environment: the patient *(A)*, the family *(B)*, and the health care team *(C)*.

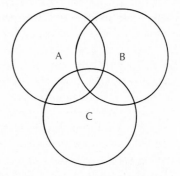

Table 1-2. Manifestations of stress

Affective	Motor-behavioral	Cognitive	Physiologic
Anxious	Agitation	Decreased attention	Increased heart rate and increased blood pressure
Depressed	Rapid movements	Selective inattention	Increased respiratory rate
Fearful	Crying	Joking	Cool extremities (peripheral vasoconstriction)
Joyful	Wringing hands	Altered judgment	Pupil dilation
Angry	Lip smacking	Delusions	Sweaty palms

may begin to sweat and we may have heart palpitations. At times, the physical reaction may precede our conscious awareness of the feeling.

Selye[55] defines stress as a specific syndrome that consists of all the nonspecifically induced changes within a biologic system. This consistent physiologic response is noted to produce both short- and long-term changes in body functions. Enhanced sympathetic tone and adrenal stimulation mark the activation of the body's defenses and are detectable very early in the stress response. With prolonged stress, long-term changes such as shrinkages of lymphatic organs, gastrointestinal ulcers, and loss of body weight may be seen.

Lazarus' theory of stress[43] augments Selye's concepts by justifying a mental appraisal of a stimulus. Lazarus defines stress as anything that is cognitively appraised to be threatening to the body or its ego structure; this may be merely the anticipation of a future confrontation with harm. The potency of the threat is relative to its imminence and the availability of adequate coping resources. The manifestations of stress, often called stress reactions or responses, become a product of the transaction between a person and a stimulus. It is therefore necessary to account for factors influencing the stimulus configuration and the psychologic makeup of the person when making an assessment of stress and coping. There are numerous manifestations of stress; these manifestations can be classified as affective, motor-behavioral, cognitive, or physiologic (Table 1-2).

The fight vs flight response, as described by

Cannon[10] and popularized by Selye,[55] postulates that humans have an inherent capacity to survive in the presence of stressful stimuli by either avoiding the stimulus or by organizing the body's defenses to fight. The latter response is characterized by the General Adaptation Syndrome (GAS), a term coined by Selye, which outlines the physiologic response of the body to stress in three stages: (1) alarm, the initial stage during which the body's defensive forces such as adrenal stimulation are mobilized; (2) resistance, the second stage that reflects the adaptive efforts of the body; and (3) exhaustion, which occurs when adaptational energies are fully expended and ineffective in reducing the stress, with the result being death.

The elicitation of the alarm reaction in response to actual or perceived threat produces both hypothalamic- and humoral-mediated responses. As early as 1914, Cannon[10] described the humoral or adrenal medullary response to pain and major emotions as a sympathomimetic response to catecholamines. Alterations identified by Cannon included "a cessation of the activities of the alimentary canal, a notable shifting of the circulation from the great vessels of the abdomen to the lungs, heart, limbs, and central nervous system, an increased cardiac vigor, and an augmentation of the sugar content of the blood."[10] Manning and Piess[48] showed that a vagotomized cat, unable to respond to circulating catecholamines, responded to direct hypothalamic stimulation with a remarkably augmented force of myocardial contraction and lesser degrees of vasoconstriction and cardiac acceleration. Manning and Piess have suggested that the hypothalamus, along with the reticular activating system (RAS), mediate a barrage of parasympathetic and sympathetic stimuli that contribute to increased ventricular automaticity and increased frequency of sinoatrial discharge. The alarm response, whether it be hypothalamic- or humoral-mediated, produces psychophysiologic responses including increased heart rate (tachycardia), blood pressure, respiratory rate, oxygen consumption, and increased myocardial excitability, as well as sweating, peripheral vasoconstriction, nervousness, and increased skeletal muscle tone—all of which contribute to an increased metabolic demand. Survival depends on successful adaptation to this increased metabolic demand. The hypothalamic-mediated response to stress is merely postulated in humans because of obvious research limitations. Therefore the alarm response is most easily measured by the amount of serum catecholamines in the body and directly affects the intensity of the autonomic reaction.

The adaptational response of the resistance phase of the GAS is the body's attempt to preserve vital processes while minimizing the impact of the stressor. The body accomplishes this by optimizing the functions of essential organs such as the heart, lungs, and brain while concomitantly "shutting down" nonessential functions. During this stage the body adapts to the compensating mechanisms activated in the alarm reaction. At the physiologic level, adaptational changes may include (1) intrapulmonary shunting in response to ventilation-perfusion mismatches at the alveolar level; (2) increased ventilatory drive in the patient with acidemia; (3) alterations of kidney function in response to hypovolemia, acid-base imbalance, and inflammatory processes; and (4) stimulation of bone marrow that produces red blood cells in people living at high altitudes. This response produces a functional polycythemia—a true adaptational response of the human organism. Psychologic adaptations in response to the anxiety, fear, or grief that trigger the alarm reaction include all the defense mechanisms but most commonly

feelings of denial, anger, depression, and resolution. These feelings are generally accompanied by cognitive and motor-behavioral cues.

Effective adaptation will promote the return of wellness in the person. Ineffective adaptation leads to the prolongation of the alarm reaction, ultimately producing exhaustion of the affected area, and can result in the death of a cell, target organ, or the entire organism. Based on this postulate, stress is measured by the resultant strain imposed on the body, which can be viewed as the residual alarm response after adaptation has been maximized. It must be kept in mind that maximal adaptation may be ineffective in reducing the alarm response in some instances. Lazarus recognizes this physiologic response as one type of reaction to stress and views cognitive appraisal as the mechanism of activation.

The fight/flight response is also thought to be caused by activation of the ergotropic zone in the anterior hypothalamus (Hess[35]). Gellhorn[29] noted that stimulation of the ergotropic zone produced pupillary dilation, increased blood pressure, increased heart and respiratory rates, and heightened motor excitability consistent with the sympathetic activity of the fight/flight reaction. The role of perception on hypothalamic-mediated responses to stressors has yet to be identified specifically.

Correlations between sudden death and emotions have been observed for centuries; in fact, emotions have been induced purposefully to cause death, as in the case of voodoo.[11,52] Engel[25] observed that sudden death occurred during and after strong emotional stress. Three common denominators observed in patients just before sudden death were overwhelming excitation; loss of control; and a sense of giving up, helplessness, or hopelessness.

Sudden cardiac death from ventricular fibrillation is the leading cause of death in the 35 to 65-year-old age group, according to epidemiologic data from the United States and Western Europe.[46]

The concepts underlying the fight/flight response and the associated neurochemical activity are particularly cogent in the discussion of ventricular fibrillation. Electrophysiologic studies by Ganong[27] and Marshall[50] indicate that sympathetic stimulation increases heart rate, force of contraction, and conduction velocity in atria, atrioventricular nodes, and ventricles. Further studies by Lown, Verrier, and Rabinowitz[46] have shown that enhanced sympathetic stimulation predisposes the laboratory animal to ventricular fibrillation by markedly lowering the cardiac vulnerable period threshold. They report, "We have recently demonstrated that when subpressor doses of norepinephrine are given or when the pressor response to large doses of the drug is controlled by exsanguination, norepinephrine produces significant and sustained reduction in the vulnerable period threshold" (p. 892).

In addition to examining the effects of catecholamines, considerable research has been done on the effects of hypothalamic and autonomic stimulation, as well as the effects of stellate ganglion innervation on cardiac vulnerability. Dikshit[23] demonstrated that cardiac irregularities could be produced by injecting acetylcholine, caffeine, and nicotine into the cerebral

Fig. 1-2. Physiologic responses to stress.

Adapted from Underhill, S.L.: Cardiac nursing, Philadelphia, 1982, J.B. Lippincott Co.

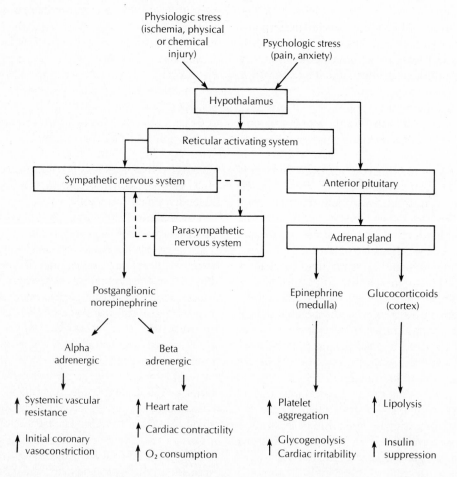

ventricles of cats and that sodium barbitone, administered intracerebrally or intravenously, lessened or abolished these cardiac irregularities. Later studies implicated the posterolateral hypothalamus and reticular formation in the genesis of repetitive junctional and ventricular arrhythmias.[3,6] Verrier, Calvert, and Lown[59] noted that stimulation of the posterior hypothalamus in dogs produced a 40% reduction in the ventricular fibrillation threshold and that the effects of hypothalamic stimulation on the ventricular fibrillation threshold persisted when heart rate acceleration and pressor response were prevented. Research confirms that ventricular arrhythmias in animals can be provoked with brain stimulation, as well as with direct sympathetic stimulation. The available literature indicates that in humans, ventricular arrhythmias result from both elevated serum catecholamines and increased activity from higher neural centers. Myocardial ischemia does not appear to be a necessary prerequisite, but neural activity alone may be sufficient to induce cardiac electrical instability.[46]

Lown, Verrier, and Rabinowitz[46] and De-Silva, Verrier, and Lown[22] have noted a correlation between stress-induced neural chemical activity and myocardial excitability; however, the precise neural pathways mediating psychologic inputs to the heart remain undefined. It has been well established that sympathetic stimulation can provoke ventricular arrhythmias. Conversely, Lown et al.[45] observed that there is a significant reduction in the number of premature ventricular extrasystoles during sleep in ambulatory patients. This reduction correlates with a lower level of sympathetic tone and increased vagal tone associated with sleep. These changes occurred regardless of the presence, type, and extent of heart disease. Fig. 1-2 summarizes the physiologic responses to stress.

Coping and adaptation

Stress is a part of living regardless of a person's life situation.[37,55] To survive, human beings must use whatever adaptational or cop-

ing resources are at their disposal, whether these resources are crude or sophisticated. A discussion of adaptation and coping follows.

Adaptation is considered by most theorists to be a permanent change in a living system that is essential to the survival of the system within a given environment. According to Murphy,[54] "Adaptation involves (1) reflexes and instincts; (2) coping efforts (to deal with a situation not adequately managed by reflexes); (3) mastery, which results from effective and well-practiced coping efforts; and (4) competence, which is seen as the development of skills resulting from cumulative mastery achievement" (p. 77).

Murphy provides a comprehensive method for classifying adaptational strategies, all of which contribute to the survival of humans in their environment. Reflexes and instincts are innate and limited, but the other three forms of adaptation are learned. To maximize learning is to maximize the potentials for adaptation.

"Coping came to include all those efforts to deal with environmental pressures that could not be handled by reflexes or organized skills, but involved struggles, trials, and persistent found energy directed toward a goal" (Murphy,[54] p. 71). Therefore coping is a part of adaptation; it can be learned, evaluated, and revised as necessary, implying a cognitive process. Reflexive reactions precede coping because they occur much more rapidly. If the reflex or instinctual reaction (such as rapidly withdrawing one's finger from a hot stove) is not sufficient to alleviate the threat, then coping efforts are employed. Lazarus identifies two classes of coping: (1) action tendencies, aimed at eliminating or mitigating the anticipated harmful confrontation that defines the threat, and (2) purely cognitive maneuvers, through which appraisal is altered without action directed at changing the objective situation (for example, defense mechanism). Action tendencies (attack, avoidance, and inaction) require an object; without an identifiable harm agent, there is no object. Therefore the person who perceives an ambiguous threat is unable to take action or prepare defenses. A state of anxiety ensues as the person experiences fear and helplessness in coping with the threat.

Defensive activity alters a person's perception of reality as that person attempts to reduce the degree of perceived threat. However, the situation is not changed with this mode of coping. The person using a defense mechanism must adapt to the stressor, wait for the stressor to become innocuous, or use the defense mechanism indefinitely. Prolonged use of defense mechanisms produces patterns of distortion and a lack of growth; the person never masters new and difficult situations.

The concept of mental rehearsal—that is, practicing counterharm tactics before the threat presents itself—is essential to the development of effective coping resources. This technique is particularly useful to the hospitalized patient and nurse in terms of preparing for procedures and tests. Mental rehearsal is the essence of patient education.[39]

The helping person, particularly the nurse, is in a position to enhance coping skills and minimize stress reactions in hospitalized patients and their families by providing information that is usable in mental rehearsals. This information is most helpful when it is concretely structured, when it tells of the nature of potential dangers and how the dangers can be surmounted, and when it tells of the mitigating or protective features of the environment.[39]

The regular elicitation of the relaxation response as a coping strategy has been found to be particularly effective against the stress responses of nonobjective anxiety. According to Benson et al.,[5] the relaxation response appears to be an integrated hypothalamic response that results in generalized decreased sympathetic nervous system activity and perhaps increased parasympathetic activity. Hess[35] identified the relaxation response as stemming from the trophotropic zone, located in the anterior hypothalamus. Electrical innervation of this zone results in decreased skeletal muscle tone, blood pressure, and respiratory rate and in pupillary constriction. Further studies by Gellhorn[29] showed that decreased oxygen consumption, decreased heart rate, increased skin resistance, and increased EEG alpha wave activity accompanied the relaxation response (trophotropic response). This state of wakeful low arousal is contrasted with the ergotropic response previously described as the stress response.

ASSESSMENT

The gathering of psychologic data remains an integral part of the nursing process and patient care planning for the critically ill patient. However, this activity is often ignored. Several studies dealing with this phenomenon have linked critical care nurses' avoidance of psychologic assessments to the following emotional issues: (1) a sense of inadequacy when dealing with the emotions of critically ill patients or their families, (2) difficulty being objective and empathic simultaneously, (3) lack of gratification from obtunded patients, and (4) defensive distancing to protect themselves from repeated loss. To extend themselves as an emotional support system to patients and their families puts nurses at risk. The nurse has offered a new source of coping energy from which the patient can draw; the nurse is now open to a new stressor: specifically, the patient at an emotional level. The conflict between wanting to be a helping, empathic nurse and needing to be a nurse who reduces emotional input to perform task-oriented functions can lead to the distancing so often seen in a critical care nurse. Other situational stressors that impede the nurse's use of psychologic data-gathering techniques include an already excessive workload, too much responsibility, and the lack of a functional psychologic assessment tool.

The purpose of a psychologic assessment tool is to aid in the nurse's psychologic evaluation of the patient, from which a therapeutic psychologic nursing care plan can be employed. This will maximize the psychologic coping resources of the critically ill patient and reduce conflict within the nursing staff by offering consistent approaches to the patient's behavior.

There are a variety of psychologic assessment tools available in the literature, but many are cumbersome to use. The Chrisman-Riehl[16] systems developmental stress model is an excellent prototypical assessment tool. It can be used in its entirety or selectively. It is divided into content segments and uses open-ended questions. During the patient interview, questions are asked concerning diet, sleep and relaxation, elimination, activity, normal health, medication, perceptions on health, and perceptions of self. The second part of the interview is done with family and friends to seek their perceptions and validate patient information. Nursing observations are compiled in the areas of appearance, communication pattern, interaction pattern/feeling tone, environment, and the patient's activity-rest schedule. A situation analysis is done, examining the interface between systems and the environment. Finally, a stress analysis is done, linking stressors with stress and coping responses found in the patient.

The concept of interpersonal and intrapersonal dynamics in the critical care unit environment was alluded to earlier in this chapter but requires further discussion as we examine assessment tools. For the purposes of this discussion, the patient (A), the patient's family (B), and the health care team (C) all function as separate but interdependent systems. The configuration of the systems relative to each other is dynamic and ever changing. As a stimulus exerts a force on any one of the systems, a coping response is formed. This response alters the intrapersonal or interpersonal dynamics of the affected system, thereby affecting other interdependent systems (Fig. 1-3). People do not exist in a vacuum (except perhaps catatonic individuals). They are surrounded by an environment, and to some degree they affect and are affected by other people, places, and things in that environment.

The stimulus configuration in Fig. 1-3 represents a critically ill patient in a critical care unit (A) whose dependence on the health care team has increased dramatically. Having only limited coping resources, this patient has responded to

his worried family members by not increasing his dependence on them (system B). He has sought support more from the health care team (C) than from his family. This patient could very well be a 38-year-old businessman, married and with young children. Let us imagine that he has suffered an acute myocardial infarction with an uncomplicated recovery. Intrapersonally he is frightened and somewhat depressed. He loves his wife and doesn't want to worry her with his fears about such issues as death, disability, troubled finances, and change in life-style. His self-image as a man is in jeopardy. This man, according to the stimulus configuration, has reacted by increasing his dependence on the health care team without increasing his dependence on his family. In this way the patient can seek information, verbalize his fears in a nonthreatening atmosphere, seek option clarification with "expert" advisors, and subsequently practice new coping responses before returning home to his family, with whom he must interact to maintain the relationship.

The patient is not the only subsystem of the critical care unit environment that can affect the stimulus configuration. For instance, the example seen in Fig. 1-4 demonstrates a lessen-

---

Fig. 1-3. This figure demonstrates a shift in the configuration of the systems within a critical care unit. The leftward shift of System *C* (the health care team) reflects an increased interdependence between Systems *A* and *C,* thus limiting the available energy for exchange with System *B* (the family) and System *C.*

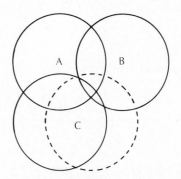

ing of mutual interdependence. The question might be asked: which subsystem has initiated the change in the stimulus configuration? Some possible answers are that the patient may have become more withdrawn; he may be reaching a higher level of wellness and may be in less need of support from interacting subsystems. Or, the nurse may be very tired intrapersonally and have little to give interpersonally on a given day. As a result, she may have initiated the withdrawal and change of the stimulus configuration. Finally, it is possible that the family may have reacted to an aspect of the health care, leading to conflict and avoidance behavior. The disastrous potential of the last possibility is the splitting apart of all three subsystems from each other, producing chaos and crisis.

The need for ongoing psychologic assessments becomes apparent. Not only the stimulus configuration's morphology but also its dynamics must be considered to predict coping strengths and intervene as necessary.

Stress is the result of any change within a system. When a stressor exerts a force, altering the stimulus configuration of the system, that system must generate a coping and, if needed, adaptational response. If the stressed change is

no longer cognitively appraised to be threatening, then the coping response is said to have been effective. The stressor-stressed change is then stored in memory for future use. If coping is appraised as ineffective, the system more closely approaches death. The system is unable to adapt to future stressors with a practiced coping repertoire. In extreme cases death may actually be perceived as adaptational; this may be seen in the case of suicide. A person suffering repeated myocardial infarctions may be physiologically unable to maintain effective adaptational responses and subsequently may die (Fig. 1-5).

As a part of the complete nursing care plan, the nurse is obligated to perform psychosocial assessments at the time of a person's admission to the unit and subsequently on a daily basis. A lack of time, feeling of inadequacy, and lack of a skill base seem to impede the critical care nurse's efforts in the area of psychologic assessments. The need exists for a brief psychologic evaluation tool in which all three systems of the stimulus configuration in the critical care unit environment can be assessed. This requires nurses to be aware of their own interactions with and reactions to patients and their families.

The tool should contain the following assessment areas: (1) a general psychologic history, including activities of daily living, perceptions of self and of health, and identification of support systems and coping resources; (2) reaction to illness and hospitalization; and (3) expectations about the future, including transfer from the critical care unit or going home. The questions are most useful when structured in an open-ended format (see Psychosocial Assessment Tool on pp. 16 and 17).

Observation by the nurse should include the following:

Appearance	Does the patient appear depressed? Euphoric? Catatonic?
Communication pattern	Does the patient speak haltingly? Does he listen, or is his attention span limited? Are

Fig. 1-4. In contrast with Fig. 1-3, the rightward shift of System *C* reflects an enhanced interdependence between the family and the health care team, with less energy being exchanged between the patient and the health care team member(s). An example of this configuration might be seen in the case of a dying comatose patient and his grieving family.

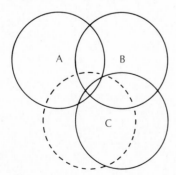

	his thought processes logical? Does he have difficulties expressing his feelings?
Interaction pattern	Does the patient initiate interaction; is she friendly? Does she seem angry or foreboding?
Environment	Is the patient attached to equipment with noisy alarms? Does he have privacy?
Activity-rest schedule	Is the patient confined to bedrest? If not, does she voluntarily get out of bed?

From these subjective and objective data, the presence of specific stressors and stress responses can be identified, producing alterations in affect, motor-behavioral cues, cognition, and physi-ology. The written psychologic nursing care plan is individually tailored with therapeutic interventions that are intended to maximize the patient's own coping resources and minimize the stress response.

Case study

Mrs. M. is a 29-year-old white female, 7 months pregnant, who is admitted to the coronary care unit at a large midwestern university medical center. Status: postcardiac arrest. Mrs. M's husband reports that they were in the hospital on their way to their first prenatal class when Mrs. M. passed out, became pulseless, and stopped breathing. Medical records indicate that CPR was initiated immediately and Mrs. M. was transferred to the emergency room, where she required multiple defibrillation for recurrent ventricular tachycardia/fibrillation. When Mrs. M.'s condition was stabilized, she was transferred to the coronary care unit of the university medical center. Admission history and physical revealed no history of previous car-

---

Fig. 1-5. This model (an adaptation of Selye's model of stressed change and the developmental-stress model of Chrisman and Riehl) examines the effect(s) of a stressor on a human system. Stressed changes resulting in effective coping are reintegrated into the coping repertoire of the individual. Ineffective coping, which is maladaptive by nature, causes the individual to move closer to death. This form of death may be characterized by a shutdown of the interpersonal, intrapersonal, or biologic subsystems, or a combination thereof.

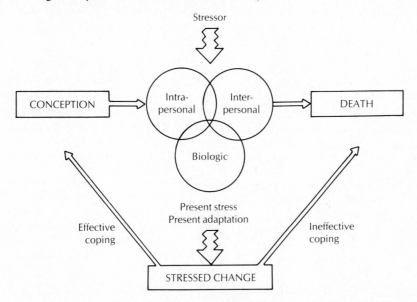

diac disease or illness during pregnancy. However, Mrs. M. now has a cardiomegaly with S_3 and S_4 gallops, sinus tachycardia with frequent salvos of ventricular ectopic beats, and severe pulmonary congestion with rales. Subsequent cardiac catheterization reveals congestive cardiomyopathy without coronary artery disease. Electrophysiologic studies confirmed the diagnosis of recurrent ventricular tachycardia. Mrs. M.'s condition was stabilized sufficiently to carry the fetus to 36 weeks, at which time the baby was delivered by cesarean section. The neonate was born with a low APGAR score, labored respirations, no gag reflex, and spastic extremities consistent with cerebral palsy. The child was also determined to have moderate mental retardation due to anoxic injury.

Mrs. M. spent the next 24 months in and out of the coronary care unit, but mostly in. Her ventricular tachycadia was unresponsive to both conventional and experimental antiarrhythmic drug therapy. During this time, she had multiple cardiac arrests at home. Her husband had taken paramedic training and had successfully resuscitated his wife on numerous occasions. Their house had a direct emergency line to the local fire station's paramedic squad. The lives of both Mr. and Mrs. M. centered around Mrs. M.'s illness. Hospitalization fees were enormous, as was their debt. To add to this situation, the baby had remained hospitalized for over 18 months because of recurrent problems with aspiration. Managing the infant at home would require full-time nursing care.

During Mrs. M.'s fourth hospitalization, she began expressing her outrage with the nurses, her husband, her friends, her child, and herself. Before this time, she had coped by relying on her faith and hope. She was an extremely religious woman who read her Bible daily and attended prayer meetings when she was able. During previous admissions, the nursing staff would always remark about the unusual coping strengths of Mr. and Mrs. M. They seemed to be the perfect couple. Initially, Mrs. M.'s anger was so subtle that only retrospective observation made it apparent. However, following a cardiac arrest during the fourth hospitalization, she reported that she could see herself and Mr. M. during the code. In her "dream," Mr. M. was standing on top of the earth looking into outer space and was swinging Mrs. M. by her hair around in a circle. She recalled, "I was going around and around flying through the air, and I wished he would let me go . . . leave me in outer space!"

This experience gave the nursing staff the oppor-

tunity to assist Mrs. M. in sorting out her fears and desires—an opportunity to verbalize thoughts that a "good Christian woman" should not.

Using the psychologic assessment tool, the following subjective and objective data were collected from Mrs. M. The problem list and related coping strategies from this data are identified in Table 1-3.

Mrs. M. disclosed feelings of inadequacy as a wife and mother and feelings of anger toward her husband for resuscitating her, toward friends who were too afraid to stay with her or take her out shopping, toward her infant daughter who cried when she held her, toward the nursing staff who delivered her pills late, and toward God. Most of this anger seemed to be directed internally in the form of guilt.

The nursing staff spent time daily, usually in the evening, encouraging Mrs. M. to ventilate and reassuring her of the normalcy of her responses. Oftentimes, Mrs. M. just wanted someone to sit with her. However, communication between her and her husband continued to deteriorate. In an effort to provide continuity of care, Mr. and Mrs. M. were offered professional counseling services through the university hospital, which could be continued in their hometown at the local community mental health clinic. The service was offered as an opportunity for Mr. and Mrs. M. to examine their relationship, which had gone from husband/wife to husband/patient, and to explore available coping strategies as Mrs. M. attempted to reassert herself as a wife and mother. The desired outcome was to minimize sources of stress in their lives, which were already saturated with unchangeable stressors including Mrs. M.'s illness, a handicapped child, and financial difficulties.

Mrs. M.'s ventricular tachycardia remained unresponsive to conventional and experimental antiarrhythmic drug therapy. After discharge she received a constant infusion of intravenous lidocaine with potassium at 2 mg/min via an indwelling subclavian catheter. During the remaining 9 months of her life, she had two hospitalizations for catheter sepsis but was able to remain at home most of the time. Six months before Mrs. M.'s death, her daughter was released from the hospital, and Mrs. M. began mothering her child for the first time. Mrs. M. died at home with her husband at her side, according to her wishes.

Alterations caused by stress

As noted previously, stress may manifest itself in a variety of ways, depending on the per-

Table 1-3. Nursing care plan

Manifestations of stress	Coping strengths	Coping needs/interventions
INITIAL ASSESSMENT Anxiety/fear: Response to lack of information; no previous experience with hospitalization, critical care equipment, or regimen; uncertain future; displacement from hometown, family, and friends. Denial: Response to survival needs at emotional level. No orientation to future.	Alertness. Ability to communicate verbally; not intubated. Seeks information. Faith in God. Active support system, including husband and aunt, is well used.	**INITIAL PHASE** Encourage patient to verbalize feelings, providing an environment of confidentiality, acceptance, warmth, and honesty. Use active listening skills. Provide information about procedures, equipment, critical care routines, and illness in small increments tolerable to patient's anxiety level. Clarify threatening situations with patient, pointing out consistencies/inconsistencies of threats to facilitate a realistic and accurate perception.
10 DAYS AFTER ADMISSION Anger/guilt: Response to loss of control, altered body image; ambivalent feelings about self, family, health care team, God, and the unexpected in a previously normal pregnancy Denial/depression: Response to the internalization of the emotional impact of illness and an uncertain future; denial gives way to episodes of depression. **4 MONTHS AFTER ADMISSION/ PREDISCHARGE** Resolution/acceptance: Beginning to look at illness in a long-term fashion. Continues to experience periods of anxiety/fear, anger/ guilt, and denial/depression.	Positive denial; limits scope of awareness to minimize disorganization and crisis.	Clarify discrepancies between patient's verbal and nonverbal communication. Validate with the patient the normal responses to illness and hospitalization and the use of positive coping mechanisms. **INTERIM PHASE** Gradually increase patient's control over self-care. Encourage patient to participate in making decisions about own care, as this is feasible. Encourage patient's expression of ambivalent feelings. Encourage patient to interact with support systems not directly involved in patient care delivery; this may aid in the expression and understanding of ambivalent feelings related to the health-care team. **PREDISCHARGE PHASE** Validate patient's and husband's understanding of illness. Clarify coping options related to going home. Provide an opportunity for patient and husband to practice coping strategies. Validate social service discharge plans.

Table 1-4. Alterations of anxiety

	Mild anxiety	Moderate anxiety	Severe anxiety	Panic anxiety
Perceptions and observations	Senses alerted; Sees, hears more. Noises seem louder.	Perceptual field narrowed. Sees, hears less. Can see and hear more if object is called to subject's attention.	Perceptual field greatly reduced. Focuses on a detail or on scattered details.	Perceptual field limited to one detail that is blown out of proportion, or rapid observation of scattered details.
Attention	Alert attention promotes skill in seeing relationships or connections.	Attention lessened or of shorter duration. Can attend if notice is called; selectively inattentive.	Attention limited to detail or scattered details.	Attention to one detail; grossly distorted.
Modes of experiencing	Syntactic; sees proper relationships.	Parataxic; sees relationships only in the past.	Parataxic and prototaxic; sees relationships to the past or present only.	Prototaxic; sees only the present.
Thought processes	Logical critical thinking available for use in solution of problems at hand.	Slower or more scattered. Can use logical critical thinking if attention is called to the need.	Illogical noncritical thinking. Control by emotions takes over. Defense mechanisms more apparent.	Natural thought processes blocked; bewilderment apparent.
Learning and adaptation	Process of learning occurs.	Learning occurs but with more difficulty and time involved.	Learning not likely. Adaptive behavior, not requiring logical thought, takes over.	Learning impossible. Adaptive behavior at maximum.

son and her interaction with the stressor and environment. The stimulus-response configuration is in constant flux; that is, the patient will respond differently to the same type of stressor depending on factors such as imminence of threat, environment and interpersonal interactions, and coping reserves. The remainder of this chapter will focus on (1) clarifying the four major categories of stress response—affective, motor-behavioral, cognitive, and physiologic; and (2) use of the nursing process when providing patient care to people with alterations in these four areas.

Affective

The affective realm includes altered feeling states such as fear, anxiety, anger, depression, and denial. When elicited, these emotions may be transient, isolated, or compounded by other types of stress responses, such as motor-behavioral responses or by complicated defense mechanisms. These emotions may be responses to internal or external stressors that are either adaptive or maladaptive (that is, self-destructive).

Fear and anxiety. Both fear and anxiety produce a physiologic and psychologic response.

The physiologic response for both emotions is the activation of the alarm response of the general adaptation syndrome. Catecholamines are released with a subsequent increase in heart and blood pressure. The hypothalamic-mediated response results in pupillary dilation and peripheral vasoconstriction.

The psychologic response to fear and anxiety is not as simple. A person must perceive impending danger by tangible threat for the evocation of the fear response. The potency of the threat depends on its imminence; however, the mere anticipation of harm has been shown to evoke a significant rise in autonomic nervous system activity. For example, Nurse A. approaches Mr. B.'s bedside with his preoperative injection. Mr. B. begins trembling; his heart rate increases as indicated by the monitor. Nurse A asks Mr. B. why he is trembling. He states that he is afraid the shot will hurt. Further clarification reveals that Mr. B. is fearful of anesthetics because his uncle had surgery and "did not wake up." Mr. B.'s anticipation of pain before receiving his preoperative medication serves to activate his alarm response. The prominent threat to Mr. B. is obviously anesthesia and surgery, but the injection signals death, or the "point of no return." The threat has become imminent and the danger real, and his ability to maintain control has been removed by sedation. The result can be an experience of helplessness and despair that, because of societal norms, may not be expressed verbally. More frequently, the patient is sedated enough to be unable to express his fears.

Anxiety, in contrast to fear, is the perception of a threat from an unidentifiable harm. Like fear, anxiety may be the mere anticipation of a future confrontation with a harm agent. The anxious person is often described as being tense, nervous, fidgety, inattentive, and moody. Janis[39] describes anxiety on four levels: mild (1+), moderate (2+), severe (3+), and panic (4+). Janis' research supports the idea that mild anxiety serves an adaptive function by sharpening the senses. Subjects observed while mildly anxious were found to be more attentive; the heightened level of alertness promoted skill in seeing relationships and connections; logical critical thinking was available for use in problem solving; and learning appeared to be maximized. As anxiety progresses to moderate levels and beyond, the senses gradually become more dulled. At the point of panic-level anxiety, perception is limited to a single detail that is often distorted; natural thought processes are blocked with the onset of bewilderment; and learning is impossible (Table 1-4).

Anxiety can be classified as either state or trait (Johnson and Spielberger[40]). State anxiety refers to anxiety associated with a particular situation. For example, a student tells the psychology researcher, "Every time I sit down to take a chemistry test, I get sweaty palms and my thoughts all seem to run together." The student denies experiencing these symptoms while taking other examinations. The student is apparently experiencing a moderate level of state or situational anxiety during chemistry tests. On the other hand, trait anxiety is found in people who are anxious constantly. These people characteristically tend to have nervous tics and complain of "nerves" unrelated to a particular situation. For example, the nurse asks a patient, "How would you describe yourself?" The patient replies, "Well, I guess that I'm one of those nervous types."

Both anxious and fear-ridden people will exhibit similar cognitive and motor-behavioral alterations; therefore it is essential to determine if there is an identifiable harm agent. Fear is a self-limited emotional response; once the harm agent is identified, coping resources can be tapped or learned to minimize or eliminate the threat. On the other hand, anxiety is a permeating and enveloping emotional response that, in the presence of inadequate coping, can lead a person to emotional or physical exhaustion. Because the source of threat is ambiguous, it is difficult to direct coping strategies toward the elimination of the threat. Therefore coping strategies tend merely to be palliative in the anxious person.

This perception of threat is often enhanced or limited by (1) previous experience, (2) stim-

PSYCHOSOCIAL ASSESSMENT TOOL

What the patient does What the patient says	The meaning to the patient The meaning to the nurse

Situation: General questions to ask the patient

I. History—prior to hospitalization

What's home like for you?	Check out statements with the patient that are confusing to you. Check out statements that seem inconsistent.
Tell me about your family.	Check out patient feelings toward the family.
Who do you go to when you have a problem?	Check out specific support systems.
Describe a typical day for you when you are not in the hospital.	
What have past hospitalizations been like for you?	Check out specific good and bad points of past hospitalizations.
Do you know anyone else with the same illness?	Check out how the patient responds to the person with the same illness.
If so, what was the illness like for the person, and how was he affected?	
When things are bugging you (or bothering you), what do you do?	Check out specific things the person does to take care of concern or discomfort. Check if what they do makes them more comfortable.

II. Impact of hospitalization and illness

What do you understand about your illness?	Check out patient misconceptions about the illness and its treatment.
How does it feel to be in the hospital?	Check if feelings are related to present situations or to past experiences.
What is the greatest change you believe will occur in your life as a result of this illness?	Check how the patient feels about changes. Check out specific details of the greatest change.
What is the most pressing problem for you now?	Check out specific details of the pressing problem. Check if the patient has a clear picture of this problem.
How does the most pressing problem cause discomfort for you?	

PSYCHOSOCIAL ASSESSMENT TOOL—cont'd

What the patient does What the patient says	The meaning to the patient The meaning to the nurse
How does the greatest change in your life cause discomfort for you?	Check out what specific feelings the patient can identify about the problem or change.
What steps have you thought about taking or have you taken to care for your most pressing problem? Your greatest change?	
How are you taking care or have you thought of taking care of the concerns or problems you have about your illness?	Check if what the patient does makes her more comfortable.
What could you tell us that would help the nurses understand you better?	Check out specific things the nurses could do for the patient.
Normal Emotional Responses to Illness	
It is not uncommon for patients to feel helpless in the hospital. Is that how you are feeling?	Check out if the patient's feelings are getting in the way of his taking care of the problems he has identified.
Patients often get angry for many reasons while in the hospital. I wonder if that fits with what you are feeling?	Check out the person's feelings and attitudes about expressing emotions.
It is normal for patients to have some fear while in the hospital. I wonder if you might be feeling that way?	
Frequently our patients feel uncomfortable with being in the hospital. Is that how you are feeling?	

III. Anticipatory questions—predischarge/pretransfer

How do you feel about leaving the hospital.	Check out feelings about being out of the hospital and away from nursing care.
What do you think will happen when you go home with your illness?	Check out specific ways the person sees herself at home, recovering.
How do you see your family responding to your illness?	Check out how the patient would like to see his family respond to his illness.
Do you have any questions that you and your family want answered before you go home?	Check out if the expectations for family members are probable.

ulus configuration, and (3) availability of adaptive coping reserves. With each life experience, the human mind has a tremendous capacity to store imprints of a person's psychologic and physiologic response to an event. These imprints may identify such responses to stimuli as joy, pain, fear, sweaty hands, pounding heart, and pleasure. Vicarious experiencing may also occur, expanding the information available to the person. With each new experience, the imprints are reviewed, although not always within the realm of the person's awareness. This process is elemental to Lazarus' concept of cognitive appraisal of threat. The degree of threat is appraised based on a person's past and present experience with a specific stimulus configuration.

As earlier discussed, the stimulus configurations within the critical care unit environment contain three human systems: the patient, the family, and the nurse. These three systems maintain a shifting level of interdependence that is contingent on the stressor and the associated target system (Fig. 1-1). If the stressor is aimed primarily at the patient—for example, surgery—the need exists for increased dependence on the nurse and the family (Fig. 1-2). As patients become stronger physically, their dependence on the nurse may decrease, and the stimulus configuration will again change (Fig. 1-3). Each time the stimulus configuration changes, the process of cognitive appraisal must be repeated to finely tune the system's coping efforts.

Mrs. G., who is hospitalized, begins to experience chest pain. She reaches for her call bell but cannot find it. She becomes restless and begins crying for the nurse. She perceives a sense of panic, helplessness, and fear that this episode of pain "might be the big one." The nurse enters the room and asks what is wrong. Mrs. G. replies, "I'm having chest pain; thank you for coming so quickly. I could not find my call bell and became frightened. But everything is all right now; you are here."

The pain is still present; the imminence of the threat has not changed. Yet Mrs. G. is calmed by the nurse's presence. A mere alteration in the stimulus configuration has altered the target system's response.

A third influence on the cognitive appraisal of threat is a person's awareness of his own coping resources. Lazarus notes that the perception of threat is lessened in the presence of effective counterharm resources.

Mrs. G. again has chest pain. However, she has now had the opportunity to learn that nitroglycerin will relieve her chest pain. She reacts to the pain by taking a nitroglycerin tablet without becoming restless or crying, although the nurse is not present in her room at the time. She subsequently reaches calmly for her call bell and rings for the nurse.

Mrs. G. now has an effective counterharm/coping resource that allows her to minimize her perception of threat during chest pain, reducing the stress response physiologically and psychologically.

Anger. Anger is described as a strong emotional response characterized by such feelings as resentment, dislike, and a desire for vengeance. This emotion can be directed toward oneself or others; however, when self-directed it is often labeled *guilt*. Anger has been said to cause the "juices to flow," and indeed anger does stimulate the autonomic nervous system, producing a sympathomimetic response. The subsequent activation of the general adaptation syndrome accounts for the tissue damage in target organs such as the heart and stomach in those people with sustained feelings of anger.

Anger is a function of loss or grief. The Latin root of the word anger means "to grieve." The loss may be internal, such as declining mental capabilities, poor body image, and decreased self-esteem, or it may be external, such as disfiguration or the imminent death of self or a significant other. The relationship between loss and anger has been discussed by many theorists in recent years; however, Elizabeth Kübler-Ross's work on death and dying remains the most prominent.

In her model of grief and loss, Kübler-Ross[41] postulates that the breakdown of the denial defense mechanism is followed by a stage of anger during which the person asks, "Why me?" She stipulates that with this natural progression to anger comes internalization of the loss. Many researchers have since argued that the stages of grief are not as well defined or sequential as Kübler-Ross presents them. They do agree, however, that anger is a part of the grief process.

Anger is also a component of the widely discussed coronary behavior pattern commonly referred to as the Type A personality. People with Type A behavior invariably feel angry toward themselves or others, although defense mechanisms such as denial or projection often block their awareness of the anger. These people tend to be highly perfectionistic and time- and efficiency-oriented. Relaxation becomes a challenge or a feat performed with great intensity. When confronted with inefficiency, failure to meet an objective, or errors, regardless of how trivial they might be, the person with Type A behavior tends to explode with anger either visibly or (more often) internally. The anger may be directed at others but frequently is self-directed (Friedman and Rosenman[26]).

The transactional analysis model (Harris[32]) works well to examine the behavior patterns of someone with a Type A personality. The "OK corral" contains four life positions: (1) I'm OK, you're OK; (2) I'm OK, you're not OK; (3) I'm not OK, you're OK; and (4) I'm not OK, you're not OK. The winner position—"I'm OK, you're OK"—is the only life position typical of Type B (noncoronary) behavior. The "I'm not OK, you're OK" person is covertly Type A and tends to internalize anger, as well as other life stressors. The "I'm OK, you're not OK" person is an overt Type A person, tending to be very selfish, egocentric, hurried, and "a martyr." The "I'm not OK, you're not OK" person is someone who chooses to be an onlooker in life, standing in the wings rather than being onstage.

Depression. Depression is nearly a universal finding among patients in critical care units, particularly when their hospitalizations are prolonged. These patients are often confronted with situations that stimulate feelings of anger resulting from changes in body image, unmet expectations, and depersonalization. When there is no longer sufficient psychologic energy to maintain anger, depression ensues.

Depression as a feeling state is a natural sequel to anger, particularly if the anger is self-directed. Like anger, depression has been identified by Kübler-Ross as a stage of mourning. When depressive symptoms are in response to a loss, it is important to allow the person to grieve, providing empathic support to that patient. Depression of this nature serves an adaptive function, allowing patients to use their available coping resources economically until their coping reserves can be replenished.

Pathologic depression is different from the feeling of being depressed. Both forms of depression are marked by decreased self-assurance, decreased sexual interest, decreased appetite (or sometimes its opposite, increased appetite and constant eating), constipation, loss of initiative, decreased energy, constriction of interests, lack of pleasure from usually pleasurable activities, and overall pessimism. Chronic fatigue and chronic pain are often considered to be depressive equivalents. When depressive symptoms become persistent and are inappropriate to the extent of the illness, pathologic depression is likely to have taken root. This form of depression is marked not only by the previously mentioned depressive symptoms but also by saddened facial expressions, tearfulness, motor retardation (or occasional agitation), insomnia, weight loss (or occasional weight gain), preoccupation with death and dying, self-critical statements, and suicide attempts or suicidal thinking. Depression of this type requires psychotherapy. With the advent of psychiatric liaison departments, qualified people now perform psychotherapeutic interventions in the critical care unit.

Denial. Denial is the refusal to accept the reality of a situation cognitively or affectively. Kübler-Ross identifies denial as the initial human response to loss. This loss may be perceived or actual. It may occur in the grief reaction of death and dying, following a divorce, following a change in body image, or even in response to an anticipated change in body image. This anticipatory grief can be seen in the dying patient, as well as in the person recently diagnosed as having an early form of a chronic disabling disease such as multiple sclerosis or rheumatoid arthritis. Rather than accepting the loss as real, these people often cope with their situations by denying the existence of the loss or by verbalizing their cognitive awareness of the loss without any affective or emotional internalization of what the loss means to them.

Recent stress theorists including Lazarus[43] have suggested that this denial process, particularly affective denial, may actually be a positive coping response during situational crises that result in grief and loss. When a person is confronted with the sense of loss and inadequate coping strengths, denial may provide the necessary time to develop new coping strategies.

Hackett[30,31] has shown repeatedly that when the postcoronary patient ceases to deny, the subsequent affective responses are fear and depression. This chain of events can be correlated to the fight/flight mechanism. Denial for the critically ill patient may actually represent the fight response. As the GAS is activated, mental energy is conserved to maximize physiologic potentials and the fight response. The alternative to fighting is to "flee" into the mind, activating particularly the affective and cognitive responses to stress, thereby depleting the available energies for physiologic coping. Depressed people often describe themselves as "too tired to fight" and are perceived as giving up. Engel[25] suggests that the person who responds to loss with feelings of hopelessness and despair is more prone to sudden death.

Motor-behavioral

Body language. Alterations in body language are often the first signs that someone is stressed. Rarely are these signs present without alterations in one of the other areas of stress responses (affective, cognitive, or physiologic). People complaining of feeling stressed may report that their hands tremble, that their muscles feel tight, or that they have nervous tics such as urges to wring their hands, smack their lips, or ruminate. They may walk very slowly or very rapidly, or they may be unable to maintain eye contact when engaged in conversation. Stress may cause people to have spontaneous episodes of crying or agitation with minimal or no provocation. Agitation and crying are frequent observations in the critical care unit environment, often causing the caregiver to feel frustrated and inadequate to intervene. This sense of inadequacy may stem from the caregiver's lack of time to assess the observed problem and intervene effectively, or it may be related to a lack of confidence in using psychotherapeutic techniques. Chemical and physical restraints become a simplistic way of managing motor-behavioral responses to stress.

Stress may alter speech patterns in the areas of style, rate, quality, and content. Style and rate are closely related and refer to the confidence expressed during delivery of speech and the rapidity with which someone speaks. Quality refers to the tone of the voice, its loudness or softness, and whether or not it quavers. The alterations in content are closely linked to Janis'[39] model of anxiety, in which thought processes are disrupted with the higher levels of anxiety (Table 1-4). Without well-connected thought processes, a clear and logical message cannot be communicated.

Cognitive

Thought and intellectual functioning. The critical care environment, with all of its stimulation, is likely to produce at the very least some sleep deprivation in a normal, healthy young adult. Studies have shown that sleep deprivation alone is a sufficient stressor to disorganize a person's thought and logic; it is a technique used in brainwashing. Place a sick young adult in a critical care unit on a ventilator and after a couple of weeks she is likely to be labeled confused but mentally normal. Place an elderly woman in the same critical care unit on a ventilator for a couple of weeks, and she is likely to become confused. The difference, however, is that her confusion will be labeled senility or organic brain syndrome.

Thought and intellectual functioning are not age dependent; declining years do not bring automatic senility. However, altered physiology, for example, poor oxygenation and brain atrophy, will produce cognitive alterations. Within the intensive care environment, anxiety flourishes. As a patient decompensates physically or psychologically, the anxiety of the caregiver often increases. If effective coping strategies are not employed swiftly, the anxiety level of the patient can rapidly escalate. Anxiety has the quality of a virus; as it moves from host to host, it gains strength. Anxiety in these proportions is quite capable of producing alterations in thought and intellectual functioning. These alterations are exhibited as confusion, loss of memory (usually short-term memory), diminished attention span, and confabulation.

Judgment. Critical logical thinking is impaired by the same stressors capable of altering thought and intellectual functioning. Judgment refers to human comprehension, the ability to see proper relationships, and problem solving using critical logical thinking. Moderate anxiety alter's a person's judgment without significantly altering intellectual functioning. However, severely impaired thought and intellectual capacities most certainly will severely alter judgment. For example, Mr. J. is a 62-year-old man in the coronary care unit. It is 2 days after he has had an acute anteroseptal myocardial infarction. He has a Swan-Ganz catheter in his right subclavian and left radial arterial line. Mr. J. suddenly experiences the need to defecate. He sees a small room with a toilet in it, which doesn't seem very far away to him. Mr. J. thinks to himself, "I won't bother the nurse, she's so busy." So Mr. J. lets his side rail down and begins to get out of bed to go to the bathroom, totally unaware of his catheter and arterial lines. Mr. J. later explains his rationale fully to the panicked nurse

---

STRESSORS AFFECTING THE MONITORED PATIENT

Monitoring itself—being "hooked up"
Immobility (restraints)
Altered body image—grief
Dependence—reliance on others for maintenance of basic physical needs
Isolation
Sensory overload
Fear of the unknown—"am I going to die?"
Lack of control—powerlessness
Change in role from supporter to supportee
Realization of own vulnerability
Pain
Physiologic disruption
Communication difficulties
Previous experience with hospitalizations

---

who rushed in when the alarms sounded. However, he is unable to see the relationship between the tubes and wires that surround him and his need to stay in bed—a clear error in judgment.

Sensory integration. Alterations in sensory integration frequently occur in the critical care environment because of sensory deprivation, sensory overload, and sleep deprivation. Sensory deprivation is defined as the lack of sufficient stimuli necessary to activate the sensory-integrated response associated with one or more of the five senses. Held and Hein[34] and Blakemore and Cooper[8] demonstrated that cats whose visual field was obstructed from birth were unable to integrate spatial relationship when their visual field was normalized. However, with repeated exposure to the experimental environment, the cats could learn spatial relationships. Neonates who lie in a critical care unit with their eyes covered respond in a manner similar to that of the cats. These infants will integrate spatial relationships more slowly than infants whose eyes were not covered. Patients who are placed in isolation receive a markedly decreased quality and quantity of stimuli and are likely to report distorted interpretations of their sensations and perceptions. According to Walsh,[61] brain-damaged people function in a deprived environment—that is, the quality and quantity of integrated stimuli are decreased. Arousal levels tend to be low in these people, making stimulus integration difficult. Furthermore, Walsh suggests that brain damage can actually be reversed or at least minimized by the optimization of arousal levels with the use of amphetamines. With higher arousal levels, brain-damaged people are more able to integrate complex environmental stimuli; for example, they are more able to actively explore an object and simultaneously describe what they feel. This state of brain damage may occur secondary to trauma, anoxia, stroke, or birth defects.

Sensory overload refers to the polar extreme of sensory deprivation. With sensory overload, people are bombarded with stimuli at a rate greater than they can integrate. Frequently the loud noises, alarms, and bright lights of the critical care unit are responsible for the excessive stimulation. Patients, families, and health care team members are all equally vulnerable to sensory overload. Once someone's integrative capacities have been maximized, additional sensory input is processed selectively and erratically, with the mind blocking all remaining stimuli. The result is distortion of sensory and cognitive perceptions and responses.

Mrs. K. is a 62-year-old white woman admitted to the surgical critical care unit following removal of a ruptured gallbladder. After 72 hours, Mrs. K. is noted to be extremely anxious and hypervigilant. A fire bell rings in the hallway and Mrs. K. screams, "They are after me and if they catch me, they'll kill me." The nurse attempts to determine the source of Mrs. K.'s anxiety. Mrs. K. states, "They never let me sleep; they wake me up for that breathing machine just as I fall asleep; if they catch me, they'll kill me."

The human capacity to integrate sensory stimuli often is determined by the presence of other stressors. Mild anxiety promotes integrative abilities; however, severe anxiety produces selective inattention and distortion of cognitive and sensory input.

Sleep deprivation is a decrease in quality and quantity of rapid eye movement (REM) sleep, producing a relative state of sensory overload. The critical care environment undoubtedly produces a degree of sleep deprivation in all its patients. The fact that REM sleep is diminished because of disruptions of circadian rhythm and sleep patterns, increased environmental stimuli, patient care, hypoxemia, and altered respiratory cycles with ventilatory assistance contributes to the state of sleep deprivation.

Cerebrovascular insufficient states. Senility, cerebrovascular arterosclerotic disease, and organic brain syndrome are terms that refer to the disorders, diseases, or symptoms of a group of patients often found in the critical care unit whose behavior is marked by gross confusion, disorientation, confabulation, crying, and depression. These people suffer from chronic cerebral vascular insufficiency, producing cerebral atrophy of the affected area. Frequently, the intensity of these symptoms is enhanced by the critical care environment, which is disruptive to the patient's normal living structure. These patients are particularly sensitive to sensory deprivation, sensory overload, and sleep deprivation. Alterations in thought processing and judgment are common for this population, often making it difficult for families, nurses, and doctors to communicate with a patient on a rational level.

Psychosis. At a more intense level of psychophysiologic stress, the critically ill patient may exhibit paranoid or delusional thoughts, often triggered by auditory or visual hallucinations. This pattern has been labeled "ICU psychosis" and indicates that the level of stress has exceeded the person's coping or adaptational limits. As critical care units came into prominence in the 1960s and early 1970s, it was recognized that there was a need to determine ways of assessing, preventing, or limiting both physiologic and psychologic stress responses in the critical care environment. Understanding the interaction between the perception of threat and the sympathomimetic stress response, nursing directed much research toward the recognition and minimization of the psychologic stress response in the critically ill patient. If the perception of threat could be eliminated or the patient supported with more effective coping, the cardiovascular responses to catecholamines, such as increased heart rate, blood pressure, and vasoconstriction and decreased fibrillatory threshold potential, could be minimized.

Much of the research in this area has been directed toward the postcardiotomy patient because of the reportedly higher incidence of psychotic behavior in this critically ill population (Lasater and Grisanti[42]). The term "post-pump psychosis" has become generally accepted and refers to a syndrome with neuropsychologic changes, as well as changes in other autonomic-controlled end organs. Alterations of thought and judgment are reflected behaviorally as confusion or disorientation, which may be accompanied by agitation, combativeness, or either auditory or visual hallucination. Associated autonomic-mediated (sympathomimetic) responses include alterations of blood pressure, rapid shallow respirations, and peripheral vasoconstrictions, as evidenced by cool pale skin and decreased peripheral pulse.

A combination of physiologic and environmental factors is thought to contribute to the development of postpump psychosis. Physiologic factors discussed in the literature include inadequate cerebral perfusion, microembolic phenomena, length of time on cardiopulmonary bypass, and age of the patient. Environmental factors seemingly inherent to critical care units include sensory deprivation, sensory overload, and sleep deprivation.

Inadequate cerebral perfusion is thought to occur in the patient on cardiopulmonary bypass because of diminished blood flow and decreased oxygen availability at the tissue level. Once patients are being supported on bypass, not only are their cardiac outputs decreased by approximately 30% to 40%, but also blood flow is changed from a pulsatile to a nonpulsatile force. The second factor of decreased oxygen availability at the tissue level occurs secondary to hemo-

dilution and damage to the red blood cell. Hemodilution results from the priming of the extracorporeal circulation with isotonic solution prior to its use. The result is a lower hematocrit with diminished oxygen availability. Once the blood is bubbled through the membrane oxygenator, structural damage can occur to the red blood cells, impairing their ability to release oxygen to the tissues.

The occurrence of microemboli secondary to the formation of platelet and protein aggregates, fibrin split products, and other precipitates participating in the extracorporeal circulation have been implicated in the genesis of transient neurologic deficits status after open heart surgery. Improved filtering of the extracorporeal circulation over the past 10 years has reduced the risk of vascular blockade intraoperatively and postoperatively in the cardiac surgical patient.

Some researchers have examined the patient's length of time on cardiopulmonary bypass and age; however, no conclusive data have been cited to support these factors as causative agents in the development of post-pump psychosis.[24]

Physiologic

Selye's General Adaptation Syndrome addresses the physiologic response to stressors in a systematic approach. With the activation of Stage 1—*the alarm reaction*—the body's defenses are mobilized. There is adrenal stimulation and a marked increase in sympathetic tone because of the elevated serum catecholamine levels. Elevated catecholamine production leads to increased heart rate (tachycardia), blood pressure, respiratory rate, oxygen consumption, and increased myocardial excitability, as well as sweating, peripheral vasoconstriction, nervousness, and increased skeletal muscle tone. The hypothalamic-mediated physiologic stress response includes pupillary dilation, increased blood pressure, increased heart and respiratory rates, and heightened motor excitability consistent with the sympathetic activity of the fight/flight reaction. The second stage, *resistance,* is character-

PSYCHOSOCIAL ASSESSMENT TOOL

Subjective data	Objective data

SITUATION: General questions to ask the patient.

I. History—prior to hospitalization

What's home like for you?

We have a good Christian home now. My husband is a good provider; we have everything we need. . . . My first husband drank too much. . . .

Mrs. M. physically exhausted; attached to cardiac monitor; frequently glancing at monitor. Respirations slightly labored; occasional deep sigh; clenches jaw periodically; eyes glassy, palms sweaty.

Tell me about your family.

We are ordinary folks. I'm from southern Indiana, and my husband is originally from Kentucky. My husband works in a factory. . . . I hope our baby is going to be OK; I want it so much.

Speech a little jerky; sitting up in bed; hands clasped around stomach.

Who do you go to when you have a problem?

I pray a lot; I have some good friends in my church. My faith is very strong.

Eyes becoming red as if trying not to cry. Tone of voice more intense. Expression withdrawn.

Describe a typical day for you when you're not in the hospital.

Oh just the usual; wash clothes, iron, cook, and clean. I used to work in an office, but haven't been able to work in recent weeks.

What have past hospitalizations been like for you?

I've never been in the hospital before. . . . This seems so weird; I never thought this would happen to me.

Glances around the room; grips bedrails firmly and repositions self.

Do you know anyone else with the same illness?

I've known old people with heart trouble, but no one in my family has a bad heart, and I don't smoke or drink.

Staring at the foot of the bed.

(If the answer is yes) What was the illness like for the person, and how was he or she affected?

My husband's father had heart trouble a long time, but he kept on working the farm. He never complained. The obituaries are full of old people who have died of heart trouble.

Talking past tense; seems more distant in awareness and eye contact. More fidgety; increased anxiety.

PSYCHOSOCIAL ASSESSMENT TOOL—cont'd

Subjective data	Objective data

When things are bugging you (or bothering you), what do you do?

Sometimes I eat more, other times I cry. But reading the Bible seems to comfort me best. I always seem to find answers in the Bible.

Very religious; didn't mention talking to significant other for help; Bible sitting on bedside table. Need to contact chaplain's service.

II. Impact of hospitalization and illness (assessed 10 days after admission)

What do you understand about your illness?

Nothing except that I pass out without warning; I know that I have been resuscitated; and I ache all over. . . . But why is my baby less active. . . . I'm scared to death.

Speech jerky; tears in eyes; holding my hand very tight. Skin cool, hands sweaty. Fetal heart monitor to be attached later today. Cardiac monitor shows that Mrs. M. has frequent bursts of ventricular ectopy.

How does it feel to be in the hospital?

I'm so mixed up, I don't really know. I've seen so many doctors and nurses, I can't remember all their names. But I'm glad they are here. I don't like being left alone in this room; everything happens so fast.

What is the greatest change you believe will occur in your life as a result of this illness?

(pause)
I don't know. . . .

Unable to answer the question. Forehead furrowed and seems unable to concentrate.

What is the most pressing problem for you now?

I don't care what happens to me, but you must help me save this baby for my husband.

Speech emotionally charged but no tears at present. Seems like she is ready to explode.

How does the most pressing problem cause discomfort for you?

(pause) I've not told anyone this before . . . you may think this sounds rotten; I feel so guilty; and I've prayed for strength; but sometimes I feel this is all the baby's fault. If I had not been pregnant, maybe none of this would have happened.

Beating fist on bed; tearful.

How does the greatest change in your life cause discomfort for you?

(Interviewer choose to delete question at this time.)

PSYCHOSOCIAL ASSESSMENT TOOL—cont'd

Subjective data	Objective data
What steps have you thought about taking or have you taken to care for your most pressing problem? Your greatest change?	
All I can do is pray and do what the doctors tell me to do.	*Stares out window; no eye contact with nurse.*
How are you taking care or have you thought of taking care of the concerns or problems you have about your illness?	
(pause) *I guess it is out of my hands.*	*Continues to stare out the window; appears helpless to deal with her emotions at present. Has not mentioned husband as a significant other today.*
What could you tell us that would help the nurses understand you better?	
I am used to taking care of myself; this is so terribly awkward for me. . . . I love music.	*Eye contact resumed; tries to regain composure.*
Normal Emotional Responses to Illness	
It is not uncommon for patients to feel helpless in the hospital. Is that how you are feeling?	
Yes, and I don't like it, but how can you help it when you are hooked up to all these machines?	*Voice louder and more intense; fists clenched.*
Patients often get angry for many reasons while in the hospital. I wonder if that fits with what you're feeling?	
Sometimes . . . but then I feel guilty because I know everyone is trying to help me.	
It is normal for patients to have some fear while in the hospital. I wonder if you might be feeling that way?	
Sometimes I get afraid, especially when no one is in the room or all the lights are out. I sometimes catch myself thinking very strange thoughts.	*Fidgeting with sheet and blanket. Glances at cardiac monitor and nurses' station.*
Frequently our patients feel uncomfortable with being in the hospital. Is that how you're feeling?	
The nursing staff is very nice here. They are all so helpful . . .	*Avoids answering the question directly. Emotions appear to be shut off at this point.*

PSYCHOSOCIAL ASSESSMENT TOOL—cont'd

Subjective data	Objective data

III. Anticipatory questions—predischarge/ pretransfer (assessed 4 months after admission)

How do you feel about leaving the hospital?

I'm really scared. What happens if I go into VT at home? I'm so sad about leaving our baby in the hospital.

Able to express fears and concerns. Apparent increase in knowledge of disease process. Looking at future. Affect anxious but less fearful.

What do you think will happen when you go home with your illness?

I don't know . . . I just keep on praying and offering to do the Lord's work once I'm feeling better.

Bargaining.

How do you see your family responding to your illness?

I don't think they will want to come near me. They are frightened.

Facial expression is sadder.

Do you have any questions that you and your family want answered before you go home?

What can be done if I have VT at home . . . When will my baby be able to come home so that we can be a family?

---

ized by increasing adaptive efforts of the body and can be likened to the mobilization of reserve troops during battle. The development of coronary collateral circulation after an acute myocardial infarction exemplifies these adaptive capabilities of the body. As long as the stressor exists and there are adaptive mechanisms available, the body will remain in this stage of resistance; however, when these adaptive energies are depleted, exhaustion and death to the target cell, tissue, organ, or organism ensues. This final process of *exhaustion* is the third stage of Selye's General Adaptation Syndrome.

Common physiologic alterations thought to be caused by prolonged exposure to stressors include coronary artery disease, hypertension, and ulcers. Diseases that are exacerbated by stress include asthma, allergies, neuromuscular disorders such as myasthenia gravis, and peripheral vascular disorders such as Raynaud's disease.

Recently there have been studies discussing the role of stress in the production of cancer cells.[57] There are no definitive data proving that exposure to prolonged psychological stress produces cancer, although a positive correlation exists between cancer and numerous physiologic stressors such as cigarettes and asbestos. Studies by Simonton,[57] using psychologic imaging techniques with children stricken with leukemia, have had positive results in eliciting remission in these children. In the studies the children were asked to conjure up images of their cancer and its destruction; for example, they might imagine the cancer as tiny little ants and then imagine themselves stepping all over the ants. The research is limited but suggests a possible neural-humoral link between stress and cancer.[57]

INTERVENTIONS

The biopsychosocial approach to the nursing process encourages the nurse to assess the interconnectedness of various bodily functions and to intervene at dependent and independent levels with that same interconnectedness. Like assessments, interventions may be directed at patients, their families, health-care team members, or the environment. The interventions may be as simple as silencing an alarm or as complex as engaging in ongoing stress counseling with dying patients and their families. The stimulus configuration may be so stressed that multiple interventions may be required for relief of symptoms and augmentation of coping strengths. Some factors that have an impact on the effectiveness of psychotherapeutic nursing interventions include the level of trust between the patient, family, and nurse; physician support of nursing interventions; frequency of evaluation of the stimulus configuration; nurses' awareness of their own stressors, feelings, behaviors, and communication styles; and nurses' awareness of cultural and value differences among the patient, the family, and the nurse. Ongoing assessment of the stimulus configuration, implementation of carefully selected psychotherapeutic drug therapy, and appropriately directed psychotherapeutic interventions followed by evaluation of individual behavior are elemental in providing effective nursing care to the critically ill person.

Psychotherapeutic drugs

The efficacious use of psychotherapeutic drugs in the critical care environment requires both the nurse and physician to be familiar with the drug's desired action, possible adverse reactions, and contraindications. For the purposes of this discussion, psychotherapeutic drugs will be limited to the following classifications: antianxiety, sedative-hypnotic, antidepressant, and anti-

psychotic agents. Many psychotherapeutic drugs depress neurologic function, decrease myocardial contractility, depress respirations, or diminish cardiac output, all of which may be undesirable side effects in selected patients.

Antianxiety agents

The benzodiazepines, such as diazepam (Valium) and chlordiazepoxide hydrochloride (Librium), are the most common antianxiety agents used. These agents produce the least amount of cardiac and respiratory depression when compared to other available antianxiety agents. Drowsiness is the most commonly reported side effect. Other less common adverse reactions include tremors, ataxia, postural hypotension, lightheadedness, mental confusion, skin eruptions, and abdominal pain. The usefulness of benzodiazepines in the anxious person is well documented; however, the question of judicious dispensing of benzodiazepines is being raised throughout the literature.[18,36,49] The widespread use and abuse of benzodiazepines, especially Valium, has been documented in the literature, as well as in mass media. Before administering Valium and other benzodiazepines, the physician and nurse must consider whether pharmacologic treatment of anxiety and other manifestations of stress is the most appropriate intervention. Issues such as the person's previous drug history, prescribed or illicit, should be assessed. Some people may benefit more from individualized counseling or psychotherapy than from pharmacologic therapy.

Sedatives/hypnotics

The barbiturates, including phenobarbital and secobarbital, are used less frequently in the critical care environment because they cause severe respiratory depression. In addition, barbiturates frequently have been found to be the cause of fatal accidental or intentional overdoses. Adequate liver functions are essential to the complete metabolism of barbiturates. Poor liver function allows barbiturate metabolites to circulate, producing prolonged sedation and depression of central respiratory centers. Furthermore, barbiturates compete with warfarin and digitoxin for the same metabolic enzyme, making it difficult to stabilize therapeutic plasma levels of these drugs. Barbiturates do have selective usefulness in the critically ill patient requiring a drug-induced state of unconsciousness. Phenobarbital is used to induce coma and reduce cerebral metabolism in the head-injured patient with lethal elevations of intracranial pressure. Methohexital sodium (Brevital) is used to induce a short-term anesthetized state for elective cardioversions.

Antidepressants

There are two classes of antidepressant drugs: tricyclics and monoamine-oxidase (MAO) inhibitors. However, they are rarely administered to patients in critical care units because of the severe adverse reactions and toxic symptoms associated with them. The lethal potential of these drugs should not be underestimated. Tricyclic antidepressant overdose produces severe toxic effects on the cardiac conduction system, leading to a variety of arrhythmias, particularly ventricular tachycardia and fibrillation. These arrhythmias do not respond to epinephrine and other sympathomimetic drugs used in cardiopulmonary resuscitation without the reversal of the drug-induced cholinergic blockage with neostigmine. Tricyclics also have a wide range of adverse reactions including central nervous system excitation or depression, peripheral anticholinergic effects, cardiovascular toxicity, skin reactions, excessive sweating, and less commonly agranulocytosis. The ingestion of both tricyclics and MAO inhibitors can produce profound hypertension resulting from simultaneous cholingergic blockade and an inability to reduce norepinephrine and epinephrine into their inactive metabolites. Monoamine oxidase is the enzyme responsible for the catabolism of catecholamines.

Although the critically ill patient is often depressed, the use of antidepressants may in fact intensify the physiologic manifestations of

stress. Therefore antianxiety and sedative-hypnotic agents are used more frequently in the critical care environment.

Antipsychotics

Phenothiazines including chlorpromazine (Thorazine) have long been the backbone of antipsychotic drug therapy. Like antidepressants, phenothiazines produce a wide variety of adverse reactions that are undesirable in the critically ill patient. These adverse reactions include cardiac conduction disturbances, hypotension, hepatic dysfunction, decreased gastric motility, and photosensitivity. The administration of butyrophenones, especially haloperidol (Haldol), in critically ill patients with psychotic reactions has become more widely accepted because of limited adverse and toxic reactions, particularly to the cardiovascular system. Haloperidol does produce some motor retardation and central nervous system depression but tends to positively affect the patient's cognitive processing abilities.

Psychotherapeutic interventions

The art and science of nursing are found in the performance of therapeutic interventions developed from scientifically based nursing assessments and interpretations of a patient's biopsychosocial stimulus configuration. The development of psychotherapeutic nursing interventions requires that the nurse be aware of mindbody interactions such as the stress response. These interventions are tailored to unique stimulus configurations, yet there is a universality observed among psychotherapeutic interventions, particularly those aimed at stress reduction. The stress response, whether it is found in the patient, family, or nurse, is apt to be reduced by the following interventions: (1) active listening, (2) information giving, (3) option clarification, (4) identification and use of resources, (5) regulation of sensory stimulation, (6) maintenance of personal control, (7) relaxation training techniques, (8) touch, and (9) optimization of physiologic functioning (see box on p. 30).

INTERVENTIONS

Employ active listening
Provide information
Help clarify options
Optimize identification and use of resources
Regulate sensory stimulation
As soon as possible, return as much control of
    self and environment to the person as pos-
    sible
Employ relaxation techniques
Use touch as a therapeutic device
Optimize physiologic functioning

Active listening

Active listening is a participatory form of communication that requires practice. It is the careful processing of incoming information without the formation of a response or judgment before the completion of the message. When employing active listening, the intended receiver listens to the entire message before formulating a response. This type of listening requires the message receiver (listener) to filter out extraneous noises and thoughts, which may confuse or block cognitive appraisal of the input.

Information giving

Because inadequate knowledge is known to breed fear and anxiety, providing information can reduce the stress reaction to fear of the unknown. Newly graduated nurses in the critical care unit are frequently frightened by their lack of technical skills. As they gain knowledge, experience, and confidence, the same nurses may perform these technical skills with unfaltering certainty. It is important to keep in mind that the readiness of the learner (patient, family member, or nurse) must be assessed before the presentation of new information. Too much information (input) can produce sensory overload in the learner, whose processing skills may be unable to keep pace with the input load.

The family of the critically ill patient tends to respond favorably to information about the critical care environment, the patient's condition and progress, anticipated procedures and therapy, visitation policies, and family waiting room facilities. Individual nurses can relay this type of information as part of their patient care activity and evaluate the family's coping responses. An alternative to this form of disseminating information is the use of critical care unit family conferences. These conferences are generally prescheduled on a routine basis, for example, daily, biweekly, or weekly, for a specified length of time ranging from 20 minutes to 90 minutes. Ideally, these family conferences are facilitated by a critical care nurse and a professional skilled in counseling, such as a social worker, chaplain, or clinical nurse specialist. Together they respond to families' needs for information, emotional support, and identification of supplemental resources. One family on a particular day merely may be interested in where to find a decent restaurant, whereas another family may need to verbalize anger toward the medical team. The group conference may be able to offer empathic understanding to the distressed family by allowing the sharing of insights and feelings. The sharing process between families is one way of validating normal human responses to stress and crisis. The facilitators' function is therefore to provide information and needed support, as well as to generate new coping strategies within distressed families. This method of family education, although initially more difficult to organize and structure than a one-to-one education format, seems to provide the most consistency for families. An ongoing confidential relationship can develop between families and the group facilitator(s), allowing the families to ventilate any concerns they may have without fear of that communication negatively influencing the level of patient care delivered.

Patient education comprises the bulk of nursing information-giving efforts. Nearly every hospital today has some sort of formalized patient education program dealing with topics such as diabetes, arthritis, heart disease, hypertension, pregnancy, and delivery. When they are given sufficient time, nurses are able to effect patient education very well. How well, however, does nursing provide information to the critically ill patient? Patient education is often at the bottom of the intervention priority list as nurses organize patient care. "If I get some time at the end of the shift, I will sit down with Mr. D. to talk with him about his heart attack," thinks the busy critical care nurse. The premium on nursing time is high; too often, patient teaching must be sacrificed. Patient teaching must be incorporated into the nursing care plan of every patient and evaluated as a nursing intervention. By providing clear, concise, and understandable information to the patient, anxiety and fear can be minimized with a subsequent reduction in the stress response. Nurses sometimes catch themselves talking to a family member, another nurse, or a physician while standing at the foot of the patient's bed; this nursing behavior contributes to patient fear and anxiety, as well as sensory deprivation. The patient perceives knowledgable people talking about him but not including him. He may therefore interpret the situation as follows: "They must be trying to keep something from me, or they think I'm already dead." To compound this situation, the type of noninteraction just described diminishes the quality and quantity of incoming stimuli for the patient, producing sensory deprivation and its associated perceptual distortions. The appropriate intervention is to include the patient in discussions within his room; discussions that necessarily exclude the patient should take place away from his perceptual field (auditory or visual). Hopefully, discussions pertaining to the patient's medical and nursing care will at some point include patient or family input.

Another type of patient may benefit from receiving less information. For example, a patient is admitted to the respiratory critical care unit for evaluation of a right upper lobe mass. Upon admission, the physician orders the insertion of an IV and preparation of the patient for an open-lung biopsy in the morning. A short,

simple explanation before the insertion of the IV is usually sufficient to ease patients to a tolerable level of stress. However, since signing the operative consent, this particular patient has been very restless, she occasionally sobs and is increasingly short of breath. The patient subjectively reports being fearful of cancer; angry at herself for not taking her doctor's advice to quit smoking; and fearful of not waking up from surgery. The nurse makes the decision to assist the patient in ventilating her fears and concerns but provides her with a limited amount of information regarding her scheduled surgery and its potential outcomes. The nurse has assessed this patient to be highly stressed, with limited coping strengths; to give her more information would only stress her further.

A contrasting situation occurs with the presurgical cardiac patient who, after 4 months of planning, enters the hospital for coronary artery bypass graft surgery. This type of patient often requires a great deal of information and is generally ready to learn. Patient teaching is usually done on the patient's disease process, the anticipated operative procedure, the critical care recovery phase, and rehabilitation. The explanations are often detailed, explaining various tubes and wires that the patient will experience. If possible, the open-heart recovery room nurse does the patient teaching to establish a relationship with the patient before admission to the critical care unit. Janis[39] demonstrated that people who are slowly desensitized to stressors and have an opportunity to anticipate a threat will spend time in the "work of worry." During this time, they review their coping strengths and practice their coping responses for different stimulus configurations.

Option clarification

The process of option clarification employs a combination of active listening, information giving, and reflective communication. The nurse assists the patient in processing the new information and putting it into context with old experiences and insights. This communication pattern results in the identification of specific coping options and their consequences. The selection of coping options belongs to the patient. This selection encourages patients to take responsibility for their own behavior and enhances patients' sense of control over their personal situation. Nurses are responsible only for providing sufficient information to patients and for validating their understanding of this information.

For example, Mr. S. is recovering from an uncomplicated subendocardial myocardial infarction. In spite of his obvious physiologic improvement, Mr. S. is extremely withdrawn. After caring for him for several days, Nurse B. remarks to Mr. S. that he seems very sad and withdrawn and offers him her time if he would like to talk. Mr. S. begins to talk about his family, and a complicated story unravels. Mr. S. is involved in a long-standing extramarital affair of which his wife is unaware. He describes his wife as an overweight, diabetic woman who has been hospitalized frequently for complications of her diabetes. When asked if he still cares for his wife, he states that he has not been responsive to her for a number of years but because of her frequent bouts of illness, he cannot bring himself to leave her. Mr. S. is asked why this situation has suddenly caused him to respond with such sadness. He verbalizes that he is trying to decide whether to leave his wife for his longtime girlfriend. Mr. S. voices conflict between what he should do as an honorable man and what he wants to do as a sensual, loving person. Nurse B. spends several days with Mr. S., acting as his mirror and discussing feelings and various coping strategies. After discharge from the hospital, Mr. S. decides to divorce his wife and marry his girlfriend. Sadly, Mr. S. dies of a massive myocardial infarction 2 weeks after his decision.

Identification and utilization of resources

Basic human survival needs such as shelter and food may be jeopardized not only by the existence of a catastrophic illness, but also by the economic and emotional crises that follow it. Family, business, and personal affairs may falter in the wake of a critical illness. The critically ill patient and more frequently the family and significant others may become immobilized by the stress response and unable to identify resources. The critical care nurse's assessment of the stimulus configuration should include these data so that the patient or family can be assisted with appropriate identification and use of available resources.

For a variety of reasons, the critical care nurse must sometimes consult auxiliary services personnel, including social workers, chaplains, and psychiatric liaisons, to deal with highly stressed patients and their families. The critical care nurse's time is valuable and in short supply. When factors such as time, high nursing stress levels, or nurse-patient-family conflicts impinge on the stimulus configuration, the appropriate intervention is to seek consultation.

Regulation of sensory stimulation

The sensory stimulation needs of humans vary daily. Therefore, to regulate the sensory input needs of patients in the critical care environment, nurses must perform both subjective and objective ongoing assessments of patients' perceptual fields and abilities to integrate sensory input (simple or complex), along with other manifestations of stress. Patients with an acute myocardial infarction or cerebral aneurysm will require decreased sensory input, including low light and noise levels. These patients preferably should be placed in a private room and should be kept at rest and sedated. Conversely, patients recovering from a cerebrovascular accident may require carefully planned sensory stimulation to maximize the return of function. These patients may need short activity periods several times a day to exercise specific muscle groups or to engage in speech retraining.

Maintenance of personal control

The fear of losing control and of permanent dependence, with all of their legal and social implications, becomes a powerful source of stress to the critically ill patient and family. Gradually returning control to the patient during morning care—for example, by letting the patient use a bedside commode (instead of the bedpan) or scratch his own nose—is often sufficient to reduce the threat of permanent dependence. Patients begin to view themselves as regaining personal power and control. Patients who avoid personal power or control and perceive that they cannot control their own life situation will become overly dependent. These patients may require a variety of interventions, ranging from gentle persuasion to behavior modification, but the expected outcome should be the same: the acceptance of responsibility for one's behavior as a means of controlling one's life situation.

Relaxation training techniques

Theoretically, the regular elicitation of the relaxation response as described earlier in this chapter should decrease the sympathomimetic response associated with psychic and physiologic stress. Benson[5,7] has identified four basic conditions necessary for the achievement of deep relaxation: (1) a mental device, such as a continuous thought, word, or phrase; (2) a passive attitude; (3) decreased muscle tonus; and (4) a quiet environment. Many of the Eastern, Oriental, and mystical religions, including early Christianity and Judaism, describe a process by which to obtain inner peace and harmony that is similar to deep relaxation, particularly that achieved through transcendental meditation. This form of relaxation has been extensively researched by physiologists and psychologists, who have documented significant decreases in oxygen consumption, carbon dioxide elimination, lowered heart rate, respiratory rate, minute ventilations, and arterial lactate; however, no significant changes have been noted in blood pressure.[7]

In contrast to deep relaxation based on imagery, Jacobson[38] describes a technique called progressive muscle relaxation, which involves the alternate tensing and relaxing of specific muscle groups. Jacobson hypothesizes that mus-

cle tension and relaxation cannot coexist and that by making people acutely aware of tension and subsequently directing them to "let go," or relax, they will learn with practice to achieve deep muscle relaxation. Electromyographic data corroborates this assumption; however, there are no other physiologic correlates documented in the literature.[5] Studies by Johnson and Spielberger[40] and others[53,58] have shown progressive muscle relaxation to be effective in reducing situational anxiety in stress reactions, particularly in introverted personality types. However, maturational anxiety is not apt to be affected by this relaxation method.

Practical application of this therapeutic intervention in the critical care environment is somewhat limited. The patient must be able to cognitively focus on what is being said by the nurse-therapist. If an imagery technique is being used, patients must be able to direct their attention to a predetermined auditory or visual image. For example, the nurse might say,

"I want you to envision yourself at the top of a staircase. Now I want you to slowly begin descending this staircase, one step at a time. At the bottom of the stairs you see the most beautiful green meadow with deer and squirrels. You want to rush to the meadow, but you can't because your arms and legs are becoming so heavy; all you can do is to walk slowly . . . ."

This exercise will probably benefit the active person, who needs to learn how to slow down and relax, but the critically ill patient is already feeling heavy and tired. This demonstrates the need to pick relaxation exercises that are compatible with individual personalities and physical capabilities. Progressive muscle relaxation requires a moderate amount of muscular control in addition to a cognitive ability to process the directions of the therapist. For example, the nurse might say, "I want you to tighten the muscles of your right leg as tight as you can. Do not let go until I tell you. Feel the tension . . . . Now, let go; let all the tension flow out of your leg through your toes. Enjoy relaxation." Some patients report that they enjoy controlling their own body through the activity associated with the performance of relaxation exercises. Other patients become acutely distressed and are unable to complete the relaxation exercise. For those patients who have an altered body image because of disfigurement, obesity, or gross cachexia, the enhanced awareness of their own body during progressive muscle relaxation may be intolerable.

Possibly the most universal relaxation exercise with the highest degree of tolerance is deep breathing. Slow inhalation and exhalation using the abdominal muscles for breathing will elicit a relative degree of relaxation. This type of abdominal breathing must be mastered before successful relaxation can be achieved with other methods.

Touch—the laying on of hands

Following deep breathing, the art of touch runs a close second as the most natural form of stress reduction. As children, we turn to our mothers so that we can be held when we are sad or frightened. As adults, we may long for the tender, caring arm on the shoulder or pat on the head, but it often seems to elude us.

Lynch[47] showed that heart rate and the frequency of cardiac arrhythmias decreased in a coronary population when the nurse remained in a patient's room longer than 5 minutes; however, when the nurse stayed less than 5 minutes in the room and had no human contact with the patient, the monitor showed increased heart rate and cardiac arrhythmias.

Touch includes a wide range of activities such as the holding of a hand, a backrub before bed, wiping a sweat-laden brow, giving a bath, physically assessing a patient, administering interventions, and exercising flaccid extremities. Touch transcends all barriers to communication regardless of age, sex, race, or nationality. The "laying on of hands" is the essence and art of nursing.

Optimization of physiologic functioning

The preceding text has attempted to clarify the balances and counterbalances among the in-

terpersonal, and biologic subsystems of the human organism. For critically ill patients to maximize their physiologic potential, they must be able to cope adequately with the interpersonal and intrapersonal stressors of the critical care environment.

SUMMARY

Stress is represented by any change in the stimulus configuration of a system. Stress may be physiologic or psychologic and situational (state) or maturational (trait). There exists a mutual interdependence of the intrapersonal, interpersonal, and biologic subsystems of the human organism so that one subsystem cannot experience a change without affecting another subsystem. When stress levels or the quantity of change exceeds the system's ability to adapt or cope to a new stimulus configuration, disorganization and crisis result.

The critically ill patient's demands on a nurse exact great amounts of time, technical skill, and physical and emotional energy. Stress reduction can be achieved in the critical care environment, but it requires skillful assessments, interpretations, interventions, and evaluations.

REFERENCES

1. Adler, D.C., and Shoemaker, N.J.: AACN organization and management of critical care facilities, St. Louis, 1979, The C.V. Mosby Co.
2. Anderson, R.E., and Carter, I.: Human behavior in the social environment, a social systems approach, Chicago, 1978, Aldine Publishing Co.
3. Attkar, H.J., Guitterreg, M.T., Bellet, S., and Ravens, J.R.: Effects of stimulation of hypothalamus and reticular activating system on production of cardiac arrhythmias, Circulation Research 12:14, 1963.
4. Barchas, J.D., Berger, P.A., Ciaranello, R.D., and Elliott, G.R., editors: Psychopharmacology, from theory to practice, New York, 1977, Oxford University Press
5. Benson, H., Beary, J.F., and Carol, M.P.: The relaxation response, Psychiatry 37:37, 1974.
6. Benson, H.: The relaxation response, New York, 1975, William Morrow and Company, Inc.
7. Benson, H., Kotch, J.B., and Crosswiller, A.B.: The relaxation response: a bridge between psychiatry and medicine, Medical Clinics of North America 61:929, 1977.

8. Blakemore, C., and Cooper, G.F.: Development of the brain depends upon the visual environment, Nature **228**:477, 1970.

9. Cadmus, R.R.: Intensive care reaches silver anniversary, Hospitals, p. 98, Jan. 1980.

10. Cannon, W.B.: The emergency function of the adrenal medulla in pain and the major emotions, American Journal of Physiology **33**:356, 1914.

11. Cannon, W.B.: "Voodoo" death, Psychosomatic Medicine **19**:182, 1957.

12. Cassem, N.H.: The nurse in the coronary care unit. In Gentry, W.D., and Williams, R.B., editors: Psychological aspects of myocardial infarction and coronary care, St. Louis, 1975, The C.V. Mosby Co.

13. Cassem, N.H., and Hackett, T.P.: Psychiatric consultation in a coronary care unit, Annals of Internal Medicine **75**:9, 1971.

14. Cassem, N.H., and Hackett, T.P.: Psychological rehabilitation of myocardial infarction patient in the acute phase, Heart and Lung **2**:382, 1973.

15. Claus, K.E., and Bailey, J.T., editors: Living with stress and promoting well-being, a handbook for nurses, St. Louis, 1980, The C.V. Mosby Co.

16. Chrisman, M., and Riehl, J.: The systems developmental stress model. In Riehl, J., and Roy, C., Sr., editors: Conceptual models for nursing practice, ed. 2, New York, 1980, Appleton-Century-Crofts.

17. Coehlo, G.V., Hamburg, D.A., and Adams, J.E.: Coping and adaptation, New York, 1974, Basic Books.

18. Cooper, J.R., editor: Sedative-hypnotic drugs: risks and benefits, 1977, U.S. Dept. of Health, Education, and Welfare, Rockville, MD.

19. Corbalan, R., Verrier, R.L., and Lown, B.: Psychological stress and ventricular arrhythmias during myocardial infarction in the conscious dog, Americal Journal of Cardiology **34**:692, 1974.

20. DeSilva, R.A., and Lown, B.: Ventricular premature beats, stress and sudden death, Psychosomatics **19**:649, 1978.

21. DeSilva, R.A., and Lown, B.: Fatal arrhythmias: role of psychophysiologic events, Primary Cardiology p. 31, Feb. 1980.

22. DeSilva, R.A., Verrier, R.L., and Lown, B.: The effects of psychological stress and vagal stimulation with morphine on vulnerability to ventricular fibrillation (VF) in the conscious dog, American Heart Journal **95**:197, 1978.

23. Dikshit, B.B.: The production of cardiac irregularities by excitation of hypothalamic centers, Journal of Physiology **81**:382, 1934.

24. Dubin, W.R., Field, H.L., and Gastfriend, B.S.: Post cardiotomy delerium: a critical review, The Journal of Thoracic and Cardiovascular Surgery **77**(4):586, 1979.

25. Engel, G.L.: Sudden and rapid death during psychological stress, Annals of Internal Medicine **74**:771, 1971.

26. Friedman, M., and Rosenman, R.H.: Type A behavior and your heart, New York, 1974, Alfred A. Knopf, Inc.

27. Ganong, W.F.: Review of medical physiology, Los Altos, 1965, Lange Medical Publishers.

28. Garfield, C.: Stress and survival, St. Louis, 1979, The C.V. Mosby Co.

29. Gellhorn, E.: Principles of autonomic-somatic integrations, Minneapolis, 1967, University of Minnesota Press.

30. Hackett, T.P., Cassem, N.H., and Wesknie, H.A.: The coronary care unit: an appraisal of its psychologic hazards, New England Journal of Medicine **279**:1365, 1968.

31. Hackett, T.P., Cassem, N.H., and Wesknie, H.A.: Detection and treatment of anxiety in the coronary care unit, American Heart Journal **78**:727, 1969.

32. Harris, T.A.: I'm OK, you're OK, New York, 1969, Harper & Row Publishers.

33. Harvey, A.M.: Neurosurgical genius—Walter Edward Dandy, Johns Hopkins Medical Journal **135**:358, 1974.

34. Held, R., and Hein, A.: Movement-produced stimulation in the development of visually guided behavior, Journal of Comparative and Physiological Psychology **56**:872, 1963.

35. Hess, W.R.: The functional organization of the diencephalon, New York, 1957, Grune & Stratton.

36. Hollister, L.E., Greenblatt, D.J., Rickels, K., Ayd, F.J., and Greiner, G.E.: Benzodiazepine 1980: current update, Psychosomatic supplement, Oct. 1980.

37. Holmes, T., and Rahe, R.: The social readjustment rating scale, Journal of Psychosomatic Research **11**:213, 1967.

38. Jacobson, E.: You must relax, ed. 4, New York, 1962, McGraw-Hill Book Co.

39. Janis, J.L.: Psychological stress, New York, 1958, John Wiley & Sons.

40. Johnson, D.J., and Spielberger, C.D.: The effects of relaxation training and the passage of time on measures of state and trait anxiety, Journal of Clinical Psychology **24**:20, 1968.

41. Kübler-Ross, E.: On death and dying, New York, 1969, Macmillan Publishing Co.

42. Lasater, K.L., and Grisanti, D.J.: Postcardiotomy psychosis: indications and interventions, Psychological Aspects of Critical Care **4**(5):724, 1975.

43. Lazarus, R.S.: Psychological stress and the coping process, New York, 1966, McGraw-Hill Publishing Co.

44. Lown, B., DeSilva, R.A., and Lenson, R.: Roles of psychologic stress and autonomic nervous system changes in the provocation of ventricular premature complexes, American Journal of Cardiology **41**:979, 1978.

45. Lown, B., Tykocinski, M., Garfein, A., and Brooks, P.: Sleep and ventricular premature beats, Circulation **48**:691, 1973.

46. Lown, B., Verrier, R.L., and Rabinowitz, S.N.: Neural

and psychologic mechanisms and the problem of sudden cardiac death, American Journal of Cardiology **39:**890, 1977.

47. Lynch, J.J., Thomas, S.S.A., et al.: Human contact and cardiac arrhythmias in a coronary care unit, Psychosomatic Medicine **39:**188, 1977.

48. Manning, J.W., and Piess, C.N.: Cardiovascular response to electrical stimulation in the diencephalon, American Journal of Physiology **198:**366, 1960.

49. Marks, J.: The benzodiazepines: use, overuse, misuse, abuse, Lancaster, England, 1978, MTA Press Ltd.

50. Marshall, J.M.: Vertebrate smooth muscle. In Mountcastle, V.B.: Medical physiology, vol. 1, ed. 14, St. Louis, 1980, The C.V. Mosby Co.

51. May, R.: The meaning of anxiety, New York, 1950, The Ronald Press.

52. McConnel, J.W.: Discussion of Yawger, W.S.: Emotions as the cause of rapid and sudden death, Archives of Neurological Psychiatric **36:**875, 1936.

53. Miller, M.P., Miller, T.P., and Murphy, P.J.: Comparison of electromyographic feedback and progressive relaxation training in treating circumscribed anxiety stress reactions, Journal of Consulting and Clinical Psychology **46:**1291, 1978.

54. Murphy, L.: Coping, vulnerability and resilience in childhood. In Cochlo, G.V., Hamburg, D.A., and Adams, J.E., editors: Coping and adaptation, New York, 1974, Basic Books.

55. Selye, H.: The stress of life, New York, 1976, McGraw-Hill Book Company.

56. Simon, N., editor: The psychological aspects of intensive care nursing, Bowie, MD, 1980, Robert J. Brady Co.

57. Simonton, O.C., Simonton-Matthews, S., and Sparks, T.F.: Psychological intervention in the treatment of cancer, Psychosomatics **21(3):**226, 1980.

58. Stoudemin, J.: Effects of muscle relaxation training on state and trait anxiety in introverts and extroverts, Journal of Personality and Social Psychology **24:**273, 1972.

59. Underhill, S.L., Woods, S.L., Sivarajan, E.S., et al.: Cardiac nursing, Philadelphia, PA, 1982, J.B. Lippincott Co.

60. Verrier, R.L., Calvert, A., and Lown, B.: Effects of posterior hypothalamic stimulation on the ventricular fibrillation threshold, American Journal of Physiology **228:**923, 1975.

61. Walsh, R.: Sensory environments, brain damage, and drugs: a review of interactions and mediating mechanisms, International Journal of Neuroscience **14:**129, 1981.

62. Weinberg, S.J., and Foster, J.M.: Electrocardiographic changes produced by hypothalamus stimulation, Annals of Internal Medicine **53:**332, 1960.

63. Weiss, T.: Biofeedback training for cardiovascular dysfunctions, Medical Clinics of North America **61:**913, 1977.

2 Circulation

LINDA ABELS

Cardiovascular diseases are one of the leading causes of death in the United States today. They are also responsible for many physical restrictions, varying from minor physical limitations to complete disability. No age group is totally exempt from these cardiovascular disorders, which impose a heavy economic burden on many people. Although the elderly are most heavily affected, approximately one fourth of cardiovascular deaths occur in people under 65 years of age, and about half of all disabling cardiovascular conditions also affect people under the age of 65.

Many changes have taken place in the last decade to help prevent, correct, or control cardiovascular disease. Experimental and clinical studies have yielded etiologic data that can be used to help prevent or interrupt some cardiovascular disease processes. Epidemiologic studies have provided impetus for intervention and control. Increased knowledge has led to the development of diagnostic tools and techniques.

Research is becoming even more complex, with continuous investigation of the relationship between cardiovascular physiology and cardiovascular disease. Critical care practitioners must continue their quest for knowledge and will undoubtedly update their skills to provide optimal care for those patients with cardiovascular disorders.

EMBRYOLOGY

The circulatory system is the first system to become functional in the fetus. Its entire development occurs between the twenty-first and fortieth days of fetal life. By the third week of embryogenesis, a single primitive cardiac tube can be identified. Its development proceeds in a caudocephalad fashion through the pericardial cavity, remaining attached to the pericardial wall at only the venous and arterial ends. This cardiac tube forms a loop with the arterial end, ultimately evolving into the ventricle forming the bulboventricular loop. The venous end differentiates into the sinus venosus, opening into the right side of the primitive atrium.

At this time, the atrium is situated above and behind the ventricle, being connected to the ventricle by means of the atrioventricular canal. As embryogenesis proceeds, the ventricle changes position, creating the tubular bulbus cordis from which arises the bulbus cordis and the truncus arteriosus. The ridge that separates the bulbus cordis from its common ventricle subsequently atrophies, dividing the truncus into the aorta and the main pulmonary artery.

The venous chambers can be seen by the end of the fourth week of fetal life. Shortly thereafter, the ventricular septum forms, separating the common ventricle into two distinct chambers. The development of the ventricular septum is complete by the end of the eighth week of gestation. Endocardial cushions, formed from a component of the ventricular septum that develops as an upward projection from the floor of the primitive ventricle, ultimately divide into the mitral and tricuspid valves. Subsequently the bulboventricular ridge, formed from another component of the ventricular septum that separates the outflow tract of the ventricles, disappears, and the aortic orifice opens into the left ventricle.

By the fifth week the single primitive atrium has been divided into the right and left atrium by the septum primum. The septum primum thins out and becomes perforated, forming the ostium secundum. This is followed by the formation of the septum secundum, which creates an opening known as the foramen ovale, a right-to-left shunt that is essential to fetal circulation (Fig. 2-1).

The venous and arterial transportation system also develop at this time. Venous blood returns to the sinus venosus, which is located in the posterior wall of the primitive atrium, via three primitive vessels that develop during the

Fig. 2-1. Development of the primitive cardiac tube.

From King, O.M.: Care of the cardiac surgical patient, St. Louis, 1975, The C.V. Mosby Co.

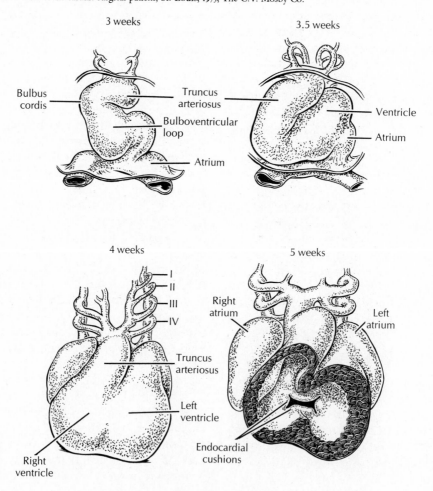

third week of fetal development. These vessels are the vitelline veins, which drain the yolk sac; the umbilical veins, which drain the placenta; and the cardinal veins, which drain the body of the fetus. The cardinal veins consist of right and left anterior divisions that drain the cephalic region and right and left posterior segments that empty the trunk and caudal regions. The right posterior cardinal vein eventually becomes the azygos vein. An anastomosis between the left and right anterior cardinal veins becomes the left innominate vein, while another portion of the left anterior cardinal vein differentiates into the first superior intercostal vein. The right cardinal vein persists as the right innominate vein and also becomes the superior vena cava. A portion of the sinus venosus remains as the coronary sinus (Fig. 2-2).

A single primitive pulmonary vein develops from that portion of the primitive atrium that eventually develops into the left atrium. This vessel subsequently divides into left and right branches, each of which subdivide again. These vessels anastomose with the pulmonary venous plexus, which later atrophies. The pulmonary veins become a part of the atrial wall as the left atrium develops from the primitive atrium (Fig. 2-3).

Arterial development proceeds simultaneously with venous development, beginning during the second week of gestation. The aorta and pulmonary artery find their roots in the septum between the bulbus cordis and the truncus arteriosus. The pulmonary artery is located anterior to the aorta and opens into the right ventricle, while the aorta opens into the left ventricle. Additional vessels that form six paired aortic arches develop between the dorsal and ventral aorta. Of these six paired arches, only the third through the sixth remain after development is complete. The third arches, with a portion of the dorsal aorta, form the internal carotid arteries. The right fourth arch differentiates into the right subclavian, and the left into the aortic arch. The left subclavian artery develops from an outgrowth of the aortic arch. The fifth arch is rudimentary. The sixth arch forms the pulmonary arteries out of the ventral segment and the ductus arteriosus from the dorsal portion (Fig. 2-4).

Fig. 2-2. Development of the great veins.

From King, O.M.: Care of the cardiac surgical patient, St. Louis, 1975, The C.V. Mosby Co.

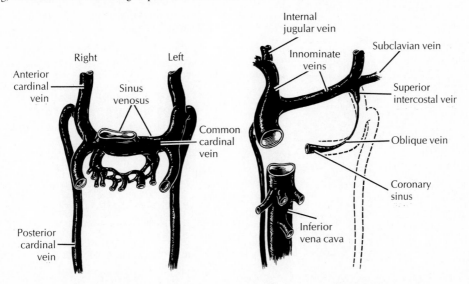

Fig. 2-3. Development of the pulmonary veins.

From King, O.M.: Care of the cardiac surgical patient, St. Louis, 1975, The C.V. Mosby Co.

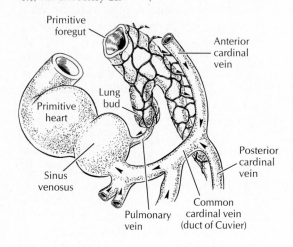

Fig. 2-4. Development of the great vessels.

From King, O.M.: Care of the cardiac surgical patient, St. Louis, 1975, The C.V. Mosby Co.

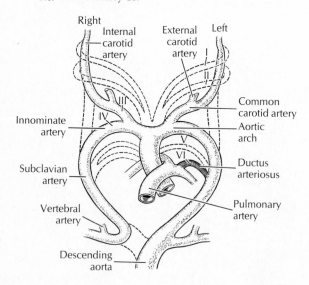

The heart begins to beat at the beginning of the fourth week of gestation. A formalized conduction system, however, does not exist until much later. It has been suggested that the sinoatrial (SA) and the atrioventricular (AV) nodes are embryologically analogous structures, arising at the junction of the right and left superior cardinal veins with the sinus venosus. As the sinus venosus becomes the medial half of the right atrium and part of the interatrial septum, the AV node migrates toward the internal position it ultimately occupies. The SA node remains near its primitive origin. The AV bundle and its proximal and distal branches are formed by convergence of fibers at the anterior and inferior margin of the AV node. Table 2-1 summarizes the development of the vascular system.

PHYSIOLOGY
Fetal circulation

Blood flow in the fetus differs from that in the adult. Fetal circulation (Fig. 2-5) receives oxygenated blood from the maternal circulation through the placenta via the umbilical vein. The umbilical vein divides into two branches, one entering the ductus venosus, which is a bypass around the liver, and the other entering the left and right branch of the portal vein continuing into the hepatic vein. Both branches reunite and enter the inferior vena cava carrying highly oxygenated blood from the ductus venosus, somewhat less saturated blood from the liver, and "venous blood" from the viscera and lower half of the body.

Approximately 66% of the well-oxygenated blood enters the right atrium through the inferior vena cava and passes through the foramen ovale into the left atrium because of the existence of a right-to-left pressure gradient. This blood bypasses the lungs. Additional blood from the right atrium, which branches from the superior vena cava, also enters the left atrium through the foramen ovale and mixes with a small amount of blood from the pulmonary system, thereby lowering the oxygen content.

Blood is then pumped into the left ventricle

Table 2-1. Development of the vascular system

Age in weeks	Size (CR*) in mm	Vascular system	Age in weeks	Size (CR*) in mm	Vascular system
2.5	1.5	Blood islands appear on chorion and yolk sac. Cardiogenic plate reversing.	7	17.0	Cardinal veins transforming. Inf. vena cava outlined. Atrium, ventricle, and bulbus partitioned.
3.5	2.5	Primitive blood cells and vessels present. Embryonic blood vessels, a paired symmetrical system. Heart tubes fuse, bend S-shape and beat begins.			Cardiac valves present. Stem of pulm. vein absorbed into l. atrium. Spleen anlage prominent.
4	5.0	Hemopoiesis on yolk sac. Paired aortae fuse. Aortic arches and cardinal veins completed. Dilated heart shows sinus, atrium, ventricle, and bulbus.	8	23.0	Main blood vessels assume final plan. Primitive lymph sacs present. Sinus venosus absorbed into right atrium. Atrioventricular bundle represented.
5	8.0	Primitive vessels extend into head and limbs. Vitelline and umbilical veins transforming. Myocardium condensing. Cardiac septa appearing. Spleen indicated.	10	40.0	Thoracic duct and peripheral lymphatics developed. Early lymph glands appearing. Enucleated red cells predominated in blood.
6	12.0	Hemopoiesis in liver. Aortic arches transforming. L. umbil. vein and d. venosus become important. Bulbus absorbed into right ventricle. Heart acquires its general definitive form.	12	56.0	Blood formation beginning in bone marrow. Blood vessels acquire accessory coats.
			16	112.0	Blood formation active in spleen. Heart musculature much condensed.
			20-40 (5-10 mo)	160.0- 350.0	Blood formation increasing in bone marrow and decreasing in liver (5-10). Spleen acquires typical structure (7). Some fetal blood passages discontinue (10).

From Arey, L.B.: Developmental anatomy, ed. 7, Philadelphia, 1974, W.B. Saunders Co.
*CR = Crown-rump.

and subsequently to the ascending aorta for distribution to the coronary arteries and aortic arch vessels, which supply the myocardium, head, and upper trunk. A small amount of blood also flows down the descending aorta to be distributed to the lower trunk. Backflow of blood through the foramen ovale is prevented because of a valve located on the left side of the septum, which closes the foramen as the atrium is ejecting blood into the ventricle.

The remaining 33% of the fairly well-oxygenated blood from the inferior vena cava continues through the right atrium, where it mixes with blood returning from the coronary sinus (from the myocardium) and superior vena cava (from the head and upper trunk). This blood is pumped into the right ventricle and subsequently to the pulmonary artery, where it is divided into three branches that go to the ductus arteriosus and both main pulmonary branches. Most of the blood is shunted through the ductus arteriosus because of the increased resistance to blood flow that exists in the pulmonary vascular bed. This blood then flows into the descending aorta, joining the blood from the left ventricle. Only a small portion of the blood enters the

Fig. 2-5. Fetal circulation. **A,** Overview. **B,** Schematic representation of blood flow. Oxygenation occurs in the placenta. Oxygenated blood enters the fetus via the umbilical vein. Most of this blood directly enters the ductus venosus, which normally constricts within 3 to 7 days of birth. From the ductus venosus, the blood enters the inferior vena cava. When this blood reaches the right atrium, it is diverted through the foramen ovale into the left atrium, through the left ventricle, and into the aorta. The foramen ovale ceases to function at birth and becomes sealed during the first postnatal month. Some blood from the umbilical vein enters the portal circulation, ultimately reuniting with highly oxygenated blood in the inferior vena cava. Venous blood from the brain and upper extremities enters the superior vena cava to return to the right atrium, mixing with blood from the coronary sinus. This blood is pumped into the right ventricle and flows into the pulmonary artery; most of it flows through the ductus arteriosus into the descending aorta. Only a small portion enters the pulmonary vascular system, returning to the left atrium via the pulmonary veins.

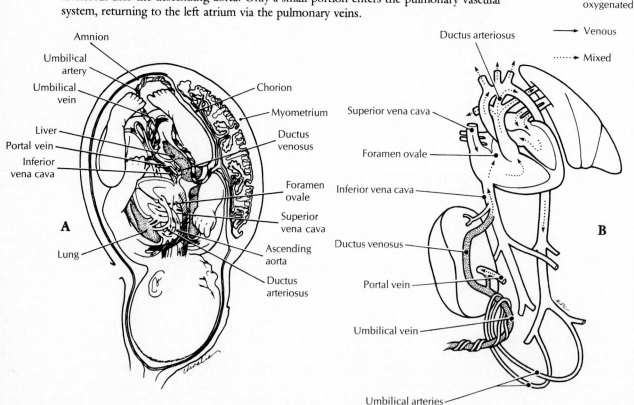

pulmonary vascular bed and returns to the left atrium via the pulmonary veins.

Approximately 60% of the blood in the descending aorta returns to the placenta for oxygenation via the common and internal iliac arteries and the umbilical arteries, with the blood that remains supplying the abdominal viscera, lower trunk, and legs.

Rather dramatic changes take place as fetal circulation adjusts to the infant's extrauterine environment. As the cord is clamped and placental circulation eliminated, the systemic blood pressure initially drops and then begins to rise. The heart rate decreases because of the increase in systemic vascular resistance. Gaseous exchange is transferred from the placenta to the lung of the neonate. The onset of ventilation is associated with an increase in pulmonary blood flow, which occurs because of the effect of oxygen on the constricted pulmonary blood vessels. As a result, pulmonary venous return and left ventricular output are increased. Over a couple of days the ductus closes as pulmonary vascular resistance decreases. A subsequent fall in pulmonary arterial and right ventricular pressures takes place, with pressures approaching those found in the normal adult. Because the foramen ovale is no longer needed, it also closes, usually by the third month of life.

General circulation

Circulation in the older infant, child, and adult travels through the systems in succession: the pulmonary system, which functions in the exchange of oxygen and carbon dioxide at the alveolar capillary membrane, and the systemic system, which carries oxygen and other nutritive materials to the tissues and removes the products of their metabolism from them (Fig. 2-6).

Deoxygenated blood in the systemic circulation returns to the right side of the heart from either the inferior vena cava (from the lower trunk), the superior vena cava (from the head and upper trunk), or the coronary sinus (from the myocardium). This blood is forced into the right ventricle through the tricuspid valve and

into pulmonary circulation through the pulmonary artery, the only artery carrying deoxygenated blood. After passing through the pulmonary semilunar valve, the deoxygenated blood enters pulmonary circulation, where the actual gaseous exchange of oxygen and carbon dioxide takes place. This blood, now oxygenated, travels through the pulmonary valve into the pulmonary vein, which is the only vein carry-

Fig. 2-6. Systemic postnatal circulation.

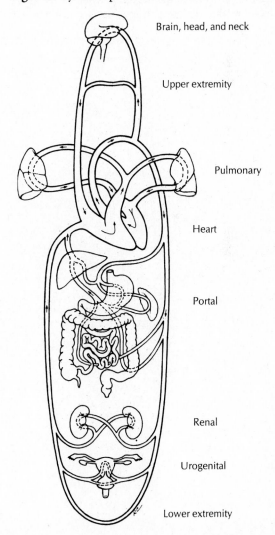

Brain, head, and neck

Upper extremity

Pulmonary

Heart

Portal

Renal

Urogenital

Lower extremity

ing oxygenated blood. It then flows into the left atrium of the heart and is forced through the mitral or bicuspid valve into the left ventricle, where it is ejected into the aorta. A portion of this blood enters the coronary arteries, which originate off of the aorta at the base of the sinus of Valsalva behind the aortic valve. These vessels provide the blood supply to the myocardium (Fig. 2-7), with the right coronary artery running in the coronary sulcus along the diaphragmatic surface of the heart before descending toward the apex, where it gives off branches to the

right atrium, the free wall of the right ventricle, and a portion of the posterior wall of the left ventricle and septum. This occurs in approximately 60% of the population, who are said to be right coronary artery dominant. In 30% of the population, the left coronary artery provides the blood supply to this area, while in the remaining 10% the blood supply to this area is evenly distributed between the right and left coronary artery. The left coronary artery, which bifurcates soon after leaving the aorta, divides into these two main branches: the left circumflex

Fig. 2-7. Coronary blood flow, illustrating blood supply to the anterior and posterior aspects of the heart.

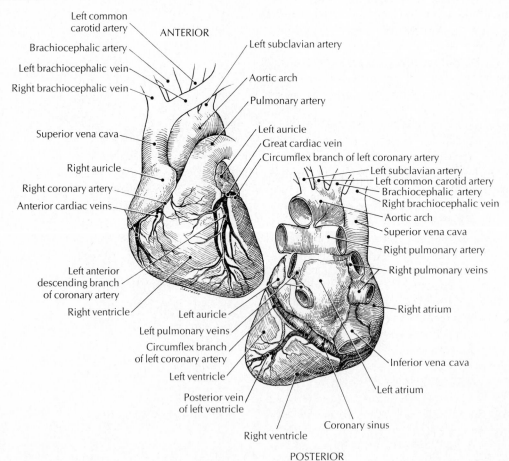

Left common carotid artery

ANTERIOR

Brachiocephalic artery

Left brachiocephalic vein

Right brachiocephalic vein

Left subclavian artery

Aortic arch

Pulmonary artery

Superior vena cava

Left auricle

Great cardiac vein

Circumflex branch of left coronary artery

Right auricle

Right coronary artery

Anterior cardiac veins

Left subclavian artery

Left common carotid artery

Brachiocephalic artery

Right brachiocephalic vein

Aortic arch

Superior vena cava

Right pulmonary artery

Right pulmonary veins

Left anterior descending branch of coronary artery

Right ventricle

Left auricle

Left pulmonary veins

Circumflex branch of left coronary artery

Left ventricle

Posterior vein of left ventricle

Right ventricle

Right atrium

Inferior vena cava

Left atrium

Coronary sinus

POSTERIOR

artery, which arises at right angles to the main vessel and flows along the atrioventricular sulcus, turning down toward the apex; and the anterior descending artery, which continues as an extension of the main branch, traveling down in the interventricular groove toward the apex. The circumflex branch provides the blood supply for the left atrium and the lateral wall of the left ventricle. The anterior descending branch supplies the free wall of the left ventricle, the ventricular septum, and to some extent the anterior wall of the right ventricle. The SA node receives its blood supply from the right coronary artery in about 60% of all people. In the remaining 40% of the population, the left circumflex artery supplies this portion of the conduction system. The AV node receives its blood supply from a marginal branch of the right coronary artery in about 90% of the population, with the left circumflex branch responsible in the remaining 10% of the population. The remainder of the blood leaving the left ventricle is distributed to the head and upper extremities via the brachiocephalic, the left common carotid, and the left subclavian arteries, which originate off the arch of the aorta; to the internal organs via the descending aorta, which continues into the thoracic aorta and abdominal aorta; and to the lower extremities via the external iliac arteries, that is, the femoral, popliteal, and tibial arteries. Fig. 2-8 illustrates the arteries that supply blood to various organs.

Blood returns to the heart from the venous system, which consists of three sets of vessels: the pulmonary, coronary, and systemic vessels. Pulmonary veins carry oxygenated blood from the lungs to the left heart. Coronary veins return blood from the myocardium and form the coronary sinus, which opens directly into the right atrium. Systemic veins of the head and neck called the external jugulars terminate in the subclavian vein, whereas the internal jugulars join the subclavian and then form the brachiocephalic vein. The brachiocephalic vein receives blood from the head, neck, mammary glands, and upper part of the thorax. The right and left brachiocephalic veins unite to form the superior vena cava. Three azygous veins form a channel between the inferior and superior vena cava. Blood can then be returned through these veins in case of an obstruction. In the abdomen and pelvis the internal and external iliac veins unite to form the common iliacs, which ultimately unite to form the inferior vena cava. Venous drainage from the upper extremities occurs via either deep or superficial veins. The deep veins are the venae comitantes of the hand, forearm, and arm; they are labeled the same as the corresponding arteries. Superficial veins are larger than the deep veins and consequently are able to return more blood from the distal part of the limb. Superficial veins consist of the cephalic vein, which begins in the dorsal network of the hand and travels to the upper arm; the basilic vein, which originates in the ulnar part of the dorsal network, extends posteriorly up to below the elbow, and is joined by the median cubital vein; the axillary vein, which is actually a continuation of the basilic vein; and the subclavian vein, which is a continuation of the axillary vein until it unites with the internal jugular vein to form the brachiocephalic. On the left side, the brachiocephalic vein is longer than on the right side. The junction of the left subclavian and left internal jugular veins receives the termination of the thoracic duct of the lymphatic system. On the right side, the junction between the right subclavian vein and the right internal jugular vein receives the short right lymphatic duct. Blood from the lower extremities is also returned via a superficial and deep set of veins. Again, the deep veins accompany the arteries. The major superficial vein of the lower extremities is the saphenous vein, which begins in the dorsum of the foot and ends in the femoral vein just below the inguinal ligament. Fig. 2-9 summarizes the venous system.

Cardiac function

The heart functions electrically and mechanically to pump blood to body tissues to meet the metabolic requirements of the cell. Varying de-

Fig. 2-8. Major arteries.

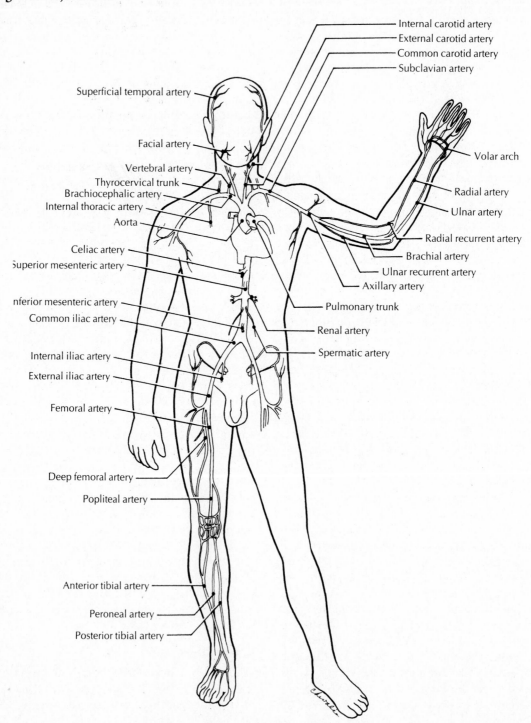

Fig. 2-9. Major veins.

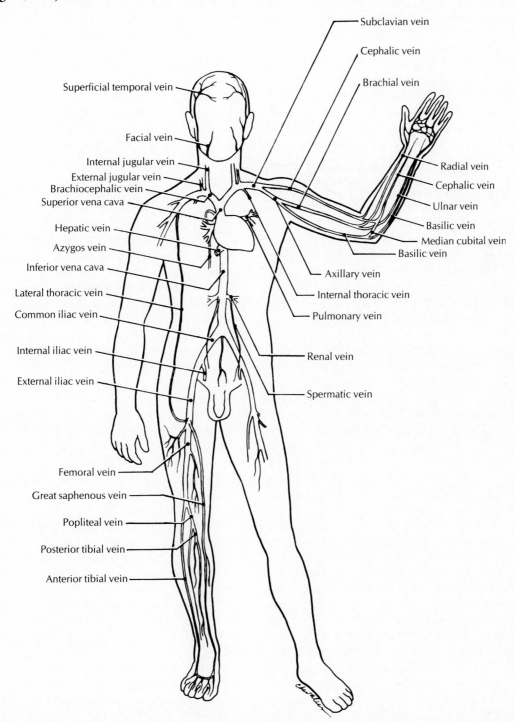

Subclavian vein

Cephalic vein

Brachial vein

Superficial temporal vein

Facial vein

Internal jugular vein

External jugular vein

Brachiocephalic vein

Superior vena cava

Hepatic vein

Azygos vein

Inferior vena cava

Lateral thoracic vein

Common iliac vein

Internal iliac vein

External iliac vein

Radial vein

Cephalic vein

Ulnar vein

Basilic vein

Median cubital vein

Basilic vein

Axillary vein

Internal thoracic vein

Pulmonary vein

Renal vein

Spermatic vein

Femoral vein

Great saphenous vein

Popliteal vein

Posterior tibial vein

Anterior tibial vein

mands are met by adjustments made in the cardiac output through changes in heart rate and/or stroke volume. A number of intrinsic and extrinsic influences affect the pumping action of the heart. Extrinsic influences on cardiac pumping are induced largely by the autonomic nervous system, which regulates heart rate and the force of contractility. Intrinsic influences affect the stroke volume by changing the end-diastolic volume and the fraction of blood ejected during systole.

Electrical control

Heart rate. Heart rate is controlled primarily by the sympathetic and parasympathetic divisions of the autonomic nervous system. Stimulation of the autonomic fibers, whether it is cardioexcitatory or cardioinhibitory, alters the rate and speed of conduction by its influence on the vasomotor center in the medulla. Sympathetic fibers are located throughout the atrial and ventricular musculature and cause postganglionic release of norepinephrine. Parasympathetic fibers are predominant in the atria, but recent investigation has shown that vagal innervation also affects the ventricles. Parasympathetic fibers, when activated, result in the release of acetylcholine. Centrally, sympathetic stimulation activates the cardioexcitatory center in the medulla and increases atrial and ventricular contractility, thereby increasing the speed of conduction and the heart rate. This action can be traced to the release of norepinephrine, which is believed to alter membrane permeability to sodium and calcium. With an increase in sodium permeability in the SA node, the membrane potential approaches threshold level for self-excitation and increases the rate of SA nodal discharge. Increased sodium permeability in the AV node also increases excitation, thereby decreasing the conduction time from the atria to the ventricles. The change in permeability to calcium enhances the contractile process of the myofibrils, ultimately leading to an increase in the contractile strength of the cardiac muscle. Parasympathetic stimulation activates the cardioinhibitory center and has the opposite effect because of the action of acetylcholine, which causes the cell membrane of the sinoatrial node to become more permeable to potassium. A rapid leakage of potassium to the exterior occurs, making the interior more negative, creating a "hyperpolarized" state. This decreases the rate of the SA node and decreases the excitability of the junctional fibers between the atrial muscle and the AV node. Ultimately, transmission of the impulse into the ventricles is slowed. Parasympathetic control predominates in the conscious state, maintaining the usual resting heart rate.

Heart rate is altered by the concentration of the cations in extracellular fluid. Decreases in the sodium (Na) levels appear to slow the heart rate and speed of conduction. The reduction in heart rate is most probably caused by a tension that develops between the sodium and calcium ions as low levels of sodium permit an increase in the binding of calcium and greater calcium influx in subsequent action potentials. The decrease in the speed of conduction can be attributed to slower upstroke and smaller amplitude of the action potential occurring with the lower sodium level.

Potassium is also important. Elevated concentrations in the serum potassium slow the heart rate and the conduction velocity. This impaired conduction can lead to heart block, especially marked in the atrioventricular node. Extremely high levels of potassium predispose to death-producing dysrhythmias—for example, ventricular fibrillation. These problems develop because an increase in the serum potassium decreases the resting potential and shortens the duration of the action potential. Calcium (Ca), also a chronotropic agent, slows the heart rate by raising the excitation threshold when the calcium level is elevated. Greatly reduced calcium levels appear to increase the heart rate because of an increase in pacemaker potential, especially in Purkinje tissue.

Cardiac action potential. A change in the membrane potential between the inside and outside of a cell, followed by a return to the resting potential, is referred to as an action potential. There exists a concentration gradient of ions across the semipermeable membrane of the cardiac cell that provides an electrochemical basis for the development of the cardiac action potential (Fig. 2-10).

The electrochemical activity of the cardiac muscle cell is regulated by four primary ions found in both the intracellular and extracellular fluids. These four ions are sodium, potassium, calcium, and chloride. Potential changes are associated with changes in the permeability of the cell membrane to sodium, potassium, and calcium. In the resting state, intracellular concentrations of potassium predominate. Sodium is dominant in the extracellular fluid. Because the cell membrane is slightly permeable to sodium, these ions begin to diffuse into the cell when the cell is stimulated. This diffusion occurs through what are called *fast channels* in the cell membrane in the direction of the concentration gradient. This change occurs because of both chemical and electrical forces, the former creating a diffusion gradient and the latter striving to balance the ionic charges. As a plateau is reached, a second inward current develops and calcium also begins to diffuse into the cell. This is referred to as the slow inward current because the current is much slower than that in the fast channel. The slow channels are more selective for calcium. As the intracellular concentration becomes more positive, potassium diffuses outward because of the same chemical and electrical forces. Sodium and calcium inward movements soon slow down. An imbalance in the overall electrical charge occurs, and potassium is pumped back into the cell with sodium subsequently eliminated in exchange for potassium. A metabolic pump is responsible for the removal of sodium from the intracellular compartment. This pump, referred to as the *sodium-potassium pump,* requires the use of energy and involves the sodium and potassium-activated enzyme adenosine triphosphase (ATPase), which is located in the cell membrane. This enzyme catalyzes the breakdown of ATP to ADP, which supplies the en-

ergy needed for active transport. There is now evidence for a bidirectional sodium-calcium exchange system that mediates the movement of calcium across the sarcolemma. Energy for this system is thought to be provided by the movement of sodium down its electrochemical gradient. The direction of movement depends on the relative concentrations of extracellular and intracellular sodium and calcium. Action potentials from cells in the atria and ventricles, from specialized cells in the intracardiac conduction system, and from distal AV nodal regions depend on both fast and slow inward currents. Rapid conduction through these regions depends on the passage of sodium through the fast channels. In contrast, pacemaker cells in the SA node and primordial regions of the AV node have a slow

Fig. 2-10. Action potential of a myocardial cell. During *Phase 0*, there is a rapid influx of sodium ions that causes the interior of the cell to become positively charged. As membrane permeability to sodium decreases, there is a sharp drop in the intracellular charge, labeled as *Phase 1*. During *Phase 2*, a plateau is reached as a small amount of sodium and a significant amount of calcium ions diffuse into the cell, and potassium ions slowly leave the cell. Repolarization occurs in *Phase 3* because of the rapid efflux of potassium ions, restoring the negativity to the interior of the cell. The inside of the cell is hyperpolarized (more negatively charged than usual) in *Phase 4*.

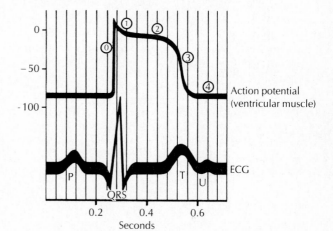

rising action potential and slower conduction and are activated by the slow inward current (Fig. 2-11).

Impulse formation. The transmembrane potential in the resting cardiac cell is approximately -80 to -90 mV. Its magnitude varies in different types of cardiac tissue, as can be seen in Fig. 2-12. When an electric impulse of sufficient magnitude stimulates the cell membrane, the transmembrane potential is lowered to a critical level, referred to as the *threshold potential,* and an action potential develops. The overall effect is that of an all-or-none response; there is either no response at all to the stimulus, or there is a maximum response. Sodium influx occurs, bringing about membrane depolarization. As the transmembrane potential increases toward zero, calcium influx occurs. Because the ionic balance has been disturbed, an attempt to balance the charges occurs, that is, potassium moves out of the cell, and the terminal phase of depolarization is completed. At this time the inside of the cell becomes positive in relation to the outside; this phenomenon is referred to as *reversal.* The overshoot (reversal of potential) is immediately followed by repolarization, which occurs in three rapid phases as the transmembrane potential returns first to zero and subsequently to that of the resting state. While this occurs, ionic transfer takes place, restoring the negative state inside the cell. Fig. 2-13 illustrates the transmembrane potential in the resting, depolarized, and repolarized states.

Although all myocardial cells have the potential to be activated by an electric stimulus, there are certain areas within the heart that are particularly developed for the generation and conduction of electric impulses. Cells in these special areas have the property of automaticity, an inherent ability that enables them to spontaneously reach threshold potential. Therefore these cells, which are located in the sinoatrial node, the atrioventricular junction, and the His-Purkinje network, can spontaneously depolarize and are responsible for the rhythmicity of the heart.

Both extrinsic and intrinsic factors control the rate of impulse formation in the automatic cells. Extrinsic influence occurs because of autonomic control. Intrinsic factors within the cell itself regulate spontaneous depolarization. Therefore cells within the sinoatrial node may have different inherent rates than those within the atrioventricular junction or His-Purkinje system because of shifts in the resting potential, threshold potential, or rates of diastolic depolarization and repolarization. Usually the inherent rate of impulse formation in the SA node is 60 to 80 beats/min. If the sinus node fails to fire or fires at a lower rate, the automatic cells in the next lower pacemaker, the AV junction, usually "take over" at an intrinsic rate of 40 to 60 beats/min. Failure of the automatic cells in the

Fig. 2-11. Schematic representation of the sodium-potassium pump.

Extracellular fluid

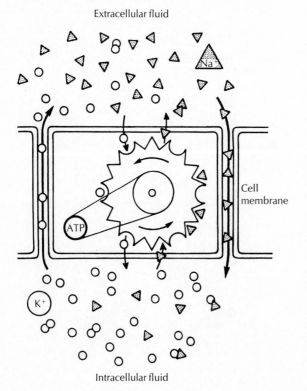

Cell membrane

Intracellular fluid

AV junction results in His-Purkinje control, at a rate of between 20 and 40 beats/min.

Conduction. Specialized conduction tissue is responsible for propagating an impulse through the myocardial tissue. An orderly sequence of activities can be identified in the normal heart. As stimulation occurs, a localized area is depolarized and serves as a stimulus for depolarization of an adjacent area. This event continues along the length of the conduction system until all of the myocardial tissue is depolarized (Fig. 2-14).

The speed of conduction varies. Beginning in the SA node, the impulse is transmitted outward in a radial fashion, simultaneously traveling through the atrial musculature, internodal tracts, and interatrial fibers. The impulse arrives at the atrioventricular junction before the atria are completely depolarized. The impulse is delayed at the AV node before proceeding slowly through the junctional tissue. It is then conducted very rapidly through the His bundle and intraventricular Purkinje system to all parts of the ventricle.

The electrical activity from excited conduction tissue can be represented by a single resultant electrical force that has finite direction and magnitude and can be transmitted equally well in all directions. This force can be recorded on the surface electrocardiogram (ECG). Its depth and direction vary with the surface lead being mon-

Fig. 2-12. Typical tracings of the cardiac action potential, recorded from different regions. The action potential of a pacemaker cell is different from that of other myocardial cells; it has a shorter, sharper prepotential and no plateau. Although all myocardial cells have the ability to depolarize spontaneously, a pacemaker cell has the most rapid rate of spontaneous depolarization because it is less negatively charged and its membrane is more permeable to sodium. Pacemaker cells can be stimulated more frequently because of a shorter absolute refractory period (no plateau).

Fig. 2-13. Transmembrane potential in the resting, depolarized, and repolarized states.

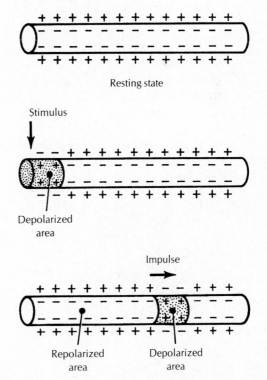

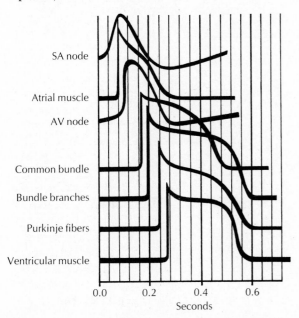

itored and depend on the distance of the lead from the point of origin of the force. If the force is perpendicular to the axis of a surface lead, no deflection will be seen on the surface lead. If the resultant force is directed toward the positive end of the axis, a positive deflection will be seen, while a negative deflection will occur if the force is directed toward the negative end of the axis.

The surface ECG, composed of waves arbitrarily named P, Q, R, S, and T waves, provides a graphic record of impulse conduction through the atrial and ventricular musculature (Fig. 2-15). Atrial depolarization is represented by the P wave. Ventricular depolarization is represented by the QRS complex. The PR interval, usually 0.12 to 0.20 second in duration, measures the time it takes for the impulse to travel through the atria, internodal tracts, and interatrial fibers to the AV node, where it is delayed approxi-

mately 0.1 second before proceeding through the remaining conductive system. Then, as the impulse spreads through the His bundle and Purkinje network in approximately 0.06 to 0.12 second, as QRS complex evolves. The QT interval represents the time it takes for complete ventricular depolarization and repolarization and is approximately 0.36 to 0.44 seconds in duration. Alterations in conduction can produce alterations in the size, shape, and configuration of the P, QRS, and T waves.

Excitability. As previously mentioned, all myocardial cells have the inherent potential to be excited. The level of excitability, although dependent on several factors, is directly related to the phase of the cardiac cycle (Fig. 2-16). Maximum excitability occurs immediately before ventricular depolarization. Excitability is zero from the instant of depolarization until midrepolarization. During this time no stim-

Fig. 2-14. Transmission of the cardiac impulse through atrial and ventricular musculature. Impulse originates in the sinoatrial node and then moves through the atrial musculature, the internodal tracts, and the atrioventricular node. It is then transmitted through the Bundle of His and down the left and right bundle branches to the Purkinje fibers, which distribute the impulse to the ventricles.

Fig. 2-15. Electrical tracing of the cardiac cycle: the PR interval, measured from beginning of the P wave to beginning of the QRS complex; the QRS interval, measured from beginning to end of the QRS complex; and the QT interval, measured from beginning of the QRS complex to end of the T wave. Longitudinal axis represents voltage; horizontal axis represents time.

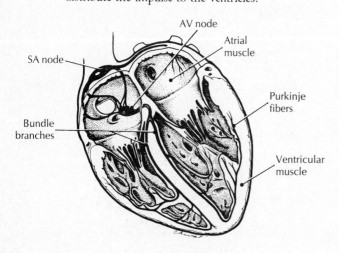

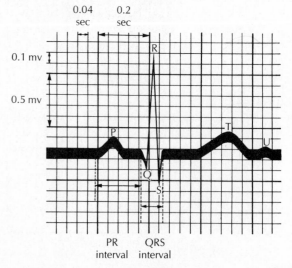

ulus, regardless of its strength, will evoke a response. The cell is absolutely refractory. Following this, the myocardium becomes less refractory such that a stimulus of sufficient magnitude could elicit a response, but a response of this type would be conducted in an aberrant or abnormal manner. This period of time is referred to as *relative refractory* and is characterized by a temporary increase in excitability, referred to as the *vulnerable period*. Following relative refractory, excitability remains normal until the ventricles are stimulated again.

Mechanical control

Stroke volume. Stroke volume, which is the amount of blood ejected with each contraction, is regulated through changes in the end-diastolic volume and ejection fraction. These changes are accomplished through alterations in the preload, afterload, and degree of contractility.

Preload. The preload can be defined as the ventricular end-diastolic volume. It is this venous filling pressure that determines the length of the muscle fiber before contraction and ultimately the contractile force volume. Preload is influenced by five interrelated factors: venous return, venous tone, systemic peripheral resistance, circulating blood volume, and distribution of the blood volume.

The amount of blood returning to the heart from the peripheral vessels, the venous return, determines the preload. Venous return is increased in the presence of increased venous tone, decreased systemic peripheral resistance, and increased circulating blood volume. The converse is also true.

Changes in venous return can occur as a result of alterations in the venous tone. As the veins fill to capacity, they are able to hold larger and larger quantities of blood because of their high distensibility. Venous pressure will be increased because of increased venous blood volume and tone and therefore will result in increased venous return.

Venous tone is of prime importance in the regulation of venous return. The smooth muscle

in the walls of the veins reacts to a variety of neural and humoral stimuli.

Transient adjustments in venous tone occur as a result of innervation of the sympathetic or parasympathetic divisions of the autonomic nervous system. Sympathetic stimulation produces a generalized venoconstriction, thereby increasing venous pressure and venous tone. Parasympathetic stimulation, on the other hand, results in dilation of the veins, permits pooling of the blood, and lowers the venous pressure and the venous tone.

The resistance to blood flow in the systemic circulation will affect the rate at which blood flows and ultimately the venous return. Venous return varies inversely with the systemic peripheral resistance.

A relationship can also be drawn between the circulating blood volume and the preload.

Fig. 2-16. Cardiac action potential and ECG tracing of refractory periods.

From Guzzetta, C.E., and Dossey, B.M.: Cardiovascular nursing: bodymind tapestry, ed. 1, St. Louis, 1984, The C.V. Mosby Co.

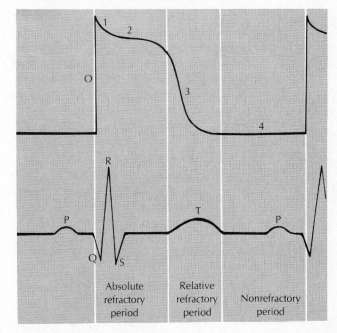

An increase in the blood volume will increase the degree of filling in the systemic circulation. This will then increase the mean systemic pressure, the average force that pushes blood from the vessels toward the heart and decreases the resistance to venous return. The overall effect will be a rapid flow of blood into the heart—an increase in the preload.

The circulating blood volume is regulated primarily by two internal mechanisms. First, the kidneys play a primary role in regulating the circulating volume by controlling the amount of angiotensin II that is produced. The juxtaglomerular cells in the vessel walls of the kidneys secrete the enzyme renin, which converts angiotensin I to angiotensin II (see Unit 5). Angiotensin II provides the stimulus for the release of aldosterone, which controls extracellular fluid volume by regulating the reabsorption of sodium by the distal kidney tubules.

Alpha and beta receptors in the right and left atria also play a regulatory role in controlling the circulating blood volume. The alpha receptors are sensitive to atrial pressures, while the beta receptors are sensitive to atrial volumes. Normally these receptors prevent the release of the antidiuretic hormone ADH (vasopressin), which enhances renal absorption of water from the distal and collecting tubules. Decreased stimulation of these stretch receptors as a result of low pressure or low volume states will have an inhibitory effect and will result in the secretion of vasopressin.

The distribution of the total blood volume also influences the preload. Venous pooling, for example, will diminish blood return. The distribution of blood is a function of body position and intrathoracic pressure. Gravity forces blood in dependent body positions. Standing, therefore, results in venous pooling in the extremities and increases the extrathoracic blood volume while decreasing the intrathoracic volume, ultimately affecting the cardiac output.

Negative intrathoracic pressure increases thoracic blood volume, thereby improving the preload. The negative intrathoracic pressure is greatest during inspiration. As a result, the gradient for venous return rises during inspiration. Increased intrathoracic pressure, on the other hand, reduces the intrathoracic blood volume and impedes venous return.

Afterload. Ventricular ejection and performance and ultimately stroke volume are influenced by the arterial pressure during ejection. This resistance to ventricular emptying is referred to as afterload. The greater the afterload, the less the stroke volume because ventricular ejection and performance will be hampered. For the left ventricle, the main factors that influence afterload are the aortic impedence, the peripheral vascular resistance, and the mass and viscosity of the blood. The corresponding factors for the right ventricle include pulmonary impedance and pulmonary vascular resistance.

Aortic and pulmonary impedance will increase the afterload in the left and right ventricle, respectively. This impedance may be caused by anything that obstructs the flow of blood through the ventricle. As the ventricular pressure rises, the performance will fall.

Vascular resistance, either in the peripheral or pulmonary vasculature, is controlled to a great extent by the autonomic nervous system. Sympathetic stimulation will produce a generalized vasoconstriction, thereby increasing the vascular resistance and afterload, while parasympathetic innervation will result in vasodilation and decreased afterload.

Increased viscosity of blood will also increase the afterload because the resistance to the viscous blood flow will be greater. Blood circulation time will be delayed, causing resistance to ventricular emptying.

Myocardial contractility. The force with which the myocardium will contract, or myocardial contractility, is a function of several factors, perhaps the most important of which is muscle fiber length. Under equivalent states of responsiveness, the degree of fiber stretch is influenced by the initial ventricular volume and increases progressively with the volume as long as the total volume does not exceed the physiologic capacity of the ventricle. The force of contraction and amount of energy released will be proportional to the degree of stretch. This rule, known as the *Starling principle,* can be simply stated: the greater the volume, the greater the stretch and subsequent force of contraction.

The sequence of atrial and ventricular activation will also influence the force of contraction. It has already been shown that myocardial fibers contract in sequence. Once an impulse is formed, it is propagated through atrial and ventricular musculature in a sequential manner. Because the atria, like the ventricles, will respond to an increase in fiber length by increasing their force of contraction, a greater volume of blood will ultimately be pumped into the ventricles. This will result in an increase in the ventricular end-diastolic volume, an increase in fiber length, and a subsequent increase in the force of contraction. This phenomenon has been referred to as the *atrial kick.* The same sequence of events can be described within the ventricular conduction system because the earlier-contracting ventricular fibers will influence the stretch and force of the later-contracting fibers. Collectively, this mechanism is described as the *idioventricular kick.*

A change in the contractile or inotropic state of the muscle can also occur without changing fiber length. In addition, neural and neurohumoral influences can alter the contractile state. Sympathetic stimulation enhances myocardial contractility with the release of norepinephrine, which appears to increase the permeability of the cell membrane to calcium, resulting in a greater influx of calcium during the plateau phase of the action potential. Norepinephrine also potentiates the interaction of calcium.

Indirectly, norepinephrine results in a shortening of the duration of ventricular systole and more rapid ventricular relaxation, therefore permitting more time for ventricular filling. Not only does norepinephrine permit more time for ventricular filling, but it also allows more rapid filling at any given atrial filling pressure. Both of these factors enhance contractility and are especially important with rapid rates, also an outcome of sympathetic stimulation. Norepinephrine, as well as epinephrine, are also released by the adrenal medulla. These catecholamines augment contractility during stress.

Changes in the heart rate itself can increase the force of contraction. Either through sympathetic stimulation and catecholamine release or through other mechanisms, an increase in contraction frequency (heart rate) will increase the force of contraction proportionately until a plateau is reached. This effect is known as the *treppe,* or *Bowditch, phenomenon* and can be described as a staircase response. It occurs as a result of a gradual rise in intracellular calcium, which plays a major role in the excitation-contraction activity by assisting in both the initiation and regulation of a contraction. The rhythm of contraction will also influence the contractile state. Extrasystoles, which alter the cardiac rhythm, augment contractility for several cycles.

The concentration of cations in the plasma will also affect the contractility of the myocardium. It has been pointed out that sodium, potassium, and calcium assume a vital role in the action potential. Sodium is a prerequisite for the beating of the heart; without it, little action will occur. An increase in the extracellular sodium concentration, however, appears to have a negative inotropic effect, thereby reducing myocardial contractility. Calcium, on the other hand, seems to have a positive inotropic effect such that an increase in the extracellular concentration of calcium leads to an increase in the maximum force of contraction. Contractility is enhanced because an increase in extracellular calcium produces a greater calcium influx during the action potential. Very low extracellular calcium levels have the opposite effect, reducing myocardial contractility until there may be no response at all.

Peripheral circulation

The blood levels form a transportation system that delivers oxygen and other nutritive materials to body cells and removes the waste products of their metabolism. In addition, these vessels distribute hormones manufactured by specialized tissues or organs and carry fats and carbohydrates from storage depots to areas where they can be used. The blood vessels also transport defense mechanisms, leukocytes, immune antibodies, and materials involved in coagulation to regions of injury or trauma. In addition, the blood vessels assist in the control of body temperature by carrying heat generated by body metabolic processes to areas where it can be given off.

Arteries and veins

Blood is distributed by the arterial system through pulmonary and systemic circulation where, at the capillary beds, actual exchange takes place. Waste products are returned via the venous system and lymphatics.

The arterial system consists of large elastic vessels (that is, the aorta and its major branches), smaller nutrient arteries, and arterioles. The larger arteries, which are easily distensible, can accommodate the volume of blood ejected during systole. In addition, these vessels can store energy for potential use in their elastic walls. The quality of elasticity permits these vessels to distribute the pulsated volume in a more even manner. The nutrient arteries, which arise off of the larger arteries, serve to carry the blood to each organ or vascular bed. The nutrient arteries are subdivided into smaller arterioles that are

richly innervated with sympathetic fibers. The fibers provide primarily alpha but also some beta adrenergic stimulation, and they assist in regulating the volume and pressure of blood in the arterial system by controlling the outflow. These vessels, which are chiefly responsible for regulating blood flow throughout the body, are labeled *resistance vessels* because they offer the greatest resistance to blood flow pumped to the body tissues.

The capillaries and their associated structures comprise the microcirculation. Capillary vessels, which provide a network for connecting the arterial and venous systems, are responsible for the exchange of fluids, dissolved gases, and small particles between the blood and the interstitial fluid.

Blood drains from the capillary system into the venous system, which consists of venules and veins. Venules are slightly larger in diameter than arterioles and appear to be similar to the capillaries in structure and function. Therefore they are, along with the capillaries, referred to as *exchange vessels*. Venules form veins with progressively larger diameters. They are also innervated with sympathetic fibers, which cause venoconstriction because of the effect of norepinephrine, or venodilation, which is secondary to the inhibition of these nerve fibers responding to local or regional stimuli. There is little resistance to blood flow in the venous system beyond the venules. The venous system has a large capacity that enables it to serve as a low pressure storage reservoir. These vessels are collectively labeled *capacitance vessels*. Fig. 2-17 illustrates the blood flow through the microcirculation.

The lymphatics can be viewed as a second circulatory system because they collect fluid and other materials that might normally accumulate in the interstitial space. These materials are transmitted to the vascular system via the thoracic ducts.

Distribution of blood flow

Total blood flow is limited and must be distributed to various tissues in appropriate

---

Fig. 2-17. Overall structure of the capillary bed.

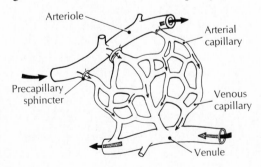

Arteriole

Arterial capillary

Precapillary sphincter

Venous capillary

Venule

amounts when the need arises. In actuality, flow distribution is quite unequal. It is influenced by both the size and vascularity of different organs, as illustrated in Fig. 2-14, which shows the average values for tissue blood flow and oxygen consumption in a 70-kg adult at rest. It becomes obvious when analyzing the graph that the liver, kidney, and skeletal muscle receive approximately 66% of the total blood flow. However, the vascularity (blood flow per unit weight) of selected tissues is very different. The kidney, liver, heart, and brain all exhibit a high flow per unit weight, whereas at rest, skeletal muscle and other relatively avascular tissues have a low flow per unit weight in comparison.

An examination of blood flow and blood flow per unit weight can be misleading without also looking at the O_2 extraction ratio, which is the fraction of arterial oxygen taken up by the tissues. In the kidneys, for example, there is a need for a large blood flow per unit weight to carry out clearance duties. This flow can be viewed as nonnutritional, however, because it is associated with modest oxygen consumption (Fig. 2-18). Stress can alter both the total blood flow and flow distribution. Without extreme exercise the cardiac output can rise to as much as 10 to 12 L/min in a healthy adult. The percentage of total blood flow shunted to tissues in need can be increased substantially to meet the oxygen demand, as seen in Fig. 2-19.

Rate of blood flow

The rate of blood flow can be determined by Poiseuille's law, which states that the rate of flow, Q, of a homogenous fluid through a cylindrical tube of length L and radius r is directly proportional to the driving pressure, ΔP (the

Fig. 2-18. Blood flow, organ weight, vascularity (blood flow per unit weight), and AV oxygen extraction of main organs in normal adult at rest. Body weight, 70 kg; cardiac output, 5400 ml/min; mean vascularity, 7.7 ml/min/100 g; mean AVO_2 difference, 5 ml of O_2/dl. (Liver flow includes that of the intestines and other organs draining into the portal vein and therefore actually refers to hepatosplanchnic flow.)

From Smith, J., et al: Circulatory physiology, the essentials, Baltimore, MD, 1980, Williams and Wilkins.

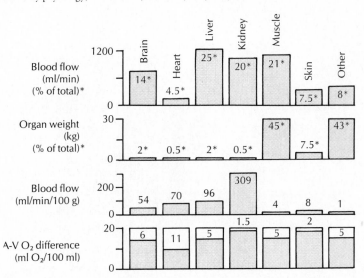

difference in the pressure between the beginning and end of the tube) and to the fourth power of the radius, and inversely proportional to the length of the tube, L, and to the viscosity of the flow liquid, n.

$$Q = \frac{\Delta P\ r^4\ \pi}{8^*\ n\ L}$$

Although blood is a nonhomogenous fluid, its pulsatile flow through a series of branching distensible tubes can be approximated well by Poiseville's Law. In the above equation, ΔP can be viewed as the driving pressure while the nonconstant factors that remain $\frac{r^4}{nL}$ can be considered impediments to flow. Mathematically, this formula can be simplified by collecting and

---

*The constants arise from geometric considerations in the equation's derivation.

inverting the residual factors $\frac{nL}{r^4}$ and labeling them R, or resistance to flow. Then:

$$Q = \frac{\Delta P}{R}$$

Therefore the rate of blood flow is determined by two factors: (1) the pressure difference, which pushes blood through the vessel; and (2) the impediment to blood flow through the vessel, or vascular resistance.

Regulation of blood flow

Each tissue can regulate its own blood flow based on its individual needs. This is accomplished via changes in the caliber of the vessel, which may occur as a passive response to transmural pressure or by active contraction or relaxation of circular smooth muscle. Although arterial or arteriolar constriction or dilation can influence peripheral vascular resistance, it is the

---

Fig. 2-19. Regional blood flow at rest (dark areas) and at maximal dilation (lighter areas) per organ and per 100 g of tissue.

From Mellander, S., and Johansson, B.: Pharmacological Reviews 20:117, 1968; adapted from Smith, J., and Kampine, J.P.: Circulatory physiology: the essentials, Baltimore, MD, 1980, Williams and Wilkins.

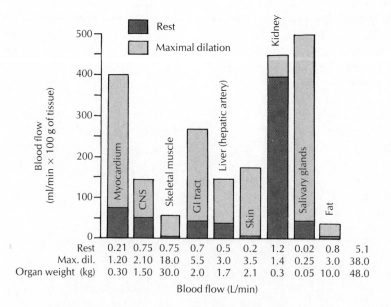

	Myocardium	CNS	Skeletal muscle	GI tract	Liver (hepatic artery)	Skin	Kidney	Salivary glands	Fat	
Rest	0.21	0.75	0.75	0.7	0.5	0.2	1.2	0.02	0.8	5.1
Max. dil.	1.20	2.10	18.0	5.5	3.0	3.5	1.4	0.25	3.0	38.0
Organ weight (kg)	0.30	1.50	30.0	2.0	1.7	2.1	0.3	0.05	10.0	48.0

Blood flow (L/min)

capacitance of the peripheral bed or distensibility of the small veins and venules that influences the diameter of these vessels.

Vessel caliber is regulated both centrally and locally in an effort to meet varying metabolic demands. The regulation of blood flow can be either neurogenic, humoral, or chemical.

Neural control. Neural control is maintained by the autonomic nervous system, or ANS, which includes the thoracolumbar (sympathetic) outflow and the craniosacral (parasympathetic) outflow. Transmission in the ANS occurs via self-propagating action potentials that are transmitted across synapses and junctions with other tissues by means of chemical neurotransmitters, which combine with specific alpha and beta receptors on effector cells to activate the end organ. The primary neurotransmitters of the ANS are acetylcholine and norepinephrine. Acetylcholine is formed in a multistep synthesis in which acetate combines with acetyl coenzyme A, forming a product that subsequently combines with choline. Acetylcholine is released by the preganglionic fibers of the entire autonomic system, parasympathetic postganglionic neurons, and some postganglionic sympathetic fibers, while norepinephrine, which is synthesized from the amino acid tyrosine, is released by most postganglionic neurons in the sympathetic nervous system. Nerve fibers that release acetylcholine are said to be *cholinergic,* while those that release norepinephrine are referred to as *adrenergic.* The term adrenergic is derived from noradrenaline, another name for norepinephrine.

Sympathetic control. The circulatory effects of sympathetic innervation are mediated by descending fibers from the cardiac and vasomotor center in the medullary portion of the brainstem, which synapse with cells of the intermediolateral cell column of the cord. Preganglionic fibers from the spinal cord travel to the sympathetic chain via the anterior spinal roots. Impulses from the cerebral cortex and hypothalamus may proceed in a similar fashion to elicit a sympathetic vascular response. Sympathetic postganglionic fibers from the cervical chain and first

four thoracic ganglia innervate the heart and entire peripheral circulation. Additional postganglionic sympathetic fibers join with other autonomic nerves to influence most of the arteries and veins in the body. Sympathetic preganglionic fibers activate the adrenal medulla, which releases epinephrine and norepinephrine directly into systemic circulation.

Sympathetic stimulation activates alpha-adrenergic receptors, leading to a generalized vasoconstriction that is most noticeable in the skin, skeletal muscle, splanchnic beds, and renal vascular beds. Vasoconstriction increases the resistance of the vessels, thereby changing the rate of flow. There is some evidence that sympathetic innervation may result in skeletal muscle vasodilation secondary to beta receptor activation. This could decrease peripheral resistance, although the constrictor effect is much stronger. The adrenal medullary response to sympathetic activation is the release of the catecholamines, epinephrine and norepinephrine. These compounds reinforce the action of postganglionic sympathetic fibers except for those in the sweat glands and those that elicit cholinergic vasodilation. Both the circulatory and noncirculatory effects of sympathetic stimulation are summarized in Table 2-2.

Parasympathetic control. The influence of the parasympathetic nervous system on circulation is mediated by preganglionic fibers that originate in either the motor nuclei of the brain stem exiting from the cranial nerves or in the sacral division of the spinal cord. A majority of all parasympathetic fibers are in the vagus nerves, which pass to the entire thoracic and abdominal regions of the body. Postganglionic parasympathetic fibers are located in the walls of the effector organ.

In general, parasympathetic innervation leads to dilation of most blood vessels, especially those in the abdominal viscera and the skeletal system. The effects of parasympathetic stimulation in skeletal muscle fibers may be short-lived because of the enzymatic action of cholinesterase on acetylcholine. Cholinesterase causes destruc-

Table 2-2. Autonomic effects on various organs of the body

Organ	Effect of sympathetic stimulation	Effect of parasympathetic stimulation
Eye: Pupil	Dilated	Constricted
Ciliary muscle	Slight relaxation	Contracted
Glands: Nasal	Vasoconstriction and slight	Stimulation of thin, copious
Lacrimal	secretion	secretion (containing many enzymes
Parotid		for enzyme-secreting glands)
Submaxillary		
Gastric		
Pancreatic		
Sweat glands	Copious sweating (cholinergic)	None
Apocrine glands	Thick, odoriferous secretion	None
Heart: Muscle	Increased rate	Slowed rate
	Increased force of contraction	Decreased force of atrial contraction
Coronaries	Dilated (β_2); constricted (α)	Dilated
Lungs: Bronchi	Dilated	Constricted
Blood vessels	Mildly constricted	? Dilated
Gut: Lumen	Decreased peristalsis and tone	Increased peristalsis and tone
Sphincter	Increased tone	Relaxed
Liver	Glucose released	Slight glycogen synthesis
Gallbladder and bile ducts	Relaxed	Contracted
Kidney	Decreased output	None
Bladder: Detrusor	Relaxed	Excited
Trigone	Excited	Relaxed
Penis	Ejaculation	Erection
Systemic blood vessels:		
Abdominal	Constricted	None
Muscle	Constricted (adrenergic α)	None
	Dilated (adrenergic β)	
	Dilated (cholinergic)	
Skin	Constricted	None
Blood: Coagulation	Increased	None
Glucose	Increased	None
Basal metabolism	Increased up to 100%	None
Adrenal cortical secretion	Increased	None
Mental activity	Increased	None
Piloerector muscles	Excited	None
Skeletal muscle	Increased glycogenolysis	None
	Increased strength	

From Guyton, A.C.: Textbook of medical physiology, ed. 6, Philadelphia, 1981, W.B. Saunders Co.

tion of the neurotransmitter within seconds after its release. Table 2-2 lists the effects of parasympathetic innervation.

Baroreceptor reflexes. Circulatory reflexes provide another mechanism by which the nervous system controls circulatory flow. Baroreceptors located in the walls of the large systemic arteries respond to a rise in pressure and send signals to the central nervous system, which responds by sending messages to the circulation to lower arterial pressure and hence peripheral vascular resistance. These pressure receptors are found in the walls of the internal carotid arteries, slightly above the carotid bifurcations, and in the walls of the aortic arch. Nerve impulses are transmitted from the carotid sinus through Hering's nerve to the glossopharyngeal nerve and finally to the medulla oblongata. Impulses from the walls of the aorta are transmitted via the vagus nerve to the medulla. Baroreceptor stimulation inhibits the vasomotor center of the medulla and excites the vagus, leading to vasodilation throughout peripheral circulation. Low pressure has the opposite effect. The baroreceptor system functions as a control for only short periods of time.

Humoral control. Humoral regulation of blood flow is mediated through hormones and other organic substances and may occur locally or centrally.

Catecholamines. Earlier, the role of the adrenal medulla was mentioned. Stimulation of the sympathetic nervous system results in activation of the adrenal medulla and the release of both catecholamines, norepinephrine and epinephrine. Norepinephrine has a vasoconstrictor effect on most vascular beds, whereas epinephrine, although it also is a vasoconstrictor in some areas, causes vasodilation in both skeletal and cardiac muscle. Basically, the catecholamines differ from each other in the degree to which they stimulate different effector responses.

Angiotensin. Angiotensin is a hormone that is formed in the blood through the action of renin. The renin-angiotensin mechanism of the kidney is activated (1) reflexly by a decrease in central blood volume or arterial pressure, (2) by a reduction in plasma sodium, or (3) secondarily to decreased distention of renal arterioles. Renin, an enzyme produced by the juxtaglomerular cells of the kidney, acts on a circulating alpha$_2$-globulin and splits off angiotensin I. A converting enzyme subsequently catalyzes a reaction that results in the removal of other amino acids to produce angiotensin II. Although its primary effect is on the zona glomerulosa (see Unit 5), angiotensin II is a potent vasoconstrictor. Angiotensin has little effect on the veins.

Vasopressin (antidiuretic hormone—ADH). Synthesized in the hypothalamus, vasopressin is a hormone released by neurohypophysis. It has a powerful constrictor effect on the arterioles and, like angiotensin, has almost no effect on the veins. Vasopressin functions primarily in the reabsorption of water from the kidney tubules and has little to do with the regulation of peripheral vascular resistance.

Kinins. Kinins are small polypeptides that have been broken away from an alpha$_2$-globulin in the plasma or tissue fluids; they can cause a powerful vasodilation. One of these kinins is called bradykinin. Kinins can develop anywhere in the circulatory system but are short-lived, being rapidly destroyed by the action of the digestive enzyme carboxypeptidase.

Serotonin. Serotonin (5-Hydroxytryptamine) is a compound synthesized from the amino acid tryptophan. It is found in large concentrations in the chromaffin tissue of the intestine and abdominal structures. Serotonin can act as a vasodilator or vasoconstrictor, depending on the area and situation. The role of serotinin in the regulation of circulation is still being investigated.

Histamine. The role of histamine in the normal regulation of circulation is not known. Histamine, however, is released in response to injury or antigen-antibody reactions. It exerts a powerful vasodilator effect on the systemic arterioles at the same time that it constricts the veins. These actions increase capillary pressure to the point where quantities of fluids leak out into the body tissues.

Prostaglandins. Prostaglandins are a group of physiologically and pharmacologically active compounds that are synthesized from polyunsaturated 20-carbon fatty acids. These compounds in minute quantities can effect great changes. Prostaglandins influence other organ systems through their effect on the cardiovascular system, serving as potent vasodilating and vasoconstricting agents. Prostaglandins also stimulate the release of renin.

Chemical control. Many chemical substances are factors in the production of local vasodilation or vasoconstriction. Although the exact role of these substances in the overall regulation of circulation has not been established, their effects can be summarized as follows.

An increase in the arterial carbon dioxide concentration triggers a slight vasodilation in most tissues, although its influence is most pronounced in the brain. This most likely can be attributed to chemoreceptor stimulation and reduced stimulation of the vasoconstrictor area. The effects of CO_2 on the vasomotor center indirectly elicit a powerful vasoconstriction.

A decrease in the pH resulting from an increase in the hydrogen ion concentration leads to arteriolar dilation if the reduction is significant. A slight reduction produces constriction of the arterioles. An elevation in the pH also causes dilation.

Because calcium stimulates smooth muscle contraction, an elevation in the concentration of this ion cause arteriolar constriction.

Vasodilation occurs in the presence of increased concentrations of potassium, magnesium, sodium, and glucose or of decreased PAo_2. The effects of potassium and magnesium can be traced to their roles as inhibitors in smooth muscle contraction. The influence of sodium and glucose can be attributed to the occurrence of a change in osmolality. Increased osmolality causes dilation, whereas decreases result in vasoconstriction. The effects of hypoxia occur secondary to chemoreceptor stimulation, as with Pao_2 elevations.

ASSESSMENT
The cardiovascular history

The diagnosis and treatment of circulatory disorders depends to a great extent on information obtained from the patient's health history. To take an accurate and relevant cardiovascular history may be a difficult task. Although it is important to permit the patient to describe her chief complaint and to review the history of her present illness using her own words, such an account may be verbose, irrelevant, and inaccurate. A leading question is often inappropriate because of the power of suggestion. However, it may be necessary to ask such a question to analyze a symptom sufficiently because the average person usually fails to mention all of the available information, unless pressed to do so. Often a negative answer provides the practitioner with additional invaluable information.

Although the patient with cardiovascular disease may have few, if any, symptoms, each one must be thoroughly investigated. Frequently, this necessitates a review of information about the prenatal, neonatal, infant, or childhood period of development. Symptoms may not parallel the severity of the disease process; they may be mild and the disease severe, or vice versa. Symptoms may vary culturally, as well as individually; what one person complains about, another may not. Symptoms may also be described inaccurately, a frequent occurrence when the historian is someone other than the patient. And finally, symptoms thought to be caused by cardiovascular disease may in fact arise from another body system.

The cardiovascular history should include mention of symptoms commonly associated with circulatory disorders such as chest pain, shortness of breath, palpitations, edema, hemoptysis, syncope, and peripheral pain. In the infant or pediatric patient, it may be necessary to investigate respiratory problems at or shortly after birth or a failure to thrive during early growth and development.

The chief concern

Chest pain. Chest pain or discomfort is a subjective sensation that must be evaluated in depth to determine its origin, which may or may not be pathologic. Because pathologic chest pain can be related to the cardiovascular, respiratory, gastrointestinal, or musculoskeletal system, it is necessary to describe its quality, location, duration, and any precipitating or aggravating factors, as well as accompanying symptoms. Sometimes therapeutic interventions, such as the use of nitroglycerin, are instituted to aid in a differential diagnosis, but their use can be confusing because, for example, nonischemic chest pain is also often relieved by nitroglycerin.

In assessing the quality of the chest pain or discomfort, it is wise to allow patients to use their own words. Functional or psychogenic chest pain is usually described as a dull, persistent ache. Chest discomfort resulting from coronary artery disease can also be described as dull or aching but is frequently described as crushing or squeezing in nature or as a heavy or tight sensation. Pain associated with a dissecting aneurysm of the aorta is often described as an excruciating, tearing sensation, whereas the inflammatory pain associated with pericarditis is persistent and is perceived to be sharp and stabbing or dull and aching.

The location of the discomfort is also helpful in establishing a cause. Because the heart is located in the midline, pain caused by cardiac ischemia is characteristically felt substernally or across both sides of the chest. It is frequently said to radiate to the shoulders, arms, elbows, fingers, jaw, or scapula. Pain of aortic dissection is most pronounced in the anterior chest and usually radiates to the midposterior, back into the abdomen, or into the neck, while pain caused by pericarditis is left-sided and frequently radiates to the neck or flank. If the pain can be localized to the skin or superficial structures, it usually arises from the chest wall. Pain located beneath the left nipple is most often noncardiac in origin. It may be functional or related to gastrointestinal or musculoskeletal disorders.

Although the duration of the chest pain or discomfort can shed some light on the pathophysiology, it is not always of diagnostic value. Anginal pain is usually short in duration, lasting from approximately 2 to 10 minutes. More severe angina, however, can last longer. Pain caused by myocardial infarction, pericarditis, or dissecting anneurysm, on the other hand, usually lasts much longer—for a matter of hours. Gastrointestinal-related pain is relatively short in duration, whereas musculoskeletal pain or func-

tional discomfort may be either short- or long-term.

Information about factors that aggravate or precipitate episodes of chest pain should be pursued in detail. Anginal pain characteristically occurs with exertion or on exposure to emotional stress, with the exception of pain caused by Prinzmetal's (variant) angina, which usually occurs at rest. Anginal pain is aggravated by cold weather and made worse after a heavy meal. In contrast, pain related to myocardial infarction can occur at any time. Gastrointestinal-related chest pain most frequently is associated with eating or positioning after eating. It may also be associated with protracted vomiting, whereas chest discomfort resulting from musculoskeletal pathology is most often noted when the patient bends, changes position, or moves. Pain and discomfort associated with such activities as breathing, coughing, and sneezing are often caused by respiratory pathology but may be related to cardiovascular disorders, such as pericarditis, or to musculoskeletal inflammation. Chest pain that occurs with or is aggravated by exhaustion, while most likely functional in origin, may also occur with cardiovascular disorders.

Accompanying symptoms also need to be evaluated. Chest pain or discomfort associated with coronary heart disease is often associated with complaints of shortness of breath, profuse sweating, nausea, and vomiting. The additional presence of palpitations suggests an associated dysrhythmia. Chest discomfort accompanied only by shortness of breath can often be traced to respiratory disorders such as pneumothorax or pulmonary embolism, whereas pain occurring with hemoptysis usually indicates the presence of a pulmonary embolism or a lung tumor. The addition of fever suggests an inflammatory disorder such as pneumonia or pericarditis. Functional chest pain and discomfort are most often accompanied by sighing and anxiety or depression.

Many people attempt to alleviate their pain by using a variety of remedies, some of which have been prescribed previously by a physician.

Questioning a patient in regard to the success or failure of such treatments often provides additional diagnostic information. Nitroglycerin, for example, characteristically relieves the pain of angina pectoris within approximately 5 minutes. Its failure to do so in the presence of a headache strongly suggests unstable angina or myocardial infarction. The headache is a secondary side effect caused by cerebral vasoconstriction, a finding that helps the practitioner establish the stability of the pharmacologic agent. Anginal pain is also usually relieved by rest. A recumbent position often makes anginal pain worse, thereby providing an additional diagnostic clue for the practitioner. Pain caused by pericarditis is relieved when the person leans forward, whereas pain secondary to pleurisy is reduced when the person holds his breath or lies on the involved side, thus creating a splinting effect. Gastrointestinal-related chest pain is usually alleviated with food or antacid therapy.

Shortness of breath. Shortness of breath (*dyspnea*) can be defined as an uncomfortable awareness of breathing. To determine its etiology, it is necessary to review the factors that may cause or relieve the unpleasant sensation, as well as the body position associated with its development.

Sudden onset of shortness of breath occurs most often with respiratory-related disorders such as pulmonary embolism, pneumonia, pulmonary edema, or obstructive disease. A myxoma must be considered, however, when there is a sudden onset of shortness of breath in a sitting position. Slow, insidious onset of breathlessness that becomes progressively worse, being more pronounced with exertions, usually indicates the existence of heart failure or chronic obstructive lung disease but may also occur with severe anemia and thyrotoxicosis, whereas the development of shortness of breath at rest, if it is the only symptom, may indicate a functional disorder. However, shortness of breath may also be associated with respiratory diseases such as pneumonia, pulmonary embolism, or pulmonary edema.

Chest pain associated with shortness of breath can be traced to cardiovascular, respiratory, or functional-related disorders. If relieved by sedation and deep breaths, the origin is often functional. If prolonged, cardiovascular pathology is usually the cause.

Breathlessness, occurring at night in paroxysms approximately 2 to 5 hours after the onset of sleep, is usually the result of left ventricular failure and is frequently associated with diaphoresis and wheezing. This type of breathlessness is characteristically worse when the patient is in a supine position and may be relieved by sitting upright.

Shortness of breath that is relieved with the institution of bronchodilator therapy suggests asthma, while breathlessness relieved by rest, digitalis, and diuretics is characteristically caused by heart failure.

Palpitations. Palpitations, defined as a disagreeable awareness of the heartbeat, are often described as racing, pounding, skipping, or jumping sensations and may be attributed to a variety of cardiovascular disorders, endocrine abnormalities, or functional alterations. Although diagnostic studies are necessary to determine the exact nature of the problem, a review of the mode of onset, associated symptoms, and method of termination often provides valuable information that is needed to identify the problem.

It is not possible to establish the exact dysrhythmia from a description of the altered heartbeat. In addition, the complaint may not be related to the seriousness of the dysrhythmia because the degree of unpleasantness is a subjective perception.

Palpitations may be the result of ectopic beats, in which case they are usually described as "skipped beats" or "flip-flop" sensations. Ectopic beats followed by a compensatory pause are associated with a feeling that the heart has stopped beating. A feeling that the heart is beating very slowly often accompanies heart block or sinus node disease, whereas a racing sensation that starts and stops abruptly is often caused by paroxysmal atrial tachycardia, atrial fibrillation, or atrial flutter. A gradual onset and cessation of a pounding heart frequently occurs with sinus tachycardia.

A history of palpitations precipitated by strenuous exercise is abnormal. Palpitations that are "physiologic" usually disappear with exercise. Frequently, they are caused by PVC's. The mechanism is uncertain. Palpitations occurring with mild exertion often suggest an underlying disorder such as heart failure, severe anemia, or thyrotoxicosis. Palpitations associated with anxiety, dizziness, and a tingling sensation may be functional, triggered by a hyperventilation episode. They may also be traced to hypokalemia and consequently should be investigated to find the cause. Palpitations accompanied by a throbbing sensation in the neck often indicate valvular heart disease, specifically aortic insufficiency. Palpitations following a syncopal episode usually indicate heart block or severe bradycardia, while the presence of chest pain with palpitations frequently occurs in coronary heart disease. Palpitations terminated by vagal maneuvers suggest paroxysmal atrial tachycardia.

Patients who count their pulse during an episode of palpitations are able to provide the practitioner with a heart rate, thus giving data that enable the practitioner to differentiate between sinus tachycardia (rate between 100 and 140 beats/min), atrial flutter (rate between 150 and 160 beats/min), and paroxysmal atrial tachycardia (rate greater than 160 beats/min).

Fluid retention (edema). Patients with some cardiovascular disorders often describe a history of swelling in the ankles, weight gain, and enlarging girth. To determine the etiology of the fluid retention, or edema, causing these complaints, it is necessary to identify the location of the problem and any associated symptoms.

Peripheral edema found in dependent positions is usually cardiovascular in origin resulting from chronic venous insufficiency or heart failure. With the latter, the edema ascends with increasing failure. If localized in only one extremity, the problem most likely can be attributed to

venous thrombosis or lymphatic obstruction. More generalized edema can be found in heart failure, valvular heart disease, the nephrotic syndrome, or hepatic cirrhosis, while edema limited to the face and upper arms suggests superior vena cava obstruction. Edema located in the face and around the eyes (periorbital edema) occurs in heart failure in children, the nephrotic syndrome, acute glomerulonephritis, and myxedema.

Edema can be associated with several other symptoms. When combined with shortness of breath it most often suggests heart failure, pulmonary embolism, or pleural effusion. Edema associated with jaundice is usually hepatic in origin, whereas edema occurring with ascites can be attributed to cardiac or renal alterations. Edema with prolonged standing or with a history of skin ulcerations or pigmentation suggests venous insufficiency.

Spitting up blood (hemoptysis). Expectoration of blood (hemoptysis) can be a symptom of cardiovascular or pulmonary pathology. It is possible to shed some light on the exact cause of the problem by reviewing the characteristics of the expectorated material.

Initially, the volume and color of the blood that is expectorated should be described. A large volume of $\frac{1}{2}$ cup or more indicates brisk bleeding and can be attributed to mitral stenosis, a ruptured thoracic aneurysm, or pulmonary infarction, while smaller quantities of dark clotted blood are usually associated with venous bleeding. Expectoration of pink frothy mucus classically suggests pulmonary edema, whereas clear to gray blood-tinged sputum usually indicates chronic obstructive lung disease. A pulmonary infection is usually the cause of blood-tinged, yellowish-green mucus.

Factors that appear to precipitate or aggravate the hemoptysis are also important. Mitral stenosis is most often suspected when hemoptysis accompanies physical exercise and excitement and is associated with shortness of breath. A history of hemoptysis with pleuritic chest pain suggests the presence of a pulmonary embolus with an infarct. Hemoptysis accompanied by increased sputum production, unexplained weight loss, and anorexia often indicate the presence of carcinoma, although tuberculosis is a possibility until ruled out by tests.

Blackout spells (syncope). The assessment is very important in establishing the cause of syncopal episodes. To determine the etiology of these episodes, it is important to examine the frequency with which they occur, the length of time of the attacks, the associated symptoms, and the position of the patient when they occur.

Syncopal episodes that occur frequently, often several times a day, are associated with Stokes-Adams syndrome, cardiac dysrhythmias, or seizure disorders. Those that last for only a few seconds can frequently be attributed to vasodepressor syncope or postural hypotension, whereas those of longer duration suggest aortic stenosis, left ventricular failure, hypoglycemia, or hysteria.

The patient's behavior before and during a syncopal episode may enable the practitioner to make a more definitive diagnosis. For example, syncopal episodes that occur abruptly suggest Stokes-Adams syndrome, cardiac dysrhythmias, or seizure disorders, whereas those with a gradual onset often indicate vasopressor syncope secondary to hyperventilation. The additional description of a prodromal aura suggests a seizure disorder, while the presence of emotional stress or painful stimuli along with giddiness, nausea, and diaphoresis is associated with vasopressor syncope. Hysterical syncopal episodes are frequently accompanied by numbness, tingling, shortness of breath, chest pain, and hyperventilation, whereas confusion, perhaps aphasia, and a unilateral weakness occur with syncopal episodes associated with transient ischemic attacks. The presence of chest pain with syncope often correlates with an acute myocardial infarction, while syncopal episodes in the infant or child who becomes cyanotic may indicate the presence of a congenital disorder associated with a right-to-left shunt, right ventricular outflow obstruction, or reduction in systemic vascular resistance. Those syncopal episodes occurring with activity or exertion in later childhood or in adulthood may be associated with aortic valve disease. Syncope in bleeding patients may occur if they become hypovolemic.

The position that the person is in when syncopal episodes occur can also be significant. Although there appears to be no relationship among Stokes-Adams syndrome, hyperventilation, and seizure-related syncopal episodes, those episodes that occur in previously upright people who suddenly bend, lean, or assume another position suggest a left atrial myxoma or ball valve thrombus, while those occurring just as a person sits or stands from a supine position are usually related to postural hypotension. Syncope associated with a sudden change in head position commonly indicates carotid sinus syncope but may also be caused by vertebral artery compression, vertebrobasilar insufficiency, or subclavian steal.

The length of the attack, as well as the rapidity of recovery, may be of value in identifying the cause. A rapid recovery from a syncopal attack is associated with cardiovascular problems, whereas central nervous system disorders are followed by a slower recovery.

Leg pain. Peripheral leg pain is a relatively common complaint that can be attributed to a variety of problems. It may be caused by circulatory aberrations, nervous system disorders, or alterations in musculoskeletal integrity.

Leg pain occurring with peripheral circulatory disorders caused by venous alterations, such as thrombophlebitis, is often described as being generalized over widespread areas of the affected leg, whereas that associated with arterial insufficiency is isolated in the calf. Leg pain with venous thrombosis is ever-present, while that caused by arterial insufficiency secondary to atherosclerosis or arteriosclerosis is precipitated or aggravated by exercise (intermittent claudication). The pain of arterial insufficiency tends to be aggravated by cold, while most venous disorders tend not to be.

Women with a history of using birth control

pills have a greater risk of developing peripheral circulatory disorders. These young women can develop either venous or arterial problems caused by thrombus or embolis development. Therefore a history of leg pain in any individual should not be ignored.

Failure to thrive. The mother of an infant or child whose problem ultimately labeled as a "failure to thrive" usually has rather general concerns when describing the child's problems. Frequently the mother will compare the child to a sibling and notice a difference in growth patterns. Often the mother will say that the infant eats poorly and cries a lot. Sometimes she describes the child as having frequent colds. With toddlers, it's not unusual to hear that they require frequent rest after limited activity or prefer to sit rather than play, while older children are described as having an inability to keep up with their peers. Consequently, developing a differential diagnosis is a difficult task because these problems can be attributed to either pathologic or nonpathologic conditions. It is helpful to pursue the feeding problems to ascertain whether they originate with the mother or reflect effort intolerance on the part of the baby. In addition, it is wise to inquire about any physical symptoms that might occur during feeding.

The development of diaphoresis or of cyanosis, which is a blue or grayish hue during feeding, suggests inadequate oxygenation and provides the practitioner with additional information (Unit 3). Ultimately, however, a complete physical examination and laboratory evaluation will be necessary to establish the presence of a cardiovascular abnormality.

Past history

In addition to the information obtained about the current problem, there are several questions that must be answered to have a thorough cardiovascular history. When the practitioner obtains the past medical history, it is important for her to review the prenatal period of life because certain environmental factors may adversely alter fetal growth

and development. For example, tobacco use has been known to be associated with babies that are small for their gestational age; the same holds true for maternal dietary inadequacies. In addition, in some areas studies have revealed that high altitudes can result in altered fetal size. It is also necessary for the practitioner to ask about the mother's health during gestation. Maternal viral disorders such as cytomegalo and rubella have been known to cause congenital anomalies during the early gestational period, as has the presence of chronic disease such as diabetes mellitus. Medications taken early during gestation should be documented because their ingestion can be associated with certain cardiac malformations. Maternal alcohol abuse is important to note because the alcoholic mother runs the increased risk of having a baby with congenital heart disease.

The childhood period must not be overlooked. It is important to check for the presence of any unusual childhood illnesses. Specific questions about the occurrence of streptococcal infections during childhood can provide the practitioner with clues leading to the diagnosis of rheumatic heart disease.

During adolescence and adulthood the occurrence and treatment of syphilis should be documented because it is known to produce heart disease. Any serious accident involving chest trauma must be noted because this may later precipitate cardiac problems. In women, a review of pregnancies, their outcome, and any complications may be important and provide information about symptoms of valvular heart disease that are often suppressed until the stress of pregnancy.

Social history

The social history must also be reviewed in detail because it can provide data that reveal the patient to be at greater risk for the development of coronary artery disease or can provide a clue for the etiological agent in certain cardiovascular problems. A stressful occupation or a smoking history, for example, increase the risk of coronary artery disease. Dietary habits are also important from the standpoint of risk. Questions are asked about general dietary habits, the fat content in the diet, and the amount of caffeine normally consumed. Questions about alcohol intake are also relevant.

Family history

An accurate family history is also necessary because several cardiovascular disorders can be linked to hereditary factors. The recurrence risk can be quite high with congenital cardiac disorders when two or more family members have been affected. In addition, a strong family history creates a greater individual risk with coronary artery disease.

The cardiovascular physical examination

A systematic and complete examination of the patient is very important because a selective or limited examination may result in the loss of valuable information. In this chapter, emphasis

will be placed on findings that influence circulation.

Vital signs

The patient's blood pressure, pulse, respirations, and temperature should be obtained before beginning the physical examination. Determination of the vital signs is a routine procedure on admission that provides a means for rapidly evaluating the patient. The data that are obtained serve as a baseline of information; subsequent changes can be used to predict both favorable and unfavorable changes in the patient's condition. The significance of these individual measurements will be discussed.

Hemodynamic monitoring

The electrocardiogram. Heart rate and rhythm can be assessed continuously in most hemodynamic monitoring systems. Although the components of the electrocardiogram (ECG) monitoring system may vary, most con-

Fig. 2-20. Electrode systems used to monitor the electrocardiogram. Three electrodes are used to simulate one of the bipolar leads, depending on where the positive and negative electrodes are placed. In Lead I, the positive electrode is placed on the right, with the negative electrode across from it on the left. The negative electrode is moved to the lower left chest in Lead II. In Lead III, the positive electrode is positioned on the upper left chest, while the negative electrode remains on the lower left chest. A 5-electrode system is used to monitor a modified chest lead by placing the positive electrode in the V_1 to V_6 position. The MCL provides an easily recognizable sequence of ventricular activation.

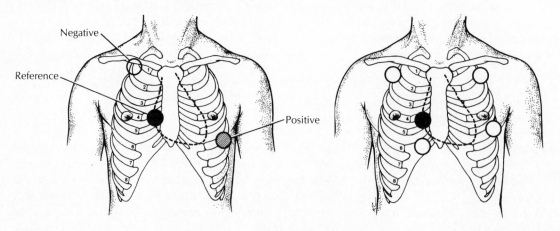

sist of an audio and a visual component. The audio component emits an audible sound with each ventricular contraction, whereas the visual component, which may have a flashing rate indicator, digital display activated by each QRS complex, and an oscilloscopic display, permits a continuous recording of the heart rate with a display of the rate and rhythm. In most monitoring systems the rate indicator and oscilloscopic display are relayed to a central console, making it possible to silence the bedside audio component so that the patient does not hear it.

Many ECG monitors are equipped with a memory loop that stores a portion of the patient's ECG. This tape can be recalled as necessary and will provide a strip recording of the cardiac rhythm for the preceding 60 seconds.

All ECG monitoring systems should have an alarm system that will alert the staff should the heart rate fall below or rise above a predetermined level. In such cases, both audio and visual alarms notify the staff, who must immediately evaluate the situation. Some monitors will initiate an automatic "write-out" when the alarm is activated; this write-out, or memory loop, provides a record of the ECG activity before the alarm and for a varying time after the alarm. Even though false alarms do occur frequently because of electrical interference, patient movement, or loose electrodes, the alarm system should never be turned off.

The ECG is monitored using external chest or extremity electrodes.* In the adult, three to five chest electrodes are applied to obtain an ECG tracing (Fig. 2-20). Three electrodes are used to monitor one of the bipolar limb leads, depending on where the positive and negative electrodes are placed. A lead that displays upright QRS complexes and P waves should be selected. Five electrodes are used to monitor one of the precordial leads by rotating the chest electrode from the V_1 to the V_6 position and by

placing the remaining four electrodes on the chest close to the upper and lower extremities. The modified chest lead, or MCL, with a subscript designating the precordial position (for example, MCL_1), clearly records the conduction sequence through the ventricles, making it possible to identify beats originating in the left or right ventricle, to detect left and right bundle branch block, and to differentiate ventricular ectopy from aberrant conduction. A modified chest lead can also be obtained with three electrodes by placing the positive electrode in the desired precordial position with the negative electrode under the left shoulder and the ground beneath the right clavicle. The configuration of the QRS complex will vary with the MCL, resembling the QRS complex in the precordial lead selected.

The skin should be thoroughly cleansed with alcohol before the electrodes are applied. It may be necessary to shave the chest in selected areas. Electrode paste is used if the electrodes are not pregelled, and the electrodes are placed over a bony prominence according to the lead that is to be monitored. Large muscle masses should be avoided because they create undesirable interference. Electrodes are changed as necessary to maintain a clear tracing. Unnecessary changes should be avoided, especially in infants, who have extremely sensitive skin. The site should be rotated slightly to avoid skin excoriation.

Arterial blood pressure. Complementary modules can be added to the basic monitoring system to monitor several other parameters such as arterial blood pressure, venous blood pressure, and pulmonary artery pressure.

Direct arterial pressure monitoring is carried out by attaching an intra-arterial catheter to a strain gauge transducer and pressure monitor that is precalibrated according to the manufacturer's requirements. The mechanical pressure of the pulse is converted to an electrical impulse and is recorded on the oscilloscope and on a pressure meter with digital display. Systolic, mean, and diastolic pressure can be read. The arterial waveform, visible on the oscilloscopic

---

*The electrodes used for infants should be 1.5 cm in diameter because adult-sized electrodes will give an electrocardiogram with abnormal voltage and configuration.

display, consists of an upstroke during systole that can be correlated with the QRS complex of the ECG and of a downstroke with a dicrotic notch, occurring with the onset of diastole and closure of the aortic valve. The peak of the waveform represents the systolic pressure, whereas the lowest point is the diastolic pressure. Waveform variation can be seen in the presence of cardiac dysrhythmias or alterations in cardiac output or vascular resistance. It can also be found with the use of artificial cardiac pacemakers. The intra-arterial catheter can also be attached to a sphygmomanometer gauge for simple continuous pressure monitoring, with pressure readings correlated with cuff inflation and deflation. Intra-arterial catheters can be used to obtain arterial blood samples for analysis. If frequent arterial samples are being drawn, the catheter may be kept patent with the heparinized flush technique or solution even after it is no longer needed for blood pressure monitoring.

The intra-arterial catheter can be inserted into one of several peripheral arteries. The radial, brachial, or femoral arteries can be used; the umbilical artery can also be used in the neonate. When this vessel can no longer be used, the radial artery serves as a suitable alternative. Insertion into the temporal or pedal arteries is also possible. The radial artery is chosen most frequently in adults because it is easily accessible and relatively easy to cannulate. It is most valuable for short-term therapy (24 hours or less). Before the insertion of a catheter into the radial artery, a test is performed to ascertain whether collateral arterial blood flow would be adequate in the event of a thrombosis to the radial artery. Either a Doppler ultrasound device must be used, or the Allen test must be done. The latter test is performed by completely occluding both the radial and ulnar arteries and then raising and exercising the hand. The hand is lowered, and the ulnar artery is released. The hand should blush rapidly once the artery is released. This reactive hyperemia occurs with capillary refill and indicates adequate collateral circulation. Its failure to do so necessitates the selection of another site. The brachial artery is also easy to cannulate and associated with few complications in adults. It is used infrequently in children. The femoral artery, although easy to use, is less desirable because of the increased incidence of contamination, limitation of movement, difficulty in applying a dressing, and lack of control of bleeding. The dorsalis pedis artery has been used most recently and seems to be associated with relatively few problems. Regardless of the site that is selected, it is necessary to monitor the extremity below the catheter's insertion, checking for pulse, color, and warmth. Any changes should be reported immediately because they may indicate the presence of an arterial obstruction, necessitating removal of the catheter and arteriotomy.

Good technique must be observed at all times while working with intra-arterial catheters. Strict asepsis must be maintained. Dressings should be kept clean and dry and changed as often as necessary. Extraneous equipment and tubing should be kept away from the arterial catheter to minimize the risk of contamination. Periodic flushing with a heparinized solution is necessary to minimize clot formation and prolong the life of the intra-arterial catheter. The procedure may be performed manually or may be carried out using a continuous arterial infusion pump designed to flush the system with approximately 3 ml/hr. The amount of flush used can be added to the intake and output record if necessary. Manual flushing is necessary after withdrawing blood samples from the intra-arterial catheter. It may also be useful in eliminating damping of the arterial waveform, a problem that often occurs when the catheter is up against the wall of the artery. It is important to note that damping of the arterial waveform can also occur with heart failure or cardiac tamponade; therefore the intra-arterial pressure should be checked with the cuff pressure when the waveform is damped.

The intra-arterial monitoring module should be equipped with an alarm system. This system can be set around systolic and diastolic readings so that it will be activated by significant increases above or decreases below the preset readings.

There are several potential sources for error. Improper calibration of the equipment can yield erroneously high or low readings. To validate readings, the intra-arterial pressure should be checked with the cuff pressure. Normally the cuff pressure is slightly lower than the intra-arterial pressure; significant discrepancies should therefore be checked. Consequently, it is advisable to check calibration at periodic intervals to prevent errors in readings. Erroneously low readings can also occur with an obstruction in the intra-arterial catheter. Obstruction may be indicated by the presence of a dampened arterial waveform or a backup of blood in the intra-arterial catheter. Sometimes the problem can be corrected simply by repositioning the extremity in which the catheter is inserted. If this fails, flushing the line may help. Flushing, however, is contraindicated in the presence of a suspected thrombus. In such a case, it is necessary to gently aspirate in an attempt to remove the clot. If flushing does not alleviate the obstruction, it may be necessary to reposition the catheter; if this also fails, it may be necessary to insert a new catheter. Air in the catheter transducer system can also yield erroneous readings. This problem, which gives inaccurately low readings, can be corrected by expelling the air and recalibrating.

A number of complications can occur in patients with intra-arterial catheters. One of the significant dangers that can occur is the development of a thrombus in the artery into which the catheter is inserted. The risk of thrombosis, however, can be reduced to some extent by monitoring the extremity below insertion for any unusual changes and promptly removing the catheter in the presence of impaired circulation. Air embolism poses another significant threat to patients with intra-arterial catheters. The possibility of injecting air into the catheter can be reduced by using good technique and thoroughly understanding the operation of the equipment. Hemorrhage and subsequent exsanguination can occur if there is a leak in the system or the equipment is used improperly. Constant monitoring and the use of an alarm system will help minimize the risk of this complication. The

presence of a leak is a potential emergency and must be handled immediately. If the leak occurs distal to the stopcock at the site of insertion, it will suffice to turn off the stopcock to the patient. If the leak is higher up in the system, direct pressure must be applied over the artery to control the bleeding while attempts are made to locate the leak and reestablish a closed system. It may ultimately be necessary to remove the catheter if the problem cannot be corrected. The possibility of an infection poses another threat; using good aseptic techniques should help reduce the risk of this complication.

Left atrial pressure. Left atrial pressure can be monitored using a catheter inserted surgically into the left atrium. The catheter, which is attached to a strain gauge transducer, is usually inserted after cardiac surgery. A heparinized flush system is used to maintain catheter patency. The catheter can also be used to withdraw arterial blood samples for analysis, but it cannot be used for infusion.

Pressure readings are taken with the patient in a supine position and the transducer positioned at midchest level.

The greatest hazard associated with left atrial catheters is the risk of an air embolus. This risk can be minimized by maintaining a closed system.

Venous pressure. Venous pressure can be monitored using either noninvasive or invasive techniques. Noninvasively, the venous blood pressure is monitored using the veins in the dorsum of the hand or the internal or external jugular veins. The patient must be in a sitting position when the veins in the dorsum of the hand are used. With the hand held below the heart, the veins are permitted to fill. Then, as the arm is raised, the practitioner notes the point at which the veins collapse. This will normally occur when the dorsum of the hand reaches a point just above the sternal angle.* In the presence of an elevated venous pressure, the veins will re-

---

*The sternal angle is used as a reference point because it is relatively easy to locate. Ideally, the reference point is the midpoint of the right atrium. Because this point is difficult to locate, the sternal angle, which is anastomically close to the midright atrium, is used.

main distended above the sternal angle. The distance above the sternal angle at which the veins collapse provides an estimation of the venous pressure.

The patient must be in a recumbent position if the jugular vein is used. The external jugular is used most often because of its accessibility. It is, however, less accurate than the internal jugular vein in estimating venous pressure because it is smaller and follows a less direct route to the superior vena cava. In addition, the external jugulars have valves that could decrease the accuracy of the measurements, whereas internal jugulars have no valves. To estimate venous blood pressure using the external jugular vein, the head of the bed of the recumbent patient is raised to a point where venous distention is visible. The external jugular vein is occluded by applying gentle pressure on the patient's neck slightly above the parallel to the clavicle. After waiting for the vein to fill and then releasing the pressure, the practitioner can estimate the venous blood pressure by measuring the degree of jugular venous distention above the suprasternal notch when the head of the bed is elevated to 45- and 90-degree angles. Normally, the vein will be distended no more than 1 cm above the suprasternal notch at 45 degrees, but it should collapse when the patient is upright at 90 degrees. Distention above the suprasternal notch at 90 degrees indicates a marked elevation in the venous pressure. The pressure can be estimated by measuring the distention above the suprasternal notch in centimeters. When using the internal jugular, the practitioner follows a similar procedure except that degree of distention is measured above the sternal angle. The angle of the patient must also be noted.

Invasive techniques measure the central venous pressure, or CVP. These measurements are obtained by attaching an indwelling catheter, positioned in the superior vena cava or midright atrium, to a precalibrated plastic or glass manometer or strain gauge transducer. Several approaches can be used. Either the internal or external jugular vein can be used, but because of their locations they are difficult to dress and uncomfortable for the patient. The subclavian vein is also satisfactory. The femoral vein is suitable, but because of its location and the possibility of contamination, it is used less frequently. The most preferred approach uses the median antecubital, or basilic, vein because it is easy to puncture and thread.

Measurements can be made in centimeters of water, using a precalibrated manometer, or in torr (mmHg), using a strain gauge transducer. Mercury is 13.6 times heavier than water. One torr (mmHg) equals 1.36 cm of water. Consequently, to convert from centimeters of water to torr, it is necessary to divide by 1.36. Conversely, it is necessary to multiply by 1.36 to convert from torr to centimeters of water.

The patient should be in a supine position when the CVP readings are made. If this is intolerable, the patient's head can be elevated slightly, but subsequent readings must be made in the same position. The patient should be disconnected from mechanical ventilation if spontaneous respirations are present because the inspiratory pressure of the ventilator will cause an erroneous elevation in the CVP. In the absence of spontaneous respirations, readings should be made with ventilatory assistance, but notation to this effect must be made. When the precalibrated manometer is used, its zero level is held at the midpoint of the right atrium. This point can be located by measuring 5 cm down from the top of the chest in the fourth intercostal space. This level is approximately equal to the midaxillary line and should be marked so that future readings can be obtained in the same place. The manometer can be attached to the bed or a portable intravenous pole for greater accuracy in making future readings. The reading is taken after the manometer is flushed with fluid and all air bubbles are removed. With the manometer open to the catheter, the fluid level will fall rapidly, fluctuating with respiration. The reading is taken at the highest point of fluctuation. After the reading has been taken, it is important to return the stopcock to the intravenous infusion position.

Measuring the CVP with a strain gauge

transducer is less complicated. Initially, the transducer is positioned at the level of the mid-right atrium. It is calibrated according to manufacturer's instructions on the venous mode. The patient is placed appropriately in a supine position and removed from assisted ventilation if possible. The reading is taken with the transducer open to the intravenous catheter. Once the CVP has been obtained, the stopcock is returned to the intravenous infusion position.

Caring for a patient with a central venous infusion catheter requires strict aseptic techniques to prevent infection. Frequently, an antimicrobial ointment is applied over the insertion site. The area should be dressed and the dressing changed as often as necessary. The rate of infusion should be monitored closely to avoid fluid overload. Before obtaining a reading, the flow rate of the intravenous infusion line is increased rapidly for a few seconds to evaluate catheter patency. Consequently, after the CVP, is read, it is necessary to reestablish the correct infusion rate. If this procedure is forgotten, fluid overload can occur in a short period of time. Using an infusion pump minimizes the risk of this occurrence.

Several complications can occur in patients with CVP catheters. Thrombophlebitis can develop because of the mechanical irritation of the catheter. In addition, poor technique, leading to contamination, can result in bacterial infection and subsequent thrombus formation. Improper forceful technique during catheter insertion or removal can lead to a broken, jagged catheter and hence an embolus. Inadequate patient monitoring can lead to fluid overload in a system that has been "left open" and is infusing too rapidly after measuring the CVP. Finally, cardiac dysrhythmias can occur if the CVP catheter is improperly positioned in the ventricles.

Pulmonary artery pressure. Pressures within the pulmonary artery can be monitored using a multilumen, flow-directed, balloon-tipped catheter that is passed intravenously through the right side of the heart into a branch of the pulmonary artery. Using a technique developed by Swan and Ganz, it is possible to measure pulmonary artery pressure (PAP), pulmonary capillary wedge or pulmonary artery wedge pressure (PCWP or PAWP), and cardiac output, using thermodilution techniques. These pressures and cardiac output measurements provide invaluable data that are used in the treatment of cardiac patients. There apparently is a direct correlation between the pulmonary artery end-diastolic pressure (PAEDP), the PCWP, and the left ventricular end-diastolic pressure (LVEDP).

Several multilumen, balloon-tipped catheters are commercially available. Style and size chosen depend on the type and age of the patient being monitored. The triple-lumen catheter can be used to monitor PAP and CVP, with the third lumen reserved for balloon inflation. The four-lumen catheter, about 100 cm in length, is used primarily for adults. The distal lumen is used to monitor PAP. A second lumen is attached to a balloon for PCWP, whereas the third lumen is attached to a thermistor for thermodilution. The fourth lumen, located approximately 30 cm from the distal end of the catheter, empties into the right atrium and is used for CVP measurement. Intravenous infusion is permitted only through the right atrial lumen in three- and four-lumen catheters.

The catheter is inserted intravenously through the internal or external jugular, subclavian, basilic, or femoral vein. Although fluoroscopic equipment was necessary to guide insertion in the past, currently the catheter is advanced using pressure waveforms to monitor its position and progress. The catheter is passed through the right atrium and through the tricuspid valve into the right ventricle, at which time the balloon is inflated to minimize ventricular wall stimulation during insertion. The circulating blood enables the catheter to float through the pulmonary valve into the pulmonary artery, where it becomes wedged in a distal branch. Once the catheter tip is positioned properly and confirmed by x-rays, it is sutured in place. The PA portal is attached to a strain gauge transducer and pressure module that has been precalibrated on the venous mode according to the manufacturer's directions. Catheter patency is maintained with a heparinized solution of 5% dextrose in water or lactated Ringer's solution that, when attached to the intraflow setup, delivers about 3 ml/hr.

Pulmonary artery pressures can be read on the systolic and diastolic modes of the pressure monitor. Right ventricular contraction is represented by the pulmonary artery systolic pressure, whereas the diastolic pressure can be correlated with the resistance to blood flow in the small pulmonary arterioles and capillaries. The pulmonary artery diastolic pressure is about the same as the pulmonary capillary wedge pressure in the absence of pulmonary vascular obstruction. A difference of 6 mmHg or more between these two readings indicates the presence of pulmonary vascular disease.

Pulmonary capillary wedge pressure is obtained by inflating the balloon, using approximately 0.8 to 1.5 cc of carbon dioxide or air to occlude a branch of the pulmonary artery. The use of air is usually satisfactory, but carbon dioxide is indicated in the presence of a right-to-left shunt to reduce the risk of air emboli in the systemic circulation. Balloon inflation should never be maintained for a long period of time because prolonged inflation can lead to necrosis or pulmonary artery rupture and hemorrhage. Overinflation should be avoided because it can rupture the balloon. The amount of air or carbon dioxide required for inflation is usually imprinted on the catheter near the balloon portal and should be used as a guide by the person instilling the air or carbon dioxide. By inflating the balloon and occluding a branch of the pulmonary artery, the practitioner is able to measure existing pressures beyond the wedge. Therefore the PCWP reflects the presence and degree of any pulmonary hypertension. PCWP also provides a good estimation of the mean left atrial pressure, and because the left atrial pressure is a good indicator of left ventricular filling, it is a good indicator of early left ventricular impairment.

A four-lumen pulmonary artery catheter can be used to monitor cardiac output using ther-

modilution techniques. This procedure can safely be done at the bedside by the critical care practitioner. It is carried out by quickly injecting, in less than 4 seconds, a 10 cc bolus of 5% dextrose in water or normal saline solution* through the right atrial portal located at the proximal end of the catheter. The injectate should be cooled to between 0° and 15° C. It is important to make sure that the injectate is free of any air bubbles. The infusate mixes with venous blood in the right atrium, flowing into the right ventricle and pulmonary artery past the thermistor lead located on the distal tip of the catheter. The thermistor, which serves as a small thermometer, measures the temperature of the blood mixture as it flows past it. A cardiac output computer connected to the thermistor portal can calculate cardiac output, using the temperature change that has occurred between the cooled solution and the circulating blood. The computer senses the temperature of the blood and measures the time it takes for the blood flowing past the thermistor to return to the normal temperature. In essence, this permits quantitation of cardiac pumping because the less time it takes to return to a normal temperature, the greater the cardiac output. Several measurements are usually made with the average cardiac output in liters per minute, using the patient's height and weight to calculate the cardiac index, which is equivalent to $\frac{\text{cardiac output}}{\text{body surface area}}$. This value correlates with the ejection fraction. Ordinarily, the first value is discarded. The subsequent measurements should be made at $1\frac{1}{2}$-minute intervals with cooled injectate and at 1-minute intervals with room temperature injectate.

Several precautions should be taken to ensure accuracy and safety while the procedure is being performed. Initially, it is important to make sure that the solution to be injected is ade-

---

*Room temperature infusate is used with late-model computers. Chilled infusate, however, is necessary in some conditions when a greater temperature differential between the blood and infusate is needed to calculate the cardiac output.

quately cooled. The amount of time sufficient for chilling is usually 30 to 45 minutes. Then the solution is injected rapidly, with the practitioner handling the syringe as little as possible to avoid warming. The PA waveform should also be checked immediately before beginning the procedure. A damped waveform may indicate that the distal tip of the catheter is in a small pulmonary artery vessel; this must be corrected because the thermistor would not permit unimpeded flow and consequently would interfere with the accuracy of the measurements. If the waveform is damped, it may be necessary for the physician to reposition the catheter. To ensure patient safety, it is important to make certain that drugs are not being infused through the line before injecting the cooled solution. If drugs are being given, it is necessary to clear the line slowly to avoid any rapid infusion. In addition, to preclude the possibility of introducing contaminants directly into the heart, aseptic techniques must be carefully observed; even the ice that is used to cool the injectate should be sterile because the end of the syringe comes into direct contact with the right atrial portal.

Pulmonary artery lines are associated with a number of potential problems. The risk of thrombophlebitis increases with prolonged use because of mechanical irritation from the catheter. Pulmonary hemorrhage or infarction can occur with continuous or prolonged wedging with the balloon and may also be traced to overinflation with wedging. Ventricular ectopy can develop if the catheter is excessively looped in the right ventricle or if it slips from the pulmonary artery back into the right ventricle.

General appearance

It is important to observe the patient's overall appearance. It is possible to pick up immediate clues regarding the degree of distress, exercise tolerance, and disease status of the patient. The general body configuration should also be noted and pertinent measurements obtained so that comparisons can be made between patient information and information on standard growth and development charts. These observations will provide the practitioner with objective data, which can be used to establish a diagnosis or evaluate a chronologic problem. They can also be helpful in monitoring clinical progress after therapy has begun. Motor coordination, muscular development, and emotional maturity are observed to make some assessments about the individual's developmental maturity.

Skin

The entire body surface should be inspected for obvious color changes, skin lesions, or changes in hair growth. Color changes may be subtle but need to be investigated further. Deoxygenated hemoglobin imparts a bluish tone to the skin. In general, the darker the skin pigmentation, the greater the amount of deoxygenated hemoglobin necessary before cyanotic changes are visible. Patients with minimal oxygen desaturation may appear rather ruddy or plethoric. Pallor or paleness is evident in anemia and shock. Both pallor and cyanosis are most evident in the palpebral conjuntiva, fingernail beds, lips, oral mucous membranes, palms of the hands, and soles of the feet. Blanching can be used to check for pallor. Exerting pressure on the fingernail bed of a white person will cause whitening, which disappears when pressure is released. The difference in color change is slight in the individual with pallor. Dark-skinned people can be assessed by gently applying pressure to their lips or gums. Localized pallor or abnormal patches of hair loss can develop with arterial insufficiency. Petechiae, or distinct pinpoint hemorrhages, are commonly found on the fingers and fingernail beds but may also be noted on the conjunctivae or other body surfaces.

Neck

Examination of the venous and arterial pulses in the neck may provide the practitioner with invaluable information leading to the establishment of a cardiac diagnosis. These pulses should be inspected, palpated, and auscultated to obtain as much information as possible.

Neck veins. To examine the neck veins, the patient should be in a semirecumbent position at approximately a 45-degree angle. Modifications may be needed for people with substantial elevations or reductions in venous pressure. Both the level of venous pressure and the type of venous wave pattern should be noted.

These neck veins will fill during expiration and empty during inspiration as the venous pressure rises and falls. To estimate venous pressure, the height of the distended proximal portion of the internal jugular vein must be determined. This height, which is reflective of right atrial pressure, should be recorded in reference to the sternal angle located slightly above the right atrium (Fig. 2-21). If the right atrial pressure is within normal limits, jugular venous distention should be less than 4 cm above the sternal angle. Increased jugular venous distention indicates venous hypertension and can be found in heart failure, reduced right ventricular compliance, pericardial disease, hypervolemia, or conditions in which the superior vena cava is compressed. Jugular venous distention can be increased in some instances by placing the patient in a semirecumbent position with the jugular vein partially filled and applying firm pressure over the right upper quadrant of the abdomen. The patient should be instructed to breathe normally. Sustained engorgement after compression is removed indicates right-sided failure; this is referred to as the *hepatojugular reflex.* A paradoxical rise in the venous pressure during inspiration, referred to as *Kussmaul's sign,* and also occur secondary to a restriction to diastolic filling. This finding generally occurs in constrictive pericarditis.

The jugular venous pulse pattern varies with the volume of blood in the jugular veins. This variation directly reflects pressure changes developing within the right atrium during the cardiac cycle. Jugular venous pulse patterns have three positive waves, the *a, c,* and *v* waves, and two negative components, the *x* and *y* descents, each of which can be correlated with the events of the cardiac cycle. The *a* wave is produced by right atrial contraction and is followed by the *x* descent, correlating with atrial relaxation. The *c* wave is apparently related to tricuspid valve closure and is followed by the *x* descent, whereas the *v* wave, associated with atrial filling, is followed by the *y* descent and is closely related to the decline in right atrial pressure occurring as the tricuspid valve opens (Fig. 2-22). Abnormalities in the size or shape of the venous pulse patterns most often can be traced to obstructive dis-

Fig. 2-21. Measurement of jugular venous pressure.

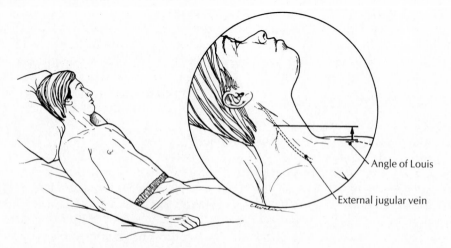

Angle of Louis

External jugular vein

orders, cardiac dysrhythmias, conditions leading to diastolic overload, incompetent valves, or restrictive disorders.

Arterial pulsations. The size and shape of arterial pulsations are determined by a number of factors, which include left ventricular stroke volume, rate of ejection, distensibility of the systemic arteries, peripheral resistance, pulse rate, systolic and diastolic pressures, size and pressure-volume characteristics of the vessel, and distance of the vessel from the heart. Because of the influence of all of these factors, it is possible to evaluate arterial pulsations effectively, employing the parameters of inspection, palpation, and auscultation.

The carotid arterial pulse is best examined with the patient in a reclining position, elevated to approximately 15 to 30 degrees. The patient's head must be turned either slightly away from or toward the examiner for maximal observation. After the practitioner has inspected the vessel, she must simultaneously palpate and auscultate it. Only one side is examined at a time to prevent excessive carotid sinus stimulation. Simultaneous auscultation facilitates usage of the heart sounds as reference points and also enables the practitioner to identify the presence of a bruit, which is a blowing sound created by interference with blood flow. Initially the practitioner applies more and more pressure while palpating the vessel. Then, as pressure is slowly released, the pulsation can be broken down into three components: ascending limb, peak, and descending limb.

Carotid arterial pulsations are normally synchronous and of equal amplitude, with a brisk upstroke and downstroke. These pulsations are commonly visible. Prominent pulsations in the carotid arteries tend to occur when there is an increase in pulse pressure. Prominent pulsations visible in the suprasternal notch can sometimes be traced to an aneurysm of the aortic arch. Carotid artery palpation, revealing reduced or unequal pulsations, occurs in the presence of carotid atherosclerosis or aortic arch disease. Audible and palpable vibrations of turbulent blood flow over the carotids are found in carotid artery atherosclerosis, kinking of the carotid arteries, and aortic valve disease. Table 2-3 summarizes some of the arterial pulsations that can be detected.

Chest

Inspection. A systematic approach must be used to carefully examine the entire precordium. Fig. 2-23 illustrates the areas to be evaluated. Initially, it is important to evaluate the shape and contour of the chest. The thorax is relatively elliptic in an adult but cylindric in an infant. The ribs are attached at approximately a 45-degree angle. In an adult, the anterior-posterior diameter is normally less than the transverse diameter. Posteriorly the scapular prominences appear symmetrical, with a slight depression between the medial scapular border and the spine. Structural deviations in the chest can be associated with cardiovascular anomalies. For example, thoracic deformities such as kyphosis and scoliosis can alter the shape and position of the heart. The thoracic deformities found in Marfan's syndrome are also frequently accompanied by cardiac abnormalities. In addition, the patient with severe emphysema, who has a barrel-shaped chest resulting from an increased anterior-posterior diameter, is often a candidate for heart problems because of the shape of the chest.

Fig. 2-22. Jugular venous pulse pattern.

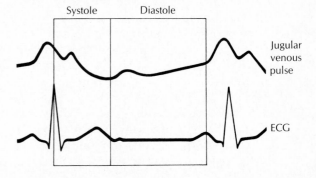

Table 2-3. Arterial pulsations

Name	Description	Significance
Pulsus alternans	Pulse pattern that remains regular in rhythm but irregular in volume, alternating between strong and weak pulsations.	Occurs in the presence of left ventricular failure and severe myocardial disease.
Pulsus bigeminus	Pulse pattern that alternates in rhythm and volume, with every other beat irregular and weaker in volume. The irregular beats are coupled with the normal beats because the interval between them is fixed.	Found in the presence of cardiac dysrhythmias; most often seen with ventricular extrasystoles that occur regularly after a normally conducted beat. Irregular volume is caused by the reduced stroke volume of the premature beat because contraction occurs before ventricular filling is completed.
Pulsus bisferiens	Pulse pattern in which dicrotic element approaches almost the same height as the primary element, therefore appearing as two beats.	Occurs in aortic valvular disease, hyperthyroidism, and severe anxiety states.
Pulsus Corrigans (water-hammer pulse)	Pulse pattern that is strong and bounding and has a wide pulse pressure.	Associated with conditions characterized by an increased stroke volume, such as aortic insufficiency, anemia, essential hypertension, patent ductus arteriosus, and thyrotoxicosis.
Pulsus paradoxus	Pulse pattern characterized by a decrease in volume during inspiration.	Occurs as a result of pooling of blood in the pulmonary circulation during inspiration, which decreases blood return to the left heart.
Pulsus parvus	Pulse pattern that is small and weak and has a narrow pulse pressure.	Occurs in severe left ventricular failure because of a decrease in the stroke volume or moderate to severe aortic stenosis as a result of slow ejection.

The chest should also be inspected for any visible pulsations. It is necessary to identify the time of their occurrence in the cardiac cycle, either by palpating the carotid arterial pulse or simultaneously auscultating the heart. These pulsations can occur during systole, diastole, or both.

The exact location of the point of maximal impulse (the PMI) can sometimes be found on inspection of the anterior chest. Often referred to as the apical impulse, this point is important in terms of its location, size, and character. Normally about 2 cm or less in diameter, the impulse is located in the fifth intercostal space in the midclavicular line in an adult and in the third to fourth intercostal space to the left of the midclavicular line in an infant. The apical impulse moves outward in early systole as the left ventricle contracts. As systole progresses, the impulse moves inward, returning to its original position before systole ends. Deviations in the location, size, and nature of the PMI do occur in pregnancy but can also be attributed to either pulmonary or cardiovascular disease. For example, an atelectasis on the right can shift the PMI to the right, whereas a massive right pleural effusion will displace the PMI to the left. In left ventricular hypertrophy, the PMI becomes much more prominent and forceful and can be deviated to the left.

Palpation. Palpation of the chest is employed to confirm findings observed during inspection. It may also be used to identify those pulsations not visible during inspection. Palpation can also be used to identify the presence of thrills or friction rubs. Thrills are defined as palpable vibrations of disturbed blood flow and are produced as a result of stenotic valves or septal defects. Thrills should be described in terms of location and transmission, as well as the point in time in the cardiac cycle at which they occur. Occasionally, it is possible to note the presence of a pericardial friction rub on palpation. This finding, produced by the rubbing together of the two layers of the pericardium, is perceived as a grating sensation and can be felt, unrelated to breathing, during either systole alone or during both systole and diastole.

Auscultation. Cardiac auscultation is carried out sequentially. It may follow inspection in the infant and young child to preclude interruption of findings because of possible crying brought on by palpation. On the other hand, some practitioners prefer to palpate the chest before auscultation. To auscultate, a practitioner must use a good stethoscope. It should be equipped with earpieces that fit snugly in the examiner's ears so that extraneous room noises are blocked out; in addition, the tubing should be made of flexible rubber or plastic and must be thick enough to ward off extraneous sounds. The tubing should be approximately 12 inches in length because tubes that are longer can damp the auscultatory sounds. The stethoscope must have a chestpiece equipped with both a diaphragm and bell. The diaphragm is applied firmly to the chest to appreciate high-pitched sounds, whereas the bell is applied lightly to auscultate low-pitched sounds. Pediatric stethoscopes are available but not always necessary because the bell, if small enough,

Fig. 2-23. Anatomic locations for auscultation of the heart. *Sternoclavicular area* includes the sternoclavicular joints, the manubrium, and the upper part of the sternum; the *aortic area* is the right second intercostal space; the *pulmonic area* is the left second intercostal space; the *anterior precordium* includes the (right ventricular) lower half of the sternum and intercostal spaces, both on the left and right; the *apical area* is the fifth left intercostal space, in or slightly medial to the midclavicular line; the *epigastric area* is inferior to the xiphoid; and the *ectopic area* includes the left cardiac border, midway between the pulmonary and apical areas.

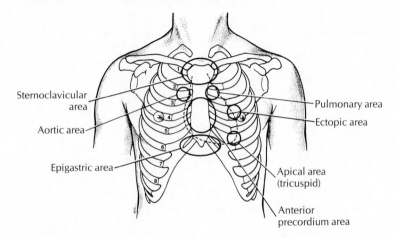

Table 2-4. Adult cardiac abnormalities detected by inspection and palpation of the precordium

Physical finding	Location*	Abnormality
Thrill	URSB 2nd to 3rd intercostal space	Aortic stenosis
	ULSB 2nd to 3rd intercostal space	Obstruction of right ventricular outflow tract
	LLSB LRSB	Ventricular septal defect
	Apex 4th to 6th intercostal space or beyond	Mitral valve disease
Forceful pulsation	URSB 2nd to 3rd intercostal space	Rheumatic heart disease, systemic hypertension, ascending thoracic aortic aneurysm
	ULSB 2nd to 3rd intercostal space mitral stenosis, pulmonary embolism	Essential pulmonary hypertension, left-to-right intracardiac shunt, mitral stenosis, pulmonary embolism
Lift or heave	LLSB LRSB	Obstruction of right ventricular outflow tract, mitral stenosis, left-to-right intracardiac shunt, skeletal deformities
Strong apical impulse or abnormally large PMI	MLSB 4th to 6th intercostal space or beyond	Left ventricular hypertrophy, aortic valve diseases
Dyskinetic apical impulse	Apex	Left ventricular aneurysm
Gallop	Apex	Myocardial dysfunction, mitral valve or aortic valve disease, hypertensive cardiovascular disease

*URSB = Upper right sternal border.   LRSB = Lower right sternal border.
ULSB = Upper left sternal border.   MLSB = Midleft sternal border.
LLSB = Lower left sternal border.

can be applied firmly to the chest wall to create a diaphragm effect.

The patient must be examined in sitting, supine, and left lateral positions, if possible, to appreciate all possible auscultatory findings. Each of the areas identified in Fig. 2-23 must be examined with the diaphragm and the bell. The practitioner can proceed either from the base to the apex or from the apex to the base, as long as all areas are evaluated.

Initially, the examiner should listen to the heart sounds produced by the opening and closure of the heart valves and by the vibrations of blood against the walls of the heart and vessels, that is, the first and second heart sounds. The first heart sound (S_1), produced by the closing of the mitral and tricuspid valves, must be differen-

tiated from the second heart sound (S_2), produced by closure of the semilunar valves. This is accomplished by timing the heart sound with carotid arterial pulsation because S_1 correlates with palpation of the upstroke of the carotid pulse. In monitored patients, the ECG can also be used because S_1 can be timed with the appearance of the QRS complex on the oscilloscopic display. Once these sounds have been isolated, they must be examined in detail in each of the illustrated areas, which depict the transmission of sound vibrations produced by the valves rather than their exact anatomic location. A description of the frequency (pitch), intensity (loudness), duration, and timing should be noted.

The first heart sound is heard over the entire

Table 2-5. Pediatric cardiac abnormalities detected by inspection and palpation of the precordium

Physical finding	Location*	Abnormality
Thrill	LLSB	Ventricular septal defect
	ULSB	Pulmonary valvular stenosis, patent ductus arteriosus
	URSB	Aortic stenosis
	Apex	Mitral stenosis, mitral insufficiency
	MLSB	Tetralogy of Fallot
Quick, forceful impulse	LLSB	Atrial septal defect
	Apex	Aortic insufficiency, ventricular defect, patent ductus arteriosus, thyrotoxicosis
Slow, heaving impulse	LLSB	Pulmonary valvular stenosis, pulmonary hypertension
	Apex	Aortic stenosis, systemic hypertension
Diffuse impulse	Anterolateral precordium	Cardiac dilation (that is, myocarditis)
Weak or absent impulse		Pericardial effusion

*LLSB = Lower left sternal border. URSB = Upper right sternal border.
 ULSB = Upper left sternal border. MLSB = Midleft sternal border.

precordium but is loudest over the apex because of the blood flow and the location of the atrioventricular valves. Because the sounds produced by left-sided events are slightly louder than those on the right because of the pressure gradient, the mitral component of the sound is usually louder. In addition, left-sided events precede right-sided events, resulting in a slight asynchrony in valve closure. Although this asynchrony is slight, it is sometimes possible to hear the separate sounds of the mitral and tricuspid valve closures. Although unusual, this phenomenon does sometimes occur and is referred to as *splitting of the first heart sound*. Splitting is intensified in pulmonary hypertension because of the increased right-sided pressure. The frequency of the first heart sound is lower than that of S_2 and its duration slightly longer.

The second heart sound is loudest over the base of the heart. Closure of the aortic component of this sound is the loudest and precedes pulmonic closure. This asynchronous valve closure occurs because right ventricular systole is slightly longer than left ventricular systole. It is even more intensified during inspiration because the decrease in intrathoracic pressure that occurs increases venous return to the right side of the

heart, further delaying right ventricular ejection and pulmonic valve closure. This is referred to as *physiologic splitting* and is best heard over the pulmonary valve area when the patient assumes either a supine or sitting position.

A physiologic third heart sound, S_3, can be heard in children, adolescents, and young adults under the age of 30. It occurs during the period of rapid ventricular filling after closure of the semilunar valves and opening of the atrioventricular valves. It is a low-pitched sound best heard with the bell of the stethoscope and is produced by the forces that act at the transition between active relaxation and passive filling of the ventricle. The third heart sound is best heard at the apex with the patient in a supine or left semilateral position. In many instances, S_3 will disappear within 30 seconds after the patient has assumed an upright position.

A physiologic fourth heart sound (S_4) may be normal in adults over 50 years of age but is pathologic in infants and children. This sound, which is heard just before S_1, is related to augmentation of ventricular filling by atrial systole. It is a result of vibrations produced in an already distended left ventricle by a rapid acceleration of the chamber wall and a deceleration of the blood mass. Although two vibrations actually occur, the first is generally inaudible because of its very low frequency. The second, although still a low frequency sound, is slightly more intense than the first and is heard with the bell of the stethoscope directly on or slightly medial to the PMI, with the patient in a supine or left semilateral position. It can occasionally be heard over the base of the heart.

There are a number of abnormal sounds that can be found by auscultating the precordium. These findings may entail abnormalities of the normal first and second heart sounds or may involve the presence of extra heart sounds, clicks, or murmurs. In the pages that follow, they will be classified as abnormalities of S_1, S_2, S_3, and S_4 sounds or extracardiac sounds (Tables 2-4 and 2-5).

The first heart sound may be abnormally increased, decreased, or variable in intensity; it may also be abnormally split. To understand some of the mechanisms that produce these variations, it is necessary to review the principal factor responsible for the production of the first heart sound, that is, AV valve closure. Any alteration in the activity of these valves could affect the intensity of S_1. For example, the position of the valve leaflets will affect the intensity of S_1. S_1 will be louder in the presence of a stenotic mitral or tricuspid valve because closure of the stenotic valve results in vibration that will produce a loud sound. The first heart sound will be less intense in the presence of a regurgitant valve because of decreased velocity of valve closure.

The position of the AV valves at the time of ventricular systole and the magnitude of ventricular pressure will also affect the intensity of S_1. This effect, reflected in the duration of the PR interval, can result in either an increase or a decrease in intensity. S_1 will be loudest when the PR interval is shortened because the valves have not had an opportunity to close before ventricular systole. S_1 will be decreased in intensity when the PR interval is prolonged because the valve leaflets are almost completely closed before the onset of ventricular systole.

The existence of a left-to-right shunt or such hyperkinetic circulatory states as hyperthyroidism, fever, anemia, and tachycardia can also increase the intensity of S_1 because of the increased blood flow that results in an increase in the force and velocity of ventricular contraction, thereby augmenting S_1. On the other hand, the loudness of S_1 will be decreased in conditions such as myocardial infarction, myocarditis, cardiac myopathy, and congestive heart failure, which decrease ventricular contractility and therefore reduce the force and velocity of contraction.

In the presence of cardiac dysrhythmias that are characterized by frequent changing of the PR interval such as in first and second degree AV block, there will be an accompanying change in the intensity of S_1. This variation will also occur in dysrhythmias associated with a totally irregular atrial rhythm and some ventricular rhythm, such as atrial fibrillation and ventricular tachycardia, because the force and velocity of conduction will be so varied.

Pathologic splitting of the first heart sound can occur and suggests the possibility of left or right bundle branch block, premature ventricular contractions, or atrial septal defect. The last condition is suspected if the tricuspid component of the closure is loudest. Although the mechanism responsible for pathologic splitting is unclear, it can be differentiated from a physiologically split S_1 because it becomes more accentuated.

The second heart sound can also be increased or decreased in intensity, as well as abnormally split. It must be carefully analyzed. The second component of S_2, the pulmonic component, may be accentuated in children and adolescents.

S_2 is often increased in intensity in the presence of arterial or pulmonary hypertension. An increase in the pressure in the systemic arterial system usually results in accentuation of the aortic component of S_2, whereas increased pressure in the pulmonary artery, resulting from atrial or ventricular septal defect, patent ductus arteriosus, primary pulmonary hypertension, recurrent pulmonary emboli, mitral stenosis, or right ventricular failure, accentuates the pulmonic component. Accentuation of the pulmonary component can be attributed to increased pulmonary blood flow or increased pulmonary venous pressure. The second sound may also be accentuated in congenital or acquired aortic stenosis.

A decrease in the intensity of S_2 can be found in conditions associated with reduced valve mobility, such as aortic stenosis and pulmonic stenosis. The aortic component of S_2 is decreased in aortic stenosis, whereas the pulmonic component is decreased in pulmonic stenosis. The exception, as mentioned, occurs in congenital aortic stenosis with normal valve flexibility.

Abnormal inspiratory and expiratory splitting of S_2 may be found in a variety of pathologic conditions. Splitting is more prominent when the asynchrony between the left and right ventricular systole is accentuated. This can occur when right ventricular ejection is prolonged, leading to delayed pulmonic closure.

Prolongation of right ventricular systole delays closure of the pulmonic valve. This may occur in the presence of increased right ventricular pressure secondary to right ventricular failure or right ventricular outflow obstruction, that is, infundibular or valvular pulmonic stenosis, or may be caused by delayed right ventricular activation, which occurs in right bundle branch block. Widening of the S_2 split can occur when early aortic closure combines with late pulmonic closure and is commonly associated with congestive heart failure, ventricular septal defect, and pulmonary hypertension.

Paradoxical splitting of S_2 occurs most commonly with a left bundle branch block because delayed activation of the left ventricle would prolong left ventricular systole, permitting pulmonic valve closure before aortic valve closure. The two components move together during inspiration, often becoming single while separating on expiration, making the split appreciable. This phenomenon may also occur if the left ventricle becomes overloaded either because of excess volume or pressure.

Abnormal third and fourth heart sounds are collectively classified as gallop rhythms because their sound resembles the gallop of a horse. Both of these sounds occur in diastole, never systole. When the sound occurs in early diastole soon after S_2, it is referred to as an S_3 gallop, S_3g, ventricular gallop, or protodiastolic sound. When it occurs in late diastole, immediately before S_1, it is termed an S_4 gallop, S_4g, atrial gallop, or presystolic sound. Both of these sounds may occur in the presence of normal or slowed heart rates, although the term gallop suggests a rapid rate. The presence of both an S_3g and S_4g superimposed on one other is referred to as a summation gallop.

The ventricular gallop is a dull, low-pitched sound heard best with the bell of the stethoscope. Its sound resembles the word "Kentucky," that is:

$$\frac{S_1 \quad S_2 \quad S_3}{\text{Ken} \quad \text{tuc} \quad \text{ky}}$$

The origin of the S_3g is still debated. This sound may originate from either side of the heart. When occurring on the left, it is best heard over the apex, whereas if it originates on the right, it is best heard at the left sternal border or over the xiphoid. A left ventricular S_3g suggests right-heart failure until proven otherwise. It may also be found in mitral insufficiency, aortic insufficiency, or a left-to-right shunt. The right ventricular S_3g occurs in right ventricular failure and often accompanies tricuspid or pulmonary valve insufficiency or an atrial septal defect. An S_3g persists when the patient stands, in contrast to the physiologic S_3g, and is increased in intensity when patients assume a left lateral position or when they exercise.

An atrial gallop is a low-pitched sound produced by vibrations that result from an increased resistance to late ventricular filling during atrial systole. Its sound is imitated by the word "Tennessee," that is:

$$\frac{S_4 \quad S_1 \quad S_2}{\text{Ten} \quad \text{nes} \quad \text{see}}$$

The S_4g, which may emanate from the left or right ventricle, is heard best with the bell over the apex when it originates from the left and at the lower left sternal border when it originates from the right. It may also be audible over the base of the heart. This sound is frequently associated with conditions in which there is an impairment in end-diastolic compliance secondary to ventricular hypertrophy, fibrosis, infarction, or inflammation. Its sound is augmented with forced inspiration or following exercise and usually is abolished by a Valsalva maneuver, by sitting, or by using rotating tourniquets.

A variety of abnormal sounds can often be heard upon auscultation of the precordium. One of these, the opening snap, is produced by the opening of the AV valves soon after S_2. It occurs most commonly in mitral stenosis because the valve forms a restrictive diaphragm that bulges into the left atrium during systole and then snaps back into the left ventricle during diastole. The abrupt recoil of the valve occurs as ventricular pressure falls below atrial pressure. The opening snap is loudest at the lower left sternal border and at the apex. It is best heard with the diaphragm of the stethoscope. The opening snap is closest to S_2 in severe mitral stenosis with a high atrial pressure. It is slightly delayed in less severe stenosis because the valve opens more slowly and the atrial pressure is not as high. An opening snap related to tricuspid stenosis can occur and is best heard over the left lower sternal border or the xiphoid. The mechanism responsible for the production of this opening snap is the same as in mitral stenosis.

The ejection sound or click is an extra heart sound heard in early systole. Its timing in systole depends on its etiology. This sound is usually found in the presence of systolic overload of the left or right ventricle because of valvular obstruction, regurgitation, dilation, or systemic or pulmonary hypertension. This ejection sound is also associated with increased blood flow caused by atrial septal defects or anomalous pulmonary venous return. Many of these sounds are followed by ejection murmurs.

Most ejection sounds are high-pitched in intensity and consequently are heard best with the diaphragm. Aortic ejection sounds are loudest over the apex but may be heard over the entire precordium, as well as the neck. This ejection sound does not vary with normal respiration. It is associated with aortic stenosis, aortic regurgitation, coarctation, aneurysms of the ascending aorta, and hypertension with aortic dilation. The pulmonic ejection sound, with limited radiation, is best heard over the pulmonic area. In contrast to the aortic ejection sound, it varies with respiration, decreasing during inspiration and increasing during expiration. It suggests the presence of pulmonic stenosis, pulmonary artery dilation, or pulmonary hypertension. Other middle to late clicks are termed nonejection clicks and are idiopathic, having recently been found to be associated with a prolapse of the mitral valve, referred to as Barlow's syndrome. The click appears to be caused by the abnormal distribution of tension in the valve, which results from the prolapse of one or both of the mitral leaflets into the left atrium during late systole. This sound is heard best at the apex and is not well transmitted.

The presence of a pericardial friction rub is also an abnormal finding. It can be found in any condition that produces a serofibrinous, fibrinous, or bloody effusion in the pericardial sac, leading to the development of a rubbing of the pericardial surfaces. It may also be heard in pericarditis without effusion. Pericardial friction rub typically is characterized as a grating to-and-fro sensation most often heard between the apex and the left sternal border, although it can be audible over the entire precordium. This sound often frustrates the practitioner because it is transient; it may remain audible for several days or disappear within hours. The pericardial friction rub is heard either during systole alone or during both systole and diastole with the diaphragm; it is not related to respiration, which differentiates it from a pleural friction rub. It is associated with pericarditis.

Cardiac murmurs are abnormal sounds produced by structural alterations or hemodynamic events occurring in the heart and great vessels. Fig. 2-24 illustrates some of the mechanisms responsible for the alterations in blood flow. Murmurs are described according to their location, transmission, timing, quality, pitch, and intensity. Patients must be examined in a supine, sitting, and left lateral decubitus position to accurately evaluate a murmur.

The location of a murmur is defined as the specific area where it is heard the loudest; although it may be heard over the entire precordium, it is most intense over one or more areas. The location often facilitates the determination of the murmur's origin because many murmurs are classically found in specific areas.

Transmission describes the radiation of a murmur to sites other than the primary location. Transmission depends to some extent on the loudness of the murmur. It occurs through the bloodstream, vascular wall, myocardium, or the soft tissue and bones. Transmission is also valuable in determining the cause of the murmur.

Murmurs must be timed with the cardiac cycle in which they occur. Murmurs can by sys-

tolic, diastolic, or both. Systolic murmurs can be heard in early, mid, or late systole. They also may be audible throughout, in which case they are referred to as holosystolic or pansystolic. Diastolic murmurs are timed similarly but are labeled as *protodiastolic* if they occur in early diastole, *presystolic* if they occur in late diastole, and *holodiastolic* if they can be heard throughout diastole. To accurately time a murmur, the practitioner can either palpate the carotid pulse or monitor the QRS complex on the oscilloscope. Auscultatory findings that occur simultaneously with the carotid pulsation or QRS configuration are timed with systole; on the other hand, if they occur after collapse of the carotid pulse or after the T wave, they are timed with diastole.

The quality of a murmur can also be of value in determining its origin. Quality refers to the auditory characteristics of the murmur. Terms such as harsh, blowing, musical, rumbling, grunting, and swishing are commonly used to describe the quality of murmurs.

Pitch is determined by the frequency band of a murmur and is regulated primarily by the velocity of blood flow. It varies directly with the velocity. Murmurs are described as high-, medium-, or low-pitched.

The intensity describes the loudness of a murmur. Although several grading scales currently are used, the most popular is based on a six-point scale, with grade I being the least intense and grade VI, the most intense. According to this method of classification, grade I and grade II systolic murmurs are often functional; that is, they are found in persons without organic heart disease. Grade IV through grade VI murmurs usually indicate underlying cardiovascular pathology. A grade IV murmur is frequently associated with a palpable thrill, whereas a grade VI murmur may be heard without a stethoscope.

The configuration of a murmur can be used to describe flow characteristics (Fig. 2-25). A murmur that starts softly and gradually increases in loudness is referred to as a crescendo murmur, whereas one that starts loudly and de-

Fig. 2-24. Mechanisms for the production of heart murmurs.

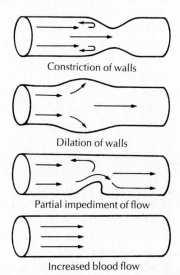

Constriction of walls

Dilation of walls

Partial impediment of flow

Increased blood flow

creases in loudness slowly is described as a decrescendo murmur. The diamond-shaped murmur, also called a crescendo-decrescendo murmur, increases and then decreases in loudness, whereas the plateau or sustained murmur remains relatively constant throughout the cardiac cycle.

The practitioner should also listen to the lungs when performing a cardiac examination because many pulmonary findings reflect cardiovascular problems; conversely, cardiovascular findings reflect pulmonary findings. For a description of a detailed pulmonary examination, the reader is referred to Unit 3.

Abdomen

The abdomen must be examined when the patient is in the proper position and in a relaxed mood. Initially, the abdomen should be inspected. In some thin patients, normal pulsations emanating from the abdominal aorta may be visible (see Unit 6) and/or palpable. Such

pulsations, however, may also indicate the presence of an aneurysm; these pulsations are usually larger in size. In addition, the practitioner should look for signs of fluid retention (ascites) manifested by taut, shiny skin and a tight, swollen abdomen with an everted umbilicus.

Following inspection, the abdomen should be auscultated. The practitioner, evaluating the cardiovascular system, first listens for a bruit over the abdominal aorta or renal arteries. The bruit, which indicates a partial occlusion of the involved vessels, is created by the turbulence in the blood flow. A bruit may also be heard in the presence of congenital vascular malformation.

Percussion of the abdomen follows auscultation and can be used to confirm some findings noted on inspection and auscultation. The tight, swollen abdomen, for example, can be evaluated for a fluid shift, which is present when there is a large amount of fluid in the abdominal cavity, such as in ascites. A fluid shift can be detected in the following manner: the practitioner places a hand palm up behind the supine patient's right flank. Then, with an assistant placing a hand palm down against the middle of the abdomen to avoid transmission of any wave through the abdominal wall, the practitioner taps the left flank of the patient. In the presence of a significant amount of fluid, a wave felt as a sharp impulse will be transmitted through the fluid.

Abdominal palpation provides a great deal of information about the cardiovascular system. It is possible to identify hepatomegaly or splenomegaly though palpation. It may be possible to identify pitting by applying pressure on patients with severe fluid retention. However, when these patients are confined to bed, the edema may shift to the sacral area. It may also be possible to palpate the abdominal aorta or renal arteries; however, to detect the presence of an aneurysm, the practitioner must also feel an expansile mass.

Extremities

Both the upper and lower extremities should be inspected, palpated, and auscultated for signs

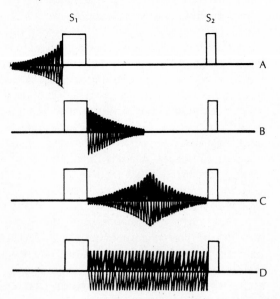

Fig. 2-25. Configuration of cardiac murmurs. *A*, Crescendo murmur. *B*, Decrescendo murmur. *C*, Diamond-shaped crescendo-decrescendo murmur. *D*, Holosystolic murmur.

of cardiovascular disorder. It is possible for the practitioner to carefully inspect the extremities while simultaneously palpating the peripheral arteries and measuring the arterial blood pressure.

Noninvasive arterial blood pressure measurement should initially be taken in both arms. To obtain accurate measurements, the practitioner must follow proper technique. The blood pressure cuff should be wrapped securely around the arm and should be 20% wider than the diameter of the extremity, or two thirds the size from the antecubital fossa to the axilla. Erroneously high readings will be obtained if the cuff is too small, whereas erroneously low readings will result if the cuff is too large.

The cuff should be placed approximately 2.5 cm above the antecubital fossa to measure the arm blood pressure. The cuff is rapidly inflated to approximately 20 mmHg, or torr,* which is above the point at which sounds of Korotkoff disappear, and is deflated slowly. The systolic pressure is read when the sounds of Korotkoff are first heard as a tapping sound. These sounds, believed to be caused by the initial spurt of blood into the collapsed artery as deflation occurs, soon become more pronounced as additional blood rushes into the artery. They change again to a tapping, become muffled, and subsequently disappear. The diastolic pressure is read when the sound disappears.

Arterial blood pressure can also be measured using a thigh cuff placed at midthigh level. Pressure readings are obtained over the popliteal artery by placing the stethoscope over the popliteal fossa. Thigh blood pressure is approximately 10 to 40 torr higher than the arm blood pressure. The sounds of Korotkoff can be augmented if they are difficult to hear. This technique does not artificially change the arterial blood pressure but merely maximizes the pressure gradient above and below the cuff. It is carried out by placing the deflated cuff on the patient's arm and raising the arm above the head for a minute to enhance venous drainage. With the arm elevated, the cuff is rapidly inflated. Then the arm is lowered and the reading is obtained.

The systolic arterial blood pressure can be measured in the absence of audible Korotkoff sounds by placing the cuff on the arm, inflating it, and palpating the radial artery as the pressure is released. The point at which the arterial pulsation is first palpated is read as the systolic pressure. Diastolic pressure cannot be obtained using this technique.

Initially, the size of the upper extremities should be compared. Bilateral enlargement can occur in superior vena cava obstruction or anasarca because of congestive heart failure. Unilateral enlargement usually signifies venous obstruction or lymph gland enlargement. The existence of tortuous vessels should be noted because these sometimes may be associated with the presence of arteriosclerotic heart disease, especially in the elderly. The fingers and hands should also be examined. Extreme length and slenderness of the fingers (and toes and legs) occur in Marfan's syndrome and may indicate a concurrent cardiovascular problem. The fingers and toes should also be checked for clubbing, which is exhibited by proliferation of the soft tissue of the terminal phalanges and loss of the unguophalangeal angle, that is, the angle between the nail and digit. Clubbing is associated with cyanotic congenital disorders and subacute bacterial endocarditis (SBE), as well as chronic obstructive pulmonary disease (COPD) and numerous other conditions, including idiopathic clubbing, hyperthyroidism, lung cancer, and gastrointestinal disorders. The fingers should be inspected for subungual hemorrhages characterized by a linear configuration, that is, the "splinter hemorrhages" of SBE (also seen in the conjunctiva and in the retina), and for Osler's nodes, which are painful red nodules on the fingertips suggestive of bacterial embolism. If latter are not painful, they are called Janeway lesions.

The fingers and hands should also be pal-

---

*1 mmHg = 1 torricelli (torr).

pated to detect warmth. If a patient has cold hands with a normal body temperature, low cardiac output states or hypometabolism may be reflected, whereas if a patient has exceptionally warm hands and a normal body temperature, it may indicate a high cardiac output state or hypermetabolism. Exceptionally cold, pale, numb fingers when exposed to cold suggest a peripheral vascular disorder such as Raynaud's disease.

In addition, the peripheral circulation should be evaluated by testing capillary filling. Referred to as blanching, blanching involves the application of pressure against the patient's fingernail. (The toenail may also be used.) Normally the digit will whiten, or blanch, when pressure is applied and will return to normal color as pressure is released. Failure of a return to normal color may indicate arterial insufficiency or severe vasoconstriction.

The lower extremities should be inspected for size, color, and skin condition. Unilateral enlargement may indicate venous thrombosis, a peripheral arteriovenous fistula, or unilateral lymphedema, as in pelvic neoplasm. Bilateral enlargement can usually be attributed to edema but should be investigated further. Whether edema is caused by congestive heart failure or constrictive clothing, it may disappear when the extremity is elevated. The degree of pitting can be assessed by applying gentle pressure with the finger over a bony prominence, measuring the depth of indentation that remains as the finger is removed and how long it persists. Patients with poor peripheral circulation have pale, ruddy, or cyanotic extremities. The legs are pale when elevated and reddish-purple when in the dependent position. Skin that appears shiny and pits with pressure suggests fluid retention, whereas skin with ulcers, tortuous veins, and a bronze pigmentation (stasis dermatitis), is characteristic of chronic venous insufficiency.

Palpation of the lower extremities may reveal signs of venous thrombosis, which include pain and tenderness associated with swelling and redness. These findings, when accompanied by calf pain upon dorsiflexion of the foot, are considered highly suggestive of pathology.

Auscultation of the lower extremities is limited to listening for a bruit over the femoral artery. This finding, when associated with poor peripheral pulses and cool extremities, is generally consistent with localized femoral arterial disease.

Laboratory studies

Laboratory studies used to evaluate patients with cardiovascular problems include both non-invasive and invasive tests. Some of these studies are used for screening purposes; others identify particular problems. Those tests that are commonly used to evaluate acutely ill patients with cardiovascular disorders will be discussed in the pages that follow. Table 2-6 outlines additional diagnostic studies used to evaluate cardiac disorders.

The electrocardiogram

The surface electrocardiogram, or ECG, provides a graphic recording of the electrical activity of the heart. It can be obtained at rest, with normal activity, or with exercise. The ECG is valuable in the diagnosis of rhythm disorders, myocardial disease, and chamber enlargement. Whereas the resting ECG is used as a baseline, the ambulatory ECG enables the practitioner to identify abnormalities that might not be apparent at rest, and the exercise ECG facilitates an evaluation of the heart's response to stress.

The resting ECG, used for diagnostic purposes, uses 12 surface leads to monitor the electrical activity of the heart muscle. Leads I, II, and III are bipolar limb leads that measure the electrical difference between two recording sites, a positive and negative pole. Leads aVR, aVL, and aVF are augmented unipolar limb leads consisting of an extremity (limb) lead and a precordial (chest) lead. They measure the difference in electrical potential between the limb and the center of the heart, which is at zero potential. The precordial, or V, leads consist of six chest electrodes, V_1 through V_6, on a horizontal

Table 2-6. Additional diagnostic studies used to identify cardiovascular disorders

Test	Description	Indications
Drug assays	Measure blood levels of specific drugs. Currently it is possible to measure plasma levels of digitoxin, digoxin propranolol, procainamide, diphenylhydantoin, quinidine, and lidocaine.	Used to differentiate between therapeutic and toxic levels.
C-reactive protein (CRP)	Venipuncture performed to obtain blood sample that is mixed and tested for the presence of an α-globulin; this precipitates the C-polysaccharide of pneumococcus.	Used to confirm the presence of rheumatic fever and other infections. Successful treatment causes CRP to disappear, making this test valuable more for prognosis than diagnosis.
Sedimentation rate	Blood test measuring the speed with which red blood cells settle in uncoagulated blood.	Used to establish a diagnosis of inflammatory disease such as myocardial infarction, bacterial endocarditis, and Dressler's syndrome.
Antistreptolysin O (ASO titer)	Venipuncture performed to obtain blood sample, which is analyzed for the presence of antistreptolysin O antibody.	Used to establish the presence of a recent streptococcal infection.
Blood cultures	Aerobic and anaerobic blood specimens obtained through venipuncture for culture and gram stain. Serial samples from different sites are obtained for greater accuracy.	Used to identify bacterial organism in blood sample so that appropriate antibiotic therapy can be instituted.
Cardiac biopsy	Forceps are introduced percutaneously through the internal jugular vein into the right atrium and into the right ventricle to obtain a specimen from the right ventricular apex or septum.	Used to diagnose rejection in the transplanted heart. Also useful in diffuse cardiomyopathy.
Cardiac series	Posterior-anterior and lateral and oblique x-rays are taken after the patient has swallowed a bolus of barium. Enlargement in the left atrium or an enlarged aorta will displace the barium-filled esophagus.	Used to establish a diagnosis of chamber enlargement.

plane, which measure how far anteriorly or posteriorly from the frontal plane the electrical forces are traveling. The ECG is used to identify the electrical rhythm (Table 2-7), which is helpful in recognizing electrolyte imbalance and drug intoxication. It is also used to identify conduction disturbances and is of value in the recognition of congenital heart disease. The resting ECG can be helpful in evaluating coronary artery disease and valvular heart disease.

A systematic approach should be used when interpreting the ECG. First, however, it is necessary to be familiar with the graph paper used to record the tracings. ECG graph paper is divided into horizontal lines measuring voltage and vertical lines measuring time. "Little boxes" equal to 0.10 millivolt (mv) or 1.0 millimeter (mm) on the vertical axis and 0.04 seconds on the horizontal axis can be identified, as can "big boxes" equal to 0.50 mv or 5.0 mm or 0.20 seconds.

Text continued on p. 96.

Table 2-7. Summary of cardiac rhythms

Rhythm patterns	Rate	Rhythm	P waves
Sinus rhythm	Infants 120-180 beats/min* Children 80-110 beats/min* Adults 60-100 beats/min	Both atrial and ventricular rhythm are regular.	Precede each QRS complex with same configuration.
Sinus bradycardia	Infants 100 beats/min Children 80 beats/min Adults 60 beats/min	Both atrial and ventricular rhythm are regular.	Precede each QRS complex with same configuration.
Sinus tachycardia	Infants 180 beats/min Children 110 beats/min Adults 100 beats/min	Both atrial and ventricular rhythm are regular.	Precede each QRS complex with same configuration. May be superimposed on preceding T wave with very rapid rates.
Sinus arrhythmia	Increases with inspiration, slows with expiration	Irregular in a cyclic pattern varying with respiration. There is a decrease in cycle length during inspiration and an increase during expiration.	Precede each QRS complex with same configuration usually seen. Occasional variation in shape with cycles.
Wandering atrial pacemaker	Decrease slightly as pacemaker approaches AV junction; increase as pacemaker returns to SA node.	Slightly irregular because of shift in pacemaker.	Precede each QRS when pacemaker is in atrium. May be inverted or buried within QRS or may follow QRS as shift to AV junction occurs. Configuration varies with position.
Sinus arrest	Slows due to temporary suspension of electrical activity for two or more cycles.	Irregular because of periods of asystole. Labeled SA exit block if rhythm returns "as if" uninterrupted, with periods of asystole multiples of normal sinus rhythm.	Absent during periods of asystole. Others precede QRS with same configuration.
Atrial flutter	Atria-200-350 beats/min Ventricles-1/1, 1/2, 1/3, 1/4, 1/5, 1/6, and so on, of atrial rate	Regular atrial and ventricular rhythm in pure flutter. Ventricular rhythm may vary if degree of block varies.	No P waves. Sawtoothed F waves present.

*Specific age-dependent rates appear in Table 2-8.
†The PR interval in infants and children varies inversely with heart rate and increases with age.
‡The QRS complex varies only slightly with age. It is usually less than 0.04 seconds in duration in the premature infant.

PR Interval	QRS interval	Significance	Treatment
Infants† 0.10-0.15 sec Children† 0.13-0.18 sec Adults 0.12-0.20 sec	0.06-0.12 sec‡	Normal rhythm.	None.
Infants 0.10-0.15 sec Children 0.13-0.18 sec Adults 0.12-0.20 sec	0.06-0.12 sec	May reflect good cardiac reserve or be caused by pathologic conditions of the heart. Occurs with increased intracranial pressure and hypothyroidism.	None unless symptomatic; if symptomatic, atropine.
Infants 0.10-0.15 sec Children 0.13-0.18 sec Adults 0.12-0.20 sec	0.06-0.12 sec	Can be related to physiologic conditions (exercise, excitement), pathologic situations not involving the heart (fever), pathologic conditions involving the heart, or pharmacologic agents.	None unless symptomatic; treat underlying cause.
Usually normal in duration; occasional variation seen with different cycles	0.06-0.12 sec	Rarely seen in infants and young children. Common in older children and adolescents.	None.
May shorten as pacemaker approaches AV junction. R-P interval is measured if P wave follows the QRS complex.	0.06-0.12 sec	Can occur in absence of heart disease.	None.
Absent during periods of asystole. Otherwise, normal in duration.	0.06-0.12 sec when present	Can be traced to increased vagal tone, anoxia, or drugs.	None unless symptomatic.
Not measurable.	0.06-0.12 sec. May be difficult to measure because of presence of F waves.	Almost always indicates the presence of organic heart disease. Can occur during fetal life. Type I (congenital atrial flutter) occurs within the first week of life. Type II (paroxysmal atrial flutter) occurs after three weeks of age and more in males. There is no sex distribution in adults.	Synchronized electrical countershock, digitalis, quinidine, propranolol.

Continued.

Table 2-7. Summary of cardiac rhythms—cont'd

Rhythm patterns	Rate	Rhythm	P waves
Atrial fibrillation	Atria-350 beats/min Ventricles, controlled-100 beats/min Ventricles, uncontrolled-100 beats/min	Both atrial and ventricular rhythm are irregularly irregular.	No P waves. Small wavy undulations referred to as f, or fibrillatory, waves.
Paroxysmal atrial tachycardia	160-300 beats/min	Regular atrial and ventricular rhythms that start and stop suddenly.	P waves are seldom seen because of their rapid rate. They are present but buried in preceding T wave.
Atrial tachycardia with block	Atria-60-300 beats/min Ventricles-1/1, 1/2, 1/3, and so on	Atrial rhythm is usually regular but may be slightly irregular with rapid rates. Ventricular rhythm may be regular or irregular, depending on degree of block.	P waves usually differ from P waves in sinus rhythm. They may be buried in preceding T waves in rapid rates.
AV junctional rhythm	40-60 beats/min	Both atrial and ventricular rhythm are regular.	P waves may be inverted and precede the QRS complex, may follow it, or may be buried within it.
Coronary sinus rhythm			Inverted P waves may precede or follow the QRS complex or be buried within it. Occasionally, P waves are absent.
Third degree AV block (complete heart block), Type I and Type II	Type I: Atria-60-100 beats/min Ventricles-40 beats/min Type II: Atria-60-100 beats/min Ventricles-40 beats/min	Both atrial and ventricular rhythm are regular.	Same size and configuration.
Right bundle branch block	60-100 beats/min	Both atrial and ventricular rhythms are regular	Same size and configuration.

PR Interval	QRS interval	Significance	Treatment
Not measurable.	0.06-0.12 sec	Always indicates the presence of organic heart disease. Relatively uncommon in infancy and early childhood.	Digitalis, quinidine, synchronized electrical countershock.
Difficult to measure because of rapidity of rate. May be slightly shortened if measurable.	0.06-0.12 sec	Can occur without organic heart disease.	Vagal stimulation (that is, carotid sinus massage), digitalis, propranolol, tensilon, synchronized electrical countershock.
May be slightly prolonged.	0.06-0.12 sec	Occurs most frequently in patients with significant organic heart disease, such as coronary artery disease or cor pulmonale. May indicate digitalis toxicity.	Discontinue digitalis if toxic. If not toxic, begin digitalis therapy; synchronized electrical countershock.
Shortened; may be measured as R-P interval.	0.06-0.12 sec	Uncommon and usually transient in infants and children.	None unless symptomatic; if symptomatic, atropine.
Normal or slightly shortened in duration; may be measured as R-P interval.	0.06-0.12 sec	Usually transient in infants and children.	
Not measurable; no relationship between atrial and ventricular activity.	Type I 0.06-0.12 sec	May be caused by drug toxicity, degenerative diseases, or electrolyte imbalances, as well as cardiac disorders. Type I is most commonly congenital; Type II usually produces symptoms and may give rise to dysrhythmias because of slow ventricular rate. It is usually acquired in childhood and may be permanent or transient. In adults, it can also be permanent or transient.	Type I
	Type II 0.12 sec (Abnormal)		Type II pacemaker
Infants 0.10-0.15 sec Children 0.13-0.18 sec Adults 0.12-0.20 sec	0.12 sec rSR^1 configuration in leads V_1, V_2	Indicates anatomic or functional discontinuity between bundle branches. Can occur in the absence of underlying heart disease.	None

Continued.

Table 2-7. Summary of cardiac rhythms—cont'd

Rhythm Patterns	Rate	Rhythm	P Waves
Left bundle branch block	60-100 beats/min	Both atrial and ventricular rhythms are regular.	Same size and configuration.
Nonparoxysmal AV junctional tachycardia	60-200 beats/min	Both atrial and ventricular rhythm are regular	P waves may be inverted and precede the QRS complex, may follow it, or may be buried within it.
Accelerated idioventricular tachycardia	Atria-60-100 beats/min§ Ventricles-40-100 beats/min	Regular atrial and ventricular rhythm.	Present but may be buried within the QRS complex. May be produced by retrograde conduction to the atria or may be independent under SA node control.
Ventricular tachycardia	100 beats/min	Atrial rhythm is regular; ventricular rhythm in most instances may be slightly irregular.	Present but often difficult to identify. Often buried within the QRS complex. May be produced by retrograde conduction or may be independent under SA node control.
Ventricular fibrillation	Not measurable.	Irregularly irregular.	Not visible.
First degree AV block (Type I, Type II)	60-100 beats/min	Regular atrial and ventricular rhythms.	Precede each QRS complex with same configuration.
Second degree AV block Type I, Wenkebach	Atria-60-100 beats/min Ventricles-slightly less because of dropped beat or beats.	Type I-regular atrial rhythm. Ventricular rhythm is cyclically irregular unless 2:1 block is present, at which time it is regular.	Same size and configuration.
Type II	Atria-60-100 beats/min Ventricles-slightly less because of dropped beat or beats.	Type II-regular atrial rhythm. Ventricular rhythm is irregular unless block is unchanging.	

§Atrial rate may vary in the presence of sinus bradycardia, sinus tachycardia, or atrial tachycardia.

PR Interval	QRS interval	Significance	Treatment
Infants 0.10-0.15 sec Children 0.13-0.18 sec Adults 0.12-0.20 sec	0.12 sec rSR[1] configuration in leads V_5, V_6; deep slurred S waves	Indicates anatomic or functional discontinuity between bundle branches. Can occur in the absence of underlying heart disease. Prognosis is more severe when found in the presence of heart disease.	None
Shortened, may be measured as R-P interval.	0.06-0.12 sec	Occurs most often with underlying disease or after open heart surgery. Can also be caused by digitalis toxicity.	Digitalis, propranolol, synchronized electrical countershock.
Not measurable.	0.12 sec; abnormal.	Usually occurs in the presence of underlying heart disease. It is usually transient and intermittent and doesn't seem to affect the course of the disease in most instances. It can also be a sign of digitalis toxicity.	None unless symptomatic; if symptomatic, lidocaine, atropine.
Not measurable.	0.12 sec; abnormal.	Usually an indication of significant underlying heart disease. Often results in hemodynamic compromise and predisposes to ventricular fibrillation.	Lidocaine, procainamide, synchronized electrical countershock, quinidine.
Not measurable.	Asymmetrical chaotic complexes.	Death-producing dysrhythmia, necessitating immediate defibrillation.	Defibrillation.
Infants 0.15 sec Children 0.18 sec Adults 0.20 sec	Type I 0.06-0.12 sec Type II 0.12 sec	Doesn't always reflect underlying heart disease. May occur with viral infections, drug toxicity, or during heart surgery or cardiac catheterization.	None.
Type I-progressively lengthens until QRS complex is dropped.	Type I 0.06-0.12 sec	Type I is usually benign.	Type I-none unless symptomatic; if symptomatic, atropine.
Type II-constant when QRS complex present. May be prolonged	Type II 0.12 sec	Type II frequently progresses to complete heart block.	Type II-pacemaker.

Table 2-8. Texas Children's Hospital electrocardiographic criteria: normal values

Age	Heart rate	P-R interval	QRS duration	Q-T interval			
				Heart Rate	R-R Interval	Q-T	
						Min-Max	Mean
0-1 mo	100-180 (120)	0.08-0.12 (0.10)	0.04-0.08 (0.06)	40	1.5	0.38-0.50	(0.45)
1-3 mo	110-180 (120)	0.08-0.12 (0.10)	0.04-0.08 (0.06)	50	1.2	0.36-0.48	(0.43)
3-12 mo	100-180 (150)	0.09-0.13 (0.12)	0.04-0.08 (0.06)	60	1.0	0.34-0.46	(0.41)
1-3 yr	100-180 (130)	0.10-0.14 (0.12)	0.05-0.09 (0.07)	70	0.86	0.32-0.43	(0.37)
3-5 yr	60-150 (100)	0.11-0.15 (0.13)	0.05-0.09 (0.07)	80	0.75	0.29-0.40	(0.35)
5-9 yr	60-130 (100)	0.12-0.16 (0.14)	0.05-0.09 (0.07)	90	0.67	0.27-0.37	(0.33)
9-12 yr	50-110 (80)	0.12-0.17 (0.14)	0.05-0.09 (0.07)	100	0.60	0.26-0.35	(0.30)
12-16 yr	50-100 (75)	0.12-0.17 (0.15)	0.05-0.09 (0.07)	120	0.50	0.24-0.32	(0.28)
>16 yr	50-90 (70)	0.12-0.20 (0.15)	0.05-0.10 (0.08)	150	0.40	0.21-0.28	(0.25)
				180	0.33	0.19-0.27	(0.23)
				200	0.30	0.18-0.25	(0.22)

T Waves

Age	Upright	±	Inverted
0-5 days	I, II, V$_6$	III, AVF, V$_1$	AVR, V$_2$-V$_5$
5 days-2 yrs	I, II, AVF, V$_6$	III, V$_5$	AVR, V$_1$-V$_4$
2 yrs-teens	I, II, AVF, V$_5$, V$_6$	III	AVR, V$_1$-V$_4$
Adults	I, II, III, AVF, V$_1$, V$_5$, V$_6$	V$_2$-V$_4$	AVR

ST Segment

Elevation-depression > 1 mm: myocardial injury
Elevation without reciprocal depression: injury/pericarditis
Depression without reciprocal elevation: injury/digitalis/"normal" premature

Modified from Garson, A.: Pediatric cardiac dysrhythmias, New York, 1982, Grune and Stratton.

Then, to identify the cardiac rhythm, the practitioner must calculate the atrial and ventricular rates, examine the rhythm, identify the P waves, measure the PR interval, and identify and measure the QRS duration. It is unnecessary to separately calculate the atrial and ventricular rate if there is one, and only one, P wave for every QRS complex. Table 2-8 lists some ECG normal values in infants and children.

Although there are several methods that can be used to determine heart rate, the method described in the box on p. 97 can be used universally, whereas the others are limited to specific situations. Once the data has been collected, the cardiac rhythm can be identified (Table 2-7).

It is sometimes possible to determine the cause of an abnormal rhythm from the data collected. Hypokalemia can be suspected in the presence of peaked P waves; a shortened, depressed ST segment; notched, flat, or inverted T waves; prolonged QT intervals; prominent U waves; and frequent premature ventricular contractions. Hyperkalemia is suggested with a widened P wave, prolonged PR interval, widened QRS complex, depressed ST segment, and peaked T wave. Hypocalcemia is represented by a prolonged QT interval, whereas hypercalcemia is suggested with a widened, rounded T wave and shortened QT interval.

Drug toxicity can sometimes be predicted.

CALCULATION OF HEART RATE

Universal approach

1. Obtain a 6-second ECG tracing. (A 3-second tracing can be used but is less representative.)
2. Count all R-R *intervals* from the beginning to the end, estimating fraction intervals. (P-P intervals may be counted to determine atrial rate.)
3. Multiply the number of *intervals* by 10 to determine rate per minute. (A multiplication factor of 20 is used in 3-second tracings.)

Quick approach*

1. Count the number of "big boxes" between R-R intervals, measuring from the *same* point on successive R waves. (P waves may be used for atrial rate.)
2. Divide the number of "big boxes" into 300 to determine rate per minute.

*Can be used only with regular rhythms.

Digitalis intoxication is characterized by a prolonged PR interval, flattened T wave, and/or a shift in the pacemaker from a higher to a lower site. The QT interval may be shortened and the ST segment may sag with both therapeutic and toxic concentrations. Digitalis toxicity may produce no ECG abnormality or may give rise to almost any dysrhythmia. Quinidine toxicity is suspected in the presence of a widened and notched P wave, widened QRS complex, depressed ST segment, and flattened or inverted T waves. A prolonged QT interval may or may not be abnormal because it can occur with therapeutic concentrations. Large doses of Pronestyl (procainamide hydrochloride) may lead to a widening of the QRS complex or, less regularly, to prolongation of the PR and QT intervals and decreased voltage in the QRS and T waves.

The ECG of the infant can be examined for the presence of specific abnormalities suggestive of congenital heart disorders. Although these findings are not diagnostically conclusive, their presence may suggest specific anomalies and can be of great value in localizing the problem to the left or right side of the heart.

The significance of coronary artery disease can often be evaluated from the resting ECG. Changes that occur because of damage to the myocardium can be seen in the various 12 leads. Those changes that directly reflect the area of damage are referred to as *indicative changes* and can be found in the leads directly facing the damaged tissue. Changes that occur in leads that are opposite the area of damage are labeled *reciprocal changes*. Both indicative and reciprocal changes are valuable in identifying the problem because there are some areas of the left ventricle, specifically the posterior wall, that are not directly monitored in the 12-lead ECG.

Three changes can occur when the myocardium is damaged. Acute myocardial injury is characterized by an elevation in the ST segment that is greater than 1 mm in the indicative leads. Reciprocally, this injury is reflected in ST segment depression, which is significant in excess of 0.5 mm. These changes are usually transient and last approximately 1 week in time. Myocardial ischemia is represented by an inverted T wave in the indicative leads and a peaked T wave in the reciprocal leads, although one of the earliest signs of a myocardial infarct may be a peaked T in the indicative leads. Changes because of myocardial ischemia may be transient or permanent. Myocardial infarction causes a permanent ECG change that is illustrated in the indicative leads by the presence of significant Q waves,* which to be considered significant must either be one third the size in height of the entire QRS complex or 0.04 second, or one whole "little box," in width. Insignificant Q waves can be found and are produced by left to right septal depolarization and thus can be found in Leads I, II, III, AVL, AVF, and V_3-V_5. The development of a significant Q wave in anterior myocardial infarction can take several days and can be preceded by

---

*The diagnosis of myocardial infarction cannot be made in the presence of a left bundle branch block (LBBB) because LBBB alters the initial QRS vector.

Table 2-9. Electrocardiographic changes that reflect myocardial damage

Area of damage	Indicative changes	Reciprocal changes
Anterior	V_1, V_2	II, III, aVF
Anteriorseptal	V_3, V_4	II, III, aVF
Anteriolateral	V_5, V_6	II, III, aVF
Lateral	I, aVL, V_5, V_6	V_1
Inferior	II, III, aVF	I, aVL
Posterior	$V_1, V_2, V_3, V_4,$ V_5, V_6	$V_1, V_2, V_3, V_4,$ V_5, V_6

a disappearing R wave, often referred to in the precordial leads as poor R-wave progression. However, poor R-wave progression may also be associated with left ventricular hypertrophy or chronic obstructive pulmonary disease or may be normal or artifactual, the last because of erroneous lead placement. Myocardial infarction is represented by large R waves in the reciprocal leads. Table 2-9 summarizes the indicative and reciprocal changes that reflect myocardial damage.

Valvular heart disease is usually characterized on the ECG by changes that reflect dilation or hypertrophy of the respective chamber (Table 2-10). These changes can involve either the atrium, ventricle, or both, depending on the underlying problem. Atrial enlargement is suspected when the changes involve the P wave, whereas ventricular hypertrophy is suggested when changes occur in the QRS complex and T wave. Right atrial enlargement can be found in the presence of tricuspid valve disease, whereas mitral valve disease usually involves the left atrium. Disorders of the pulmonic valve affect the right ventricle, whereas aortic valve disease focuses on the left ventricle. Severe valvular heart disease can involve more than one chamber.

Ambulatory electrocardiography can be used as an extension of the resting ECG to obtain tracings during normal daily activities for a select group of patients.* By means of a portable

---

*In some special situations, this technique may be used for bedfast patients.

recorder worn on the patient's shoulder or belt, either a magnetic tape is recorded over a period of time or the ECG is transmitted to a monitoring station. The tracings are scanned with selected abnormal areas printed out. This set-up can be used to monitor high-risk patients who have been transferred from critical care or discharged from the hospital. It can be helpful in identifying dysrhythmias that do not appear on the resting ECG in symptomatic patients or in monitoring the effects of drug therapy in the patient who no longer needs to be in intensive care.

The exercise electrocardiogram is used to evaluate patient response to stress. The electrocardiogram is monitored continuously as the patient is subjected to increasing levels of exercise. Although many devices have been designed for stress testing, beginning with the development of the Masters two-step, the most popular protocols use bicycle ergometry or the treadmill. From these tests it is possible to measure myocardial oxygen consumption and to evaluate the myocardial response to stress. Patients are tested until they reach a predetermined heart rate based on their age and sex or until symptoms of ischemia or exhaustion develop. The patient is constantly monitored for signs that indicate myocardial ischemia, specifically ST segment depression, the development of chest pain, or the appearance of dysrhythmias. Stress testing is of value in establishing a diagnosis of coronary artery disease in the presence of a normal or nonspecific resting ECG. It is also useful in the diagnosis of cardiac dysrhythmias. Lately, stress testing has enjoyed widespread use as a mechanism for evaluating specific therapies. The exercise electrocardiogram is contraindicated in patients who are acutely ill with a myocardial infarction, myocarditis, a severe dysrhythmia, congestive heart failure, or drug toxicity.

The echocardiogram

Echocardiography provides a graphic recording of reflected ultrasound using a transducer placed against the chest wall. Often referred to

Table 2-10. ECG changes indicative of chamber enlargement (hypertrophy) in adults and children

Chamber	ECG alterations
Left atrial enlargement	*Adult:* P wave duration of 0.12 sec or more (normal is 0.11 sec). P wave is notched and slurred in Leads I and II (P mitral). Diphasic P waves with wide, deep, terminal component in V_1, V_2. *Children:* Lead II: P wave > 0.09 sec in duration Lead V_1: late negative deflection > 0.04 sec duration and > 1 mm deflection.
Right atrial enlargement	*Adult:* P wave duration is 0.11 sec or less. P wave is peaked and tall (P pulmonale) and measures 2.5 mm or more in amplitude in leads II, III, and AVF. P waves in V_1 and V_2 are diphasic, frequently an increase in voltage in the initial component. *Children:* Peaked P wave > 3.0 mm if child is < 6 months old or > 2.5 mm if child is > 6 months old.
Left ventricular enlargement	*Adult:* R wave or S wave in limb lead that is 20 mm or more in the amplitude; or S wave in V_1, V_2, or V_3 that is 30 mm or more; or R wave in V_4, V_5, or V_6 that is 30 mm or more. Left axis deviation. QRS interval that is 0.09 sec or more. Intrinsicoid deflection in V_5-V_6 that is 0.05 sec or more. Left atrial enlargement. *Children:* R wave in V_6 + S wave in V_1 ≥ 60 (do not use transition leads); use V_5 if R wave in V_5 > R wave in V_5. S wave in V_1 > twice R wave in V_5 Abnormal R/S ratio Abnormal amplitude R wave in V_1 or R wave in V_6
Right ventricular enlargement	*Adult:* Large tall R waves over V_1 and V_2 with deep S waves in V_5 and V_6. The R to S ratio in V_1 is greater than 1.0 QRS within normal limits. Right axis deviation. *Children:* QR pattern V_{4r}, V_{3r}, or V_1 (may be ventricular inversion). Upright T wave V_{4r}, V_{3r}, or V_1—5 days adolescence (if R/S = 1) (may be reciprocal from left chest) Abnormal R/S ratio V or V_6 Abnormal amplitude R wave in V_1 or S wave in V_6

R = right.

as ultrasound cardiography or ultrasound imaging, this technique reflects echoes from pulsed high frequency sound waves. It is used to study the movement and dimensions of several cardiac structures, especially the mitral and aortic valves, the interventricular septum, and right and left ventricular walls. It may also be helpful in evaluating the motion of the tricuspid and pulmonic valves. Echocardiography measures the sizes of the cardiac chambers and provides a graphic recording of changes taking place throughout the cardiac cycle, thereby aiding in the recognition of filling defects.

As a noninvasive procedure, echocardiography is used to confirm the diagnosis of valvular heart disease, pericardial effusion, atrial septal defect, atrial tumors, hypertrophic cardiomyopathy, and a variety of congenital anomalies. It is also helpful in evaluating the function of the left ventricle.

The chest roentgenogram

The chest roentgenogram, using posterior-anterior (PA) and lateral views, provides information about the size, shape, position, and contour of the heart and great vessels. The size of the heart is estimated by measuring the cardio-thoracic diameter. This is done by adding the midright and midleft dimensions (the distance from the midline to the right and left borders), and dividing the sum by the longest transverse diameter of the chest. Cardiac enlargement is suspected when the cardiothoracic ratio is greater than 50%. It is also possible to estimate chamber size in both the PA and lateral views. The PA view provides information about the left atrium and left ventricle. Some inference can also be made about the right atrium. A lateral view is used to evaluate the right atrium and right ventricle.

Biochemical analysis

Complete blood count. The *complete blood count (CBC),* which is discussed in detail in Unit 8, is of value in following the progress of some cardiovascular disorders.

The red blood cell count (RBC) is often elevated in cyanotic heart disease. This elevation, called polycythemia, occurs as a compensatory response because decreased tissue oxygenation stimulates erythropoiesis.

A decreased hemoglobin (Hb) and hematocrit (Hct) can explain anginal pain in patients with coronary artery disease or hemolysis in patients with prosthetic valves. Because anemia accentuates the symptoms in cyanotic heart disease, its presence can explain some of the problems associated with the cyanotic infant. In addition, it can produce heart failure in patients without other heart disease or aggravate the symptoms of underlying heart disease.

The white blood cell count (WBC) is increased in inflammatory disorders and will be elevated in infectious cardiovascular diseases. A mild leukocytosis can also be found in noninfectious inflammatory disorders related to physical and emotional stress. Therefore the WBC will be elevated in myocardial infarction and Dressler's syndrome, as well as in bacterial endocarditis or rheumatic fever. The WBC may be normal or elevated in pericarditis.

Platelet counts are frequently reduced in cy-anotic heart disease. Although the exact mechanism causing the thrombocytopenia is unclear, it occurs fairly often.

Serum electrolytes. Analysis of the serum electrolytes sodium (Na), potassium (K), chloride (Cl), and carbon dioxide (CO_2) are obtained during a routine biochemical screening and facilitate an evaluation of the patient's fluid and electrolyte balance. These analyses are helpful in monitoring the progress of heart failure and serve as a guide for the use of diuretic therapy in the treatment of this condition.

Serum lipids. The blood lipids (cholesterol, triglycerides, and phospholipids) are found bound to proteins circulating in the blood plasma. Labeled as lipoproteins, these lipids are normal constituents of the circulating blood volume. Recently lipids have been fractionalized according to their densities. Four major groups of lipoproteins have been identified that are important both physiologically and in clinical diagnosis. These include the chylomicrons, very low density lipoproteins (VLDL), low density lipoproteins (LDL), and high density lipoproteins (HDL). Triglycerides are predominant in chylomicrons and VLDL, whereas cholesterol and phospholipids predominate in LDL and HDL. Elevations of both cholesterol and triglycerides have been associated with a greater risk of coronary artery disease (CAD). An excess of VLDL, type IV hyperlipidemia, has been associated with premature atherosclerosis and the development of nonfamilial CAD. Elevations of the LDL fractions are positively correlated with CHD (type II familial hyperlipidemia), whereas there appears to be an inverse relationship between HDL levels and CHD development. Studies have shown that increases in HDL are associated with reduced blood pressure; decreased total cholesterol, cigarette use, and weight; increased exercise; and a moderate alcohol intake. HDL is thought to enhance the removal of LDL and inhibit its uptake. Its protective effect is nullified with very low or very high cholesterol levels. Blood lipids are not reliable after a recent myocardial infarction.

Cardiac enzymes. The enzymes are naturally occurring compounds that are found in body tissues. They serve as catalysts for the biochemical reactions of the body and are released into the bloodstream when the particular tissue in which they are found is significantly damaged.

Creatinine phosphokinase (CPK, or CK) is an enzyme found in skeletal, muscle, brain, and cardiac tissue. CK elevation can occur with vigorous exercise, skeletal muscle disease, brain damage, and myocardial damage and following intramuscular injections. Three isoenzymes, CK-MM, CK-BB, and CK-MB, have been isolated in an effort to identify the underlying disorder in CK elevations. The myocardium contains the MB and some MM fractions. In myocardial damage, it is the MB type that is elevated, making it possible to identify myocardial injury. The CK is the first enzyme to become elevated in the presence of myocardial damage. It rises within 2 to 5 hours of the initial attack of chest pain, peaks within 24 hours, and returns to normal after 48 to 72 hours. Elevations from 6 to 15 times the normal range are not unusual.

The serum glutamic oxalic transaminase (SGOT), also referred to as the aspartate transaminase (AST), is an enzyme found in the heart, the kidneys, red blood cells, the brain, the pancreas, the lungs, the liver, and skeletal muscle tissue. It is raised in the presence of cardiac disorders, pericarditis, myocardial infarction, and congestive heart failure. Within 6 hours after myocardial infarction, the level of this enzyme begins to rise, peaking within 24 to 48 hours and returning to normal within 3 to 4 days. SGOT may reach elevations that are 2 to 15 times the normal level.

Lactic dehydrogenase (LDH, or LD) is found in the heart, the kidneys, blood cells, the brain, lymph nodes, the spleen, the pancreas, the liver, the lungs, and skeletal muscle tissue. This particular enzyme remains elevated for a longer period of time, making it valuable in establishing a diagnosis in the patient who is seen several days after the onset of chest pain. LD isoen-

zymes can also be obtained. The LD level peaks at 2 to 8 times the normal level. It begins to elevate within 6 to 12 hours after a myocardial infarction, peaks in 48 to 72 hours, and returns to normal within 5 to 6 days.

Arterial blood gases

Arterial blood analysis (Unit 3) is useful in diagnosing some cardiovascular disorders and provides valuable information that can be used to plan, implement, and evaluate the care of patients with cyanotic heart disease, myocardial infarction, and heart failure. A knowledge of the partial pressure of oxygen (PO_2) and the oxygen saturation (O_2 Sat) should judiciously guide therapy in these situations.

Cardiac catheterization. Cardiac catheterization is an invasive procedure used to (1) measure the oxygen saturation of blood in the cardiac chambers and great vessels, (2) measure pressure changes within the chambers and great vessels, (3) measure changes in the cardiac output or stroke volume, and (4) identify anatomic abnormalities. Using one of two approaches, a catheter is inserted into the right heart via the cephalic or basilic vein in the arm, through the femoral vein in the leg, or into the left heart in a retrograde manner through the aorta via the femoral artery. Although the approach depends on just what data is needed, catheterization procedures in children use the right-sided approach most often because septal defects permit entrance into the left heart.

Once inserted, the catheter is threaded slowly, being guided through the heart with the assistance of fluoroscopy. Blood samples and pressure readings are obtained at various intervals for analysis.

Several other procedures may be carried out during the cardiac catheterization. A contrast substance can be injected through the catheter in an effort to opacify a specific area. Using concomitant roentgenograms or cineangiography, a permanent graphic record can be obtained. Referred to as angiography, this procedure can be used to examine the mitral and tricuspid valves.

It may help detect a pulmonary embolism if injected into the pulmonary artery.

Injection of a contrast medium into the coronary arteries, or coronary arteriography, can be useful in identifying coronary artery obstruction. By positioning the catheter at the coronary ostia, the practitioner can inject the contrast material and obtain roentgenographic studies. Coronary arteriography is also employed to evaluate the effects of revascularization procedures.

Invasive electrophysiology studies. Electrophysiologic studies can also be conducted during the catheterization procedure. Catheters with recording and stimulating electrodes on the tip are used at multiple intracardiac sites to stimulate the heart and record the intracardiac electrocardiogram. Electrical stimulation and mapping can determine the origin and nature of dysrhythmias. These techniques are also valuable in the examination of tachydysrhythmias and help in differentiation of supraventricular and ventricular tachycardia.

Nuclear scans

Using radioactive isotopes injected intravenously, nuclear scans examine left ventricular size and wall motion to evaluate pumping performance. The exact ejection fraction can be calculated by multiple acquisition blood pool scans. These scans are also used to check for coronary artery obstruction and myocardial infarction. Once injected, the radioactive isotopes, which have an affinity for certain healthy tissue in "cold" scanning, subsequently collect in this healthy tissue. In "hot spot" scanning, the isotopes collect in the damaged tissue. Then, gamma rays emitted by these isotopes are picked up by a scintillation camera. The information is transmitted to a computer that converts the data into a picture for interpretation.

Thallium-201 myocardial imaging is a technique used to demonstrate the presence, location, and extent of myocardial ischemia or infarction. In providing information complementary to the information obtained from stress,

electrocardiography, and coronary angiography, this procedure uses thallium-201, a radioactive isotope injected as thallous chloride. Thallium is a potassium analogue that localizes in heart muscle.

Thallium can also be injected at the point of peak stress when symptoms appear or at the point that target heart rate is reached during a treadmill test. Pictures are taken approximately 1 minute after injection and repeated in about 2 to 3 hours. This time schedule permits differentiation of ischemic vs infarcted tissue because no thallium will initially be seen in either infarcted or ischemic areas but will be deposited in ischemic areas after blood flow is redistributed. This isotope is taken up by myocardial cells immediately after the injection and accurately reflects regional myocardial perfusion at the time of injection. Areas of recent infarction or scar tissue take up little or no thallium, appearing as defects on the nuclear image.

Radionuclide angiocardiography

Nuclear medicine techniques can be employed to evaluate ventricular performance. One of the most common radionuclide procedures is multiple-gated acquisition (MUGA) cardiac imaging, which uses a minicomputer system programmed for collection and storage of multiple images recorded during the cardiac cycle. With this technique, the patient's red blood cells are labeled in vivo with technetium 99m. After a single intravascular injection, the intracardiac blood pool is imaged in multiple views with a gamma scintillation camera gated electronically to the ECG, so that counts are taken during end-systole and end-diastole. This approach permits simultaneous visualization of the contraction patterns of the right and left ventricles and atria in time. It is of value in analyzing ventricular wall motion and ventricular ejection fraction, the latter using the following formula:

Ejection fraction (%) =
$$\frac{\text{End-diastolic volume} - \text{End-systolic volume}}{\text{End-diastolic volume}} \times 100$$

Serial images can be collected over a period of several hours following injection of a single radionuclide for assessment of ventricular performance before and after therapeutic interventions. This can be done without disturbing ventricular function or inducing dysrhythmias.

ALTERATIONS—A PATHOPHYSIOLOGIC EXPLANATION

It has been pointed out that blood is circulated throughout the body to deliver oxygen and other nutrients to the cells and to remove waste products from the cells. Tissue perfusion is regulated by several mechanisms that strive to create and maintain an equilibrium along all body systems. Because the heart, brain, and kidneys play such vital roles in the maintenance of body homeostasis, these systems are protected as much as possible during pathologic states of disequilibrium. Complete protection is not always possible. A variety of signs and symptoms emerge when the physiologic processes of circulation are interrupted; these alterations are described below.

Chest pain

Pain often indicates actual or impending tissue damage. Pain occurs when fine unmyelinated nerve endings in the tissue are excited by an adequate stimulus. Stimulation of these nerve endings may evoke a variety of responses. Less intense stimuli may be perceived as nonpainful sensations such as pressure. More intense stimuli produce sensations interpreted as pain.

The severity of the perceived pain depends not only on the intensity of the stimulus but also on individual tolerance. Although the threshold for the perception of pain is about the same for all people, it may be altered by anesthetics or influenced by two factors, one of which is anatomic and the other, physiologic. For example, interference with normal anatomic pathways will affect pain perception. Noxious stimuli may not be perceived if there is an anatomic interruption of the normal pain pathway, such as that which occurs with transection of the spinal cord.

The individual will be unable to perceive stimulation from structures innervated by segments below the transection. In addition, it is possible for nerve endings to be damaged by ischemia and therefore to become insensitive to normally noxious stimuli.

Physiologic inhibition will also alter the perception of pain. Several mechanisms such as the level of relaxation and the degree of distraction can influence the patient's interpretation of the pain impulse.

Pain may also be physiologically facilitated. Such factors as fear and fatigue may result in a less intense stimulus being perceived as more noxious. The individual who overeats or has difficulty coping may respond in a different manner from the individual who is less fearful. The person who is tired can usually tolerate less pain than the person who is relaxed.

The presence of inflammation in any structure will lower the pain threshold, making less intense stimuli more painful.

Impulses produced by stimulation of nerve endings or receptors are transmitted to the brain for localization and interpretation. Stimulation of superficial receptors is more precise and easily localized than is stimulation of deeper structures. Thus visceral pain is often generalized, making a differential diagnosis more difficult. In addition, multiple structures send impulses along the same route. This explains the phenomenon of referred pain, in which pain from one structure is perceived by the nervous system to come from another structure, often adding more confusion to the diagnosis.

Chest pain or discomfort can be caused by a number of pathologic conditions. Because there is much overlap in the physiologic mechanisms responsible for the production of this symptom, it is necessary for the practitioner to perform a thorough assessment by obtaining a complete history and carrying out a thorough physical examination. Specific questions and findings that will enable the practitioner to establish a differential diagnosis must be reviewed.

Chest pain or discomfort that is coronary in

origin results from myocardial ischemia, which develops when the functional requirements of the myocardium are greater than the oxygen supply. Coronary artery atherosclerosis is usually present, creating an obstruction to myocardial blood flow. A partial obstruction results in temporary or transient ischemia, producing symptoms that are often apparent only on exertion, emotion, or exposure to cold. Complete or total obstruction causes tissue necrosis, producing symptoms that are more severe and long lasting and can occur at any time.

Several pathologic problems that do not directly involve coronary artery disease can cause chest pain or discomfort. These conditions may be congenital or acquired and often are associated with chest pain or discomfort, the etiology of which may be difficult to trace.

Valvular heart disease resulting from either stenotic or regurgitant valves often causes complaints of chest discomfort or pain. The pain, which is related to myocardial ischemia, can be produced by several mechanisms. With a stenotic aortic valve, an obstruction to the outflow of blood is created. There is basically a disproportion between the perfusion pressure and ventricular work. Mild obstruction may produce no symptoms or may produce symptoms only when the patient is exposed to stress or exertion. Severe obstruction clearly limits the amount of oxygenated blood being carried to the myocardium, causing severe chest pain and even sudden death; the latter is most likely caused by a cardiac dysrhythmia.

In addition, contracting against a stenotic aortic valve results in the development of ventricular hypertrophy. The enlarged ventricle will require more oxygen so that, even with normal coronary arteries, the oxygen demand will be greater than the oxygen supply.

Myocardial ischemia with valvular heart disease can also occur as a result of a sudden obstruction in a coronary artery that was previously found to be patent. The vessel becomes blocked with calcified fragments that are broken off from the diseased valve, creating either a partial or complete obstruction.

The descriptions of chest pain or discomfort that can be attributed to myocardial ischemia are often similar. The pain is usually described as being substernal in origin. It is frequently characterized as radiating to the arms, elbows, or fingers and is often pressing or constricting in nature. These similarities occur because the pathologic conditions that cause chest pain resulting from myocardial hypoxia directly involve the myocardium and thus sensory fibers in the left upper thoracic viscera, arising from the second to the fourth thoracic segments of the cord. Therefore, although the pathologic condition may vary, the physiologic mechanisms remain the same.

Chest pain or discomfort may be caused by irritation of serous membranes, an indirect result of an inflammatory condition. For example, the visceral surface of the pericardium is usually insensitive to pain. The parietal surface, except in a small area, is also relatively insensitive to pain. Inflammation of these structures alone therefore results in few complaints of pain. However, when the inflammation is caused by an infectious process, surrounding areas are also affected because the inflammatory process involves multiple body structures, not just the area directly attacked. Thus pericardial inflammation, specifically inflammation in the parietal surface, spreads to the adjacent parietal pleura, causing chest pain. This pain is characteristically associated with other pleuritic symptoms because of adjacent anatomic structures and is felt at the tip of the shoulder and the neck because the involved area of anatomy receives its sensory supply from the phrenic nerve, which arises from the third to the fifth cervical segments of the spinal cord.

Abdominal pain

Intraabdominal vascular disturbances may produce pain that is severe or diffuse and mild in nature. This pain, often caused by the presence of an embolism, thrombosis of the superior mesenteric artery, or impending rupture of an aneurysm in the abdominal aorta, usually is caused by tension on the nerves in the affected aortic wall or by pressure on surrounding nerves. It may also be a result of inflammation that occurs, for example, as peritoneal inflammation develops, or with hepatomegaly secondary to right-sided heart failure. Radiating pain may also occur as surrounding structures are deprived of oxygen.

Peripheral pain

Intravascular pain in the extremities is usually caused by tissue ischemia or localized inflammation. Ischemic leg pain can be attributed to arterial insufficiency. The pain, which is sharp in nature if there is total occlusion—but is often experienced as a dull ache or cramp in the more common situation of partial obstruction—occurs distal to the occluded artery. It may occur with exercise (intermittent claudication) or it may be experienced at rest. It may also be experienced only with ulceration and infection. It is frequently associated with coldness of the extremity, paresthesia, and numbness. The severity of the pain will vary with the degree of available collateral circulation.

Inflammatory leg pain is caused by venous thrombosis when superficial leg veins are involved. The thrombosed vessel is easily palpated and quite painful. Because superficial vessels are involved, the pain is easily localized. Deep venous thrombosis is not necessarily characterized by inflammation and can be positively identified only by some independent means, such as venography or fibrinogen scanning.

Palpitations

The heartbeat is rhythmic and regular under ordinary circumstances. People experiencing palpitations develop an awareness of the beating of their heart, usually because of an underlying alteration in the rate or rhythm of the heartbeat or an augmentation of its contractility. Palpita-

tions may be caused by either psychic or pathologic disorders. They often occur in the person with organic heart disease as a result of a psychic disturbance such as anxiety, creating a vicious cycle that may ultimately involve the underlying disorder and be incapacitating.

When psychically induced, palpitations are associated with stimulation of the sympathetic nervous system and a consequent increase in heart rate, rhythm, and contractility. They may occur in perfectly healthy people under certain stressful circumstances or even under no stress at all, as studies with ambulatory electrocardiography have shown. In these situations, the individual becomes suddenly aware that his heartbeat is more rapid or more forceful.

Palpitations that can be traced to underlying pathologies are not directly related to the seriousness of the disease process. Palpitations may occur when the heart rate and rhythm are entirely normal or when the rhythm is disturbed by ectopy, tachycardia, bradycardia, or heart block. They may also be a sign of an underlying organic or functional problem outside of the circulation. Some palpitations can be traced to a premature cardiac contraction out of cadence with or without a compensatory pause. Others can be attributed to a sudden slowing in the heart rate or to a rapid regular or irregular heartbeat.

Palpitations are described in many different ways. People often characterize them as skipped beats. Frequently, subjects describe a pounding or fluttering sensation. Sometimes they say their heart is doing flip-flops. An electrocardiographic examination is necessary to establish the exact identity of palpitations.

Shortness of breath (dyspnea)

Dyspnea is a symptom that means difficult breathing. Normally, breathing is an automatic process controlled by the brainstem. The cerebral cortex, however, can override the respiratory centers if voluntary control is desired. When this occurs, breathing becomes a conscious effort.

Dyspnea may or may not be precipitated by an actual physiologic alteration in the pattern of breathing. It may be functional, or it may be a symptom of cardiac or pulmonary disease. Functional dyspnea cannot be explained. Cardiac and pulmonary dyspnea are more easily understood, although the identity of the exact mechanism responsible for their production is quite controversial and not universally accepted.

Several theories attempt to explain the mechanism responsible for the production of cardiac dyspnea. Implicit in these theories is a neurophysiologic basis with receptors and neural pathways, which ultimately lead to the feeling of a conscious discomfort frequently described as a need for increased breathing. Two of the more appealing theories relate cardiac dyspnea to heart failure, which can exist either as a primary or secondary entity. Proponents of one theory identify the presence of juxtacapillary receptors, or J receptors, in the alveolar walls close to the capillaries. These J receptors, previously referred to as deflation receptors, are stimulated by pulmonary capillary engorgement and increased interstitial fluid volume in the alveolar walls. Once stimulated, J receptors send impulses to the central nervous system via vagal afferents. As the respiratory rate is increased, people develop a conscious awareness of their breathing effort. The sensation of labored breathing does not occur at any given rate but rather is a subjective function for each person.

Another theory describes the presence of chest wall receptors. These receptors sense the restrictive ventilatory effort occurring in left ventricular failure as a consequence of the air in the lungs being replaced with blood or interstitial fluid. The lungs are stiff and become an impediment to normal reflex breathing because of mechanical interference to inflation and deflation. These receptors, located in the muscle spindles, detect an inappropriate muscle tension in relation to the muscle length for the muscles involved with breathing. This results in increased afferent discharge and central nervous system stimulation of the involuntary respiratory cen-

ters. Breathing, which is already shallow because the rigid lungs permit less expansion and bring inflation and deflation closer together, becomes more rapid as efferent impulses are transmitted back to the lungs. Patients become consciously aware of their increased respiratory effort and develop an unpleasant sensation of breathlessness.

This theory can be used to explain just how dyspnea occurs with exertion, on different occasions, or in different positions. Dyspnea upon exertion (DOE) can be traced to the augmented venous return and increased pulmonary congestion that occurs with exercise. Paroxysmal dyspnea, frequently occurring at night as paroxysmal nocturnal dyspnea (PND), can be explained in relation to what occurs during sleep. With sleep, it is assumed that the diminished irritability of the central nervous system permits greater lung engorgement. In addition, there is an increase in pulmonary blood flow during sleep. There may also be such a diminution of muscular activity during sleep that venous stasis occurs within the muscle. Any sudden movement would then serve to increase venous return and subsequent pulmonary congestion. In addition, dyspnea that occurs in a recumbent position, called *orthopnea*, is more severe because of mechanical interference with ventilation caused by the shortened thoracic compartment.

It is important to note that all of these mechanisms responsible for the production of dyspnea are theories and therefore not proven in all settings. Proponents can be found for each point of view.

Fatigue and weakness

Complaints of fatigue and weakness that can be attributed to cardiovascular pathology usually occur with effort, whereas fatigue and weakness noted at rest are most often related to anxiety. The pathophysiologic mechanisms responsible for the production of these symptoms are threefold. The most common etiologic mechanisms can be traced to a reduction in the cardiac output or arterial oxygen unsaturation. This results in inadequate tissue nourishment. Initially, the area affected is the skeletal muscle. Poor perfusion and/or inadequate oxygenation of skeletal muscle produces symptomatic complaints that surface primarily with exertion because the metabolic requirements of the muscle are increased with effort.

Fluid and electrolyte imbalance can also produce symptoms of fatigue and weakness. This may occur because of a primary problem but often can be traced to secondary therapeutic interventions and the injudicious use of diuretics. The imbalance may be caused by hypokalemia, hyponatremia, or hypovolemia.

Fluid retention (edema)

Edema, an abnormal accumulation of fluid in the intercellular spaces, occurs because of a disturbance in the mechanisms of fluid interchange. The normal balance between the inward and outward flow of fluid through the capillary membrane becomes upset, resulting in transudation.

Although there are several pathophysiologic mechanisms responsible for the formation of edema, cardiac edema basically is caused by an increased capillary hydrostatic pressure. Heart failure occurring as a primary problem or a secondary entity with valvular heart disease or hypertension may involve systemic and/or pulmonary circulation.

Systemically, with right-sided heart failure there is a buildup of pressure in the right heart, which leads to an increase in pressure in the venules and capillaries. In essence, the right heart is unable to pump all of the returning blood adequately. This leads to pooling in the venous circulation and an increase in peripheral venous pressure. As the volume of blood in venous circulation is increased, hepatic congestion develops. This leads to hepatomegaly and ultimately to fluid accumulation in the peritoneal cavity, that is, *ascites*. As pooling in the periphery continues, edema becomes visible in dependent areas. The edema occurs because fluid tends to accumulate as the result of local hydrostatic factors in dependent body parts. This also explains the shift in fluid from the extremities to the sacral region in bedfast individuals.

Left-sided heart failure may exist alone, may result from progressive right-sided failure, or may lead to right-sided heart failure. Regardless of the sequence of events, when left-sided heart failure occurs, two things happen: pulmonary congestion begins to develop, and cardiac output becomes inadequate. The clinical manifestations that occur can be traced to pulmonary vascular congestion or fluid retention.

Pulmonary vascular congestion is a major problem in left-sided heart failure. The congestion occurs as a result of an increase in the volume of blood contained in the pulmonary vasculature. Consequently, both the arterial and venous pressures in the lungs are elevated. The congested lungs become inelastic, thereby impairing ventilation and increasing the difficulty of breathing. As the venous pressure in the lungs is increased, fluid is extravasated into the alveolar spaces because of a disequilibrium between hydrostatic pressure and colloid osmotic pressure.

Position changes can produce even more pulmonary vascular congestion by increasing the amount of blood in the pulmonary vascular bed. This takes place when the body changes from an erect to a supine position, leading to a reduction in the venous hydrostatic pressure in the extremities and a shift in the fluid equilibrium across the capillary membranes into the vascular space. The increased circulatory blood volume, along with the redistribution of blood returning to the right heart in a supine position, results in increased pulmonary congestion.

A cardiac output that is insufficient to meet the metabolic requirements of the body triggers a chain of events that ultimately leads to fluid retention. When the cardiac output is inadequate, arterial blood flow is altered so that the vital centers of the heart and brain receive adequate blood flow. This is accomplished through a generalized vasoconstriction, which occurs secondary to the sensing by carotid and aortic chemoreceptors of reduced blood flow to the chemoreceptor cells. As a result, renal blood flow is compromised. Impaired renal circulation leads to reduced glomerular filtration and sodium and water retention. Aldosterone production is also increased because of increased renin release by the kidney as a consequence of altered renal circulation. This mineralcorticoid also impairs sodium excretion, thereby adding to the sodium and water retained. The increased extracellular sodium and fluid volume leads to a generalized edema because of the increased capillary hydrostatic pressure. The distribution of edema will vary with the tissue pressure because fluid collects more readily in loose tissue.

Spitting up blood (hemoptysis)

Coughing up blood, or hemoptysis, can be a symptom of a number of problems. When the etiologic factor is related to circulatory pathology, the material that is coughed up is usually streaked with blood and small in quantity. Frequently hemoptysis is associated with acute pulmonary congestion and originates from the rupture of pulmonary capillaries under high intravascular pressure.

When hemoptysis is induced by exercise, it is usually caused by valvular heart disease, specifically, mitral stenosis, and comes from a break in the pulmonary veins, which have ruptured under extremely high pressure.

Fainting (syncope)

Syncope can be defined as a loss of consciousness resulting from cerebral ischemia. It may involve cardiovascular, metabolic, or neuropsychologic factors. Although usually occurring when someone is sitting or standing, syncopal episodes can also take place in a supine position. The depth and duration of the period of unconsciousness can vary. Initially, the pulse may be weak or impalpable, the blood pressure low, and breathing almost imperceptible. These alterations are the body's attempt to protect the vital organs and prevent permanent damage. These vital signs frequently strengthen when the body is placed in a horizontal position to facilitate blood flow to the brain.

A syncopal episode occurs as a direct result of a deficient amount of blood being circulated to the brain. This reduction in circulation may be caused by inadequate vasoconstrictor mechanisms, a mechanical reduction in the venous return, or a reduction in the cardiac output.

The occurrence of syncopal episodes as a result of inadequate vasoconstrictor mechanisms is not always related to an underlying disease process. Vasovagal syncope, for example, is caused by hypotension caused by sudden diffuse vasodilatation and bradycardia, often related to emotion. This type of syncope is commonly experienced in normal people but is also found in people with organic heart disease who are especially susceptible to stress.

Postural hypotension can also precipitate syncopal episodes because of inadequate pressor reflexes. Postural syncope occurs when a person attempts to stand from a recumbent position. There is a failure of the reflex hemodynamic adaptation that usually occurs with the assumption of an upright posture. Therefore the normal reflex arteriolar and venous constriction, acceleration of heart rate, mechanical pumping of the leg muscles, and decreased intrathoracic pressure that occur when someone assumes an upright posture because of the associated gravitational stresses on circulation are either inadequate or absent. This failure of adaptation is common in prolonged illnesses, after sympathectomy, or in people receiving antihypertensive or vasodilator drugs.

Massage or compression of the carotid sinus can precipitate a syncopal episode, referred to as *carotid sinus syncope*. It may occur with a hyperirritable carotid sinus, resulting in a profound fall in the arterial blood pressure and a slowing of the heart rate. Therefore the syncopal episode may be of the cardioinhibitory type or of the vasodepressor type. In the latter, there is a marked fall in perfusion pressure to the brain, and it is often more common in people with organic heart disease.

A mechanical reduction of the venous return caused by a Valsalva maneuver or coughing episode may also precipitate a syncopal attack. The intrathoracic pressure increases and consequently interferes with venous return. The blood flow to the brain is impaired because of compression of the intracranial capillary and venous beds, which occurs as the rise in pressure in the thorax is transmitted via the cerebrospinal fluid.

Cardiac syncope, brought about as a result of a reduction in the stroke volume or the development of an alteration in the heart rate or rhythm, lowers the cardiac output and is usually a symptom of an underlying disorder.

Cardiac syncope is often secondary to exertional hypotension and is a common finding in people with aortic stenosis, pulmonic stenosis, or pulmonary hypertension. It occurs because the cardiac output is insufficient to meet the demands of exercise. Usually, the cardiac output rises by increasing the stroke volume and heart rate in an effort to provide adequate tissue oxygenation with exercise. This increase occurs when the need for increased cardiac output is anticipated by cortical mechanisms, which subsequently results in increased sympathetic discharge. To redistribute blood to the needed areas, the sympathetic nervous system causes peripheral vasodilatation in the skeletal muscle.

With sustained exercise, cortically integrated activity gives way to simple reflex responses, resulting in vasodilation secondary to the local release of tissue metabolites. This produces a small decrease in arterial pressure while skeletal muscles squeeze blood out of the capacitance vessels in an effort to increase venous return. The increased preload therefore eventually increases contractility because of the Starling principle. In individuals with severe obstructive outflow lesions, the cardiac output is relatively fixed and cannot rise enough to meet the increasing demands. In addition, increased intraventricular pressure diminishes stimulation of the ventricular pressoreceptors and blunts the carotid and aortic chemoreceptor reflex, producing a generalized vasodilation. It is the combination of these two mechanisms that precipitates the syncopal episodes.

Dysrhythmia-induced syncope lowers the cardiac output because of asystole, severe bradycardias, heart block, or tachydysrhythmias. The reduction in cardiac output is produced by two mechanisms. With bradyarrhythmias, maintenance of a normal cardiac output with an increase in stroke volume is usually not possible because of the extremely slowed heart rate, although there is often a great increase in ventricular filling during diastole. With tachydysrhythmias, there is usually insufficient time for adequate ventricular filling, therefore leading to a great reduction in the stroke volume. Therefore dysrhythmia-induced syncope can be traced to a significant reduction in either the heart rate or stroke volume.

Bluish discoloration of skin and mucous membranes (cyanosis)

A bluish discoloration of the skin and mucous membranes occurs when the quantity of reduced hemoglobin or hemoglobin derivatives is increased. The actual discoloration occurs in areas perfused with blood containing these pigments, usually the lips, nails, and ears. The increased amount of reduced hemoglobin in the cutaneous vessels may occur because of an increase in the amount of venous blood in the skin secondary to dilation of the venules and venous ends of the capillaries or because of a decrease in the oxygen saturation of the capillary blood. This phenomenon, referred to objectively as *cyanosis,* is apparent at a mean capillary concentration of 4/100 ml of reduced hemoglobin.

There are two types of cyanosis: central cyanosis and peripheral cyanosis. Central cyanosis is caused by a right-to-left shunt when the shunted blood is greater than 30% of the left ventricular output or by an impairment in pulmonary function (Unit 3). The etiologic mechanism responsible for the development of peripheral cyanosis is a cutaneous vasoconstriction brought about by a decrease in cardiac output or exposure to cold. Localized peripheral cyanosis in an extremity may also be caused by arterial or venous obstruction.

Failure to thrive

Organic failure to thrive is occasionally a sign of a congenital cardiac anomaly in an infant or child. Characterized by impaired growth and development and delayed onset of adolescence, failure to thrive can be a manifestation of a cyanotic or acyanotic heart defect. The severity of the growth impairment depends on the anatomic lesion and its functional effect. Rarely is mental development impaired. Generally, children with cyanotic lesions (right-to-left shunts) usually appear to be retarded in both height and weight, whereas children with acyanotic conditions are slower in weight gain.

The mechanism responsible for the impaired growth and development in congenital cardiac anomalies cannot be attributed to any one factor. Inadequate nutrition and calorie intake can be a problem in the infant who cannot suck. Acidemia, cation imbalance, tissue hypoxemia, diminished peripheral blood flow, and chronic cardiac decompensation may all be causative factors.

INTERVENTIONS

Planning, implementing, and evaluating the care of the patient with cardiovascular disorders necessitates a working knowledge of a number of practices and procedures because a variety of therapeutic interventions currently are used to treat circulatory problems. Some interventions influence the heart rate and rhythm; some affect the heart's ability to pump; others influence the flow of blood. As these treatment modalities are reviewed in the following pages, an attempt will be made to identify the principle influence of each regimen.

Often the decision about the appropriate therapeutic modality is complicated by the fact that clinical recognition of the unstable and changing levels of cardiac function that can occur is difficult, if not impossible. Findings obtained from the physical examination and laboratory tests regarding abnormal cardiac function are helpful but sometimes limited. The testing that is necessary to detect changes is time-consuming. The use of hemodynamic monitoring devices permits more precise and more immediate assessment, allowing the exact mechanism and degree of depression of cardiac function to be established. With hemodynamic monitoring, it therefore becomes possible to judiciously select or modify a specific plan of care.

Interventions that affect rhythm

Antidysrhythmic interventions are begun in an attempt to suppress irritable foci. These interventions may include such therapeutic modalities as CPR, a precordial thump, electrical countershock, oxygen therapy, drug therapy, electrolyte replacement, and pacemaker insertion.

Cardiopulmonary resuscitation (CPR)

The abrupt cessation of effective electrical cardiac activity results in mechanical failure and the cessation of circulation. Cardiac arrest is usually precipitated by cardiac standstill (ventricular asystole) or ventricular fibrillation, the latter occasionally preceded by ventricular flutter or ventricular tachycardia. Recognized by pulselessness or absent respirations, cardiac and respiratory arrest must be treated immediately to prevent residual central nervous system damage.

Cardiopulmonary resuscitation (CPR) combines cardiac compression with artificial ventilation in an effort to deliver oxygen to the brain and other vital organs. Properly performed chest compressions can produce systolic pressures of more than 100 mmHg. The mean pressure averages about 40 mmHg, whereas the diastolic pressure remains low, resulting in a reduction in the coronary artery blood flow to between one fourth and one third of normal. Although it is possible for one person to adequately perform CPR, it is physically and mentally exhausting. Therefore it is ideal for two people to work together, with one person performing artificial ventilation and the other providing artificial cir-

Fig. 2-26. Algorithm for CPR.

Based on American Heart Association standards.

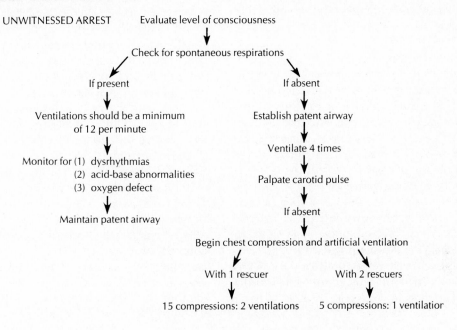

UNWITNESSED ARREST   Evaluate level of consciousness

Check for spontaneous respirations

If present   If absent

Ventilations should be a minimum of 12 per minute   Establish patent airway

Ventilate 4 times

Monitor for (1) dysrhythmias   Palpate carotid pulse
(2) acid-base abnormalities
(3) oxygen defect   If absent

Maintain patent airway

Begin chest compression and artificial ventilation

With 1 rescuer   With 2 rescuers

15 compressions: 2 ventilations   5 compressions: 1 ventilatior

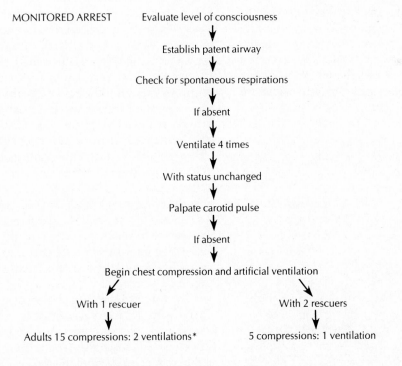

MONITORED ARREST   Evaluate level of consciousness

Establish patent airway

Check for spontaneous respirations

If absent

Ventilate 4 times

With status unchanged

Palpate carotid pulse

If absent

Begin chest compression and artificial ventilation

With 1 rescuer   With 2 rescuers

Adults 15 compressions: 2 ventilations*   5 compressions: 1 ventilation

*Compression rate for infants should be approximately 100 times per minute, while for older children it should be 80 times per minute.

culation. Fig. 2-26 describes the steps to follow in performing CPR in both a monitored and an unmonitored arrest.

To perform CPR, it is necessary to first establish a patent airway. This often can be accomplished by using the simple head tilt maneuver. If this fails or is contraindicated because of other preexisting conditions, the triple airway maneuver may be employed. These techniques, along with more advanced procedures that are used to establish and maintain a patent airway, are described in Unit 3.

Cardiac massage is necessary in the pulseless patient to restore circulation. It can be performed either externally or internally. External cardiac massage is accomplished, with the patient in a supine position on a firm surface, by compressing the heart between the sternum and spine. The sternum is compressed $1\frac{1}{2}$ to 2 inches (4 to 5 cm) in an adult, 1 to $1\frac{1}{2}$ inches (2.5 to 3.8 cm) in a child, and $\frac{1}{2}$ to 1 inch (1.3 to 2.5 cm) in an infant. The two-handed, chest-encircling method of chest compression is preferred in the newborn (Fig. 2-27). In an adult, it is necessary to use both hands, positioned one on top of the other, to apply the pressure needed to compress the heart and circulate the blood. The heel of the hand placed on the chest should be positioned midsternally, about 2 fingerbreadths above the

xiphoid process. The heel of one hand provides sufficient pressure to compress the heart in the young child, whereas the tips of the index and middle fingers are adequate in the infant. Pressure is exerted over the midsternum in infants and young children because their ventricles are located higher in the chest cavity.

The rhythm of the cardiac compressions must be regular and uninterrupted, with relaxation of equal duration following each compression. This permits the ventricles to completely refill. The following mnemonics are helpful in establishing a regular rhythm and an adequate rate of compression. When two people are performing CPR, a compression rate of 60 times/min will maintain an adequate blood flow in an adult. This rate can be attained by counting in the following manner: "One, one thousand, two, one thousand, three, one thousand, four, one thousand, five, one thousand." If only one person is performing CPR, it is necessary to increase the compression rate to 80 times/min to make up for the time lost during lung inflation. This will achieve an actual heart rate of approximately 60 times/min. It can be accomplished by counting: "One and two and three and four and five and one and two and three and four and ten and one and two and three and four and fifteen." With this rhythm, the rescuer will maintain the correct rate and will be aware of when to ventilate. Because of inherently rapid heart rates in infants and children, the compression rate for infants should be 100 times/min, and that for children should be 80 times/min.

Automatic chest compressors can be used to perform long-term external CPR. These mechanical devices provide regular rhythmic compressions with simultaneous ventilation, thereby eliminating the fatigue experienced by those giving CPR. The use of these machines is limited, however, because they are heavy, difficult to operate, and easily dislodged during movement.

To perform internal cardiac massage, it is necessary to make an incision in the fourth or fifth intercostal space that extends from the edge of the sternum to the midaxillary line. Using this

Fig. 2-27. Hand position for chest encirclement technique for external chest compression. Thumbs are together over midsternum. In the small newborn, thumbs can be superimposed.

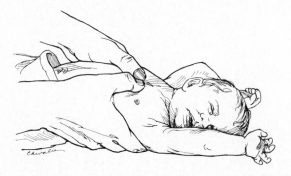

approach, the palmar surfaces of the fingertips are used to compress the heart against the sternum. If this approach proves to be ineffective, the pericardium can be opened, allowing the rescuer to compress the heart with one hand placed anteriorly and the other, posteriorly. The hands must be removed from the ventricles after each compression to allow ventricular filling.

There are several complications that can occur whether CPR is performed properly or improperly. The most common complication is a fracture or fractures of the ribs. Although fractures may occur even with the best technique, they can frequently be traced to improper hand placement. Poor compression technique in infants and small children can cause liver lacerations because of the pliability of the chest and the high position of the liver. Laceration of vital organs may lead to bleeding and hemorrhage. Fractures of the sternum, costochondral separation, pneumothorax, hemothorax, lung contusions, and fat emboli are all possible. The incidence of some of these complications can be reduced with strict adherence to good technique. CPR, however, must be continued even in the presence of complications because the only alternative for the victim is death.

Precordial thump[3]

A precordial thump delivered by the practitioner over the midportion of the sternum with the fleshy portion of the fist may restore the heartbeat in a pulseless patient, although there is growing consensus that this may be a waste of time when the arrest is unwitnessed and the patient is in critical condition. This maneuver, performed from a distance of 8 to 12 inches, is only effective within the first minute after a cardiac arrest. It is indicated in a witnessed cardiac arrest, in the monitored patient, at the onset of ventricular tachycardia or ventricular fibrillation, or in ventricular asystole caused by heart block. It is contraindicated in infants and children.

The precordial thump supposedly initiates a small electrical stimulus of about 0.2 to 0.5 joules in the heart that is reactive. Therefore it may be useful in restoring the heartbeat in ventricular asystole, in reversing ventricular tachycardia or ventricular fibrillation of recent onset, or in acting as a pacemaker in third-degree atrioventricular block.

There are potential hazards associated with the use of the precordial thump. Ventricular fibrillation may be induced in the anoxic heart that is still beating if the thump is delivered during the relative refractory period. In addition, CPR may be delayed if the practitioner persists in repeatedly delivering precordial thumps. Consequently, the precordial thump should be delivered as a single blow in limited situations.

Electrical countershock

Electrical countershock may be effective in terminating ventricular fibrillation in a cardiac arrest. Defibrillation may also be used in the treatment of ventricular tachycardia in the pulseless patient. A direct current of electricity is delivered to the heart in an effort to spontaneously depolarize it. All of the myocardial cells are depolarized simultaneously in the hope of stopping the chaotic electrical activity. Subsequently, as the cells repolarize at the same time, the SA node often is able to resume its role as pacemaker, resulting in coordinated rhythmic contractions and the restoration of an effective cardiac output. Defibrillation must be carried out as soon as possible because the fibrillating heart provides insufficient oxygen, quickly resulting in an anoxic and acidotic myocardium that is more difficult to convert.

Direct current (DC) defibrillators are equipped for both external and internal use. They have a high-voltage DC power supply that is used to charge an energy storage capacitor. The capacitor is connected to the paddles via a current-limited inductor. Newer model defibrillators are equipped with ECG monitors; some have the capacity to monitor the cardiac rhythm from paddle electrodes, as well as patient leads. All defibrillators have some mechanism for measuring energy either as stored or delivered.

Optimal paddle size has not been established. Currently, circular paddles of 10 to 13 cm in diameter are recommended for adults. Electrode paddles of 8 cm in diameter are suitable for older children, whereas paddles of 4.5 cm in diameter are suggested for small infants.

Electrode paddles are used; they are placed either anteriorly and posteriorly or anteriorly only over the base and apex of the heart, using 20 to 25 pounds of muscular pressure. The anterior approach is used most often, placing one electrode paddle in the second intercostal space to the right of the sternum and the other electrode paddle over the left precordium, left of the left nipple, in the anterior axillary line. With an anterior-posterior approach, the electrode paddles are positioned below the left scapula and over the left precordium. Studies have not shown one approach to be more effective than the other.

Standard electrode paste or saline-soaked pads are used beneath the paddles to reduce skin resistance and facilitate conduction. Care must be taken to avoid spilling saline or spreading electrode paste over the chest because the spills may conduct electricity and cause superficial surface burns. In addition, they will reduce the amount of delivered electrical energy, possibly making defibrillation ineffective. Alcohol-soaked pads should never be used because they are flammable. The paddles should be placed flat on the surface of the chest to avoid arcs of electricity and diminished effective output.

The amount of energy necessary for successful defibrillation is still controversial. Generally, 2.0 to 3.5 joules/kg of body weight are recommended for children. Electrical stimulation potentiates the effect of digitalis in infants; consequently, it is recommended that the energy dose in these patients be as low as the defibrillator will permit and cautiously increased as necessary. It is suggested that initial attempts for adults begin at approximately 200 joules. The procedure may be repeated several times. Defibrillation may be successful with repeated countershock because the transthoracic resistance is decreased each time a shock is delivered. It is advisable to use only the amount of electricity that is necessary to terminate the dysrhythmia because damage from defibrillation is roughly proportional to the amount of electricity used.

Internal defibrillation can be performed if the chest has been opened. Paddles covered with saline-soaked gauze are placed directly over the heart. Paddle placement is dictated by the dysrhythmia being converted. The paddles are positioned anteriorly, one over the atrium and one over the ventricle, for supraventricular dysrhythmias. For ventricular dysrhythmias, one is placed directly over the left ventricle on the diaphragmatic surface with the other placed inferiorly, also on the left ventricle. Only minimal amounts of electrical energy are used because myocardial damage is proportional to the amount that is delivered. Initial attempts begin with 5 to 10 joules of electricity. No more than 20 joules should be used.

Synchronized cardioversion

Synchronized countershock may be indicated for the treatment of rapid ventricular tachycardia or supraventricular rhythms associated with inadequate cardiac output. It is contraindicated in the treatment of tachydysrhythmias caused by digitalis toxicity. A synchronizing circuit permits delivery of the countershock during a specific part of the QRS complex. The procedure is similar to that followed for defibrillation. If the patient is conscious, anesthesia is accomplished with the intravenous administration of diazepam (Valium) or a similar short-acting drug. The patient is monitored to synchronize the machine. The machine is adjusted so that the R wave is at least 1 cm in height. The R wave of the ECG must be taller than the T wave; this is necessary because the machine senses the largest complex, and inappropriate sensing could result in discharge during the supercritical period and the development of ventricular fibrillation. (Should this occur, it is necessary to change modes from synchronous to asynchronous and defibrillate as soon as possible.) For synchronized cardioversion, the synchronizer switch is activated and the machine set to deliver approximately 25 to 50 joules of electricity. Immediately before discharging, the operator must recheck the patient's rhythm to make sure that cardioversion is still necessary. If it is still indicated (that is, if the rhythm has not spontaneously converted), the discharge button is depressed until the machine fires. The procedure can be repeated using more energy if initial attempts are unsuccessful.

Oxygen therapy

Oxygen therapy is indicated in the presence of hypoxia-induced dysrhythmias. The amount and type of oxygen therapy is dictated by the patient's individual needs. Unit 3 discusses oxygen therapies.

Pharmacologic agents used to treat dysrhythmias

Therapeutic interventions used in the management of the patient with disorders in the heart rate and rhythm often involve the use of pharmacologic agents. Before beginning drug therapy, however, it is important to accurately interpret the dysrhythmia and to determine its etiology if possible. Etiologic data can dictate the appropriate intervention. Ventricular ectopy, for example, may be precipitated by such factors as hypoxia, electrolyte imbalance, drug toxicity, and pain. Although lidocaine is generally accepted as the drug of choice, a knowledge of the specific cause could illustrate the need for oxygen, electrolyte replacement, analgesia, or some other therapeutic modality.

It is also necessary to identify the potential consequences for the patient with an irregularity in the heart rate or rhythm. Drug therapy can sometimes be avoided until the etiology is determined if the dysrhythmia poses no electrophysiologic or hemodynamic threat to the patient. However, in the presence of rapid ventricular rates, dysrhythmias of a long dration, and underlying heart disease, severe consequences can develop. For example, a rapid tachydysrhythmia with an increased ventricular rate will

result in decreased diastolic filling time and could lead to a subsequent reduction in the stroke volume and cardiac output. This could significantly affect the patient with a diseased heart but may have little effect on a healthy heart. Conditions such as this may need treatment while etiologic data is being obtained.

Antidysrhythmics

The classification of pharmacologic agents used in the treatment of tachydysrhythmias is based on the effect these drugs have on the action potential of the cardiac cell. In this classification, drugs are grouped as Class I, II, III, or IV agents. Class I drugs are membrane-stabilizing agents that have local anesthetic activity. They slow the rate of rise of phase O of the action potential, increase the threshold of excitability, depress conduction velocity, prolong relative refractory, and inhibit spontaneous diastolic depolarization. With the introduction of new agents, Class I drugs have been further divided into three subgroups. Class IA agents depress phase O, prolonging the duration of the action potential, whereas Class IB drugs slightly depress phase O, shortening the action potential. Class IC agents markedly depress phase O, exerting little effect on repolarization and the duration of the action potential. Class II drugs function as beta blockers through competitive inhibition. Drugs in Class III exert their effect by increasing the action potential duration. They have an antifibrillatory effect. Minor changes in the classification system in the early 1980s resulted from the introduction of verapamil. Grouped as a Class IV agent, verapamil and other similar drugs are classified as calcium channel blockers. They depress phase 4 depolarization and lengthen phases 1 and 2 of repolarization. This depression and lengthening is accomplished via a selective blockade of the atrioventricular node and its effects on calcium transport.[73]

Quinidine is a Class IA antidysrhythmic drug with a variety of electrophysiologic effects. It prolongs the atrial and ventricular effective refractory period. It also decreases pacemaker automaticity, depressing ectopic impulse formation. Myocardial excitability is decreased, which diminishes the ability of the ventricles to respond to a stimulus. Conduction time is prolonged in the cardiac muscle, Purkinje fibers, and AV conduction tissue. Quinidine also elevates the threshold to electrically induced ventricular fibrillation.

Quinidine is used in the treatment of both atrial and ventricular dysrhythmias. It is also used prophylactically following the conversion of atrial fibrillation to sinus rhythm, in the early stages of myocardial infarction, and in the management of patients with paroxysmal atrial tachycardia.

The most common side effects associated with quinidine therapy are gastrointestinal and consist of nausea, vomiting, and diarrhea. More serious and potentially dangerous toxic effects, however, can occur. Severe hypotension, respiratory depression, convulsions, and even death can occur with hypersensitivity. Thrombocytopenic purpura and exfoliative dermatitis have been reported. The development of cinchonism characterized by tinnitus, visual disturbances, vertigo, and headache can occur with large doses. Because quinidine depresses impulse formation, conduction, and contractility, it can cause SA or AV block and cardiac asystole if given in large doses or given to patients with severely damaged hearts. It can also cause "quinidine syncope." The vagolytic effect on AV junctional transmission can result in an accelerated ventricular rate in atrial fibrillation and atrial flutter.

The effect of quinidine can also be demonstrated by changes in the ECG. The Q-T interval is prolonged, as is the duration of the QRS complex. The changes take place because of the influence of quinidine on the refractory period and conduction time.[51,75,124]

Serum quinidine levels should be obtained if toxicity is suspected based on clinical symptoms. Signs of quinidine toxicity can often be obliterated by reducing the dosage. With actual toxic-

ity, molar sodium lactate or sodium bicarbonate can be used. Isoproterenol may be necessary to treat the conduction disturbances, whereas norepinephrine or metaraminol may be needed for vascular collapse.

Disopyramide (Norpace, Rhythmodan) is also a Class IA antidysrhythmic drug that has several actions. It prolongs the duration of the action potential and the effective refractory period of the Purkinje fibers. It also prolongs conduction time, decreases pacemaker automaticity, and inhibits the vagus.

Clinically, disopyramide is used in the treatment of both supraventricular and ventricular dysrhythmias. It appears to be similar to quinidine. Disopyramide is administered to adults orally. It is currently not available in intravenous (IV) form.

Side effects are attributed to the use of this drug, including dry mouth, urinary hesitancy, urinary retention, and dryness in the eyes and nose. These effects can occur because of the anticholinergic activity of the drug. Constipation and blurred vision have also been reported. ECG changes and dysrhythmias have also been documented. Prolongation of the Q-T interval has been noted with maintenance doses, as has ventricular tachycardia and ventricular fibrillation. Disopyramide should be used with caution in patients with preexisting heart failure or low ejection fractions because it exerts a negative inotropic effect and may worsen the failure.[51,75]

Lidocaine (Xylocaine) is an antidysrhythmic agent that depresses automaticity of the Purkinje fibers and shortens the refractory period and duration of the action potential. Consequently it is used to suppress ventricular ectopy. It is indicated in the treatment of premature ventricular contractions (PVCs) that occur frequently (that is, more than five times/min), that are multifocal in origin, that are paired, or that occur in short runs of three or more in succession. It is also used if ventricular tachycardia and ventricular fibrillation are unresponsive to defibrillation.

The side effects associated with lidocaine toxicity generally involve the central nervous system. Initially, they include symptoms of dissociation, paresthesias (often perioral), mild drowsiness, or mild agitation. Higher concentrations of lidocaine may cause decreased hearing, disorientation, muscle twitching, convulsions, or respiratory arrest.[51]

Procainamide hydrochloride (Pronestyl) as a Class IA agent prolongs atrial and ventricular refractory periods and depresses atrial and ventricular excitability. Conduction time is prolonged in cardiac muscle, in AV conduction tissue, and in the Purkinje fibers. The drug also decreases pacemaker automaticity, depresses myocardial contractility, and elevates the atrial and ventricular threshold to electrically induced fibrillation.

Procainamide is an antidysrhythmic drug used most often in the treatment of ventricular ectopy and ventricular tachydysrhythmias unresponsive to lidocaine therapy. It is also used when lidocaine is contraindicated. Procainamide may be used in the treatment of atrial dysrhythmias in low-dose combination with another drug or when maximal doses of other more commonly used agents have been ineffective. It is used infrequently with children.

IV administration of procainamide can result in a precipitous fall in the blood pressure if it is given too rapidly. Hypotension can occur even with judicious administration and may result in cardiovascular collapse, convulsions, and coronary insufficiency. Therefore procainamide hydrochloride should be used cautiously in patients with acute myocardial infarction. Large doses of procainamide may result in widening of the QRS complex, prolongation of the P-R and Q-T intervals, and T-wave changes. Large doses may also result in the development of AV block and ventricular ectopy, the latter predisposing to ventricular fibrillation. When used in the treatment of atrial fibrillation or flutter, the ventricular rate may increase as the atrial rate decreases and the degree of block is lessened. This is because of procainamide's anticholinergic effects. The drug may cause CNS disturbances, blood dyscrasias, bone marrow depression, signs and

symptoms of systemic lupus erythematosus (SLE), and allergic reactions. Oral administration may cause anorexia, nausea, vomiting, and diarrhea.

Procainamide should be given cautiously to patients with renal failure because it is excreted by the kidneys. It is contraindicated in patients with complete AV block and should be used sparingly, if at all, in patients with partial heart block because it may cause asystole or advance the degree of block. The EKG and blood pressure must be monitored with IV administration to monitor for signs of toxicity. The drug should be discontinued if the QRS becomes excessively widened or the blood pressure drops significantly. Vasopressors should be available for treatment of hypotensive episodes. Blood studies should also be monitored because fatal agranulocytosis has been documented.[51]

Amiodarone is the newest of the antidysrhythmics to be released for general use. It is grouped as a Class III agent. Experimental studies have shown that this drug may worsen conduction system disease and may cause sinus bradycardia and hypotension.[60] Other side effects noted include corneal microdeposits, skin discoloration, photosensitivity, thyroid dysfunction, and gastrointestinal upset.[60]

Phenytoin (Dilantin), a Class IB agent, is used as an antidysrhythmic agent and possesses electrophysiologic effects similar to lidocaine. Traditionally classified as an anticonvulsive, phenytoin depresses pacemaker automaticity and shortens the effective refractory period and action potential duration in the Purkinje fibers and ventricular muscle. It also shortens the effective refractory period and action potential duration in the atria, but its predominant influence is in the ventricles.

Phenytoin is the drug of choice for the treatment of ventricular dysrhythmias induced by digitalis. It also appears to be effective in the treatment of some digitalis-induced atrial dysrhythmias, such as atrial tachycardia with block and nonparoxysmal AV junctional tachycardia. It may also be prophylactically used with patients who exhibit a lot of ectopy and have had large amounts of lidocaine.

Central nervous system manifestations occur with phenytoin toxicity. They include ataxia, vertigo, nystagmus, seizure activity, behavioral changes, and confusion. Peripheral neuropathies, gum hyperplasia, skin lesions, nausea, and vomiting have also been reported. Hypotension can occur with rapid administration, and a poorly diluted solution can elicit extreme pain and may cause phlebitis.

Phenytoin should be used with caution, if at all, in patients with sinus bradycardia or SA or AV block. The effective dose in patients on anticoagulant therapy is less because oral anticoagulants retard the metabolism of the drug.[51]

Trocainide is one of the newer antidysrhythmic drugs to be released for general use. It is classified as an IB agent. Tocainide can cause an increase in congestive heart failure and can lead to a disturbance in conduction. Other side effects associated with its use include neurologic effects, such as tremors, dizziness, lightheadedness, paresthesia, confusion, and memory loss; gastrointestinal effects, such as nausea and diffuse rashes; immunologic syndrome; and hepatitis.

Propranolol hydrochloride (Inderal), a Class II drug, is a beta-adrenergic receptor blocking agent. Propranolol has negative ionotropic and chronotropic actions and exerts a myocardial depressant effect by decreasing the heart rate, cardiac output, and stroke volume. Consequently, it decreases the oxygen requirements of the myocardium. It also depresses pacemaker automaticity, thereby slowing the sinus rate of discharge and also suppressing ectopic beating. AV conduction is prolonged, as is the refractory period.

Propranolol is used clinically in the treatment of recurrent episodes of atrial and ventricular tachydysrhythmias. It has been effective in preventing or reducing the frequency of paroxysmal atrial tachycardia (PAT). It has also been useful in controlling the ventricular response in atrial tachydysrhythmias such as atrial

flutter and atrial fibrillation. Propranolol is mildly effective in suppressing ectopy, being second choice for use (after phenytoin) in digitalis-induced dysrhythmias. It is also of value because it can be used in combination with other pharmacologic agents for maximum effectiveness. For example, it can be used with nitrates for patients with angina, with quinidine for patients with ventricular dysrhythmias, and with digitalis for patients with supraventricular tachydysrhythmias. Dosage has only been established for adults.

Administration of propanolol is contraindicated in the presence of bradydysrhythmias and AV block. It should not be given to patients with congestive heart failure because, as a betalytic drug, it decreases myocardial contractility. It should also be withheld from patients with bronchospasm or chronic lung disease because it can cause bronchoconstriction. Propranolol can precipitate congestive heart failure and can cause hypoglycemia, the latter by blocking epinephrine-induced glycogenolysis. For some people with hypoglycemia, it blocks the symptoms so that patients often do not recognize them and therefore are in danger of syncope.[42,51,75,89]

Bretylium tosylate (Bretylol) is a Class III antidysrhythmic agent that exhibits a variety of rather complex cardiovascular actions. Initially, it causes a release in catecholamines. The release of norepinephrine from the sympathetic postganglionic fibers has a positive inotropic and chronotropic effect, thereby enhancing myocardial contractility. The initial catecholamine release is followed by a postganglionic adrenergic blocking action, interfering with the release of norepinephrine and inhibiting the uptake of catecholamine. The adrenergic blockade with bretylium in moderate doses does not depress adrenal medullary activity. Therefore centrally mediated cardiovascular pressor reflexes are not completely blocked because they are in part mediated by the release of catecholamines from the adrenal medulla. Therefore, even as the blood level of the drug increases, the release of norepinephrine predominates, ac-

Table 2-11. Antidysrhythmic drugs under investigation[60,148]

Drug	Classification	Side effects	
		Cardiac	Noncardiac
Ajmaline	IA	Intraventricular conduction delay AV block Acceleration of arrhythmias Ventricular arrhythmias (in cardio- myopathy)	Hepatotoxicity Agranulocytosis Neurologic side effects
Aprindine	IB	Prolonged conduction times Increased PR interval and QRS duration	Neurologic side effects (appear with plasma concentrations > 1 mg/ml), including tremor, dizzi- ness, vertigo, ataxia, visual dis- turbances, psychosis
Encainide	IC	Worsening of conduction system disease Prolonged H-V interval and QRS duration Worsening of ventricular arrhythmias	Neurologic side effects including dizziness, ataxia, tremor Diplopia Nausea Metallic taste Leg cramps
Ethmozin	IB		Dizziness (with IV administration) Nausea Epigastric distress Pruritus Headache
Flecainide	IC	Chest pain	Feeling of warmth Tingling in fingers
Lorcainide	IC	Prolonged PR interval and QRS duration	Insomnia with sweating and night- mares Dizziness Flatulence Dry mouth Excessive perspiration Vivid dreams
Mexilitine	IB	Prolonged conduction Bradycardia Hypotension Cardiac depression	Neurologic side effects including tremor, convulsions, dizziness Gastrointestinal side effects includ- ing nausea and vomiting Photosensitive dermatitis
N-acetylpro- cainamide	IA	Worsening of arrhythmias Worsening of conduction system disease	Gastrointestinal side effects Vasculitis

Modified from Schwartz, J.B., Keefe, D., et al.: Adverse effects of antiarrhythmic drugs, Drugs 21:23, 1981.

counting for the clinically visible ionotropic and chronotropic actions.

Clinically, bretylium is used as an antidysrhythmic agent, thus far only for adults, in the treatment of recurrent ventricular arrhythmias (ventricular tachycardia and ventricular fibrillation) that are not responsive to traditional forms of therapy. Consequently, it is not a first-line drug; rather, it is used when other forms of therapy have failed.

There are some potential side effects associated with the administration of bretylium. Initially, there is a period of hypertension resulting from the catecholamine release. This initial hypertension is often followed by a period of hypotension, particularly postural in nature. In digitalis-induced dysrhythmias, there is often a transient increase in the dysrhythmia, associated with bretylium administration. Bretylium can also interact in an adverse manner with other antidysrhythmics such as quinidine; in addition, it may cause nausea and vomiting. Prolonged oral administration of the drug may be associated with parotid pain.[51,75]

Verapamil (Calan, Isoptin) is one of the newest antidysrhythmic agents approved in the United States. As a Class IV drug, it is used to block the passage of calcium and possibly sodium across the sarcolemma. Verapamil is particularly effective in slowing the rate of discharge of the SA node. It also prolongs AV conduction. In addition, verapamil depresses myocardial contractility. It is used clinically in the treatment of ventricular tachydysrhythmias and has also been successful in terminating supraventricular tachycardia. Verapamil has slowed the ventricular response in atrial flutter and atrial fibrillation and has been given prophylactically in an effort to prevent recurrent paroxysmal supraventricular tachydysrhythmias. It has also been used in the treatment of angina pectoris, serving as a coronary vasodilator.

Although verapamil can be given orally or intravenously, it is most effective when given intravenously. It is used cautiously for children. Verapamil is contraindicated in patients with sick sinus syndrome, in conduction distur-

bances in the AV junction because of its effect on conduction, and in severe heart failure because it depresses contractility. It should also be avoided in combination with beta-adrenergic receptor blocking agents.

Side effects associated with the use of verapamil are minimal and include bradycardia, transient asystole, hypotension, worsening of heart failure, headache, dizziness, constipation, and nausea.[19,83,149]

Other antidysrhythmics currently being investigated are outlined in Table 2-11.

Parasympatholytics

Atropine sulfate is a parasympatholytic drug that inhibits the action of acetylcholine. In doing so, vagal tone is reduced. The rate of discharge of the SA node is enhanced and AV conduction improved, the latter by shortening the refractory period and increasing the speed of conduction through the AV node. Atropine is used clinically in the presence of symptomatic sinus bradycardia. It is also indicated in the treatment of sinus bradycardia accompanied by severe hypotension or frequent ventricular ectopic beats. In addition, it may be beneficial in patients with high-degree AV block, such as Wenckebach, and in the presence of ventricular asystole. Although atropine can be used with infants and children in the above situations, its most frequent pediatric use occurs in the treatment of sinus bradycardia.

Atropine administration is associated with relatively few side effects when only one or two doses are given. Atropine may cause dryness of the mouth and skin, flushing of the face, and pupillary dilation. Bronchial secretions are reduced, possibly predisposing to pulmonary complications. In men, especially those with prostate enlargement, atropine administration may be associated with a transient inability to void. Larger doses of atropine are often associated with symptoms of mental confusion and acute glaucoma.

Atropine should be given cautiously to patients who have had a myocardial infarction because the increase in heart rate caused by the drug may be accompanied by premature ventricular contractions or ventricular tachycardia.[151]

Isoproterenol hydrochloride (Isuprel) is a sympathomimetic drug that stimulates beta-adrenergic receptors. It is both inotropic and chronotropic and decreases peripheral vascular resistance. Increases in heart rate and contractility coupled with the increase in venous return raise the cardiac output. Consequently, oxygen requirements of the myocardium are increased and myocardial efficiency is decreased.

Clinically, in the presence of rate and rhythm disorders, isoproterenol enhances pacemaker automaticity. It also enhances AV conduction in the presence of heart block to increase the ventricular rate. Therefore it is indicated in the treatment of atropine refractory bradycardia resulting from heart block. It may also be beneficial in the treatment of ventricular ectopy associated with a slowed heart rate because the drug will increase the rate, possibly eliminating the ectopy.

Several side effects are associated with the use of isoproterenol. It may precipitate dysrhythmias such as sinus tachycardia, premature ventricular systoles, ventricular tachycardia, or ventricular fibrillation. Hypotension can occur in low-volume states because of the drug's vasodilating effect. It can also cause headache, dizziness, anginal pain, nausea, flushing of the skin, and diaphoresis.[51]

Sympathomimetics

Epinephrine (Adrenalin) is both an alpha-adrenergic and beta-adrenergic stimulant. In low doses, epinephrine acts directly on the beta-adrenergic receptors to increase the heart rate and force of contraction. Stroke volume increases, as does coronary blood flow. The cardiac output will also rise. Larger doses of epinephrine activate the alpha-adrenergic receptors, elevating the blood pressure and peripheral resistance, thereby reducing blood flow to the skin and kidneys.

Epinephrine is used clinically in a cardiac arrest to initiate the cardiac rhythm by stimulating the pacemaker cells. It also can be used in heart block to lessen the degree of block because it improves conduction in the AV node, bundle of His, Purkinje fibers, and ventricle.

Several potential problems occur with the use of epinephrine. Oxygen consumption is increased because of the increase in heart rate and contractility; therefore cardiac efficiency is diminished and anginal attacks may be precipitated. Ventricular dysrhythmias may also develop. The glomerular filtration rate and sodium excretion are reduced because renal blood flow is decreased. The blood sugar and free fatty acids are increased, as is the body metabolism, all of which may add additional strain to the diseased heart. The acidotic state may also reduce the effectiveness of the catecholamines. On addition, prolonged use of the drug can damage the arterial wall and the endocardium.[51]

Electrolytes

Potassium is the primary intracellular cation. It is regulated by the kidneys and can be altered by several disease states and therapeutic regimes. Potassium loss affects the cardiac muscle and is manifested by changes in the heart rate and rhythm. Hypokalemia can cause both supraventricular and ventricular dysrhythmias. It can result in conduction defects and increased automaticity, leading to tachydysrhythmias of either supraventricular or ventricular origin. Ectopic pacemaker activity also can occur with a low extracellular potassium level.

Potassium exerts several effects on the heart rate and rhythm. Initially, it enhances but then depresses the conduction velocity and excitability of the heart. Potassium suppresses automaticity, thereby depressing ectopy if the ectopy is caused by hypokalemia. It also further depresses the AV conduction produced by digitalis therapy. Potassium is used clinically to treat hypokalemia-induced dysrhythmias.

Artificial cardiac pacemakers

Many disorders of the heart rate and rhythm can be managed effectively with an artificial cardiac pacemaker. The pacemaker, whether external or internal, functions in the same way. The pacing system is a simple electrical circuit. It consists of a power source (pulse generator) with a positive terminal (anode) and a negative terminal (cathode) connected by an electrically conductive insulated wire (lead) that is implanted within the epicardium or in contact with the endocardium. Initiated by the pulse generator, pacemakers deliver electrical stimuli to the myocardial cell to spontaneously depolarize the heart. The ability of the cardiac cell to respond to the electrical stimulus is referred to as its *threshold*. Threshold is the minimal amount of current or voltage that is necessary to elicit depolarization.

Principles of operation

The principles of pacemaker operation are governed by Ohm's law, which states that the ratio of potential difference (V-voltage) between any two points in a circuit to the current (I) is constant and equals the resistance (R) between the two points.[87]

$$R \text{ (resistance)} = \frac{V \text{ (potential difference)}}{I \text{ (current)}}$$

Resistance depends on the impedance to the flow of current within the lead, both at the connection to the pulse generator and lead tip and at the interface of the electrode with the myocardium. It can be defined as the degree of nonconductivity within the pacing system. Resistance is affected by the status of the cells in contact with the electrode. It is increased when the lead is placed in contact with an area of fibrosis or ischemia. Location is also important. Resistance is higher in the atrium and in the epicardium.

Voltage and current may be variable or constant. When voltage is variable, current is constant. Voltage is internally regulated to deliver the set current. Voltage is fixed when current is variable. It is usually set from 10 to 12 mV, whereas the current output varies from 0.1 milliampers to 20 milliampers.

The most desirable pacing system is one with low resistance because such a system requires reduced voltage or current. Because the power consumed is the product of the current (I) and the potential difference (V),[121] this type of system will also use less power, prolonging the life of the pacemaker.

Power source[38,107,121,150]

Most pacemakers are battery operated. Temporary systems employ standard alkaline or mercury batteries. Implanted pacemakers use one of several battery types. These devices have been studied by engineers since the advent of permanent pacing in an effort to find a long-lasting power source.

Mercury zinc batteries were popular in the 1960s and early 1970s. The longevity of these batteries was typically limited to from 24 to 42 months. These cells have been abandoned today because of their shortened life span. In addition, the cells produced hydrogen gas, making it difficult to seal and protect the pacemaker from damaging body fluids.

Rechargeable nickel cadmium batteries were also introduced but never gained much popularity because of the necessity for recharging.

Strict government regulations limited the use of nuclear-powered pacemakers introduced in the 1970s. These units converted the heat produced by a radioactive isotope of plutonium (238 Pu) into electrical energy. Although nuclear batteries were effective and had the longest life span, they were unacceptable from an economic standpoint.

Pulse generators currently used are made with lithium batteries. These batteries, which vary in the composition of the cathode materials, include lithium iodine, lithium thionyl chloride, lithium cupric sulfide, lithium lead sulfide, and lithium silver chromate. Each exhibit similar characteristics that make them advantageous for use. They have a low internal energy drain (self-discharge); produce no gas, permitting the pulse generator to be hermetically sealed; and offer high-energy density. Lithium batteries differ in their longevity; some have lasted as long as 8 years, whereas others have lasted only 18 months.

Some antitachycardia pacemakers, powered by radiofrequency energy transmitted through the body to the pulse generator, have been used to terminate episodes of tachydysrhythmias.[107,150] When they are symptomatic, patients manually activate the system by placing a battery-operated transmitter over the receiver unit and pressing a button to activate the implanted device. This system is valuable because constant pacing is not required. It also eliminates the need for battery replacement.[150]

Data continue to be collected to identify the type of power source that reflects the most longevity.

Electrode system

The pacing electrode may be unipolar or bipolar. A unipolar system has one electrode, the cathode, in contact with the heart. The anode, usually the metallic case on the pulse generator, is placed away from the heart to complete the circuit. In a bipolar catheter, there are two electrodes located in the cardiac chamber. The distal electrode is called the cathode and is in direct contact with the heart; it is attached to the negative terminal. Approximately 1 cm above the distal electrode is the anode (proximal electrode), which is connected to the positive terminal. Although there is minimal physiologic difference between the two systems, the pacing threshold may be lower with a unipolar electrode. Bipolar catheters appear to be less susceptible to extraneous electromagnetic interference. A bipolar system can be converted to a unipolar one by disconnecting the anode from the pacemaker pulse generator, inserting a metal suture and wire into the subcutaneous tissue, and attaching this to the positive terminal of the pacemaker generator.[38,150]

Indications for pacing

Pacemakers can be inserted on a temporary or a permanent basis. Temporary pacemakers are used for both diagnostic and therapeutic purposes. Permanent pacing is always therapeutic. Table 2-12 outlines the uses of temporary and permanent pacemakers.

Classification code

A classification code for cardiac pacemakers was proposed by the Inter-Society Commission for Heart Disease as a standardized means for identifying the functional operation of a pulse generator, regardless of the model number or trade name.[106,137,150] This code has been revised and expanded to a five-letter code to extend its flexibility.[137,150] The minimum code length is three letters. O is used when the pacemaker does not have a particular function. Positions iv and v need not be included unless there are letters in that position. The current system of nomenclature appears in Table 2-13.

The first two positions indicate the chamber in which the pacemaker operates, with position I representative of the chamber paced and position II indicative of the chamber sensed. Dual chamber pacemakers, that is, those that pace or sense in both the atrium and the ventricule, are designated by the letter D (dual).

The mode of response is described in the third position. Pacemakers that are inhibited by the presence of sensed spontaneous electrical activity are represented by I (inhibited), whereas those that elicit a pacing spike after sensing spontaneous depolarization are labeled T (triggered). D is used in position III for atrial-triggered and ventricular-inhibited pacemakers. Pacing systems used to terminate a tachydysrhythmia function in reverse; they are silent at slow rates and discharge when the rate is too fast. These pulse generators are designated R (reverse).

Position IV describes the programming characteristics. These devices provide a noninvasive mechanism for altering the electronic control of the pacemaker. Programmable features vary according to the manufacturer. Numerous possibilities exist. Some of the programmable features include rate (minimum and maximum), output (pulse duration and amplitude), sensitiv-

Table 2-12. Pacing indications

	Definitely indicated	Probably indicated	Probably not indicated	Definitely not indicated
COMPLETE AV BLOCK				
Congenital (AV nodal)				
Asymptomatic				X
Symptomatic	T,P			
Acquired (His-Purkinje)				
Asymptomatic		T,P		
Symptomatic	T,P			
Surgical (persistent)				
Asymptomatic	T	P		
Symptomatic	T,P			
SECOND-DEGREE AV BLOCK				
Type I (AV nodal)				
Asymptomatic				X
Symptomatic	T,P			
Type II (His-Purkinje)				
Asymptomatic		T,P		
Symptomatic	T,P			
FIRST-DEGREE AV BLOCK				
AV Nodal				
Asymptomatic				X
Symptomatic			X	
His-Purkinje				
Asymptomatic				X
Symptomatic			X	
BUNDLE BRANCH BLOCK				
Asymptomatic				X
Symptomatic				
Normal H-V		P‖		
Prolonged H-V	P			
Distal His block at paced atrial rates <130/min	P			
LBBB during right heart catheterization	T			

From Zipes, D., and Duffin, E.C.: Cardiac pacemakers. In Braunwald, E.: Heart disease, textbook of cardiovascular medicine, ed. 2, Philadelphia, 1984, W.B. Saunders Co.

T = Temporary pacing; P = permanent pacing; X = pacing not indicated.

BBB = Bundle branch block; LBBB = left bundle branch block.

HV = Measure of His-Purkinje conduction time.

*Site and rate of stimulation may influence success.

†Atrial fibrillation with a rapid ventricular response may be a complication.

‡Prove efficacy with temporary pacing.

§May accelerate VT.

‖No other cause found for symptoms.

Table 2-12. Pacing indications—cont'd

	Definitely indicated	Probably indicated	Probably not indicated	Definitely not indicated
ACUTE MYOCARDIAL INFARCTION				
Newly acquired bifascicular BBB	T			
Preexisting BBB				X
Newly acquired BBB plus transient complete AV block	T	P		
Second-degree AV block				
Type I (asymptomatic)				X
Type II	T	P		
Complete AV block	T	P		
ATRIAL FIBRILLATION WITH SLOW VENTRICULAR RESPONSE				
Asymptomatic				X
Symptomatic	T,P			
SICK SINUS SYNDROME				
Asymptomatic			X	
Symptomatic	T,P			
HYPERSENSITIVE CAROTID SINUS SYNDROME				
Asymptomatic			X	
Symptomatic	T,P			
BRADYCARDIA-TACHYCARDIA SYNDROME				
Asymptomatic			X	
Symptomatic	T,P			
BRADYCARDIA-MISCELLANEOUS				
Asymptomatic			X	
Symptomatic	T,P			
TACHYCARDIA PREVENTION*				
Associated with bradycardia	T,P			
Associated with long Q-T, torsades de pointes	T	P		
Not associated with bradycardia, long Q-T, torsades de pointes (after drug failure)		T	P†	
TACHYCARDIA TERMINATION (AFTER DRUG FAILURE)*†				
Atrial flutter	T,P			
Atrial fibrillation				X
AV nodal reentry	T,P			
Reciprocating tachycardia in WPW syndrome	T,P†			
Ventricular tachycardia	T§	P§		

Table 2-13. Nomenclature code for cardiac pacemakers (ICHD)

First letter, chamber paced	Second letter, chamber sensed	Third letter, mode of response	Fourth letter, programmable functions	Fifth letter, special tachyarrhythmia functions
V-Ventricle	V-Ventricle	I-Inhibited	P-Programmable (rate and/or output)	B-Burst
A-Atrium	A-Atrium	T-Triggered	M-Multiprogrammability	N-Normal rate competition (such as in the "dual demand pacemaker)
D-Dual (atrium and ventricle)	D-Dual (atrium and ventricle)	D-Atrial-triggered and ventricular-inhibited	O-None	S-Scanning response (such as timed extrasystoles and others)
S*-Single	O-None	R†-Response		E-External control (activated by magnet by patient, physician, or radio-frequency)
	S*-Single	O-None		

Adapted from Parsonnet, V., Furman, S., and Snyth, N.: A revised code for pacemaker identification, PACE 4(4):401, 1981.

*When suitably programmed (usually in sensitivity, refractory period, and output), pacemakers can be used in the atrium AAI or in the ventricle VVI.

†Reverse functions, indicating that pacemaker is silent at slow rates and activated by fast rates.

ity, refractory period, mode, AV interval, hysteresis,* and polarity (universal or bipolar). Telemetry allows interrogation of the pacemaker for record keeping, pacemaker status, and physiologic information.[82] The applications of programmable parameters are listed in Table 2-14.

Antitachyarrhythmia functions are indicated by the fifth position. These systems have special units that respond specifically to a tachyarrhythmia. Control is achieved via rate maintenance, termination of tachyarrhythmias, and prevention of the onset of tachycardia.[150] These systems can be used during electrophysiologic studies as a tool for understanding normal and pathologic electrophysiology. They induce changes in the cardiac rate and rhythm using single, paired, coupled, bursts, or other groupings of stimuli. Pacemakers with this function can be used to terminate some drug-refractory tachyarrhythmias.[150]

Atrial and ventricular asynchronous pacemakers (A00 V00)

Early pacemakers stimulated the myocardium at a fixed rate. They discharged continuously at a preset rate without regard for any spontaneous beat. The interval between paced beats was consistent. These devices, which are illustrated in Fig. 2-28, are rarely used today because of the potential risk of competitive pacing.

Atrial and ventricular demand pacemakers (AAI, AAT, VVI and VVT)

Sensing circuits were added to pacemakers in the early 1970s to prevent competition between the pacemaker and any underlying intrinsic rhythm. Demand pacing systems sense spontaneous electrical activity. They either withhold

---

*Pacemakers with hysteresis are designed so that the pacemaker escape internal (measured from the onset of the last spontaneous sensed beat to the ensuing pacemaker spike) is longer in duration than the interval between two consecutively paced beats (the automatic interval). This permits the maintenance of a normal sinus rhythm over a range of rate while ensuring the resumption of pacing as needed.[150]

Table 2-14. Applications of programmable pacemaker parameters

Parameter	Patient/pacemaker optimization	Diagnostic applications	Correction of malfunctions
Rate	Improve cardiac output by allowing greater range of conducted sinus activity. Minimize angina by keeping the rate below that which produces pain. Suppress arrhythmias. Adapt pulse generator to pediatric needs (faster rates). Terminate tachycardias with short rapid bursts. Minimize "pacemaker syndrome" (caused by AV dissociation) by selecting low rate.	Suppress pacing to access underlying rhythm by ECG. Test AV conduction with an atrial pacemaker by determining rates at which AV-nodal Wenckebach behavior occurs. Test sinus function with an atrial pacemaker by using bursts of rapid pacing to determine SA node recovery times. Confirm atrial capture by altering pacemaker rate and observing concomitant ventricular rate change.	
Output, amplitude, or duration	Maximize pulse generator longevity by selecting output energy that provides the minimal level of stimulation consistent with reliable maintenance of pacing. Provide increased energy for high threshold patients. Avoid extracardiac stimulation (pectoral muscle, phrenic nerve).	Evaluate pacing threshold.	Regain capture following threshold increases caused by infarcts, electrolyte disturbances, drugs. Eliminate diaphragmatic or pectoral muscle stimulation.
Amplifier sensitivity	Establish appropriate sensitivity to detect intracardiac electrogram while avoiding sensing of extraneous signals (pectoral muscle potentials, electromagnetic interference). Increase sensitivity for atrial sensing applications.	Alter sensitivity to evaluate possible sources of oversensing or undersensing.	Compensate for changes in intracardiac electrogram amplitude. Resolve oversensing of T waves, muscle potentials, electromagnetic interference.

From Andreoli, K.G., et al.: Comprehensive cardiac care: a text for nurses physicians and other health professionals, St. Louis, 1983, The C.V. Mosby Co.

Continued.

Table 2-14. Applications of programmable pacemaker parameters—cont'd

Parameter	Patient/pacemaker optimization	Diagnostic applications	Correction of malfunctions
Refractory period	Extend duration for atrial applications to avoid sensing conducted R waves. Shorten duration in ventricular applications to detect closely coupled ectopic events.	Alter duration to evaluate possible causes of oversensing or undersensing.	Lengthen duration to avoid T-wave sensing. Shorten duration to eliminate failure to sense closely coupled ectopic events.
Hysteresis	Minimize pacemaker syndrome by allowing sinus rhythm over widest possible rate range while establishing adequately high pacing rate when needed.		
Unipolar/bipolar		Evaluate lead fracture (bipolar → unipolar). Enhance stimulus artifact visibility on ECG (bipolar → unipolar). Evaluate oversensing (unipolar → bipolar).	Convert to unipolar operation to regain capture in case of lead fracture Change mode to adapt to altered electrogram causing sensing failure. Convert to bipolar to eliminate sensing of myopotentials. Convert to bipolar to avoid extracardiac stimulation.
Mode	Select optimum mode (for example, VDD for patients who have normal sinus function and impaired AV conduction.) Alter mode if patient's needs change (for example, VDD → DVI if patient develops sinus bradycardia).	Establish triggered mode to enable external control of pacemaker from chest electrodes and external stimulator to perform noninvasive electrophysiologic studies of sinus function. AV conduction, efficacy of antiarrhythmic agents. Confirm oversensing signal source by selecting triggered mode.	Change to backup mode (for example, VVI) if atrial portion of dual-chamber system is nonfunctional (for example, lead displacement). Prevent oversensing by selecting asynchronous mode.

Table 2-14. Applications of programmable pacemaker parameters—cont'd

Parameter	Patient/pacemaker optimization	Diagnostic applications	Correction of malfunctions
AV delay	Maximize hemodynamic efficacy. Control or prevent tachyarrhythmias.		
Atrial-rate—tracking limit	Maintain widest range of sinus rate control without incurring angina. Control ventricular response to atrial arrhythmias. Prevent rapid synchronization to dissociated atrial activity during ventricular escape pacing in VVD mode. Prevent occurrence of retrograde atrial activity that would result from a long delay between the triggering event in the atrium and the resultant stimulus in the ventricle. This retrograde activity can continuously trigger the pacemaker, causing "pacemaker tachycardia."	Select high rate limit for stress testing.	Reduce tracking rate limit if pectoral muscle activity triggers rapid pacing.
Telemetry		Compare programmed settings to actual device operation. Use marker channel indicators to determine which events pacemaker is causing and which events are being sensed. Use electrogram to evaluate causes of undersensing or over-sensing. Use electrogram to evaluate drug effects on myocardium.	

Fig. 2-28. Atrial and ventricular asynchronous pacemakers (AOO, VOO). On the left is a schematic diagram of the heart, with the right and left atria on the top and the right and left ventricles on the bottom. The name of the type of pacemaker is given. The term output circuit connected to an asterisk indicates the chamber stimulated (Fig. 2-29). A circle connected to an arrowhead labeled *amp* indicates the sensing portion of the pacemaker and identifies the chamber in which spontaneous activity is sensed (Fig. 2-29). A circle surrounding an asterisk indicates that both pacing and sensing are performed in that chamber. The letters in the middle panel conform to the first three positions of the pacemaker code, as indicated in Table 2-13. Panels on the right indicate an ECG example produced by that particular type of pacemaker.

In the top panel, an example of an atrial asynchronous pacemaker (AOO) is displayed. In the left panel, the asterisk indicates that the atrium is paced. The ECG demonstrates pacemaker stimuli preceding each paced P wave. The asynchronous mode of operation cannot be seen in this ECG example because spontaneous P waves do not ocur.

The format in the bottom panel is the same. The asterisk indicates that the ventricle is paced. On the right, ventricular asynchronous pacing is seen following the third paced QRS complex. A spontaneous QRS complex occurs, and yet a pacing stimulus falls in the ST segment of this complex. The next pacemaker stimulus occurs during the QRS complex of the following beat, producing a fusion complex. Finally, the last QRS complex is initiated by the pacemaker spike.

From Andreoli, K.G., Fowkes, V.K., et al: Comprehensive cardiac care, ed. 1, St. Louis, 1983, The C.V. Mosby Co.

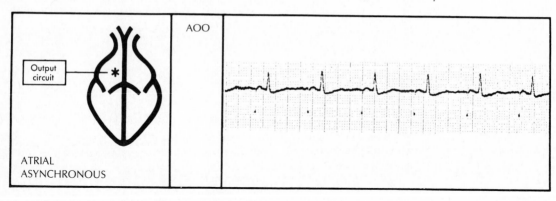

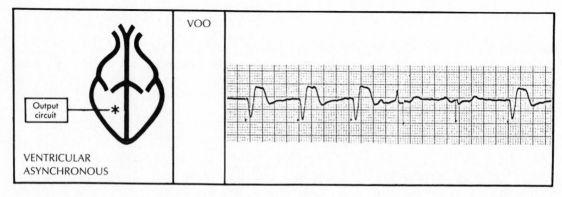

their stimulus (that is, they are *inhibited*), or they deliver their stimulus immediately after spontaneous depolarization during the absolute refractory period of the myocardium, when there is no cardiac response (that is, they are *triggered*). Both demand-inhibited and QRS-triggered pacemakers reset their timing cycle following discharge or on sensing spontaneous electrical activity. Each deliver a stimulus at the end of the pacemaker escape interval if no intrinsic activity is sensed. The triggered mode was developed because of concerns that demand-inhibited units would sense extraneous electrical activity, leaving the patient asystolic. Modern technology has reduced the chances of this happening. Consequently, triggered systems, which create artifact distorting the ECG and have high energy requirements, have become less popular. They continue to be useful in the treatment of some tachydysrhythmias and in situations when it is necessary to determine when or if the pacemaker senses spontaneous activity.[137,150] Fig. 2-29 shows the ECG for atrial and ventricular demand-inhibited and QRS-triggered pacemakers.

Atrial synchronous ventricular pacemakers (VAT VDD)

Atrial triggered synchronous ventricular pacemakers were designed to closely approximate the normal electrical sequence of the cardiac cycle. These dual-chambered units have a sensing electrode in the atria that senses the voltage of an atrial contraction and, after a preset simulated PR interval, elicits a ventricular contraction through a stimulating electrode located in the ventricle. These units do not normally pace the atria. Asynchronous pacing occurs only if the pacemaker fails to sense any intrinsic atrial activity; if the atrial activity becomes subthreshold, such as occurs in low voltage atrial fibrillation; or if the atrial rate becomes less than the base rate. If the atrial rate becomes excessively rapid, this type of pacemaker has an upper escape limit that protects the ventricle from direct stimulation in atrial tachycardia and that will introduce an AV response similar to type I

or type II AV block. This mode of pacing preserves the atrial contribution to ventricular filling, maintains sinus control of the ventricular rate, and permits a variation in the ventricular rate according to changing physiologic demands. It also preserves sequential AV conduction. A very recent development has been the addition of a ventricular sense amplifier to this pacemaker to create atrial synchronous ventricular inhibited units, referred to in the ICHD code as VDD.[150] These pacing systems are described in Fig. 2-30.

AV sequential pacemakers (DVI)

The AV sequential pacemaker senses ventricular activity only, but it can pace both the atrium and the ventricle via two bipolar electrodes, one in the atrium and one in the ventricle. This unit monitors for ventricular depolarization. In the absence of ventricular activity during a prescribed pacemaker escape interval, a stimulus is elicited to the atria. The ventricle is subsequently paced after a period of AV delay if no ventricular activity is detected. (Some AV sequential pacemakers do not wait for normal AV conduction but rather stimulate the ventricle immediately, following atrial stimulation.[4,7] The pulse generator is inhibited should spontaneous ventricular activity occur. Atrial stimulation is suppressed if the ventricular rate is sufficiently rapid. The timing mechanism is reset each time pacemaker output is inhibited.[150] Fig. 2-31 illustrates this mode of pacing.

Optimal sequential stimulation (DDD)

A dual chamber (atrioventricular sequential, atrioventricular sensing) pacemaker has been introduced that operates in four modes. This system can be used as an atrial pacemaker (atrial bradycardia with normal AV conduction), an AV sequential pacemaker (atrial bradycardia with impaired AV conduction), or an atrial synchronous ventricular pacemaker (normal sinus rhythm with impaired AV conduction), or it can be totally inhibited (normal sinus rhythm with normal AV conduction). This pacemaker is contraindicated in patients with atrial tachycardia and in patients with retrograde conduction to the atria concomitant with a long VA interval.[150] This system is shown in Fig. 2-32.

Pacemaker malfunction

The design characteristics of artificial cardiac pacemakers make them vulnerable to failure. Malfunction of the electronic and mechanical factors must be distinguished from physiologic

Fig. 2-29. Atrial and ventricular demand pacemakers (AAI, AAT, VVI, VVT). Top left, the asterisk and circle in the atrium indicate that the pacemaker stimulates the atrium and senses atrial activity. In the bottom panel the circle and asterisk in the ventricle indicate that the pacemaker stimulates the ventricle and senses spontaneous ventricular activity.

In the top ECG of the upper panel, an example of an atrial-inhibited (AAI) pacemaker is illustrated. Note that the pacing spike is inhibited from discharge until the fifth and seventh complexes, when the atrial rhythm slows down slightly and allows escape of the atrial demand pacemaker. In the second ECG example, each sensed P wave elicits a pacing spike delivered within the P wave (third, fourth, fifth P waves). A pacing spike initiates the P wave of the first, second, sixth, and seventh P waves. This is an example of AAT pacing.

In the bottom panel, upper ECG, an example of a ventricular demand pacemaker (VVI) is illustrated. Note that spontaneous ventricular activity inhibits pacemaker discharge, and pacing spikes are delivered only when the ventricular rate becomes slower than the escape interval of the pacemaker. In the lower ECG, pacing spikes are delivered into the QRS complex of each QRS complex (VVT).

From Andreoli, K.G., Fowkes, V.K., et al: Comprehensive cardiac care, ed. 1, St. Louis, 1983, The C.V. Mosby Co.

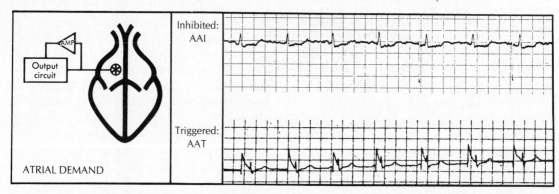

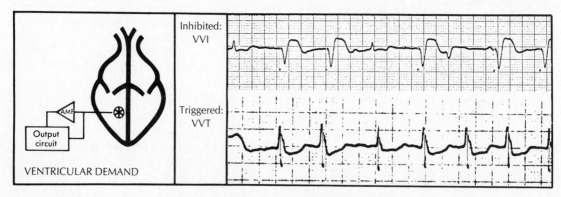

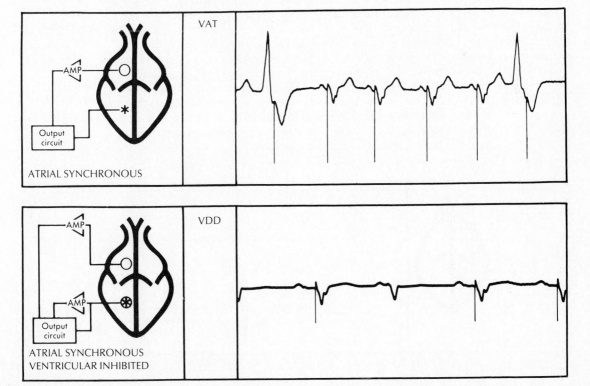

problems that develop. A thorough understanding of the physiologic and bioengineering principles involved in pacemaker therapy is necessary to differentiate normal from abnormal functions. Misinterpretation can occur with anti- tachycardia and synchronous pacemakers, as well as with hysteresis. Rational management of problems depends on careful investigation and interpretation of the symptoms.

Fig. 2-30. Atrial synchronous pacemakers (VAT, VDD). For the VAT pacemaker *(top panel)* the circle in the atrium and the asterisk in the ventricle indicate that the pacemaker senses atrial activity and paces the ventricle. In the lower panel the circle in the atrium and the circle and asterisk in the ventricle indicate that the pacemaker senses both atrial and ventricular activity and paces the ventricle (VDD).

In the midportion of the top ECG, the pacemaker delivers stimuli following each sensed P wave and produces a paced QRS complex. The first and last QRS complexes are spontaneous premature ventricular complexes (PVCs) that are *not* sensed by the pacemaker. The sinus P wave (hidden within the QRS complex) is sensed by the pacemaker and triggers it to deliver a pacing spike to the ventricle. Conceivably, such a response can deliver a stimulus into the T wave of the PVC. To avoid this problem, the VDD pacemaker has been equipped with a sensing circuit to sense spontaneous ventricular activity. Note in the lower ECG (VDD pacemaker) that the second P wave conducts to the ventricle with a PR interval shorter than the P-stimulus interval of the pacemaker. This conducted QRS complex is sensed by the pacemaker and the pacing spike is inhibited, thus eliminating problems of pacemaker competition with spontaneous ventricular activity.

From Andreoli, K.G., Fowkes, V.K., et al: Comprehensive cardiac care, ed. 1, St. Louis, 1983, The C.V. Mosby Co.

History

A thorough history of the symptomatology is necessary. Information regarding the newness of the symptoms should be elicited. Is the presenting symptom the same as or similar to the one that caused the initial implant? The return of syncope suggests failure to capture. Intermittent orthostatic hypotension may indicate the pacemaker syndrome.* Does the patient complain of palpitations? Ectopy of atrial or ventricular origin may be spontaneous or pacemaker in-

duced and may indicate a sensing abnormality and competitive pacemaker rhythms.[46]

Physical examination

The site of implantation should be assessed. Local pain can occur in the presence of infection or may be caused by the skin pocket being too tight. Careful examination is required because a pulse generator implanted in the axilla or anterior axillary fold can normally cause discomfort.

Laboratory examination and equipment

A full 12-lead electrocardiogram permits evaluation of pacemaker sensing, capture, approximate rate, electrode positioning by vector analysis, and appropriate function of the pacing mode being used.

---

*Pacemaker syndrome is a term used to describe new or persistent symptoms of lightheadedness, vertigo, syncope, or hypotension that occur in patients with ventricular pacemakers. It is believed that these complaints are caused by low cardiac output, cerebral insufficiency, functional labyrinthities, or vasovagal reflex.[88]

Fig. 2-31. AV sequential pacemaker (DVI). In the diagram the asterisk in the atrium and the asterisk and circle in the ventricle indicate that the pacemaker paces the atrium, paces the ventricle, and senses spontaneous activity in the ventricle. The ECG example demonstrates this operation. The first three sinus-initiated QRS complexes occur at a rate faster than the escape rate of the pacemaker, and the pacemaker is completely inhibited. At this point, SA node discharge rate slows and the pacemaker delivers a stimulus (upper spike) to the atrium. Because the paced P wave does not conduct to the ventricle within the escape interval of the pacemaker, the pacemaker then paces the ventricle (downward directed spikes). This occurs for three beats. Then the PR interval shortens slightly, inhibiting ventricular pacemaker discharge. The last two beats in the top strip and first three beats in the lower strip indicate pacing in the atrium and ventricle. Then a PVC occurs and is sensed, and the pacemaker activity is inhibited. The pacemaker then resumes delivery of spikes to atrium and ventricle. In the terminal portion of this ECG, the atrial rate speeds slightly. Because atrial activity is *not* sensed, pacemaker spikes "march" through the P wave but ventricular spikes are inhibited.

From Andreoli, K.G., Fowkes, V.K., et al: Comprehensive cardiac care, ed. 1, St. Louis, 1983, The C.V. Mosby Co.

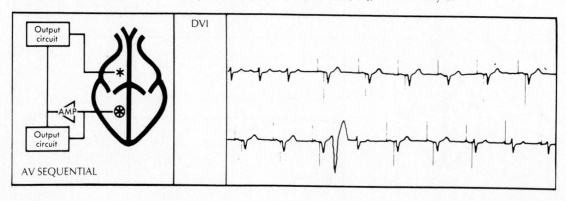

The pacing rate and pulse width can be accurately interpreted with a digital counter. This device may be provided as a special patient monitor or a part of a pacemaker programmer or may be purchased as a separate entity. It is important in the investigation of changes in the pacing rate and pulse width, which may be caused by battery depletion, component failure, or reprogramming.[4,150]

A magnet should be available to convert the pacemaker to the asynchronous mode. This permits evaluation of capture in inhibited units and can be used to identify oversensing by disabling the sensing function. Magnets should be used carefully to avoid reprogramming or the induction of tachydysrhythmias.[4,150]

The patient's intrinsic rate may be slower to induce pacing via carotid sinus massage (p. 139) or a Valsalva maneuver. This can be used to evaluate capture, especially in the absence of an asynchronous magnet mode. Exercise may be used to increase the intrinsic rate to evaluate sensing efficacy.[150]

Sensing ability may also be evaluated with a chest wall stimulator that has an external stimulator connected to precordial surface leads. This stimulator can also be used to identify rate tracking limits for atrial tracking pacemakers.[4,150]

Manipulation of the implanted pulse generator may be useful in eliciting ECG changes that confirm the presence of a loose connection or damaged lead close to implantation site.[4,150]

A baseline x-ray film should be compared to x-ray and fluoroscopic studies of the chest and

Fig. 2-32. Optimal sequential pacemaker (DDD). The diagram on the left indicates that the DDD pacemaker both senses and paces in the atrium and ventricle. The ECG on the right illustrates this feature. In the first five complete complexes, spontaneous atrial activity (P waves) is not followed by a spontaneous QRS complex within an appropriate PR interval. Therefore a pacemaker spike is delivered to the ventricle following each sensed P wave. The third QRS complex from the end occurs in time to be normally conducted from the P wave but not quite early enough to inhibit the pacemaker spike. The next QRS complexes follow a normal PR interval and thus inhibit pacemaker output. In the lower strip the development of sinus bradycardia triggers atrial pacemaker discharge, and pacemaker spikes precede the onset of P waves. Finally, in the bottom right portion, an atrial stimulus paces the atrium, and a ventricular stimulus paces the ventricle.

From Andreoli, K.G., Fowkes, V.K., et al: Comprehensive cardiac care, ed. 1, St. Louis, 1983, The C.V. Mosby Co.

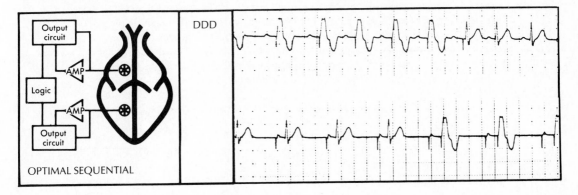

pacemaker system, using multiple views to identify lead position, gross lead fractures, and disconnections at the pulse generator site.[4,150]

Multiple functions can be evaluated noninvasively, using a pacemaker programmer. This permits variation in stimulus strength, amplifier sensitivity rates, refractory modes, and pacing modes. Some newer systems can be used to record intracardiac ECGs to evaluate sensing function; in addition, many are equipped with the capacity to provide digital telemetry of the programmed settings to permit comparison of the actual and expected performances. A marker channel (Fig. 2-33) is part of the most sophisticated system; this provides a noninvasively telemetered tracing that can be used with the surface ECG to evaluate pacemaker operation.[4,150]

Invasive procedure may be necessary when noninvasive approaches are unsuccessful. A pacing system analyzer is employed to evaluate generator functions (sensing, refractory periods, rates, pulse widths, and amplitudes), to check the position and integrity of the lead, and to provide electrophysiologic information about the patient (stimulation thresholds, ECG amplitude, sinus function, and conduction patterns).[4]

Classification of problems

Pacemaker problems can be classified into five general categories: failure to pace, failure to sense, oversensing, pacing at an altered rate, and undesirable patient-pacemaker interactions.

Failure to pace. Failure to pace (Fig. 2-34) can be defined as the inappropriate nondelivery of a stimulus or the delivery of an ineffective stimulus that fails to depolarize or capture the myocardium at a time when it is fully excitable.[4,150]

A faulty connection between the lead and the pulse generator, broken lead wires, "cross talk" between atrial and ventricular electrodes in a dual-chambered device, failure of one of the generater components, loss of power, or oversensing can result in failure to deliver a stimulus. Failure to capture can be attributed to lead displacement, failure of lead insulation and/or wire fracture, changes in threshold secondary to drug therapy, electrolyte imbalance fibrosis, or infarct and/or inappropriate programming of the pacemaker stimulus. A stimulus delivered during the relative refractory may be misinterpreted as failure to capture.

Failure to sense. Failure to sense (Fig. 2-35) results in a pacemaker that discharges without regard for any inherent spontaneous activity. Competing rhythms may develop, predisposing the patient to ventricular tachycardia or ventricular fibrillation if the pacing stimulus falls within the vulnerable part of the T wave. Multiple etiologies can be described. The most common causes of lack of sensing include lead displace-

Fig. 2-33. Lower tracing is Lead III surface ECG from patient with normally functioning Medtronic "Enertrax" atrial synchronous ventricular inhibited pacemaker. Upper tracing is marked channel transmitted by implanted pacemaker, indicating detection of atrial activity (small positive deflection) an pacing in ventricles (larger negative deflection). Right half of panel was recorded during exercise to show utility of marker channel in identifying atrial activity in presence of interference.

From Andreoli, K.G., Fowkes, V.K., et al: Comprehensive cardiac care, ed. 1, St. Louis, 1983, The C.V. Mosby Co.

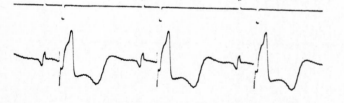
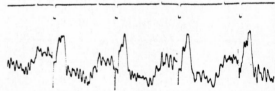

ment, lead fracture or insulation defect, pulse generator failure, improper programming of amplifier sensitivity or refractory period, inadequate ECG amplitude (because of fibrosis, infarct, drug therapy, or electrolyte imbalance), or reversion to asynchronous pacing (because of electromagnetic interference or erroneous programming). The development of fusion beats, while perfectly normal, may be misinterpreted as a sensing failure. These beats occur when spontaneous activity takes place simultaneously with the delivery of the pacing stimulus. Similar ECG findings can be recorded when stimulation occurs into refractory tissue (AAT or VVT pacing). These beats are labeled as *pseudofusion* beats because they have no effect on the electrical sequence of conduction but rather distort the waveform configuration.[150]

Oversensing. Oversensing occurs when a pacemaker senses extraneous cardiac or noncardiac signals that aren't supposed to be detected. T waves may be sensed by ventricular sensing pacemakers if the pacemaker amplitude is too sensitive or if its period of refractory is too short. Peaked or delayed T waves, characteristic of hyperkalemia or hypercalcemia, may also activate the sensing mechanism. Inappropriate atrial sensing can occur with a dislodged ventricular lead that localizes in the ventricular outflow tract. Atrial sensing pacemakers may sense ventricular activity when the atrial amplifier refractory period is shortened or atrial signals are too small. "Cross talk" in AV sequential devices may cause the ventricular sensing mechanism to sense atrial activity and inhibit the ventricular stimulus if the atrial and ventricular electrodes are too close together.[150] Skeletal muscle activity may be sensed in unipolar systems, leading to unneces-

Fig. 2-34. ECG tracing illustrating pacemaker out of capture. Arrows indicate pacemaker activity.

From Abels, L.F.: Mosby's manual of critical care, ed. 1, St. Louis, 1979, The C.V. Mosby Co.

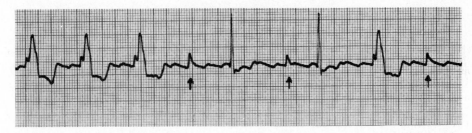

Fig. 2-35. ECG tracing illustrating pacemaker failing to sense. Arrows indicate non-sensed impulses.

From Abels, L.F.: Mosby's manual of critical care, ed. 1, St. Louis, 1979, The C.V. Mosby Co.

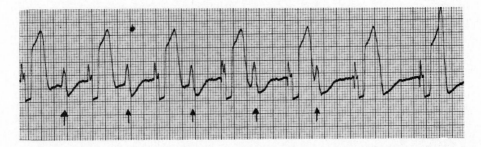

sary inhibition or triggering of the pacing stimulus. And finally, changes in voltage (caused by lead fracture or faulty connections) and electromagnetic interference may precipitate oversensing of the latter, especially common to unipolar devices.

Pacing at altered rates. Pacing at altered rates can occur with oversensing and battery or circuitry failure. Oversensing can slow the pacing rate because of inhibition or increase it because of triggering. Battery failure causes a gradual slowing in rate (rate drift). Rate change may also occur in older pacemakers that do not use digital timing circuits in the presence of temperature extremes. Rate reduction is built into many current models to warn of impending generator failure. Circuitry failure may inhibit stimulus delivery or cause rapid firing, referred to as a *runaway pacemaker*. A malfunctioning timing clock results in the rapid rate, with extremes of less than 150 to 180 pulses/min caused by the inclusion of a "runaway" protective device.[46]

Undesirable patient-pacemaker interactions. Undesirable patient-pacemaker interactions, although infrequent, can occur. The lead insertion site or pacemaker pocket may become infected. A hematoma may develop and can result in decreased arterial perfusion distal to it. With the insertion of a temporary epicardial or transthoracic endocardial electrode, bleeding into the pericardial sac leading to cardiac tamponade can occur. The pulse generator may erode through the skin. And finally, patients who "twiddle" or "play with" the implanted generater may rotate it and retract a lead, resulting in system failure.

Most pacing systems are insulated to protect them from extraneous electromagnetic interference. Microwave ovens are constructed to prevent leakage of an electrical current when operating properly. Citizen's band radios, if used according to Federal Communications Commission guidelines, are safe. Airport metal detectors may be activated by the metal encasing the generator but will not interfere with its operation. The taking of diagnostic x-ray films does not endanger pacemaker operation.

Some signals may interrupt pacemaker operation. An electric razor may be used on the face but should not be used under the arm if the generator is implanted nearby. Diathermy is contraindicated near the pacemaker because it can cause tissue burns and damage the pacemaker wires or components. Electrocautery can inhibit or trigger pacemaker output and can change the mode of operation. Interference depends on the amount of current delivered, the location of the cautery probe, and the duration of current delivered. Transcutaneous electrical nerve stimulators can also interfere and should only be used with an ECG monitor.[46] Defibrillation can be damaging when the paddles are placed too near the pulse generator. Although most manufacturers contend that pacemakers are protected from damage by currents of up to 400 watt seconds (joules), interference has been reported and total generater failure documented with repeated defibrillation. And finally, stimulation of the pectoralis muscles or diaphragm can generate an electric current (myopotential) that can simulate a cardiac potential and result in pacemaker inhibition or triggering. An isometric exercise test should be performed in pacemaker-dependent patients who lack an intrinsic rhythm to ascertain whether the device will respond to a myopotential.[150]

Pacemaker education

Patients with pacemakers must be evaluated to determine exactly what their educational needs will be. Because people react differently to having an implantable life-sustaining device, close attention must be given to their individual responses. In general, they should be made aware of their disorder and its cause, the type of implanted pacemaker and its mode of operation, and any restrictions placed on them. They must be taught to take their pulse daily, counting for a full minute. Any changes in the rate or symptoms of pacemaker malfunction should be reported immediately. The patient should be instructed to call about dizziness, syncopal episodes, palpitations, hiccoughs (caused by stimulation of the chest wall), chest pain, or shortness of breath. They must also be alert to any signs of infection over the implantation site. Because people vary in their ability to comprehend what is being taught, reinforcement should be ongoing.

Carotid sinus massage

Stimulation of the carotid sinus serves as a valuable diagnostic aid and therapeutic tool. Located at the bifurcation of the common carotid arteries just below the angle of the jaw at the upper level of the thyroid cartilage, the carotid sinus is manipulated with digital pressure to diagnose a cardiac dysrhythmia, to determine its etiology, and in some situations to terminate it. The massage slows the heart rate, therefore making it possible to identify the underlying mechanism responsible for the production of an abnormality. Carotid sinus massage is seldom used in infants because it is usually ineffective.

Carotid sinus massage is performed on one side of the carotid sinus at a time, with digital pressure applied posteriorly and medially for a maximum of 5 seconds. It may be repeated on the other side, but at no time should bilateral compression be attempted. ECG changes should be documented before, during, and after the maneuver.

Patients often complain of feelings of nausea and lightheadedness and may experience a syncopal episode during the procedure because of the interference with cerebral blood flow. With prolonged slowing of the rate, they may exhibit ECG changes consisting of sinoatrial arrest, AV junctional escape beats, and AV conduction defects, leading to a prolongation of the PR interval and changes in the duration and morphology of the P wave. Ventricular fibrillation and asystole can also occur.

Interventions that affect contractility

Therapeutic interventions implemented to augment cardiac pumping operate directly on the myocardium by increasing the force of contraction or indirectly by reducing the preload and afterload. Direct influences exert a positive inotropic effect, making each contraction more efficient either through drug therapy or direct cardiac compression. Indirect influences reduce the workload of the heart, thereby reducing oxygen requirements. Preload is reduced by decreasing the amount of blood that the ventricle must eject. Afterload is decreased by lowering the pressure the ventricle must generate to eject blood. Both direct and indirect interventions are important.

Pharmacologic agents used to improve contractility

Cardiac glycosides.[16,28,116,131] Digitalis is a cardiotonic that is capable of increasing the force and velocity of each myocardial contraction in the normal and the failing heart.[16,30] It acts at the cellular level, blocking sodium and potassium transport across the cell membrane by inhibiting the enzyme sodium potassium ATPase. Inhibition of this transporter enzyme results in potassium efflux from the myocardium. Glycoside interaction with the sodium potassium ATPase leads to an increase in membrane-bound calcium, which enters the cell to increase contractile protein function.[16,131]

In the normal heart, digitalis increases contractility and wall tension, thereby increasing oxygen consumption. In the failing heart, myocardial oxygen consumption is decreased with digitalis administration because the augmented contractility decreases left ventricular end-diastolic pressure, reduces the end-diastolic volume, and leads to a decline in wall tension.[28]

Digitalis also exerts a number of other electrophysiologic effects. The exact effect depends on the type of myocardial fiber. It shortens the refractory period of the atria but prolongs that of the AV node. This is manifested by a prolonged PR interval. After atropine is given, digitalis has a reverse effect of prolonging atrial refractory and shortening ventricular refractory periods. Digitalis decreases the refractory period of the ventricle, as evidenced by a shortened Q-T interval on the ECG. It increases automaticity,

Table 2-15. Digitalis toxicity

Body locus	Clinical indicators
Cardiovascular system	Conduction disturbances (AV block)
	Ventricular dysrhythmias
Gastrointestinal system	Anorexia, nausea, vomiting, diarrhea, abdominal pain, bloating
Central nervous system	Fatigue, confusion, lethargy, insomnia, apathy, drowsiness, psychotic episodes, headaches, neurologic facial pain, paresthesias
Eyes	Blurred vision, altered or indistinct color perception, amblyopia, diplopia, scotomas, halos, flickering, retrobulbar neuritis
Endocrine system	Gynecomastia in men (rarely)
Skin	Allergic reactions, urticarial or scarlatiniform (rarely)

*Adapted from Michaelson, C.R., editor: Congestive heart failure, St. Louis, 1983, The C.V. Mosby Co.

especially in the Purkinje fibers. Both excitability and conduction velocity are increased with small doses of digitalis and decreased with larger doses.

Systemically, digitalis has been shown in normal subjects to increase the tone of peripheral resistance vessels.[116] This increase in afterload is thought to be a transient effect.[16] The cardiac glycosides cause venous constriction in the normal subject but lead to venodilation in persons with failing hearts. This paradoxical response is believed to be caused by the lowering of catecholamines that occurs as cardiac function is improved.[28]

Digitalis also augments some vagal activity. A reduction in the chronotropic effects of epinephrine and sympathetic stimulation have also been shown with high doses of these drugs.[28]

Clinically, digitalis is used in the treatment of congestive heart failure to increase myocardial contractility and efficiency and in the management of supraventricular dysrhythmias such as atrial fibrillation, atrial flutter, and paroxysmal atrial and AV junctional tachycardia, as long as they are not precipitated by digitalis toxicity.

Digitalis can be administered parenterally or orally. Intravenous administration is usually preferred for emergencies, whereas intramuscular and oral routes are used for digitalization and maintenance therapy. In digitalizing a patient, the size of the dose may be difficult to determine. The digitalization dose is given daily as a loading dose until the desired therapeutic effect

is visible. The full digitalizing dose may be much less than the dose that is likely to cause toxicity, or it may be almost equal to it. Once the patient is digitalized, the dosage is reduced slightly for maintenance therapy.

The loading and maintenance dosage must be individualized for each patient and clinical situation. Younger patients tolerate high levels better than people in older age groups. Serum levels of digitalis should be monitored to guide drug therapy. Digitalis should be given cautiously to patients with a disturbance in renal function because the drug is normally excreted by the kidneys. It should be administered with care in hypothyroidism because toxicity occurs at lower levels. Hypoxia and acid-base alterations may also decrease digitalis tolerance. Serum electrolyte levels should be followed because hypokalemia, hypercalcemia, and magnesium deficiency may make the heart more sensitive to the toxic effects of the drug.

There are several potential toxic effects associated with digitalis therapy. They classically involve the cardiovascular system, the nervous system, or the gastrointestinal tract. The signs and symptoms of digitalis intoxication are summarized in Table 2-15.

Electrolytes

Calcium is a potent inotropic agent involved in excitation-contraction coupling. Although traditionally it has been known for its direct ef-

Table 2-16. Some sympathomimetics and their "mixed" effects

Drug	Trade name	Receptor stimulation			Generalized effects		
		Alpha (vasoconstrictive)	Beta (B_1) contractility	Beta (B_2) vasodilatory	Cardiac output	Heart rate	Total peripheral resistance
Dopamine	Intropin	O/++++*	++++	++	↑	+/++*	↑/↓*
Dobutamine	Dobutrex	O/+	++++	++	↑	O/+*	↓
Epinephrine	Adrenalin	++++	+++	++	↑	+++	↓
Isoproterenol	Isuprel	—	++++	+++++	↑	++++	↓
Norepinephrine	Levophed	+++++	++++	—	O/↓	++†	↑

*Dose dependent.

†↓ HR secondary to reflex mechanism.

fect on myocardial contractility, it also affects the heart rate and rhythm. Calcium slows spontaneous rhythm and can block impulse conduction. It can also increase automatic discharge. Basically, its actions are in opposition to those of potassium. Calcium also influences the effects of digitalis on the sodium pump. Elevated calcium levels potentiate the effects of digitalis, often leading to digitalis toxicity. The opposite is true for low calcium levels. Current investigation suggests that calcium is important in impulse formation and conduction in cells in the sinus and AV node or in cells during certain pathologic conditions (the so-called *slow response*).[19]

Clinically, calcium is used in a cardiac arrest to increase myocardial tone or contraction. It is also used in the presence of ventricular fibrillation to make the fibrillatory waves coarser or of larger amplitude.

Calcium therapy may cause a moderate fall in the blood pressure because of vasodilation. Painful tissue sloughing can occur with extravasation of calcium chloride. Excess calcium may also cause shortening of the S-T segment and Q-T interval.

Sympathomimetics[28,75]

Other "mixed" pharmacologic agents also increase myocardial contractility. These drugs exert their effect through alpha- or beta-adrenergic receptor stimulation. Alpha-receptor stimulation causes vasoconstriction. Activation of different beta (B) receptors elicits different responses. B_1 receptors found in the heart in the heart are inotropic. Located in the arterioles and bronchi, B_2 receptors have a vasodilatory effect. The effects of these drugs are summarized in Table 2-16. The major differences of these drugs are in the magnitude of alpha- or beta-receptor stimulation.

Diuretics

Diuretic therapy plays an integral role in the treatment of heart failure as a preload reducer. The exact mechanism by which this is accomplished is reviewed in Unit 5. Other drugs used in failure that decrease preload or afterload are discussed in the pages that follow.

Rotating tourniquets

Rotating tourniquets are employed to reduce the volume of blood returning to the heart. This temporarily reduces the preload and is necessary when the alveoli become engorged as a result of a sudden rapid transudation of fluid from the pulmonary capillaries. Congestion is reduced by decreasing the right atrial inflow of systemic venous blood and increasing left ventricular output. Right atrial outflow is decreased by pooling blood in the peripheral venous system. Often referred to as a dry phlebotomy, this process is accomplished by placing cuffs on all four extremities sequentially, inflating and deflating them to control the flow of venous blood. With the patient in a semi-Fowler's position to promote pooling in dependent portions of the body, the cuffs are applied. They must be placed high enough on each extremity to trap large amounts of blood. All of the outlet valves are closed and the timer is set to the desired cycle length, which is determined individually and prescribed by the physician. The cycle length is multiplied by 3 to identify the individual cuff inflation time. The inflation pressure is dictated by the patient's diastolic blood pressure. This permits impedance to venous return without compromising arterial flow to the limbs. The valves can be reopened and the machine activated. The machine should automatically inflate and deflate cyclically in rotation. The alarm system should be activated to monitor for failure in the rotation system or for an air leak. Continuous observation of the patient and the patient's blood pressure must be maintained. Blood pressure can be obtained when one of the arm cuffs is deflated by closing the valve, disconnecting the air tube, and attaching an aneroid sphygmomanometer. The cuffs should be released one at a time at the completion of the procedure.

Manual tourniquets can also be used, in the same manner. They are applied and removed in a clockwise manner approximately every 15 minutes. If blood pressure cuffs are used, one always remains deflated. When tourniquets and pads are used, they are placed on three extremities. The fourth is left next to but not on the remaining extremity. As rotation proceeds, the first tourniquet and pad are removed before the fourth ones are applied. Rotation continuity should be maintained, with a diagram kept at the bedside.

Several complications can occur with the use of rotating tourniquets. Although some discoloration and temperature change may be visible in an extremity while the cuff is inflated or the tourniquet is in place, peripheral ischemia can develop if the tourniquet is inflated too long or the inflation pressure occludes the intra-arterial pressure. Cuffs should never be inflated, nor should tourniquets be left in place, for longer than 45 minutes under any circumstances. The integrity of the skin can be interrupted with improperly applied tourniquets. Hypotension may occur secondary to the circulatory changes that take place while rotating tourniquets are used. Circulatory overload can be precipitated with sudden simultaneous removal of all of the tourniquets. Cardiac and respiratory arrest may also develop. As an adjunct to the use of rotating tourniquets, left ventricular output can be increased with drug therapy.

Phlebotomy

A therapeutic phlebotomy can be performed to decrease venous return and subsequently to reduce right ventricular output. This decrease is usually indicated when alveolar engorgement develops as a result of overadministration of blood and/or infusion fluids. Intravascular volume is reduced by withdrawing approximately 250 to 500 ml of blood from a peripheral vein. Red blood cell mass is also reduced. Although phlebotomy may be an elective procedure in the treatment of polycythemia, it is usually an emergency intervention in a critical care setting.

Anticoagulated vacuum bottles are used to collect the blood. Sterile technique is mandatory. A large vein should be selected and a large bore needle used to prevent clotting and reduce lysis of red blood cells. The blood withdrawn can then be used for autotransfusion if necessary. Once the procedure is completed, the blood must be transferred to the blood bank for refrigeration and storage if autotransfusion is anticipated.

Patients should be monitored continuously throughout and following this procedure for changes in their cardiopulmonary status. Hemodynamic alterations may lead to hypovolemia, syncopal episodes, convulsions, and even cardiac or respiratory arrest. Hematoma and infection can develop at the phlebotomy site.

Circulatory-assist devices

Circulatory assistance can be provided by a number of devices when myocardial function is significantly altered because of increased pre-load, increased afterload, or impaired contractility. These fundamental determinants of myocardial mechanics can be manipulated by mechanical devices that reduce the preload, reduce the afterload and augment diastolic pressure, or directly compress the heart. Although support provided by circulatory-assist devices is categorized according to the primary effect it exerts, changes often will be noted in another parameter because there is constant interaction among the preload, afterload, and contractile states of the myocardium.

Currently, circulatory support can be provided by both invasive and noninvasive devices.

Internal assistance is accomplished with the intra-aortic balloon pump (IABP) and the Anstadt cup. Noninvasive support is obtained with an external counterpulsation device and an external counterpressure. Two other left-heart-assist devices, a left atrial-arterial bypass unit and a left ventricular-arterial bypass unit, are undergoing extensive clinical evaluation.

The intra-aortic balloon pump. The intra-aortic balloon pump (IABP) is a circulatory-assist device that uses a balloon-tipped catheter inserted retrograde through the femoral artery into the descending thoracic aorta, where it is positioned distal to the left subclavian artery and proximal to the renal arteries. The balloon is

Fig. 2-36. Counterpulsation with hypothetical reservoir; illustrates correlation between balloon inflation, deflation, and ECG waves.

Courtesy Datascope Corporation, Paramus, NJ. From Abels, L.F.: Mosby's manual of critical care, ed. 1, St. Louis, 1979, The C.V. Mosby Co.

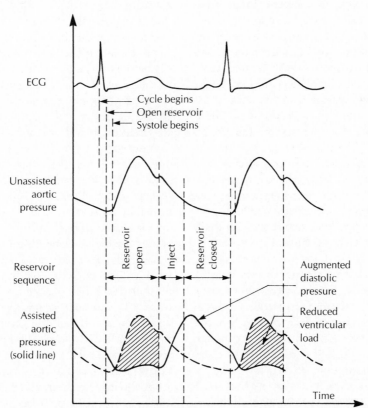

synchronized with the cardiac cycle to inflate with air during diastole and deflate during systole (Fig. 2-36). The R wave of the ECG is used for timing. Because timing of the balloon's inflation and deflation is opposite to normal ventricular activation, the technique is referred to as *counterpulsation*. It serves a dual purpose: to augment the diastolic pressure and to reduce the afterload.

Initially, as the balloon is inflated at the end of ventricular ejection, intra-aortic volume is increased, which also raises aortic pressure. This augments the diastolic pressure. Diastolic augmentation is a valuable tool for increasing coronary artery perfusion pressure and ultimately coronary artery blood flow and oxygen supply, principally when the need is great because the myocardium has been underperfused. Actual coronary blood flow may be elevated, unchanged, or even reduced. An internal autoregulatory process maintains a precise balance between the myocardial oxygen supply and demand. With counterpulsation, the work of the myocardium and oxygen demands can be reduced. When this occurs, autoregulated vasoconstriction may actually reduce coronary blood flow in spite of an elevation in the aortic diastolic pressure because tissue hypoxia and need for oxygen are the most potent stimuli for increasing coronary blood flow. The IABP supplements the autoregulatory process, serving as a reserve in the absence of need. In low pressure states the pump increases the supply of oxygen to the myocardium, improves the coronary blood flow to potentially ischemic areas, and improves peripheral tissue perfusion.

Deflation of the balloon just before systole reduces the intra-aortic volume, thus decreasing intra-aortic pressure. This decrease lowers the resistance to left ventricular ejection and decreases the afterload. Cardiac work is reduced because the ventricle does not have to generate as much pressure during systole, therefore decreasing the consumption of oxygen.

The IABP can be used in a variety of clinical settings. It can be used in cardiogenic shock as-sociated with myocardial infarction, regardless of the etiology, and often can serve as a means of reversing myocardial ischemia. It has been used to reverse resistant postcardiotomy shock and to protect the myocardium after preoperative insertion in the presence of high-risk coronary artery lesions. Counterpulsation is contraindicated in the presence of aortic aneurysm and aortic dissection because of the danger of progressive aortic wall damage and potential rupture. It is avoided in an insufficient aortic valve because balloon inflation would increase the retrograde flow into the left ventricle. It is not used with severe peripheral vascular disease because of the increased risk of arterial trauma and peripheral embolization. Extensive atherosclerotic disease could also interfere with passage of the balloon catheter, although an alternate approach is possible via the aortoiliac system or through the ascending aorta into the descending aorta.

Caring for the patient with the IABP requires continuous observation and monitoring. A thorough cardiovascular assessment is essential before catheter insertion. The patient's case history must be reviewed; pertinent questions about any bleeding abnormalities should be asked. Medication allergies should be noted because anticoagulant and antibiotic therapies are routine components of counterpulsation techniques. A physical exam should be conducted close to the time of insertion of the IABP, with special attention given to the status of the peripheral pulses.

Once the above information is obtained, hemodynamic monitoring can be implemented. Because the R wave of the ECG serves as the stimulus for balloon activation, the electrode must be positioned to obtain a tracing with an R wave of maximal amplitude; the remaining waves should be of minimal amplitude. The twelve-lead ECG should be reviewed, with the appropriate lead simulated using chest electrodes. If none of the conventional twelve leads are adequate, the chest electrodes can be rotated until the appropriate placement is identified.

Failure to monitor the ECG accordingly can lead to asynchrony between the balloon and cardiac cycle.

An intra-arterial catheter must also be inserted, preferably into the left radial artery. Because the balloon is positioned distal to the left subclavian artery, using this site will permit accurate monitoring with minimal waveform delay and distortion. The femoral artery can be used but is associated with greater distortion because of the increased distance from the central aorta.

A pulmonary artery balloon-tipped, flow-directed, thermodilution catheter should also be in place to evaluate the effect of the balloon on the left side of the heart. This catheter permits continuous measurement of the pulmonary artery pressure with periodic determinations of the right atrial pressure, pulmonary capillary wedge pressure, and cardiac output.

Both a central and a peripheral intravenous line should also be established. A central site is necessary for the infusion of vasopressors if they are needed during balloon insertion. Solutions of these drugs should be mixed and on standby. The peripheral site is needed if a large volume of fluid must be infused. Volume expanders should be readily available, with blood typed and crossmatched in the blood bank.

The balloon can be inserted in the critical care setting with the patient under a local anesthetic. Accurate placement can be facilitated by estimating the length of catheter needed and marking the proximal end with a tie. Measurement is made over the chest, with the distal end at the angle of Louis and the proximal end over the insertion site. An incision is made and the catheter is advanced up the iliofemoral system into the descending thoracic aorta, where it is positioned distal to the left subclavian artery. The left radial intraarterial waveform can also serve as a guide. Damping of this waveform usually indicates upward displacement of the catheter. A sidearm graft that has previously been placed around the catheter is anastomosed to the arteriotomy. The balloon catheter must be threaded through the graft into the femoral ar-

tery because any contact with metal objects could disrupt the antithrombogenic surface. Fluoroscopy or a chest roentgenogram is used to confirm the position of the balloon immediately after insertion.

Pumping is initiated once the balloon's position has been confirmed. Timing is adjusted by synchronizing balloon inflation with the dicrotic notch on the arterial waveform. Pressure elevation produced by balloon inflation should begin precisely on the dicrotic notch so that the balloon is inflated as the aortic valve closes. Balloon inflation should continue until just before the next systole. At that time, the balloon will rapidly deflate, reducing the intra-arterial pressure to a level consistent with the end-diastolic pressure without balloon assistance. The arterial waveform will exhibit an elevated diastolic pressure and a reduced systolic pressure.

Anticoagulant therapy is often implemented with counterpulsation to reduce the possibility of thrombus formation. If anticoagulation is to be instituted, baseline clotting studies should be obtained before therapy is initiated. The initial dose of heparin is administered approximately 3 minutes before catheter insertion. Anticoagulation is maintained via continuous infusion or individual bolus doses. Rheomacrodex (low-molecular-weight dextran) is also administered, either alone or with heparin therapy; if administered alone, it decreases platelet aggregation. It is administered at a rate of 10 to 20 ml/hr.

Antibiotic therapy is usually instituted for 24 to 48 hours after insertion and is reinstituted ½ hour before balloon removal. Broad-spectrum antibiotics are used because the number of indwelling catheters and procedures associated with IABP therapy predisposes the patient to infection. To reduce the likelihood of infection and sepsis, antibiotic coverage is combined with strict aseptic technique that must be observed throughout insertion, line management, dressing changes, and removal.

Patient care regimens may be continued as long as they do not interfere with balloon pumping. Most modifications are positional. The head of the bed should not be elevated more than 45 degrees, and the involved leg should not be flexed at the hip. Flexing could kink or crack the catheter at the insertion site or could displace the catheter proximally into the aortic arch, causing further damage. The patient can be turned from side to side very carefully with only mild angulation of the involved leg. Chest physical therapy can and should be carried out during IABP therapy. The introduction of artifact to the ECG should be avoided because the electrocardiogram is synchronized with balloon inflation.

The effects of counterpulsation should be reviewed at regular intervals. Hemodynamic parameters should be monitored every 15 to 60 minutes. Pulmonary capillary wedge pressures should fall and cardiac output should rise as ventricular function improves. Improvement in ventricular function may be associated with an increase in the urine output of not less than 30cc/hr. A reduction in urine output could also be caused by embolization during insertion. As the cardiac output increases, the level of consiousness should be improved or unchanged. A disturbance in mentation may signify a reduction in cerebral blood flow that, aside from a reduction in cardiac output, can be attributed to embolization, hypoxia, or psychosis. Efforts to minimize extrasensory input and sleep deprivation help prevent psychosis. Failure to respond to counterpulsation, evidenced by a falling cardiac output, a reduced urine output, and a reduced level of consciousness, carried a poor prognosis.

Bleeding studies should be monitored closely for indications of abnormal ties. The hematocrit should be followed and may fall after insertion because of blood loss and blood sampling or excessive anticoagulation. All blood losses should be recorded on a cumulative record. Packed cell replacement may be necessary. The platelet count should also be evaluated. Thrombocytopenia may occur because of interruption of platelet integrity by the balloon surface. The risk of thrombocytopenia is minimized by the institution of Rheomacrodex infusion.

Weaning the patient from IABP therapy is considered when hemodynamic parameters indicate an improvement in cardiac function. Removal before that time occurs only because of ischemia in the involved extremity. The weaning process is characterized by a gradual reduction in balloon support. Typically, the ratio of patient to balloon cycles is reduced from 1:1 to 1:8 over a period of hours, as specified by the physician. Criteria necessitating resumption of balloon pumping at a higher ratio should be predetermined. Intolerance to the weaning process is evidenced by a fall in the mean intra-arterial pressure, a rise in the pulmonary capillary wedge pressure, a fall in cardiac output, a reduction in the urine output, the development of cardiac dysrhythmias, or the development of chest pain. Should these occur, conventional modes of support such as vasopressors and volume expanders are often instituted before balloon pumping is resumed at a higher frequency. The balloon catheter is removed after weaning only when the patient's hemodynamic stability is confirmed. Removal is carried out in the critical care unit under local anesthesia, using strict asepsis. Any accumulated clots are removed. The incision is monitored for bleeding for 24 hours initially every 15 minutes, then every 30 minutes, and finally hourly.

IABP counterpulsation is associated with several potential complications. Septicemia and wound infection are potential problems that can be prevented with strict adherence to aseptic technique and the institution of broad-spectrum antibiotics. Hematopoietic abnormalities can occur secondary to bleeding or trauma. Blood loss should be monitored and recorded, with packed cell replacement carried out as necessary. The use of Rheomacrodex helps reduce the risk of platelet adhesion. Prophylactic anticoagulant therapy minimizes the chance for thrombus formation and embolization but increases the risk of bleeding. Bleeding can be evidenced by guaiac-positive stools and nasogastric aspirant, petechiae, or oozing from incisions. Partial thromboplastin studies should be evaluated regularly. Prolonged balloon deflation should be avoided because venous pooling occurs and stagnant blood predisposes the patient to clot formation. The balloon should never remain deflated for over 15 to 30 minutes. The risk of arterial trauma or dissection can be reduced by closely evaluating the peripheral vascular status before insertion. Obstruction to catheter passage in one femoral artery may necessitate the use of the opposite vessel. Force should never be used. Difficult insertion may be handled by using a smaller catheter or considering another approach, either directly into the iliac artery or the ascending aorta. Machine malfunction can occur but is highly unlikely because all current models have a sophisticated alarm system that will cause the machine to cease operation in the presence of unsafe pumping. If a machine malfunction does occur, a 20-ml syringe can be used for periodic quick inflation to prevent pooling and minimize clot formation.

Anstadt cup. The Anstadt cup is used to provide direct cardiac compression, therefore improving the force of contraction. This device is placed directly over the ventricles and pneumatically compresses the heart. Its current principal use is for the preservation of organs for transplantation because it necessitates a thoracotomy and can traumatize the myocardium.

External counterpulsation. External counterpulsation uses a noninvasive approach to temporarily assist circulation. Pressure is applied and released in synchrony with the cardiac cycle. Similar to the mechanism involved in the IABP, positive pressure is applied to the lower extremities during diastole to increase pressure within the arterial and venous circulations. The increase in arterial pressure is transferred in a retrograde manner to the aorta, thus elevating aortic diastolic pressure. Cardiac function improves in response to increased coronary blood flow and enhanced perfusion of collateral coronary vessels. The latter occurs as pressure changes open collateral channels for blood flow. Changes in venous circulation lead to an increased venous return and subsequent increase in preload be-

cause of the unidirectional valves in the peripheral venous vasculature. Cardiac output increases proportionally to the increased preload, according to Starling's law. The positive pressure is removed and negative pressure may be added during systole. Blood is displaced toward the periphery, thereby reducing the aortic volume and pressure. The reduction in the afterload decreases arterial resistance to ventricular ejection and reduces the work of the heart.

The mechanics of external counterpulsation are accomplished with a leg unit and control console. The leg unit serves as a pumping chamber and consists of two parallel cylindric leg cavities with plastic bladders filled with water (temperature 95° F, or 35° C) to obliterate the air space between the unit and the legs. Contoured leg padding can be added to fill in excessive space between the legs and leg unit. The control console contains the electronic and hydraulic controls, as well as an oscilloscopic display, recorder, and pressure module.

Counterpulsation is synchronized with the ECG. The R wave of the electrocardiogram is used as a triggering stimulus. The chest electrodes should be positioned to obtain maximal R-wave amplitude with minimal amplitude of all other waves. Both the ECG and the intra-arterial waveform are observed to adjust the timing and duration of leg pressure. The onset of diastolic augmentation must coincide with the dicrotic notch. Visual markers on the oscilloscopic display correlate the timing of pressurization with the cardiac cycle. The ECG visual marker should coincide with the end of the T wave, whereas the small arterial marker should coincide with the onset of the systolic upstroke and the large arterial marker with the dicrotic notch. Positive pressure up to 250 mmHg can be applied during diastole to raise the diastolic pressure by as much as 40% to 50%. Pressures of 150 to 180 mmHg are usually adequate and are best tolerated. During systole, the positive pressure is removed and negative pressure of up to −50 mmHg applied. A pressure blanket must be placed over the leg unit and lower torso if pressures less than atmospheric pressure are desired. This creates an airtight pumping seal so that pressure within the unit can be reduced.

External counterpulsation has been used so far in the treatment of patients with cardiogenic shock, severe chronic angina pectoris, and acute uncomplicated myocardial infarction. Its use in cardiogenic shock is still controversial. In patients with severe angina, it has provided relief and improved exercise tolerance; the latter improvement is probably related to the development of collateral channels. Currently, its value in salvaging the area of ischemia in an acute myocardial infarction is being evaluated.

The patient must be closely monitored throughout this procedure. Peripheral circulation should be checked before application of the leg unit and every hour thereafter. The patient's vital signs can be monitored frequently. Counterpulsation may result in a slight increase in the CVP and PAP because of the increased venous return. Long periods of pumping should be interrupted for short periods, if possible. Skin care can be carried out during this time, especially over pressure points. Foot and leg exercises should also be started at this time. Voiding of the bladder should be encouraged during the intervals of pumping interruption.

This form of counterpulsation is contraindicated in patients with insufficient aortic valves and peripheral arterial or venous disease. Although the noninvasive nature of this technique reduces the risk of complications, it has been associated with the development of systemic and pulmonary emboli and pulmonary edema.

External counterpressure. External counterpressure can be applied with an antigravity suit or G-suit, which is designed to minimize blood loss from intra-abdominal bleeding and redistribute intravascular volume to vital organs during hypotensive episodes. This mode of counterpressure is temporary and is used preoperatively, to control subdiaphragmatic bleeding until surgical intervention is possible, and postoperatively, to control hemorrhaging until the etiology can be determined and remedied. It has been used preoperatively in patients with ruptured abdominal aortic aneurysms or in those who have suffered massive trauma; it has been used postoperatively in patients with diffuse bleeding or clotting abnormalities.

The G-suit, consisting of double-layered clear plastic sheets, is placed beneath and above the patient, closed securely from bottom to top, and inflated with a noncombustible gas such as nitrogen or air. The amount of pressure is inversely proportional to the volume of gas. The suit is filled through a gas inflow tube connected to the gas source. It is removed via an outflow tube attached to a plastic chamber that is filled with distilled water to a predetermined level. The fluid level regulates the amount of pressure exerted by the G-suit by creating a resistance to gas outflow. The fluid chamber is calibrated in markings that indicate equivalents in torr (mmHg). Approximately 20 to 30 torr (mmHg) should be sufficient to achieve the desired effect. It is considered dangerous to use 40 torr (mmHg) or more. Pressure should be reduced gradually at a rate of about 5 torr (mmHg) every $\frac{1}{2}$ hour by removing fluid from the drainage port.

Continuous assessment of the patient's cardiovascular status must be maintained while the G-suit is being used. Vital signs and the peripheral circulatory status should be evaluated and recorded at least every 30 minutes. Arterial blood gases should be drawn before therapy and repeated every 15 to 30 minutes to monitor pulmonary status. Respiratory function also should be watched closely.

This procedure is associated with relatively few complications when used for short-term purposes. The G-suit does restrict chest and diaphragmatic movement. Atelectasis, pneumonia, and pulmonary edema have been reported resulting from reduction in the vital capacity, immobilization, and fluid redistribution. These problems can be minimized by positive-pressure assisted ventilation. Skin necrosis or blistering can also occur because of the unremitting local pressure.

Left-heart assist devices. Left-heart devices are designed to provide temporary mechanical support for the failing ventricle, allowing it additional time to recover. These devices have been used in patients who cannot be weaned from cardiopulmonary bypass after cardiac surgery despite intra-aortic balloon support, positive inotropic drug therapy, and pacing and in patients in whom a satisfactory cardiac output cannot be maintained during the initial 24 hours following surgery. The devices divert oxygenated blood from either the left atrium or left ventricle through the assist device back to the aorta, thereby reducing the preload and the volume work of the heart and augmenting total systemic blood flow. Currently, there are two types of left-heart-assist devices being used. The left atrial-arterial bypass unit is being used at Mt. Sinai in New York under the direction of Dr. Robert S. Litwak. The left ventricular-arterial bypass unit is being used by Dr. William Bernhard at Children's Hospital in Boston, Dr. John Norman at the Texas Heart Institute, and Dr. William C. Pierce at Hershey Medical Center in Pennsylvania.

The left-heart-assist device used by Dr. Litwak and his associates, the left arial-arterial unit, consists of two internal cannulas, inserted into the left atrium and ascending aorta, connected to an extracorporeal tubing loop and calibrated roller pump. The distal ends of the cannulas cross the mediastinum and diaphragm and terminate in the subcutaneous tissue of the right upper abdominal quadrant. The roller pump is affixed to the abdominal wall and is connected to a central console.

Left atrial-arterial units can shunt approximately 25% to 50% (up to 5 liters) of the total systemic blood flow around the left ventricle, thus providing conditions more favorable for left ventricular recovery. Hemodynamic stability occurs promptly as the bypass unit reduces left ventricular preload while continuing to maintain adequate peripheral arterial pressures. Some units can also reduce afterload with a pulsatile flow. The unit is synchronized with the cardiac cycle to fill during ventricular systole and to divert blood into the arterial circuit during diastole. These units necessitate the use of cannulas with larger diameters, creating a potential problem of insertion in patients with multiple bypass grafts and aortic valve replacement. Most commonly used is the system that provides a nonpulsatile flow. Blood return to the arterial system is continuous throughout both systole and diastole. As a result, afterload is increased because the left ventricle must eject against the resistance produced by the continuous flow of blood.

Management of the patient undergoing left ventricular bypass requires continuous observation. Routine hemodynamic, physiologic and hematologic parameters are measured. The flow rate is adjusted according to the total systemic blood flow (left ventricular output plus left-heart-assist device flow) and the left ventricular filling pressures. The thermodilution method is used to measure total systemic blood flow. The flow rate is manipulated to maintain total systemic blood flow at approximately 2.5 L/min/ square m, with mean left atrial pressures below 20 torr (mmHg). Satisfactory urine output is also used as a guide. Discontinuance is considered when the flow rate has been reduced to 500 ml/min or less. The flow through the left-heart-assist device is gradually reduced. Once the weaning process is completed and separation is possible, the subcutaneous distal ends of the cannulas are exposed and completely obliterated with angular obturators, using a small right subcostal incision while the patient is under local anesthesia. Thus, reentry into the thorax is unnecessary, and general anesthesia is avoided. The cannulas are subsequently buried *in situ*. The design of the cannulas and obturator minimizes the risk of thromboembolism from stagnant blood and infection. Maintenance anticoagulation is continued throughout therapy.

Eligibility for left atrial-arterial assist is determined by failure to withstand separation from cardiopulmonary bypass despite adjuvant therapy including drugs, pacing, and intraaortic balloon counterpulsation, whenever possible. At Mt. Sinai, patients must also exhibit an elevated left ventricular filling pressure (left atrial pressure greater than 25 mmHg), systemic hypotension (systolic pressure under 90 mmHg), and visibly impaired contractility in the left ventricle.

The left ventricular-arterial assist devices also provide temporary mechanical circulatory support for patients who cannot be weaned from cardiopulmonary bypass. The intracorporeal device used by Dr. John C. Norman is implanted within the abdomen and diverts blood from the left ventricle into the descending thoracic aorta. Because of its position, removal of the device can be accomplished without a thoracotomy. Referred to as an auxiliary left ventricle, it is capable of delivering a unidirectional flow up to 6 L/min, assuming over 80% of total cardiac work. Units designed by Dr. Bernhard and Dr. Pierce are extracorporeal devices. Dr. Bernhard uses an external unit secured to the right anterolateral chest with an inflow tube at the left ventricular apex and the outflow tube sutured to the ascending aorta. Dr. Pierce uses an external pump attached to the left ventricular apex and the thoracic aorta.[10,110] One of several modes is used. A low-rate asynchronous mode (35 to 45 beats/min) is used during the initiation of assistance and in the recovery period when only partial assistance is necessary. Asynchronous pumping at a rate of 45 to 140 beats/min has been used routinely for long-term assistance during experimentation. A stable ECG is not necessary because there is no synchronization. Synchronous counterpulsation is accomplished using the synchronous counterpulsation mode at 20 to 140 beats/min or the intermittent synchronous counterpulsation mode at a ratio of 1:1, 1:2, . . . 1:10, and so on. The intermittent mode is used during recovery for weaning. The R wave of the ECG is used as the triggering stimulus. Filling occurs during left ventricular systole, whereas ejection takes place during left ventricular diastole. Consequently, left ventricular work is reduced, myocardial oxygen consumption is decreased, and diastolic systemic perfusion is increased with this counterpulsation technique. Preload and afterload reduction permits maximal "resting" of the heart. The weaning process is begun after test periods reveal that satisfactory left ventricular function has returned. This is evidenced by mechanical recovery (linear increase in left ventricular pressure, flow, and work generation) and electrical recovery (decreases in QRS duration). The unit is removed within 14 to 30 days, with the inflow and outflow tubes remaining *in situ*.

As with left atrial-arterial assist, indications for left ventricular-arterial circulatory assistance include (1) failure to withstand removal from cardiopulmonary bypass despite adjuvant therapy, including drugs and the intra-aortic balloon pump; and (2) persistent low output states, even with balloon support.

The ultimate success of these devices depends on the degree of reversibility of the failing ventricle.

Pharmacologic agents that alter blood pressure

An arsenal of drugs is available today to prevent the sequelae associated with acute hypertensive and hypotensive disorders. The mode of action of the antihypertensive agents varies greatly. Some act to block alpha-adrenergic receptors and to antagonize circulating catecholamines (alpha-adrenergic blocking agents). Others bind to the beta receptors, thereby inhibiting the beta response (beta-adrenergic blocking agents). Still others exert their effect centrally, inhibiting sympathetic outflow, or directly on the peripheral vascular system.

Drugs used to treat hypotensive states are sympathomimetic, simulating the effects of sympathetic nerve stimulation. Three types of receptors are stimulated: alpha-adrenergic, beta-adrenergic, and dopaminergic. The antihypotensive agents stimulate alpha receptors that reside primarily in the resistance vessels of the skin, mucosa, intestines, and kidneys. Some of them also affect beta receptors, but when used to ameliorate low blood pressure, the alpha effect is dominant.

Alpha-adrenergic blocking agents

Alpha-adrenergic blockers bind to the alpha receptors, thereby inhibiting excitatory responses mediated by epinephrine and norepinephrine. This leads to vasodilation of the vascular beds, reducing the peripheral vascular resistance and the afterload.

Prazosin hydrochloride.[51] Prazosin hydrochloride (Minipress) is both an arterial and venous dilator that seems to act predominantly as an alpha-adrenergic blocking agent on the vascular smooth muscle. Its hemodynamic effects are similar to those of nitroprusside. Prazosin decreases the afterload, making it advantageous in the treatment of mild to moderate hypertension. Cardiac output, heart rate, glomerula, filtration rate, and renal blood flow remain unaltered. Plasma renin activity is unchanged, but peripheral vascular resistance is reduced. Prazosin is also being used in the treatment of severe chronic congestive heart failure in adults. The effects of prazosin begin within 2 hours after therapy is instituted and last for 24 hours after administration is discontinued. The dose recommended for pediatric therapy is being evaluated.

The toxic effects of prazosin include lethargy, lightheadedness, headache, mild nausea, and syncope.

Phenoxybenzamine.[28,75] Phenoxybenzamine (Dibenzyline) is an alphalytic agent. It reduces sympathetic tone, leading to an increased blood flow to the kidneys, viscera, and skeletal muscles. Blood flow to the brain and coronary vessels is unchanged.

Clinically, phenoxybenzamine is used to reverse pressor responses resulting from sympathomimetic amines. It increases vasodilatation, being useful in the presence of emboli, hypertension, and pulmonary congestion or edema. In patients with cardiogenic shock, it may counteract some of the effects of alpha-adrenergic stimulating agents.

The administration of phenoxybenzamine may result in production of significant hypotension with a reflex tachycardia. This occurs during standing (postural hypotension) and may be especially dangerous in hypovolemic patients. The hypotensive effects of narcotics may be magnified during phenoxybenzamine therapy because compensatory vasoconstriction is blocked. Miosis, nasal congestion, sedation, weakness, inhibition of ejaculation, and nausea and vomiting may develop.

Phentolamine (Regitine) is another alpha-adrenergic blocker with effects similar to phenoxybenzamine.

Beta-adrenergic blocking agents[42-45,76,89]

Beta-adrenergic blockers (Table 2-17) constitute a group of pharmacologic agents that are antagonistic to beta-adrenoreceptors in the heart. These drugs can produce wide-ranging effects because stimulation of beta receptors increases contractility and heart rate and accelerates AV conduction, and stimulation of beta receptors leads to bronchial relaxation and vasodilation in peripheral arterioles.

In addition to inhibiting the beta response, some beta blockers also stimulate the receptor. This partial agonist activity is referred to as *intrinsic sympathomimetic activity (ISA)* and results in reduced lowering of the heart rate, lessening the risk of excessive bradycardia.

Beta blockers are *selective* or *nonselective* depending on their ability to antagonize beta receptors in some tissues at lower doses than others. Cardioselective beta blockers inhibit beta-1 receptors but have little influence on bronchial and vascular beta receptors. Such agents would therefore be safe and valuable for patients with bronchial asthma and hypertension.

Clinically, beta blockers are used in the treatment of angina and hypertension. The exact mechanism by which these drugs reduce blood pressure is still being studied. Most likely, they slow the heart rate and decrease myocardial contractility, leading to a decrease in cardiac output that ultimately results in a reduction in blood pressure. Therefore their value is greatest in hy-

Table 2-17. Beta-adrenoreceptor blocking agents: pharmacologic and pharmacodynamic properties

Drug	Synonyms	Beta-blockade potency ratio (propranolol-1)	Cardioselectivity*	Partial agonist activity	Membrane stabilizing activity
Acebutolol	Sectral	0.3	+	+	+
Alprenolol	Aptin‡	0.3	0	+ +	+
	Betaptin‡				
	Betacard‡				
Atenolol	Tenormin	1	+	0	0
Metoprolol	Lopresor	1	+	0	±
	Betaloc‡				
Oxprenolol	Trasicor‡	0.5-1	0	+ +	+
Pindolol	Visken	6	0	+ + +	+
Practolol	Eraldin‡	0.3	+	+ +	0
Propranolol	Inderal	1	0	0	+ +
Sotalol	Betacardone‡	0.3	0	0	0
	Sotacor‡				
Timolol	Blocadren	6	0	±	0
Isomer: d-propranolol		0.1	0	0	+ +

Modified from Frishman, W.: Clinical pharmacology of the new beta-adrenergic blocking drugs. Part I. Pharmacodynamic and new beta-adrenergic blocking drugs. Part II. Physiologic and metabolic effects, American Heart Journal, 97(6):797, 1979.
*Cardioselectivity of certain beta blockers is only seen with low therapeutic concentrations of drugs. With higher concentrations,
†Effects of d-propranolol occur with doses in humans well above the therapeutic level. The isomer also lacks beta-blocking activity.
‡Not available in the United States.

pertension associated with a high output state. They do not lower peripheral vascular resistance, and although some do possess membrane stabilizing effects, this does not affect blood pressure. There is considerable controversy about the effects of beta blockers on plasma renin. Although it is known that these drugs can antagonize sympathetically mediated renin release, it is also generally accepted that there are other mechanisms that mediate renin release. Although questions still exist, some studies have shown that "high renin" patients respond to some beta blockers, whereas "low renin" patients do not. The response is less predictable with "normal" renin patients. There is also a question about the role of reduced plasma volume and venous return in the control of blood pressure by beta blockers; investigation continues in this area.

Central acting agents

Some pharmacologic agents exert a sympatholytic effect directly on the central nervous system. They may also act directly on the peripheral vascular system.

Clonidine (Catapres) is a newer antihypertensive agent that stimulates alpha-adrenergic receptors centrally, thereby decreasing sympathetic outflow from the central nervous system. Peripheral vascular resistance is also lowered, suggesting a peripheral affect. Clonidine reduces cardiac output, heart rate, and plasma renin activity while leaving the glomerular filtration rate and renal blood flow unchanged. It acts within 30 to 60 minutes after administration and persists for 6 to 8 hours after therapy is discontinued.[75]

Methyldopa (Aldomet) is an antihypertensive drug whose primary site of action is the brainstem, but it may act on the peripheral vascular system as well. The hypotensive effect of this drug can be seen within 4 to 6 hours after the institution of therapy. Its effect can persist for as long as 24 hours after administration. Because cardiac output, heart rate, glomerular fil-

and cardiac effects

Resting heart rate	Rate of heart rate increment in response to exercise	Myocardial contractility	Resting blood pressure	Resting atrioventricular conduction	Antiarrhythmic effect
↓	↓	↓	↓	↓	+
↓ ↔	+	↓ ↔	↓	↓ ↔	+
↓	↓	↓	↓	↓	+
↓	↓	↓	↓	↓	+
↓ ↔	↓	↓ ↔	↓	↓ ↔	+
↓ ↔	↓	↓ ↔	↓	↓ ↔	+
↓ ↔	↓	↓ ↔	↓	↓ ↔	+
↓	↓	↓	↓	↓	+
↓	↓	↓	↓	↓	+
↓	↓	↓	↓	↓	+
↔	↔	↔ ↓ +	↔	↔ ↓ +	+ − +

pharmacokinetic properties, American Heart Journal **97**(5):663, 1979; and Frishman, W., and Silverman, R.: Clinical pharmacology of the

cardioselectivity is not seen.

tration rate, and renal blood flow are unaffected, methyldopa is useful in the treatment of moderate to severe hypertension in patients with coronary artery disease or congestive heart failure or in the presence of impaired renal function. Methyldopa should not be given to patients with pheochromocytoma because it interferes with urinary catecholamine excretion; nor should it be given to patients with hepatic disease or hemolytic anemia.[51]

Unloading agents (vasodilating agents)

Drugs that decrease the blood pressure by direct relaxation of vascular smooth muscle are referred to as *vasodilators*. Their effect is similar to alpha-adrenergic blockers, but the mechanism differs. These drugs also decrease afterload and/or preload.

Nitroglycerin[51,52]

Nitroglycerin, or glyceryl trinitrate (Nitroglyn) is a rapid-acting nitrate that dilates arterial and venous smooth muscle. It reduces myocardial oxygen requirements by decreasing the preload and afterload. Preload is reduced by dilating the venous capitance vessels, thereby decreasing venous resistance and venous return to the heart. As previously discussed, the ventricular end-diastolic pressure and volume is reduced, as is oxygen consumption. Afterload is reduced by decreasing the peripheral arteriolar resistance and reducing the ventricular work. This also decreases the myocardial consumption of oxygen. Nitroglycerin also increases collateral coronary flow, thus increasing myocardial oxygen in the ischemic areas of the myocardium. The increased collateral coronary flow occurs either by creating a selective vasodilation of collateral vessels bypassing constricted regions or by altering the mechanical factors exerted on them to reduce their resistance to flow.

Clinically, nitroglycerin is used in the treatment of heart failure because it reduces the preload and afterload. It also increases the ejection fraction, stroke volume, and ultimately the cardiac output. By decreasing the peripheral vascular resistance, the intrinsic adrenergic response that raises the peripheral vascular resistance in the filling heart is reversed to allow perfusion of vital organs. This latter effect is temporary and protective only to a certain degree because it does not correct the underlying problem. Although it has no direct effect on the inotropic or chronotropic state of the heart, nitroglycerin is particularly useful when conventional therapy fails. It is also beneficial in the treatment of angina pectoris, either because of its effect on collateral coronary circulation or its role in reducing the oxygen requirements of the myocardium. It does not relieve the pain of acute myocardial infarction; in addition, it should be used cautiously in the presence of a myocardial infarction because studies have shown that it can cause hypotension and actually decrease coronary blood flow.

Nitroglycerin can be administered sublingually, orally, topically, or intravenously. The sublingual approach is avoided in the treatment of heart failure because its effects are so short lasting.

The most common side effect associated with the use of nitroglycerin is the development of a headache that can be severe. Although it usually diminishes in a few days if treatment is continued, the headache's severity can also be controlled by decreasing the dosage. Transient dizziness and weakness may also occur and are usually attributed to the postural hypotension that may develop.

Hydralazine[51]

Hydralazine (Apresoline, Rolazine, Dralzine) is a potent vasodilator that directly relaxes the vascular smooth muscle. Peripheral vascular resistance is decreased, whereas the heart rate, stroke volume, and cardiac output are increased. Coronary, cerebral, renal, and hepatic blood flow are increased unless the fall in blood pressure is extreme.

Because it is an afterload reducer, hydralazine is used clinically in the treatment of congestive heart failure and hypertension.

Sodium nitroprusside[28,51,75]

Sodium nitroprusside (Nipride) is a potent vasodilator that relaxes both arteriolar and venous smooth muscle, thereby decreasing both preload and afterload. Normally its administration is associated with an increase in heart rate and a mild reduction in peripheral vascular resistance. A decrease in cardiac output occurs except in myocardial disease, in which cardiac output and stroke volume increase with the administration of nitroprusside. Renal blood flow and glomerular filtration are maintained. Anginal pain often improves with nitroprusside therapy.

Nitroprusside is used in the treatment of acute heart failure in the presence of myocardial infarction, in heart failure associated with mitral valve disease, and in chronic heart failure secondary to myocardial disease. It can be used in conjunction with digitalis therapy with additive effects. It is most beneficial when the left atrial and pulmonary pressures are elevated, but it may be detrimental if used in the presence of normal or reduced left ventricular filling pressures. Nitroprusside is also valuable in hypertensive emergencies.

Administration of nitroprusside is done intravenously. The onset of action occurs within 30 to 60 seconds after the infusion is started, and the effects of the drug are dissipated as the infusion is discontinued. The recommended dosage ranges from 1 to 10 mg/kg/min and is increased until the pulmonary artery wedge pressure or mean arterial pressure declines. An infusion pump should be used to ensure a precise flow. Continuous monitoring of the patient's blood pressure and pulmonary artery wedge pressure is essential.

Toxic symptoms occurring with nitroprusside therapy can be attributed to excessive vasodilation and hypotension and include sweating, restlessness, headache, palpitations, and substernal discomfort.

Sympathomimetic agents

As mentioned previously, sympathomimetics simulate sympathetic nerve stimulation. These drugs have both alpha and beta effects, but the alpha effects are what make them useful in the treatment of hypotensive emergencies.

Dopamine[51,75]

Dopamine (Intropin) is a chemical precursor of norepenephrine with both alpha- and beta-receptor stimulating actions (Table 2-16). Its alpha-adrenergic stimulating effect produces mild vasoconstriction, primarily in the skeletal muscle. Its beta-adrenergic-receptor stimulating action results in an increase in myoardial contractility. Dopamine also dilates renal and mesenteric blood vessels, increasing the blood flow to these regions. Dopamine is used clinically in shock and congestive heart failure to correct the hemodynamic imbalance. It causes diuresis and natriuresis in patients with congestive heart failure. Dopamine can be useful when digitalis is contraindicated. It is also more advantageous than isoproterenol when peripheral vascular resistance is low because dopamine will increase the peripheral vascular resistance. Oxygen consumption is less with dopamine than with isoproterenol, and the tachydysrhythmias associated with isoproterenol therapy are usually avoided.

Dopamine may cause ectopic dysrhythmias. It may also be associated with anginal pain, dyspnea, headache, hypotension, and nausea and vomiting. It is contraindicated in patients with uncontrolled dysrhythmias, those receiving monoamine oxidase inhibitors because they potentiate its effect, or those who have a pheochromocytoma. Low volume should be corrected before initiating dopamine therapy. Therapy should be tapered gradually, not terminated abruptly.

Dobutamine[51,75]

Dobutamine (Dobutrex) is a synthetic sympathomimetic that was developed by modifying the chemical structure of isoproterenol to avoid some of the side effects of the latter. Dobutamine stimulates beta-adrenergic cardiac receptors, thereby increasing the contractile force of the myocardium. It produces little systemic arterial constriction, making it superior to norepinephrine and dopamine in this regard. Dobutamine is used in the management of refractory pump failure and is intended only for short-term use. This drug is particularly successful in reversing pump failure when it is caused by temporary depression of ventricular function and myocardial contractility.

Clinically, metaraminol is a first-line drug when immediate blood pressure elevation is desired. It is used frequently in the treatment of hypotensive states and has also been effective in terminating supraventricular tachycardias by reflex vagal stimulation.

Mephentermine[51,75]

Mephentermine (Wyamine) is a sympathomimetic drug that primarily stimulates beta-adrenergic receptors but also has a weak alpha-adrenergic effect. It acts almost totally by release of norepinephrine (indirect), as does metaraminol. Mephentermine increases peripheral resistance in normal patients but may decrease resistance or exert no effect in hypotensive patients. Centrally, it increases the force of cardiac contraction and may lead to an increased cardiac output. It is used principally in the treatment of hypotensive states.

Mephentermine is given parenterally, as a single dose intramuscularly, intravenously, or in a slow intravenous infusion titrated to achieve the desired effect. The most common side effects associated with mephentermine therapy include ventricular tachydysrhythmias. Hypotension may occur in the presence of hypovolemia. Headache, flushing of the skin, nausea, dizziness, weakness, and diaphoresis have also been reported.

Methoxamine[51,75]

Methoxamine (Vasoxyl) is a sympathomimetic drug that stimulates alpha-adrenergic

Table 2-18. Actions of long-acting nitrates for anginal therapy

Name	Trade name	Effects		Formulation	Route	Side effects
		Physiologic	Therapeutic			
Isosorbide dinitrate	Isordil Sorbitrate	Relaxes vascular smooth muscle	Decreases venous return	Sublingual tablets* Tablets and capsules	SL PO	Headache Flushing Tachycardia Dizziness Postural hypotension
Pentaerythritol tetranitrate	Peritrate	Dilates arterioles; reduces peripheral vascular resistance	Decreases blood pressure; decreases net myocardial oxygen consumption	Oral*	PO	
Erythrityl tetranitrate	Cardilate	Reflex tachycardia		Oral, sublingual, and chewable tablets	SL or PO	Possibly causes tachyphylaxis to nitroglycerin with prolonged use

Modified from Braunwald E.: Heart disease, a textbook of cardiovascular medicine, ed. 2, Philadelphia, 1984, W.B. Saunders Co.
*Also available as sustained action tablets; efficacy not well documented.

Table 2-19. Actions of nitroglycerin for anginal therapy

Name	Trade name	Effects		Formulation	Route	Side effects
		Physiologic	Therapeutic			
Glyceryl trinitrate	Nitrostat	Relaxes vascular smooth muscle	Decreases venous return	Sublingual tablets	SL	Headache Flushing Tachycardia Dizziness Postural hypotension
	Nitro-Bid	Dilates arterioles	Decreases blood pressure	Sustained-release capsules	PO	
	Nitroglyn	Reduces peripheral vascular resistance	Decreases net myocardial oxygen consumption	Sustained-action tablets	PO	
	Nitrospan	Reduces mean arterial pressure		Sustained-release microdialysis cells	PO	
	Nitrol ointment			Lanolin, petrolatum	Topically	

Modified from Braunwald, E.: Heart disease, a textbook of cardiovascular medicine, ed. 2, Philadelphia, 1984, W.B. Saunders Co.

receptors. Consequently it affects only the peripheral vasculature, producing peripheral vasoconstriction. Arterial resistance and arterial pressure are increased, whereas venous return is decreased. Methoxamine is used to raise the blood pressure rapidly and is thus effective in reversing hypotension caused by the use of ganglionic-blocking agents. It is also used in the treatment of patients in shock, who develop a low peripheral resistance while maintaining a normal or elevated cardiac output. Methoxamine may also be used to terminate paroxysmal atrial tachycardia by reflex vagal stimulation.

Side effects associated with an excessive dosage of methoxamine include headache, pilomotor stimulation, and projectile vomiting. Prolonged therapy may cause reduced plasma volume, evidenced by an elevation in the hematocrit.

Phenylephrine (Neo-synephrine) is also an alphamimetic adrenergic agent with actions similar to those produced by methoxamine. Phenylephrine may cause a marked reflex bradycardia. It should be used with caution in patients with hyperthyroidism, bradydysrhythmias, heart block, or myocardial disease.

Miscellaneous agents

Diazoxide.[51] Diazoxide is useful in the reduction of systemic vascular resistance. It is most effective in combination with a "loop" diuretic that decreases sodium excretion. Diazoxide is effective within a short period of time and will usually maintain reduced pressure for several hours.

Pharmacologic agents that alter coronary blood flow: nitrates and nitrites.[28,51,104] Nitrates and nitrites relax most smooth muscles, including those in the circulatory system. This relaxation produces a generalized vasodilation, although the effect on the venous system is more profound. Venodilation decreases venous return to the heart and reduces ventricular filling pressure.[104] Systemic arterial resistance is reduced to some degree because of the influence of these drugs on the arteriolar bed. The beneficial effect

of nitrates and nitrites in the relief of anginal pain has traditionally been attributed to their role as vasodilators. However, it has become evident that coronary vessels with atheromatous plaques are not likely to dilate in response to these drugs. In addition, branches distal to an obstruction are already maximally dilated because ischemia is present.[28]* Therefore the value of nitrate or nitrite therapy is thought to lie in its reduction in myocardial wall tension as a result of an increase in the venous capacitance bed, which lowers myocardial filling pressures.[52] This effect may occur in the absence of changes in peripheral arteriolar resistance and with minimal or no change in the cardiac index.[28]

A number of different nitrate preparations are available. Long-acting nitrates are of value in the treatment of angina pectoris, especially in the presence of unstable patterns.[29] They are of little benefit in the relief of acute attacks. These drugs may be administered orally or applied externally as a sustained release ointment.

Rapid-acting nitrates are indicated in the treatment of acute anginal pain. They may be administered intravenously or sublingually. Because some parenteral preparations are absorbed into plastic, a nonabsorbing intravenous system should be used. Sublingual preparations are absorbed directly into the system; they are effective within 1 to 3 minutes and persist for 20 to 30 minutes. The dosage may be repeated in 3 to 5 minutes if pain continues, and evaluation is necessary if the pain doesn't subside after 3 doses. Tables 2-18 and 2-19 summarize some nitrate compounds currently used along with their most common side effects.

Beta-adrenergic blocking agents.[28,56,89] Beta-adrenergic blockers are useful in the treatment of effort-induced chronic stable angina.[28] These drugs appear to reduce the frequency of anginal episodes and to raise the anginal threshold via competitive inhibition of neuronally released and circulating catecholamines.[56,89] These drugs,

---

*Prinzmetal's angina, or variant angina producing coronary artery spasm, does appear to be relieved by vasodilator therapy.[28]

which are extremely useful in treating hypertension, are described in Table 2-17.

Adverse effects associated with beta-blocking drugs include fatigue, mental depression, gastrointestinal upset, intensification of insulin-induced hypoglycemia, cutaneous reactions, bronchoconstriction, and heart block.[76,104] These drugs may precipitate or intensify congestive heart failure in the patient with impaired left ventricular function. They are contraindicated in bradydysrhythmias unless a pacemaker has been inserted.[29]

Calcium-channel blockers.[5,19,77,115,126,130,135] Calcium channel blockers are of value in the treatment of vasospastic and stable (effort-induced) angina, either alone or in combination with nitrate therapy and beta-blocking agents.[19,77,126,135] Their effectiveness in abolishing or reducing attacks of angina at rest can be attributed to their potency as coronary artery dilators.[19] In addition, these drugs have often been shown to eliminate the life-threatening ventricular tachydysrhythmias that accompany ischemic episodes.[5,19] The beneficial effects of calcium antagonists in stable angina are multifactorial. These drugs appear to augment the supply of oxygen to the myocardium by increasing coronary blood flow. There is dilation of the coronary arteries and improved subendocardial perfusion with all of these agents.[19] Calcium channel blockers also reduce myocardial oxygen demand. All agents decrease peripheral vascular resistance, reducing afterload,[19,130,135] whereas verapamil decreases myocardial contractility, and verapamil and diltiazem reduce the heart rate.[19,115,130,135] When used in conjunction with beta blockers and nitrate to treat chronic stable angina, calcium antagonists reduce the dosage amounts of the aforementioned agents that are needed to control pain.[19]

Verapamil and diltiazem are contraindicated in sick-sinus syndrome with bradycardia in the absence of a pacemaker.[115] Both drugs should be used with great caution in second- and third-degree AV block and left ventricular dysfunction.[19] Nifedipine should be avoided in hypotensive patients.[19]

Side effects associated with the use of verapamil and diltiazem include nausea, constipation, dizziness, fatigue, headache, and skin rashes.[115] Adverse effects of nifedipine therapy are hypotension, flushing, and headache.[19]

Pharmacologic agents that may protect the ischemic myocardium

Glucose-insulin-potassium infusion. The administration of a solution consisting of glucose, insulin, and potassium is a controversial metabolic therapy. Proponents of this infusion suggest that it may decrease infarct size and increase survival changes.[61,118] The infusion of glucose provides additional fuel because glycogen stores are rapidly depleted in ischemic areas. Ionic gradients are restored with potassium, thereby reducing the frequency of premature ventricular beats.[117] The solution also lowers the concentration of free fatty acids by inhibiting intracellular lipolysis. As a result, free fatty acids are esterified, and triglyceride stores are increased. Ventricular performance improves because of increased myocardial perfusion and enhanced contractility.[117]

Streptokinase infusion. Streptokinase is an enzyme that activates plasmin, a fibrinolytic agent that causes dissolution of fibrin. Intracoronary streptokinase infusion has been successful in reestablishing coronary blood flow at the site of vascular occlusion.[119] The procedure is contraindicated if previous surgery has taken place within 10 days; if the patient has experienced a cerebral vascular accident in the past, a CPR trauma, subacute infective endocarditis, or significant valvular disease; or if there is a risk of hemorrhage. Additional research is necessary to evaluate the effectiveness of this therapy.

Corticosteroids. The administration of a single large dose of methylprednisolone has been shown to decrease infarct size according to enzymatic measurement, whereas multiple doses appear to have the opposite effect. Further study is required to determine whether a single large dose could reduce the size of an infarct without interfering with its healing.[83]

REHABILITATION IN CARDIOVASCULAR DISEASE

Rehabilitation of the cardiac patient begins once the vital signs are stabilized and the imminent threat of death is removed. The goals of rehabilitative efforts are to restore the patient to an optimal level of medical, psychologic, physiologic, sociologic, vocational, and recreational well-being and to prevent further complications of the disease process. These goals are accomplished with both inpatient and outpatient programs that use a multidisciplinary approach. Physician-directed rehabilitation programs use the services of a cardiac rehabilitation nurse, an exercise specialist, a dietitian, a physical therapist, an occupational therapist, and a psychiatric social worker to help manage patients and their families in the rehabilitative process. Currently, the basis of most cardiac rehabilitation consists of education and behavioral modification programs and reconditioning exercise activities designed to enhance the quality and quantity of life for patients with known cardiovascular disorders or for patients who are at risk of developing cardiac diseases. Therefore the goals of these programs are both restorative and preventive.

Early interventions have been successful in reducing some of the complications associated with bedrest and inactivity. Structural teaching begins in an effort to educate patients about their disease process. Carefully supervised exercise programs are instituted and gradually intensified during convalescence. Conclusion of inpatient rehabilitative efforts coincides with the patient's discharge from the hospital. At that point, outpatient programs are initiated and continue the rehabilitation process.

Educational programs are designed to enlighten patients and their family members about the disease process and to assist them in developing realistic expectations in regard to long-term physical and psychologic adjustment. Programs are individualized to meet patient and family needs and are implemented only after a complete assessment of their readiness to learn has been made. Inpatient programs are initially of short duration (approximately 15 to 20 minutes) to avoid tiring the patient. They may be carried out informally with patients alone or with patients and their families or may be more structured, such as those consisting of group classes. More structured programs are most often implemented during the recovery phase, after the patient has been transferred from the critical care unit. Outpatient classes are usually aimed at modifying life-styles. The information presented during informal and formal programs should be reinforced and repeated throughout the inpatient phase and later during the outpatient phase so that it can be incorporated into the patient's daily life. Topics traditionally covered include anatomy and physiology of the heart, the nature of coronary artery disease and myocardial infarction, risk factors for coronary artery disease, the healing process, medications, dietary restrictions, sexual activity, resumption of work, and prudent heart living.

An understanding of basic cardiovascular anatomy and physiology is necessary for patients to understand their disease process. Included in the review should be an explanation of the conduction system and its role in the origin of the heartbeat, as well as a discussion of the pumping mechanism of the heart. In addition, the coronary arteries can be located, and a description of their relationship with the heart muscle can be provided. An explanation of "normal" helps patients understand their own problems when a description of their disease process is given.

Drug regimens should be reviewed and must be thoroughly understood by patients to ensure their adherence to the plan. Implicit in this is the need to explain the purpose of a drug, as well as the side effects and symptoms of toxicity that can occur with overdosage.

A discussion of any modifications that must

be made in eating habits is vital. Dietary restrictions are often difficult to institute because they are confusing, often make food tasteless, and are hard to follow. A review of the rationale behind such limitations may enlist patient support. Sodium restriction may be ordered; sodium-restricted diets are implemented to decrease extracellular fluid retention by reducing the amount of free-floating sodium. The degree of modification varies and is dictated by the patient's condition. Patients need to know just what a "low-sodium" diet means. Sodium restrictions may be mild (eliminate the use of table salt alone or eliminate both table salt and salt in cooking), moderate (approximately 3 g of sodium/day), or severe (250 mg to 1 g of sodium/day). Because sodium-restricted diets may be unpalatable, patients may find meals and cooking distasteful and boring. Instructions can be given regarding the use of salt substitutes, flavorings, spices, and herbs, all of which can be used to make food more palatable and hopefully to facilitate adherence to dietary modifications. Questions about adhering to sodium restrictions outside the home can be answered by providing patients with a list of the sodium content of commercially prepared foods.

Fat-restricted diets may also be necessary. These restrictions are usually implemented after a coronary profile reveals an elevation in the serum cholesterol or triglyceride level. Cholesterol is a fat component that combines in the blood with lipoproteins. Low-density lipoproteins carry the cholesterol to peripheral tissue such as the arterial wall, where atheromatous plaques accumulate and occlude the arterial lumen. The plaques are formed from cells overburdened with cholesterol, which either die and leave collections of fat in the tissue or produce scar tissue after dividing at an increased rate. High-density lipoproteins, on the other hand, carry the cholesterol away from the tissue. Hypercholesterolemia has been associated with a greater risk of developing coronary heart disease, a process that begins in infancy. Therefore modifying the diet to reduce the risk is hoped to be advantageous.

Triglycerides are another form of serum lipids that can possibly influence atheromatous plaque formation. They also are apparently carried by the very-low-density lipoproteins in the bloodstream to the peripheral tissue. Although the influence of triglycerides is still controversial, many physicians suggest efforts to reduce the serum triglyceride level to their patients.

Dietary modifications that can be used to reduce the serum cholesterol and triglyceride levels have been suggested by the Select Committee on Nutrition and Human Needs of the United States Senate and include the following:

1. A reduction in the consumption of fat to 30% of the total caloric intake.
2. A reduction in the consumption of saturated fat to 10% of the total caloric intake.
3. A balance between the monounsaturated and polyunsaturated fats consisting of 10% (each) of the total caloric intake.
4. A reduction in the cholesterol intake to 300 mg/day.
5. An increase in the consumption of complex carbohydrates to 48% of the total caloric intake.
6. A reduction in the consumption of sugar to 10% of the total caloric intake.

Information about sexual activity should not be neglected. Often patients develop many fears and misconceptions about sex and cardiovascular problems. The goal of sexual counseling in patients with cardiovascular disease is to educate both partners about the physiologic and psychologic factors associated with sexual activity. The counselor helps to alleviate fears and correct erroneous ideas, enabling patients to make informed decisions regarding sexual activity.

Avoidance of discussions about sex can increase the patient's anxiety. Patients often feel that sexual activity must be restricted with known cardiovascular disease or that sexual function will be inadequate. They may be reluctant to discuss their fears. Discussions can help, and they should begin with a general description of the physiologic and psychologic variables associated with sexual intercourse. General information can be given about the changes that take place during sexual activity, and comparisons can be made between the energy expended during sexual intercourse and normal work activity. Individual histories can be reviewed, and information about the effects of a specific disease process or therapeutic intervention can be clarified. The influence of medications on sexual activity should be explored. In general, however, it should be pointed out that sexual activity can be safely resumed (usually within 4 to 8 weeks after hospitalization) because the physiologic demands of coitus on the cardiovascular system can usually be met safely.

Discussions about the prevention of further cardiovascular damage can be helpful. Patients need to be made aware of what factors make them at risk for developing cardiovascular disease and specifically what they can do about them. Table 2-20 lists the risk factors associated with the development of coronary heart disease and describes what modifications can be made to help control them.

Exercise programs are implemented during rehabilitation to improve the efficiency of the heart muscle and to improve oxygen extraction. Current evidence suggests that exercise regimens also enhance the development of collateral circulation; increase coronary blood flow; and, in the postsurgical bypass patient, reduce stagnation of blood, hopefully helping to keep coronary artery grafts patent.

Controversy exists about when to introduce exercise into the recovery process. In many areas, inpatient programs are begun as soon as the patient is stabilized. Postinfarction patients and postoperative bypass patients are encouraged to participate in their own care as early as 24 to 48 hours after their infarct, or surgery, beginning with low-level exercises. Most exercise programs introduce the concept of metabolic energy expenditures (METs) to describe the energy expenditure per minute per kilogram of body weight for varied activities. The exercise routine includes passive and active exercises per-

Table 2-20. Risk factors associated with coronary heart disease

Risk factors	Therapeutic interventions
PRIMARY RISK FACTORS*	
Heredity	
Hypercholesterolemia	Dietary modification
Hypertension	Dietary modification
	Pharmacologic agents
Cigarette smoking	Behavioral modification
SECONDARY RISK FACTORS	
Hyperlipidemia†	Dietary modification
	Pharmacologic agents
Diabetes mellitus	Dietary modification
	Pharmacologic agents
Morbid obesity	Dietary modification
	Behavioral modification
Sedentary life-style	Exercise regimen
Sex	
Stress	Exercise regimen
	Biofeedback

*All controllable risk factors.
†Hyperlipidemias can be classified on the basis of lipoprotein concentrations as type I (↑ VLDL and LDL both normal and low - cholesterol, ↑↑ triglycerides); type IIA (↑LDL, VLDL normal - ↑ cholesterol, triglycerides normal); type IIB (↑ LDL, ↑ VLDL - ↑ cholesterol, ↑ triglycerides); type III (abnormal cholesterol, enriched VLDL in excess - ↑ cholesterol, ↑ triglycerides); type IV (↑ VLDL, LDL normal - cholesterol normal, ↑ triglyceride); type V (↑ chylomicrons, ↑ VLDL, LDL normal or low; ↑ cholesterol, ↑↑ triglycerides).
‡Females have a lower incidence of coronary heart disease before menopause, possibly because of a protective hormonal mechanism whose process is unknown.

formed in the supine, sitting, and standing positions. Advancement is gradual throughout the hospital stay. Progression is made in a systematic fashion, based on the patient's ability to tolerate the demands of the exercise routine. Heart rate and blood pressure readings are closely monitored. The ECG is examined for development of cardiac dysrhythmias or changes in the ST and T wave. The patient's subjective evaluation is also considered. Exercises are individualized according to the disease process, length of time from the onset of the current problem, and activity level at the time of acceptance into the program. The patient's history and physical examination, resting electrocardiogram, and enzyme levels are also considered.

Outpatient exercise programs begin when the patient is discharged from the hospital. Exercise testing is carried out before discharge or within a few weeks of discharge to determine the individual's exercise prescription and also to determine whether cardiac catheterization is indicated. Patients who cannot participate in a formalized outpatient program may be given a personalized progressive home walking program, with specific instructions about pulse taking and recognition of untoward responses. These programs are monitored by the individual patient, with followup testing performed at specific intervals to reevaluate and update the exercise prescription.

The home walking program is also recommended for patients who participate in an outpatient exercise program. Exercise is begun after a complete cardiovascular evaluation, which is repeated at predetermined intervals thereafter. Individualized exercise prescriptions are determined based on the level of aerobic capacity (the maximal oxygen uptake) achieved by the subject during the exercise test. The exercise intensity is determined individually as a percentage of this level. A percentage of the maximal predicted heart rate for age and sex is most often used. The exercise effort must be greater than the patient's usual level of daily activity to produce change. The response to the program is directly related to the effort put forth by the patient. Improvement usually takes place in untrained patients when their heart rate is about 60% to 70% of maximal heart rate; it takes place in more highly trained patients when their heart rate is 85% to 90% of the maximal heart rate.

The frequency and duration of the exercise program is also important. A given level of intensity is ideally maintained for 15 to 30 minutes a day, 3 to 4 days per week. As adaptation takes place, the amount, duration, and frequency of exercise can be modified.

Exercise routines involving dynamic aerobic activities are most beneficial to cardiovascular function. They include activities such as jogging, bicycling, rowing, and swimming. Exercises that involve sudden stop-and-go aerobic activities, as well as heavy resistance and isometric exercises, are less beneficial because they are more likely to increase the oxygen demands of the myocardium. This is especially dangerous to patients whose cardiovascular function is already compromised. Isometric exercises specifically have been known to provoke dangerous Valsalva maneuvers, rhythm alterations, and pressor responses with subsequent crash of the blood pressure as soon as the activity is finished.

Ideally, exercise programs should consist of both continuous and intermittent training techniques. This combines the benefits of sustained, moderately intense activity (maintaining a steady state) and short periods of higher-intensity exercises that are interspersed with periods of less intense exercise or rest. In reality, however, most programs begin with continuous training techniques to prepare the myocardium and skeletal muscle for more intense activity. Then intermittent training can safely be introduced with varying activities to enhance total fitness. Each program session begins with warm-up exercises that prepare the body by elevating temperature and increasing circulation in an effort to enhance oxygen delivery to muscle tissue, where it is needed. This is followed by the training period, during which the target heart rate is attained, and then by a cool-down period that permits a gradual slowing of activity. The cool-down period is required to maintain sufficient cardiac output for the transportation and removal of the resynthesized high energy phosphate compounds and metabolic waste by-products. An inadequate cool-down period, or sudden termination, can result in venous pooling in the lower extremities, leading to a reduction in venous return and an increased demand on the myocardium. This leads to an elevation in heart rate that increases the oxygen uptake of the myocardium. Throughout exercise, the patient continues to be monitored for the development of chest pain, cardiac dysrhythmias, significant changes on the ECG, and alterations in the blood pressure and heart rate.

When they have completed the outpatient exercise program, patients are encouraged to participate in a supervised program within their own community. Unsupervised exercise is encouraged if supervised exercise is not available. Although these patients are not continuously monitored, they should be reevaluated at periodic intervals to measure their progress and update their exercise prescription.

Restorative, rehabilitative efforts may be difficult for patients with cardiovascular disease because these efforts frequently necessitate a change in habits that are difficult to break. Equal emphasis should be placed on prevention and healthy heart living.

REFERENCES

1. Adams, J.M., Rudolph, A.J.: The use of indwelling radial artery catheters in neonates, Pediatrics **55:**261, 1975.
2. American Heart Association: Standards and guidelines for cardiopulmonary resuscitation (CPR) and emergency cardiac care (ECC), JAMA **244**(5):453, 1980.
3. American Heart Association: Textbook of advanced cardiac life support, Dallas, TX, 1983, American Heart Association.
4. Andreoli, K.G.: Comprehensive cardiac care, ed. 5, St. Louis, 1983, The C.V. Mosby Co.
5. Antman, E., et al.: Nifedipine therapy for coronary artery spasm: experience in 127 patients, N. Engl. J. Med. **303:**1269, 1980.
6. Arey, L.B.: Developmental anatomy, ed. 7, Philadelphia, 1974, W.B. Saunders Co.
7. Bageant, R.A.: Variations in arterial blood gas measurements due to sampling techniques, Respir. Care **20:**565, 1975.
8. Barold, S., et al.: Characterization of pacemaker arrhythmias due to normally functioning AV demand (DVI) pulse generators, PACE **3**(6):712, 1980.
9. Bates, B.: A guide to physical examination, ed. 3, Philadelphia, 1983, J.B. Lippincott.
10. Berne, R.M., and Levy, M.N.: Cardiovascular physiology, ed. 4, St. Louis, 1981, The C.V. Mosby Co.
11. Bernhard, W.F., et al.: A new method for temporary left ventricular bypass, J. Thoracic Cardiovascular Surg. **70:**880, 1975.
12. Bigger, J.T.: Management of arrhythmias. In Braunwald, E.: Heart disease: a textbook of cardiovascular

medicine, Philadelphia, 1980, W.B. Saunders Company.
13. Bigger, J.T.: Mechanisms and diagnosis of arrhythmias. In Braunwald, E.: Heart disease: a textbook of cardiovascular medicine, Philadelphia, 1980, W.B. Saunders Co.
14. Birtwell, W.C., et al.: The evolution of counterpulsation techniques, Medical Instrumentation **10:**11, 1976.
15. Bloom, W., and Fawcett, D.W.: A textbook of histology, ed. 10, Philadelphia, 1975, W.B. Saunders Co.
16. Bolognini, V.: The Swan-Ganz pulmonary artery catheter: implications for nursing, Heart Lung **3**(6):979, 1974.
17. Braunwald, E., et al.: Studies on digitalis IV observation in man on the effects of digitalis preparations on the contractility in the non-failing heart and on total vascular resistance, Journal of Clinical Investigation **40:**52, 1961.
18. Braunwald, E.: Examination of the patient: the history. In Braunwald, E.: Heart disease: a textbook of cardiovascular medicine, Philadelphia, 1980, W.B. Saunders Co.
19. Braunwald, E.: Examination of the patient: the physical examination. In Braunwald, E.: Heart disease: a textbook of cardiovascular medicine, Philadelphia, 1980, W.B. Saunders Co.
20. Braunwald, E.: Mechanism of action of calcium-channel blocking agents, N. Engl. J. Med. **307**(26):1618, 1982.
21. Braunwald, E.: Regulation of the circulation, New Engl. J. of Med. **290**(20):1124, 1974.
22. Braunwald, E., et al.: Contraction of the normal heart. In Braunwald, E.: Heart disease: a textbook of cardiovascular medicine, Philadelphia, 1980, W.B. Saunders Co.
23. Buchbinder, N., and Ganz, W.: Hemodynamic monitoring: invasive techniques, Anesthesiology **45:**146, 1976.
24. Burrell, A.L., and Burell, L.O.: Critical care, ed. 4, St. Louis, 1981, The C.V. Mosby Co.
25. Castellanos, A., and Myerburg, R.J.: The resting electrocardiogram. In Hurst, J.W.: The heart, ed. 5, New York, 1982, McGraw-Hill Book Co.
26. Chameides, L., et al.: Guidelines for defibrillation in infants and children: report of the American Heart Association target activity group: cardiopulmonary resuscitation in the young, Circulation **56**(suppl.):502A, 1977.
27. Chameides, L., et al.: Resuscitation of children. In American Heart Association: Textbook of advanced cardiac life support, Dallas, TX, 1981, American Heart Association.
28. Civetta, J.M.: Intensive care therapeutics, New York, 1980, Appleton-Century-Crofts.

29. Cohn, P.F., and Braunwald, E.: Chronic ischemic heart disease. In Braunwald, E.: Heart disease: a textbook of cardiovascular medicine, ed. 2, Philadelphia, 1984, W.B. Saunders Co.

30. Covell, J.W., et al.: Studies on digitalis: effects of oxygen consumption, Journal of Clinical Investigation, 45:1535, 1966.

31. Craige, E.: Inspection and palpation of the precordium. In Hurst, J.W.: The heart, ed. 5, New York, 1982, McGraw Hill Book Company.

32. Cranefield, P.F.: The conduction of the cardiac impulse, Mt. Kisco, NY, 1975, Futura.

33. Craver, J.M., and Hatcher, C.R.: Techniques of using the intraaortic balloon pump. In Hurst, J.W.: The heart, ed. 5, New York, 1982, McGraw Hill Book Co.

34. Creed, J.D., et al: Defibrillation and synchronized cardioversion. In American Heart Association: Textbook of advanced cardiac life support, Dallas, TX, 1981, American Heart Association.

35. Davidson, R., et al.: The validity of determinations of pulmonary wedge pressure during mechanical ventilation, Chest 73(3):352, 1978.

36. DeBakey, M.E.: Left ventricular bypass pump for cardiac assistance, American Journal of Cardiology 27:3, 1971.

37. DeGowin, E.L., and DeGowin, R.L.: Bedside diagnostic examination, ed. 4, New York, 1981, Macmillan and Co.

38. Dreifus, L.S.: Pacemaker therapy, Cardiovascular Clinics 14(2):1, 1983.

39. Escher, D.J.W.: The use of cardiac pacemakers. In Braunwald, E.: Heart disease: a textbook of cardiovascular medicine, Philadelphia, 1980, W.B. Saunders Co.

40. Fozzard, H.A., and Das Gupta, D.S.: Electrophysiology and the electrocardiogram, Modern Concepts of Cardiovascular Diseases 44(6):29, 1975.

41. Fozzard, H.A., and Gibbons, W.R.: Action potential and contraction of heart muscle, American Journal of Cardiology 31(2):182, 1973.

42. Frishman, W.: Clinical pharmacology of the new beta-adrenergic blocking drugs. Part I. Pharmacodynamic and pharmacokinetic properties, American Heart Journal 97(5):663, 1979.

43. Frishman, W., and Silverman, R.: Clinical pharmacology of the new beta-adrenergic blocking drugs. Part 2. Physiologic and Metabolic Effects, American Heart Journal 97(6):797, 1979.

44. Frishman, W., and Silverman, R.: Clinical pharmacology of the new beta-adrenegic blocking drugs. Part 3. Comparative clinical experience and new therapeutic applications, American Heart Journal 98(1):119, 1979.

45. Frishman, W., Silverman, R., et al.: Clinical pharmacology of the new beta-adrenergic blocking drugs. Part 4. Adverse effects: choosing a B-adrenoreceptor blocker, American Heart Journal 98(2):256, 1979.

46. Furman, S.: Cardiac pacing and pacemakers VI. Analysis of pacemaker malfunction, American Heart Journal 94(3):379, 1977.

47. Furman, S., Hurzeler, P., et al.: Cardiac pacing and pacemakers IV. Threshold of cardiac stimulation, American Heart Journal 94(1):115, 1977.

48. Gallagher, J.J.: Mechanisms of arrhythmias and conduction abnormalities. In Hurst, J.W.: The heart, ed. 5, New York, 1982, McGraw Hill Book Co.

49. Garson, A.: Pediatric cardiac dysrhythmias, New York, 1981, Grune and Stratton.

50. Gauderer, M., and Holgersen, L.O.: Peripheral arterial line insertion in neonates and infants: a simplified method of temporal artery cannulation, Journal of Pediatric Surgery 9:875, 1974.

51. Gilman, A.G., Goodman, L.S., et al.: Goodman and Gilman's The Pharmacological basis of therapeutics, ed. 6, New York, 1980, Macmillan Publishing Company, Inc.

52. Greenberg, H., Duyer, E.M., et al.: Effects of nitroglycerine on the major determinants of myocardial oxygen consumption, American Journal of Cardiology 36:426, 1975.

53. Guyton, A.C.: Textbook of medical physiology, ed. 6, Philadelphia, 1980, W.B. Saunders Co.

54. Guyton, A.C., Coleman, T.G., et al.: Circulation: overall regulation, Annual Review of Physiology 34(1072): 13, 1972.

55. Guyton, A.C., and Jones, C.E.: Central venous pressure: physiological significance and clinical implications, American Heart Journal 86:431, 1973.

56. Harris, F.J., Low, R.I., et al.: Antianginal efficacy and improved exercise performance with timolal. Twice daily beta blockade in ischemic heart disease, American Journal in Cardiology 51:13, 1983.

57. Harvey, W.P., and de Leon, A.C.: Auscultation of the heart: gallop sounds, clicks, snaps, whoops, honks, and other sounds. In Hurst, J.W.: The heart, ed. 5, New York, 1982, McGraw Hill Book Co.

58. Harvey, A.M., Richard, J.J., et al.: The principles and practice of medicine, New York, 1976, Appleton-Century-Crofts.

59. Hecht, H.H., and Kossman, C.E.: Atrioventricular and interventricular conduction, American Journal of Cardiology 31(2):232, 1973.

60. Heger, J.J., Prystowsky, E.N., et al.: New antiarrhythmics amiodarone and encainide, Drug Therapy 12:153, 1982.

61. Heng, M.D., Norris, R.M., et al.: Effects of glucose and glucose-insulin-potassium on haemodynamics and enzyme release after acute myocardial infarction, British Heart Journal 39:748, 1977.

62. Hill, D.W., and Dolan, A.M.: Intensive care instrumentation, New York, 1976, Grune and Stratton.

63. Hoffman, B.F., and Cranefield, P.F.: The physiological

basis of cardiac arrhythmias, American Journal of Medicine **37**(5):670, 1964.

64. Holman, B.L.: Radioisotopic examination of the cardiovascular system. In Braunwald, E.: Heart disease: a textbook of cardiovascular medicine, Philadelphia, 1980, W.B. Saunders Co.

65. Hurst, J.W.: Chest pain secondary to cardiovascular disease. In Hurst, J.W.: The heart, ed. 5, New York, 1982, McGraw Hill Book Co.

66. Hurst, J.W.: The physician's approach to the patient with heart disease. In Hurst, J.W.: The heart, ed. 5, New York, 1982, McGraw Hill Book Co.

67. Hurst, J.W., Morris, D.C., et al.: The history: symptoms due to cardiovascular disease. In Hurst, J.W.: The heart, ed. 5, New York, 1982, McGraw Hill Book Co.

68. James, T.N., Sherf, L., et al.: Anatomy of the heart. In Hurst, J.W.: The heart, ed. 5, New York, 1982, McGraw Hill Book Co.

69. Johnson, P.C.: Peripheral circulation, New York, 1978, John Wiley & Sons.

70. Katz, A.M.: Physiology of the heart, New York, 1977, Raven Press.

71. Kaye, W.: Invasive monitoring techniques. In American Heart Association: Textbook of advanced cardiac life support, Dallas, TX, 1981, American Heart Association.

72. Kaye, W.: Invasive therapeutic techniques. In American Heart Association: Textbook of advanced cardiac life support, Dallas, TX, 1981, American Heart Association.

73. Keefe, Deborah, L.D., Kates, et al.: New antiarrhythmic drugs: their place in therapy, Drugs **22**:363, 1981.

74. King, O.: Care of the cardiac surgical patient, St. Louis, 1974, The C.V. Mosby Co.

75. Knoben, J.E., and Anderson, P.O.: Handbook of clinical drug data, ed. 5, Hamilton, IL, 1983, Drug Intelligence Publications, Inc.

76. Koch-Weser, J.: Beta-adrenoreceptor antagonists: new drugs and new indications, New Engl. J. of Med. **305**:500, 1981.

77. Krikler, D.M., and Rowland, E.: Clinical value of calcium antagonists in treatment of cardiovascular disorders, Journal of the American College of Cardiology **1**:355, 1983.

78. Lambrew, C.T., Guildner, C.W., et al.: Adjuncts for artificial circulation. In American Heart Association: Textbook of advanced cardiac life support, Dallas, TX, 1981, American Heart Association.

79. Leathan, A., Leeck, G.J., et al.: Auscultation of the heart. In Hurst, J.W.: The heart, ed. 5, New York, 1982, McGraw Hill Book Co.

80. Litwak, R.S., Koffsky, R.M., et al.: Support of severely impaired cardiac performance with left-heart assist device following intracardiac operation, Heart and Lung **7**:622, 1978.

81. Lown, B., and De Silva, R.A.: The technique of cardioversion. In Hurst, J.W.: The heart, ed. 5, New York, 1982, McGraw Hill Book Co.

82. Mahmud, R., Lehmann, M., et al.: Atrioventricular sequential pacing: differential effect on retrograde conduction related to level of impulse collision, Circulation **68**(1):23, 1983.

83. Maclean, E., Maroko, P.R., et al.: Effects of corticosteroids on myocardial infarct size and healing following experimental coronary occlusion, American Journal of Cardiology **39**:280, 1977.

84. Marriott, H.J., and Myerburg, R.J.: Recognition of arrhythmias and conduction abnormalities. In Hurst, J.W.: The heart, ed. 5, New York, 1982, McGraw Hill Book Co.

85. Meursing, B.T.J., Zimmerman, A.N.E., et al.: Experimental evidence in favor of a reversed sequence in cardiopulmonary resuscitation, Journal of the American College of Cardiology **1**(2):610, 1983.

86. Mierop, L.H.S., and Kutsche, L.M.: Embryology of the heart. In Hurst, J.W.: The heart, ed. 5, New York, 1982, McGraw Hill Book Co.

87. Miller, F.: College physics, New York, 1977, Harcourt Brace, Jovanovich, Inc.

88. Miller, M., Fox, S., et al.: Pacemaker syndrome: a noninvasive means to is diagnosis and treatment, PACE **4**:503, 1981.

89. Miller, R.R., Olson, H.G., et al.: Efficacy of beta-adrenergic blockade in coronary heart disease: propranolol in angina pectoris, Clinical Pharmacology and Therapeutics **18**:598, 1975.

90. Milnor, W.R.: Autonomic and peripheral control mechanisms. In Mountcastle, V.B.: Medical physiology, ed. 14, St. Louis, 1980, The C.V. Mosby Co.

91. Milnor, W.R.: Capillaries and lymphatic vessels. In Mountcastle, V.B.: Medical physiology, ed. 14, St. Louis, 1980, The C.V. Mosby Co.

92. Milnor, W.R.: Cardiovascular system. In Mountcastle, V.B.: Medical physiology, ed. 14, St. Louis, 1980, The C.V. Mosby Co.

93. Milnor, W.R.: Normal circulatory function. In Mountcastle, V.B.: Medical physiology, ed. 14, St. Louis, 1980, The C.V. Mosby Co.

94. Milnor, W.R.: Principles of hemodynamics. In Mountcastle, V.B.: Medical physiology, ed. 14, St. Louis, 1980, The C.V. Mosby Co.

95. Milnor, W.R.: The cardiovascular control system. In Mountcastle, V.B.: Medical physiology, ed. 14, St. Louis, 1980, The C.V. Mosby Co.

96. Milnor, W.R.: The heart as a pump. In Mountcastle, V.B.: Medical physiology, ed. 14, St. Louis, 1980, The C.V. Mosby Co.

97. Mondejar, E.S.: The patient with left-heart assist device: nursing management, Heart and Lung **8**:296, 1979.

98. Myerburg, R.J., and Lazzara, R.: Electrophysiologic basis of cardiac arrhythmias and conduction disturbances, Cardiovascular Clinics 5:2, 1973.

99. Norman, J.C.: Intracorporeal partial artificial heart: initial clinical trials, Heart and Lung 7:788, 1978.

100. Nutter, D.O.: Measurement of the systemic blood pressure. In Hurst, J.W.: The heart, ed. 5, New York, 1982, McGraw Hill Book Co.

101. O'Rourke, R.A.: Physical examination of the arteries and veins. In Hurst, J.W.: The heart, ed. 5, New York, 1982, McGraw Hill Book Co.

102. Parmley, W.W.: Beta blockers in coronary artery disease, Cardiovascular Reviews and Reports 2:65, 1981.

103. Parmley, W.W., and Chatterjee, K.: Vasodilator therapy. In Harvey, W.P., editor: Current problems in cardiology, Chicago, 1978, Yearbook Medical Publishers, Inc.

104. Parmley, W.W., Chatterjee, K., et al.: Hemodynamic effects of noninvasive systolic unloading (nitroprusside) and diastolic augmentation (external counterpulsation) in patients with acute myocardial infarction, American Journal of Cardiology 33:819, 1974.

105. Parsonnet, V., Furman, S., et al.: A revised code for pacemaker identification, PACE 4(4):400, 1981.

106. Parsonnet, V., Furman, S., et al.: Implantable cardiac pacemakers: status report and resource guideline, The American Journal of Cardiology 34:487, 1974.

107. Parsonnet, V., Furman, S., et al.: Optimal resources for implantable cardiac pacemakers, Circulation 68(1):227A, 1983.

108. Petty, T.L., Bigelow, D.B., et al.: The simplicity and safety of arterial puncture, JAMA 195:693, 1966.

109. Pierce, W.S., Donachy, J.H., et al.: Prolonged mechanical support of the left ventricle, Circulation 58(3):133, 1978.

110. Prior, J.A., and Silberstein, J.S.: Physical diagnosis, ed. 6, St. Louis, 1981, The C.V. Mosby Co.

111. Rackley, C.E.: Techniques of monitoring the seriously ill patient with heart disease. In Hurst, J.W.: The heart, ed. 5, New York, 1982, McGraw Hill Book Co.

112. Randall, R.C.: Neural regulation of the heart, New York, 1977, Oxford University Press.

113. Roach, L.B.: Color changes in dark skin, Nursing 77 7(1):48, 1977.

114. Roark, S.F., and Pritchett, E.L.: New therapy update, Cardiovascular Review and Reports 5(6):599, 1984.

115. Ross, J., Waldhausen, J.A., et al.: Studies on digitalis I effects on peripheral vascular resistance, Journal of Clinical Investigation 39:930, 1961.

116. Rogers, W.J., Russell, R.O., et al.: Acute effects of glucose-insulin-potassium infusion on myocardial substrates, coronary blood flow, and oxygen consumption in man, American Journal of Cardiology 40:421, 1977.

117. Russell, R.O., Rogers, W.J., et al.: Glucose-insulin-potassium, free fatty acids and acute myocardial infarction in man, Circulation (suppl. I):1, 1975.

118. Rutsch, H.: Recanalization of coronary arteries in impending myocardial infarction by means of intracoronary streptokinase infusion, Circulation 62(suppl. 3):80, 1980.

119. Sackner, M.A., Avery, W.G., et al.: Arterial punctures by nurses, Chest 59:97, 1971.

120. Samet, P., and El-sherif, N.: Cardiac pacing, ed. 2, New York, 1980, Grune and Stratton.

121. Schlant, R.C., Sonnenblick, E.H., et al.: Normal physiology of the cardiovascular system. In Hurst, J.W.: The heart, ed. 5, New York, 1982, McGraw Hill Book Co.

122. Schroeder, J.S., and Daily, E.K.: Techniques in bedside hemodynamic monitoring, ed. 2, St. Louis, 1981, The C.V. Mosby Co.

123. Schwartz, J.B., Keefe, D., et al.: Adverse effects of antiarrhythmic drugs, Drugs 21:23, 1981.

124. Sheffield, L.T.: Exercise stress testing. In Braunwald, E.: Heart disease: a textbook of cardiovascular medicine, Philadelphia, 1980, W.B. Saunders Co.

125. Sherman, G., and Liang, C.S.: Nifedipine in chronic stable angina: a double-blind placebo-controlled crossover trial, American Journal of Cardiology, 51:706, 1983.

126. Sherman, J.L., and Fields, S.K.: Guide to patient evaluation, ed. 4, New York, 1982, Medical Examination.

127. Silverman, M.E., and Hurst, J.W.: Inspection of the patient. In Hurst, J.W.: The heart, ed. 5, New York, 1982, McGraw Hill Book Co.

128. Smith, J., and Kampine, J.P.: Circulatory physiology: the essentials, Baltimore, 1980, Williams & Wilkins.

129. Smith, M.S., Chacko, P., et al.: Pharmacokinetic and pharmacodynamic effects of diltiazem, American Journal of Cardiology 51:1369, 1983.

130. Smith, T.W., and Haber, E.: Digitalis, New Engl. J. of Med. 289:945, 1973.

131. Smith, W.M., and Gallagher, J.J.: Management of arrhythmias and conduction abnormalities. In Hurst, J.W.: The heart, ed. 5, New York, 1982, McGraw Hill Book Co.

132. Soroff, H.S., Cloutier, C.T., et al.: External counterpulsation, JAMA 299:1441, 1974.

133. Sparks, H.V., and Belloni, F.L.: The peripheral circulation: local regulation, Annual Review of Physiology 40(1186):67, 1978.

134. Subramanian, V.B.: Long-term therapy of angina with calcium antagonists, Cardiovascular Reviews and Reports 4:493, 1983.

135. Subramanian, V.B.: Calcium channel blockade as primary therapy for stable angina pectoris. A double-blind placebo-controlled comparison of verapamil and propranolol, American Journal of Cardiology 50(5):1158, 1982.

136. Sutton, R., Perins, J., et al.: Physiological cardiac pacing, PACE 3(2):207, 1980.

137. Swan, H.J.C.: The role of hemodynamic-monitoring in the management of the critically ill, Critical Care Medicine 3:83, 1975.

138. Swan, H.J.C., Ganz, W., et al.: Catheterization of the heart in man with use of a flow-directed balloon tipped catheter, New Engl. J. of Med. 283:447, 1970.

139. Todres, I.D., Rogers, M.C., et al.: Percutaneous catheterization of the radial artery in the critically ill neonate, Journal of Pediatrics 87:273, 1975.

140. Vander, A.J., Sherman, J.H., et al.: Human physiology, ed. 2, New York, 1980, McGraw Hill Book Co.

141. Vassale, M.: Cardiac physiology for the clinician, New York, 1976, Academic Press.

142. Wallace, A.G.: Electrical activity of the heart. In Hurst, J.W.: The heart, ed. 5, New York, 1982, McGraw Hill Book Co.

143. Walmsley, R., and Watson, H.: Clinical anatomy of the heart, Livingstone, NY, 1978, Churchill.

144. Watanabe, A.G.: Recent advances in knowledge about beta adrenergic receptors: application to clinical cardiology, Journal of American College of Cardiology, 1: 82, 1983.

145. Weissler, A.M., Lewis, R.P., et al.: Syncope. In Hurst, J.W.: The heart, ed. 5, New York, 1982, McGraw Hill Book Co.

146. Wenger, N.K., and Gilbert, C.A.: Rehabilitation of the myocardial infarction patient. In Hurst, J.W.: The heart, ed. 5, New York, 1982, McGraw Hill Book Co.

147. Zipes, D.P., and Noble, R.J.: Assessment of electrical abnormalities. In Hurst, J.W.: The heart, ed. 5, New York, 1982, McGraw Hill Book Co.

148. Zipes, D.P., and Troup, P.J.: New antiarrhythmic agents: amiodarone, aprindine, disopyramide, ethmozin, mexiletine, tocainide, verapamil, The American Journal of Cardiology 41:1005, 1978.

149. Zipes, D.P., and Duffin, E.C.: Cardiac pacemakers. In Braunwald, E.: Heart disease, a textbook of cardiovascular medicine, ed. 2, Philadelphia, 1984, W.B. Saunders Co.

3 Respiration

JOANN BROOKS-BRUNN

To plan for optimal care of all respiratory patients, the critical care practitioner must be able to apply current knowledge of respiratory assessment and management to the needs of the individual patient.

Inpatient and outpatient care of persons with respiratory disease is an increasingly significant problem in the health care delivery system. According to 1980 statistics, respiratory disease is one of the leading causes of disability and death of adults in the United States.[9] In infants and children the most common cause of illness is infection of the respiratory tract.[8]

The outlook is discouraging for a sudden decline in the number of persons who develop respiratory problems because of the vulnerability of the lungs to numerous toxic pollutants in the environment. Furthermore, many patients in the critical care setting are hospitalized as a result of trauma, and various respiratory problems may occur secondary to the traumatic event.

In response to the need for increased knowledge of the requirements of this growing patient population, greater emphasis in health care is being placed on education, new technologic advances, and research in respiratory care. Continuing education on respiratory disease is being offered to health care professionals as well as to the public. Preventive medicine is being emphasized to reduce the number of persons developing respiratory disease. Prevention is especially important, because symptoms of many pulmonary diseases become manifest only at an advanced stage, after many years of subclinical dysfunction. Improved devices and systems are being used in the care of the critically ill patient with respiratory problems. Screening tests allow earlier diagnosis of respiratory problems in both neonates and adults. However, test sensitivity needs to be improved to allow earlier detection of changes in lung function so that remedial measures can be taken before a person is hospitalized with acute respiratory distress. Laboratory research in lung physiology and pathophysiology is being conducted, and clinical research is being done by many members of the health care team.

The physical and psychosocial management of the patient with respiratory disease is a challenge for the critical care practitioner. Because the field of respiratory care has become a distinct clinical discipline, all critical care personnel must participate in the improvement of patient care through clinical practice, continuing education, and application of research findings in routine practice.

EMBRYOLOGY

Increasing knowledge of prenatal and postnatal growth and development of the lung provides important insights into respiratory function in health and disease. Because the fetus develops in a totally aquatic environment, all oxygen (O_2) uptake and carbon dioxide (CO_2) elimination is provided by the placenta. Although the fetus is thought to make breathing motions during gestation, the lung is not allowed any practice for its ultimate role in gas exchange in the external environment.[30] The growth and development of the lung can be divided into three periods: (1) early fetal life, (2) perinatal lung maturation, and (3) postnatal life.[4]

Early fetal life

Embryologic development of the lung occurs during early fetal life. At approximately 3 weeks the epithelial structure of the lung arises as a pouch or bud from the endodermal tube or foregut (Fig. 3-1). The lobes of the lung can be structurally identified at about 12 weeks, and at 16 weeks the basic formation of the bronchial tree is complete. After 16 weeks, growth in the major conducting airways involves elongation of the existing branches and an increase in the cross-sectional area[30] (Fig. 3-2).

Goblet cells (which are mucus-secreting cells) appear in the airways at about 13 weeks, whereas cilia appear in the large airways at 10 weeks and in the more peripheral airways at approximately 14 weeks. The cartilage rings of the trachea are visible at 7 to 8 weeks, and the cartilaginous development in all bronchi can be seen by 24 weeks.

The embryologic formation of the diaphragm is completed within the seventh week of fetal life. The abdominal cavity provides a mesodermal fold that forms the major portion of the diaphragm, whereas the lateral portion of

Fig. 3-1. Development of the fetal lung from a bud of the endodermal foregut (21 to 24 days) through the initial development of the gas exchange units (24 weeks).

From Korones, S.B.: High-risk newborn infants: the basis for intensive nursing care, ed. 3, St. Louis, 1981, The C.V. Mosby Co.

Primitive lung bud
(24 days)

First branching
(26-28 days)

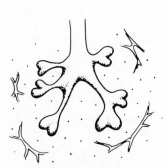

Capillaries differentiate
from mesenchyme;
respiratory bronchioles formed
(20-24 weeks)

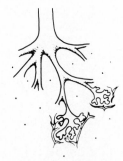

Alveolar sacs differentiated;
capillaries contact
alveolar membrane
(24-28 weeks)

the diaphragm is formed by the thoracic muscles.

Development of the major vessels of the respiratory system also occurs early in fetal life, coinciding with the development of the airways. A primitive aortic arch appears within the first month of fetal development. At approximately 5 weeks, primitive pulmonary arteries extend from the sides of the aortic sac. The development of each pulmonary artery forms a close relation with the bronchi and follows the course of the developing airways. Arising from the left atrium at about 4 weeks is the primitive pulmonary vein, which connects with the intrapulmonary capillaries. Bronchial artery circulation develops from the dorsal aorta at 2 months of fetal life and forms numerous interconnections with the pulmonary circulation.[4] Fetal systemic circulation is very different from adult circulation; for a more detailed discussion of this topic, the reader is referred to Unit 2.

Although the major bronchial and vascular development of the lung is completed by 16 weeks, the distal lung units or respiratory portion of the lung follows a different course of development (Fig. 3-2). Alveolar development begins at about the twenty-fourth week and extends until term. At birth there are approximately 25 million primitive alveoli for gas exchange. This is one tenth the amount found in the adult lung. In early development, alveoli are thick walled and shallow in depth compared to the thin-walled, cuplike appearance seen in later development.[4] The cells that line the terminal air spaces are among the last to appear in fetal development. Type I cells serve a primarily structural function in the alveoli, that is, they form the walls or structure of the alveoli and are responsible for the structural basis. Type II cells, on the other hand, are thought to be responsible for surfactant production. Type II cells, which begin to mature at about 24 weeks, appear to contain phospholipids and protein, the essential elements of pulmonary surfactant. A clinical indicator of lung maturity is the ratio in the amniotic fluid of lecithin to sphingomyelin. Lecithin levels increase with the maturation of the lung, whereas sphingomyelin levels remain constant. The absence of a mature surfactant system leads to unstable lungs, which in turn causes a variety of respiratory problems if the fetus is born at this stage of development. This is referred to as *respiratory distress syndrome* or hyaline membrane disease.

Structurally the fetus is not viable before the twenty-eighth week of life. Before that time the pulmonary bed is unable to accommodate the entire cardiac output, and the pulmonary capillary bed is not in close proximity to the alveoli for gas exchange. Furthermore, surfactant production is incomplete before the twenty-eighth week. Although fetal lung development is nearly complete early in the gestational period, certain

Fig. 3-2. Major structural features of the bronchial tree and the approximate gestational age of formation.

From Korones, S.B.: High-risk newborn infants: the basis for intensive nursing care, ed. 3, St. Louis, 1981, The C.V. Mosby Co.

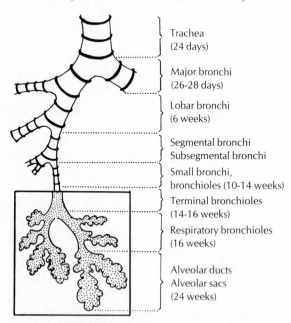

Trachea
(24 days)

Major bronchi
(26-28 days)

Lobar bronchi
(6 weeks)

Segmental bronchi
Subsegmental bronchi

Small bronchi,
bronchioles (10-14 weeks)

Terminal bronchioles
(14-16 weeks)

Respiratory bronchioles
(16 weeks)

Alveolar ducts
Alveolar sacs
(24 weeks)

Levels of airway from trachea to
alveoli and approximate gestational
week of formation

structures, such as the gas exchange units and the pulmonary circulation, must be fully functional before the fetus is able to survive in the external environment.

Although the fetal lung is not used as a gas exchange organ, it has several other important functions. The fetal lung serves a secretory function in that it is one of the major sources of amniotic fluid.[30] The production of fetal lung liquid is also an important function. The exact production site of this fluid remains unknown, but it is thought to involve most of the lung. During the early embryologic development of the lung, the lung fluid fills the developing airways and primitive alveoli. In the last 3 weeks of fetal life, the content of this fluid changes as it mixes with the surfactant produced by the type II cells of the alveoli.

Perinatal period

The second phase of fetal lung development is called the perinatal period. The period begins as the lung prepares itself for its introduction to the extrauterine environment. It is important to remember that this is indeed a critical period of fetal lung development: the total respiratory system must be ready to function in concert and to act as a gas exchange mechanism when called on to do so.

Before birth, the fetal lung is partially distended by fluid, approximately 30 ml/kg of body weight.[25] The removal of this fluid and its replacement with air is the major obstacle to be overcome during the infant's first extrauterine breaths. At birth, fetal lung liquid is removed by three mechanisms: (1) draining externally through the mouth and nose, (2) removal by the pulmonary vessels, and (3) clearance by the lymphatic system.[25] In a vaginal birth, some of the fluid is removed as the infant moves through the birth canal. During the movement through the canal, the thoracic cage of the infant is compressed by pressures up to 100 cm H_2O.[30] This pressure facilitates the movement of the liquid from the lungs. A small amount of this liquid is removed by the infant's cough or by suctioning

by the practitioner. Additional fluid is reabsorbed into the alveolar capillaries and lymphatic channels during the first hours after birth.

As the infant prepares for his first breath, several components of the respiratory system must be ready to perform in harmony. The respiratory muscles must be able to generate sufficient negative pressures for inspiration to occur, while the respiratory center of the central nervous system must be prepared to assume the control of ventilation. The alveoli must have sufficient surfactant so that alveolar collapse does not occur as ventilation begins.

During the first breaths of life, the infant's respiratory muscles must be able to generate a negative intrathoracic pressure of between -40 to -80 cm H_2O.[30] This negative pressure is necessary to draw air into the lungs against several different forces operating in the infant's lung. First, the air must be drawn into airways partially filled with liquid. Then enough force must be generated to overcome the surface tension in the lung and to distend the lung tissue.[30] Therefore the infant must work very hard to begin the process of breathing in the external environment. Air does not totally replace the lung fluid after the first breath. Over the first few breaths of life, more and more air is retained in the lung at the end of each expiration. This amount of air left in the lung at the end of a normal expiration is called the *functional residual capacity*. Over several breaths, the functional residual capacity slowly increases to 25 to 35 ml of air per kg of body weight.[4] As the functional residual capacity is established in the infant, a less negative intrathoracic pressure is necessary for the generation of each breath.

During the infant's initial breaths in the external environment, the circulation undergoes dramatic changes. Before birth, pulmonary vascular resistance is very high, because it receives virtually no blood flow (only 3% to 7% of cardiac output) and because the vascular structure is very tortuous and kinked.[25] At birth, as the lungs expand and flow increases to the pulmonary circulation, pulmonary vascular resistance decreases. This decrease results from the increasing partial pressure of oxygen in the blood and the opening up of the pulmonary circulation with blood flow. Many other changes occur in the system circulation at birth; these are discussed in Unit 2.

Postnatal growth

Although the lung is fully functional as a gas exchange system at full-term birth, it continues to grow and develop in the postnatal period. Fig. 3-3 shows the configuration of the adult tracheobronchial tree. The large and small airways do not increase in number but continue to elongate and increase their cross-sectional area. At birth the alveoli are primitive in structure; after birth the alveoli continue to develop in number and in structure. It is believed that new alveoli develop until 8 years of age, when the lung reaches its full complement of 300 million alveoli. As the alveoli develop, they change into very delicate, thin-walled sacs that provide an optimal structure for gas exchange.

The pulmonary capillaries within the gas exchange units are not well developed at birth. The number of capillaries increases enormously during the first year of life. With the increasing numbers of alveoli and pulmonary capillaries, the area for gas exchange enlarges. At birth the total surface area for gas exchange in the neonate is about 3 m², whereas in the adult it increases to 70 m².[4] Table 3-1 summarizes the development of the respiratory system.

PHYSIOLOGY

The primary function of the respiratory system is gas exchange, which allows oxygen to move from the air into the blood and carbon dioxide to move from the blood into the atmosphere. Problems of the respiratory system may be classified as abnormalities in the processes of ventilation or perfusion or a combination of the two. These processes are involved in air entering the alveoli, gases crossing the blood-gas membrane, and gases being transported to and from the cells of the body. The practitioner must also have a firm understanding of the areas of gas transport and acid-base balance to provide effective care for the respiratory patient.

Ventilation

Ventilation is the process of air moving into and out of the lungs. Many factors may interfere with the normal process of ventilation. Problems

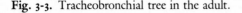

Fig. 3-3. Tracheobronchial tree in the adult.

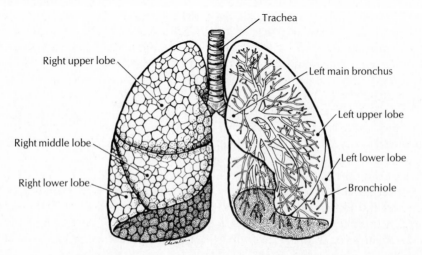

Trachea

Right upper lobe

Left main bronchus

Left upper lobe

Right middle lobe

Left lower lobe

Right lower lobe

Bronchiole

Table 3-1. Development of the respiratory system

Age in weeks	Size (crown-rump) in mm	Respiratory system
2.5	1.5	—
3.5	2.5	Respiratory primordium appearing as a groove on floor of pharynx
4	5.0	Trachea and paired lung buds become prominent Laryngeal opening a simple slit
5	8.0	Bronchial buds presage future lung lobes Arytenoid swellings and epiglottis indicated
6	12.0	Definitive pulmonary lobes indicated Bronchi sub-branching Laryngeal cavity temporarily obliterated
7	17.0	Larynx and epiglottis well outlined; orifice T-shaped Laryngeal and tracheal cartilages foreshadowed Conchæ appearing Primary choanæ rupturing
8	23.0	Lung becoming gland-like by branching of bronchioles Nostrils closed by epithelial plugs
10	40.0	Nasal passages partitioned by fusion of septum and palate Nose cartilaginous Laryngeal cavity reopened; vocal folds appear
12	56.0	Conchæ prominent Nasal glands forming Lungs acquire definitive shape
16	112.0	Accessory nasal sinuses developing Tracheal glands appear Mesoderm still abundant between pulmonary alveoli Elastic fibers appearing in lungs
20-40 (5-10 mo)	160.0-350.0	Nose begins ossifying (5 mo) Nostrils reopen (6 mo) Cuboidal pulmonary epithelium disappearing from alveoli (6 mo) Pulmonary branching only two thirds completed (10 mo) Frontal and sphenoidal sinuses still very incomplete (10 mo)

From Arey, L.B.: Developmental anatomy, ed. 7, Philadelphia, 1974, W.B. Saunders Co.

or alterations in ventilatory control or lung mechanics may cause problems in the normal process of gas exchange. Normally ventilation is caused by active changes in the size of the thorax and by the passive recoil property of the lung. The act of breathing is spontaneous and is normally accomplished without effort or voluntary awareness.

Muscles of ventilation

The muscular work of ventilation is done mainly by the diaphragm and the external intercostal muscles. The diaphragm, a dome-shaped muscle that lies between the thorax and abdomen, is innervated on each side by the phrenic nerves, which arise from the third and fourth cervical segments. Although anatomically it is considered to be one muscle, the diaphragm is divided into two hemidiaphragms, each of which is innervated separately. This allows each hemidiaphragm to act independently when one side is paralyzed by disease or trauma. With normal diaphragmatic function, both hemidiaphragms contract synchronously and automatically to initiate each inspiration.

Contraction of the diaphragm causes it to descend, with a resulting decrease in intrathoracic pressure and an increase in lung volume. The external intercostal muscles also assist in the outward movement of the rib cage on inspiration. The scalene and sternocleidomastoid muscles are the accessory muscles of ventilation; they effectively assist the inspiratory process. The scalene muscles help to elevate the first and second ribs, thus contributing a small amount to the inspiratory volume. The sternocleidomastoid muscles help to elevate the sternum, thus increasing the anteroposterior diameter of the thorax. These muscles are often actively used by patients who have severe obstructive lung disease or by any patient in respiratory distress.

In contrast to the active process of inspiration, expiration is normally a passive process. The normal elastic properties of the lungs and chest wall bring the thorax to its normal resting position when all forces are equal and in opposition. When expiration is forced or labored, the internal intercostal muscles contract and have a net effect of lowering the ribs and assisting in the expiration of air. The muscles of the abdominal wall are also powerful and function mainly on expiration. Normally these muscles are used to generate the expulsive pressure needed to produce an effective cough or a maximal expiratory effort.

Ventilatory control

Neuronal control. Ventilatory control is based on several different factors. Spontaneous ventilation depends on the neurogenic innervation of the muscles used in ventilation. The major respiratory center in the brain is located in the medulla oblongata of the brainstem. The medullary respiratory center contains two types of neurons, inspiratory cells and inspiratory-expiratory cells. The inspiratory cells are called the *dorsal respiratory group,* whereas the inspiratory-expiratory cells are called the *ventral respiratory group.*[28] It is thought that the dorsal respiratory group is the initial site for processing of all afferent (incoming) input. Activity of neurons in the dorsal respiratory group initiates neuronal impulses, which travel down the phrenic nerve and other motor tracts to cause diaphragmatic contraction for each inspiratory cycle. With an increased intensity or rate of impulse production, there is an effective increase in the ventilatory tidal volume or rate. The ventral respiratory group opposes the dorsal respiratory group and its neuronal activity. Through a complex homeostatic mechanism, the automatic or unconscious control of ventilation occurs.

In addition to the medullary control of ven-

Fig. 3-4. Control of ventilation. Interrelationships of the mechanisms involved in the control of ventilation are shown.

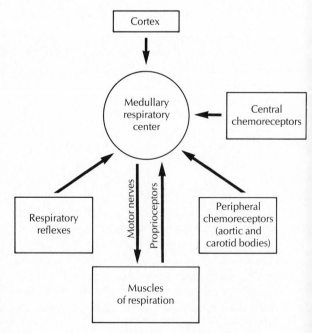

tilation, there are other areas of the brain that further influence the ventilatory process. The apneustic and pneumotaxic centers are located in the pons. The apneustic center by itself produces a prolonged inspiratory effort, interrupted by occasional expiration. Investigators believe that the apneustic center may also be the site of various types of information that can terminate inspiration.[28] The pneumotaxic center has no intrinsic rhythmicity but functions to modulate respiratory depth and frequency. It is the coordination of all the regulatory mechanisms in the brain that leads to normal ventilation. Fig. 3-4 demonstrates the interrelationships of these various control mechanisms of respiration.

Chemical control. The two primary components in the humoral control of ventilation are the central and peripheral chemoreceptors. A chemoreceptor responds to changes in the chemical composition of the blood or fluid around it. Chemical regulation of ventilation refers to the control of ventilatory activity by changes in concentration of carbon dioxide (CO_2), hydrogen ions (H^+) and oxygen (O_2) in the body fluids. In the control of ventilation there are both central and peripheral chemoreceptors, as shown in Fig. 3-4.

Central chemoreceptors. The central chemoreceptors are located on the ventral surface of the medulla in the vicinity of the exit of the ninth and tenth nerves. The central chemoreceptors in the brain are bathed in cerebrospinal fluid, which is separated from the blood by the blood-brain barrier. The blood-brain barrier is relatively impermeable to H^+ and bicarbonate ions (HCO_3^-), but CO_2 can easily diffuse across it. Carbon dioxide has a strong effect on the central chemoreceptors. When the arterial partial pressure of carbon dioxide (Pa_{CO_2}) increases, CO_2 diffuses into the cerebrospinal fluid from the cerebral blood vessels. Once in the cerebrospinal fluid, the CO_2 combines with water to ultimately produce HCO_3^- and H^+. It is this change in the H^+ that directly stimulates the central chemoreceptors. Thus for a given change in the Pa_{CO_2} there will be a change in the H^+ concentration in the cerebrospinal fluid. The stimulation of the central chemoreceptors by an increase in Pa_{CO_2} or H^+ produces an increase in ventilatory depth, followed by an increase in ventilatory rate. Conversely, a decrease in the Pa_{CO_2} or H^+ causes a depression in ventilation (decreased rate and depth).

Cerebrospinal fluid has a lower buffering capacity than blood because of its lower protein content. Bicarbonate is the major buffering component in the cerebrospinal fluid. Because of the lowered buffering capacity, any change seen in the cerebrospinal fluid pH will be greater than that seen in the blood. As stated earlier, the ventilation changes quickly in response to the H^+ concentration in the cerebrospinal fluid. Changes in the blood HCO_3^- are seen more slowly in the cerebrospinal fluid (24 to 48 hours).[25] The slow movement of HCO_3^- into or out of the cerebrospinal fluid is accomplished by diffusion and active transport mechanisms. The difference in ventilatory response of the stimuli in respiratory and nonrespiratory (metabolic) acid-base disorders is caused by this slow movement of HCO_3^-.

Peripheral chemoreceptors. Peripheral chemoreceptors are also involved in the control of ventilation. These chemoreceptors are located in the carotid bodies, which lie in the bifurcation of the common carotid artery and in the aortic bodies above and below the aortic arch. Their role in the relationship to the other control mechanisms or ventilation is shown in Fig. 3-4. The carotid bodies stimulate the respiratory center by way of the glossopharyngeal nerve. The aortic bodies increase impulse transmission in the respiratory center via the vagus nerve. These receptors are sensitive to increased partial pressure of carbon dioxide (Pa_{CO_2}) levels in the blood, but they are not as powerful as the central chemoreceptors in triggering changes in ventilation. They act primarily as a backup mechanism in case the central chemoreceptors fail.

Peripheral chemoreceptors are also highly sensitive to decreases in O_2 tension in the blood. Because of their location in the aorta and carotid arteries, peripheral chemoreceptors receive more blood flow than other tissues, so that much of their O_2 requirements are satisfied by the O_2 normally present in the blood. A decline in Pa_{O_2} will stimulate the carotid bodies and aortic receptors as will a reduction in blood flow. With peripheral chemoreceptor stimulation, impulses to the respiratory center increase and ventilation is increased. As the Pa_{O_2} rises in response to the increased ventilation, the frequency of impulses coming from the peripheral chemoreceptors decreases. In addition to the above-mentioned responses to peripheral chemoreceptor stimulation, these chemoreceptors also activate the vasomotor center in the brain in response to the low O_2 levels. This produces an increase in cardiac output and vasoconstriction, which increases arterial blood pressure.

To understand the processes that control ventilation, one must appreciate the differences and complex interrelationships of the central and peripheral chemoreceptors. The central chemoreceptors will respond to changes in the Pa_{CO_2} of 1 mmHg with extreme quickness. The peripheral chemoreceptors, on the other hand, will not respond to Pa_{CO_2} changes of less than 10 mmHg. The higher the Pa_{CO_2} above normal levels, the quicker the central chemoreceptors will respond. For the peripheral chemoreceptors to respond to lowered O_2 levels, the Pa_{O_2} must fall below approximately 60 mmHg.

The normal respiratory stimulus for ventilation is caused by changes in Pa_{CO_2}. It must be noted that extremely high arterial CO_2 levels will depress rather than stimulate the central chemoreceptors. As the Pa_{CO_2} approaches approximately twice the normal level, it begins to exert a narcotic effect that depresses the ventilatory drive.[10] The role of hypoxic ventilatory response in the normal control of ventilation is very small. However, there are two situations in which the hypoxic ventilatory response is very important.

Chronic elevation of Pa_{CO_2} is often found in the patient with severe chronic lung disease. For reasons that are not entirely clear, the ventilatory response to Pa_{CO_2} appears to become significantly diminished in these patients. In these patients hypoxemia then becomes the primary stimulus for ventilation, and the peripheral chemoreceptors are the principle regulators of ventilatory drive. In chronic CO_2 retention states, the cerebrospinal fluid pH returns to near normal because of the compensatory response of the body. The initial depression of pH is nearly abolished by buffering mechanisms in the cerebrospinal fluid. Therefore the patient with severe chronic lung disease and CO_2 retention may initially be seen with an arterial blood gas level that looks significantly abnormal. The arterial pH level may be near normal, while the Pa_{CO_2} will be elevated. One will also notice that the HCO_3^- level will be elevated because of renal compensation. Because hypoxemia is the chief stimulus for ventilation in patients with severe chronic obstructive lung disease, control of supplemental oxygen administration is of extreme importance so as not to abolish the ventilatory drive.

A second situation in which the hypoxemic response plays an important role in ventilatory control is the body's initial adaptation to high altitude. There is a large increase in ventilation in response to hypoxemia during the early stages of adaptation. Hyperventilation is caused by hypoxic stimulation of the peripheral chemoreceptors.[42] Initially at high altitude, CO_2 production is normal, whereas alveolar and arterial Pa_{CO_2} fall, causing respiratory alkalosis. After a day or so the cerebrospinal fluid pH is brought back toward normal by movement of HCO_3^- out of the cerebrospinal fluid. After a few days the arterial blood pH is returned to near normal levels by renal excretion of HCO_3^-.[28]

In summary, one can readily see that ventilation is controlled by several factors. The rate, depth, and pattern of ventilation are regulated by the respiratory center and central and peripheral chemoreceptors, which respond to changes in CO_2, O_2, and H^+ concentrations. Other factors that may influence ventilation include thermal stimuli, pharmacologic intervention, pulmonary reflexes of stretch receptors, pressoreceptors in response to blood pressure changes, and proprioreceptors in the bones and joints.[25] The practitioner must be conscious of all the factors that control and influence ventilation when caring for a patient with problems in ventilation.

Distribution of ventilation

In assessing the distribution of ventilation in the lung, the practitioner must consider the regional differences in the distribution of the gases with each breath. In the normal lungs of a standing person, alveoli in the upper portions (apices) of each lung are somewhat distended because the lower pleural pressure pulls them open. In contrast, the alveoli at the base of each lung are less distended because there is slightly less subatmospheric pleural pressure as a result of the weight of the lungs. In this case the lungs can be visualized as a soggy bath sponge that is partially supported from the top. The bottom of the sponge is compressed because of gravity, and the top of the sponge is pulled open. In the thoracic cage, the lung is held adjacent to the parietal pleura by a negative intrapleural pressure, and there is a very gradual shift from more open alveoli near the apices to more closed alveoli near the bases. Therefore the uppermost alveoli can expand less with inspiration during a normal breathing cycle than can the alveoli in the lower portions of each lung. In the supine position, the differences between the ventilation of the apical and basilar regions of the lungs become minimal. In the supine position, distribution of ventilation is equal in the apical and basilar areas. It is important to note that the dependent or bottommost areas of the lung, which are affected by gravity, are the site for optimal gas exchange, because this is the site of optimal ventilation and perfusion. Therefore the practitioner must be aware that positioning of the patient will have a direct effect on ventilation and perfusion and ultimately on gas exchange.[32]

Deadspace ventilation

A portion of ventilation may not be involved in gas exchange. In the conducting airways of the lungs, no gas exchange occurs. This part of the respiratory system is referred to as the *anatomical dead space*. When there are alveoli that are being ventilated but not being perfused by blood, this is called the *alveolar dead space*. The sum of the anatomical dead space and the alveolar dead space is described as the *physiological dead space* or wasted ventilation. In the critical care patient it is important to consider the addition of any dead space to the airway, because this may interfere with adequate gas exchange. An example of this would be the addition of ventilator tubing from the artificial airway to the ventilator circuit. This is known as the addition of *mechanical dead space*. In some instances a measurement of the dead space to tidal volume ratio (V_D/V_T) may be obtained for a patient. Therefore the percentage of the patient's tidal volume that is actually involved in gas exchange can be estimated. A normal V_D/V_T is less than 0.3.

Lung mechanics

The characteristics of the thoracic cage and lungs must be considered in a discussion of ventilation. The rib cage provides protection for the contents of the thoracic cage and also serves as a support device. Respiratory muscles generate forces or pressures that produce mechanical alterations in the dimensions of the thoracic cage. To produce these alterations, opposing forces or the resistance of the lung itself must be overcome. Furthermore, the elastance characteristics of the lung itself must be considered when discussing lung mechanics. One must understand the interrelationship of lung mechanics and the work of breathing.

Pressures within the lungs and thorax. During inspiration, air moves by bulk flow from the external environment into the lungs because of pressure differences within the system. The gas moves from an area of higher pressure to one of lower pressure. For air to flow into the lungs, the intrapulmonary pressure within the lungs and airways must reach a level lower than atmospheric pressure; thus a pressure gradient is generated.

The pressure existing within the pleural space is known as the *intrapleural pressure* or intrathoracic pressure. The elastic properties of the lungs cause them to draw inward on the relatively fixed thoracic cage; therefore a subatmospheric pressure is created in the pleural space between the parietal and visceral pleurae. It is important to keep in mind that the pleural space is normally only a potential space and that the visceral and parietal pleurae are usually in close approximation. The different pressures within the thoracic cage as well as the elastic properties of the rib cage and lung itself are shown in Fig. 3-5.

Airway resistance. Airway resistance is defined as the frictional resistance produced in the airways by the movement of air from outside the body down to the alveolar level. During nasal breathing the nose constitutes up to 50% of the total airway resistance. If one is mouth breathing at rest, the mouth, pharynx, larynx, and trachea create between 20% and 30% of the airway resistance.[28] In total, during normal breathing conditions, 80% to 90% of the total resistance to breathing results from resistance in the airways 2 mm in diameter and larger.[42]

The airway diameters are not constant; they change during the ventilatory cycle. During inspiration the airways dilate, thus causing decreased airway resistance, whereas during expiration the airways become smaller. Airway resistance is also related to lung volume. As lung volume increases, airway resistance decreases. This results from the fact that at increased intrathoracic volumes, the airways are distended. Therefore the airways cause less airway resistance at large lung volumes and during inspiration.

The intricate branching of the system of airways results in a changing combination of laminar and turbulent flow, which influences the pressure-flow relationships and the resistance. In the normal lung the bulk of resistance is in the central airways because of the small cross-sectional area and the high flows generated. The relative distribution of airway resistance is dif-

Fig. 3-5. Pressure relationships within the thoracic cage.

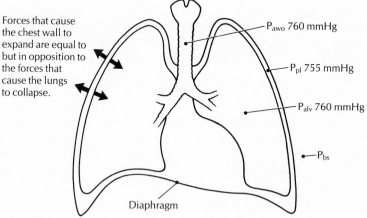

P_{awo}: Pressure at airway opening (usually atmospheric)
P_{pl}: Pressure in pleural space (syn: intrapleural or intrathoracic pressure)
P_{alv}: Pressure in terminal air spaces (syn: intrapulmonary pressure)
P_{bs}: Pressure at the body surface

ferent in the neonate and in early life, however, because the growth of the conducting airways lags behind during the period of rapid alveolar multiplication. In the neonate more of the airway resistance is located in the peripheral airways.[25] As the child grows, the major site of airway resistance moves to a more central location.

In the clinical setting several factors may cause an increase in airway resistance and thus an opposition to the airflow. Secretions in the airways or bronchospasm will narrow the airway, therefore causing an increase in airway resistance. An endotracheal tube or tracheostomy tube will also cause increased airway resistance. It is important to choose the size or caliber of artificial airway that will minimize the amount of airway resistance caused by it.

Elastic recoil. Elastic recoil is the property of the lung that allows it to return to its original shape or resting volume. During inspiration, the elastic recoil property of the lung must be overcome by the muscular forces of the chest wall for lung expansion to occur.

The elastic recoil properties of the lung are usually referred to in terms of *lung compliance*. Lung compliance can be defined as the distensibility of the lung; it is measured as the amount of volume change per unit of pressure change across the lung ($\Delta V/\Delta P$). As the elastic recoil of the lung is decreased, lung compliance is increased. This is best demonstrated in the patient with emphysema. With emphysema the structural integrity of the lungs has been diminished and there is a loss of the recoil property of the lung. It takes very little pressure change to cause a substantial volume change in a patient with emphysema. Therefore it can be said that in emphysema, the lung is very compliant.

Inversely, as the elastic recoil property is increased, lung compliance is decreased. This can be demonstrated in a patient with adult respiratory distress syndrome (ARDS) or an infant with infant respiratory distress syndrome (IRDS). In IRDS there is a surfactant deficiency that increases surface tension within the alveoli and also increases hyaline membrane formation. Because of these two factors, infants with IRDS have very noncompliant or "stiff" lungs. Therefore it takes a large change in pressure to cause a given change in lung volume.

The total compliance of the respiratory system has two components—that of the chest wall and that of the lungs. Chest wall compliance is influenced by the characteristics of the thoracic cage and respiratory muscles. Lung compliance is characterized by the elastic properties of the lung as well as the airflow resistance. The normal value for total compliance of the respiratory system in the adult is about 0.1 L/1 cm H_2O.[28]

Compliance is an important concept to consider when a patient is being mechanically ventilated. Total respiratory compliance measurements are often done on these patients as a method of evaluation. Two types of total compliance measurements may be made on the patient who is intubated and whose lungs are being mechanically ventilated; these measurements are dynamic respiratory compliance and static respiratory compliance. With a volume-controlled positive-pressure ventilator, the pressure needed to deliver a certain volume of air is shown on the airway pressure manometer. The measurement of dynamic compliance provides an estimate of total compliance and airway resistance. Dynamic compliance is measured by comparing the patient's total volume with the peak airway pressure on the pressure manometer at end inspiration.

Static compliance measurements are made under conditions of virtually no airflow. The measurement of static compliance allows a better analysis of total respiratory compliance without the influence of airway resistance. To measure static compliance, the expiratory port of the ventilator is occluded at end inspiration, and the plateau pressure is recorded on the pressure manometer after a few seconds of stabilization. Static compliance is then calculated by dividing the preset ventilator volume by the plateau airway pressure on the pressure manometer.

When either type of compliance measurement is done, two factors must be noted. First, if the patient is receiving positive end expiratory pressure (PEEP) therapy while the lungs are being mechanically ventilated, the amount of PEEP must be subtracted from the peak or plateau pressure before the compliance is calculated. Second, one must take into consideration the compliance or distensibility of the ventilator circuit. This should be subtracted from the tidal volume before calculating compliance.

Work of breathing. The act of breathing requires that the muscles of ventilation perform a specific amount of work. The body's total work of breathing can be divided into two types of work: mechanical work and metabolic work.[39] The mechanical work of breathing is proportional to the pressure change times the volume change. The volume change refers to the amount of air moved into or out of the lung during a normal ventilation (tidal volume). The pressure change refers to the pressure needed to overcome the elastic and resistive forces of the lung. The mechanical work of breathing can be divided as follows: (1) elastic work of breathing (approximately 65%), and (2) nonelastic work of breathing (about 35%).[39] Of the 35% of the nonelastic work of breathing, 28% results from airway resistance and 7% results from the viscous resistance of the lung.

The elastic work of breathing refers to the amount of work necessary to overcome the elastic recoil property of the chest wall and lung tissue and also to overcome the surface tension of the alveoli.[28] Resistive work of breathing refers to the work done to overcome airway resistance and tissue resistance.[28] Examples of patients who have increased elastic work of breathing are those with a restrictive lung disease, such as pulmonary fibrosis, or those who have a decrease in the amount of pulmonary surfactant present in the alveoli. Clinical examples of patients with increased resistive work of breathing are those with chronic obstructive lung disease (emphysema, bronchitis, cystic fibrosis), asthma, or upper airway obstruction.

The metabolic work of breathing is described as the oxygen cost of breathing. The metabolic cost of breathing is quite low during quiet breathing and increases proportional to increases in ventilation. At rest, the oxygen cost of normal, quiet breathing is less than 5% of total body oxygen uptake.[28] In a normal person this amount may increase up to 30% during maximal exercise. When a disease state is present, such as chronic obstructive lung disease or congestive heart failure, the oxygen cost of breathing may be four to ten times that for a normal person.[7]

All factors related to the work of breathing must be taken into account when caring for the critically ill patient. Any abnormality of ventilatory mechanics may result in an altered breathing pattern. If a patient has noncompliant lungs, a rapid, shallow breathing pattern may be optimal to decrease the work of breathing. If the flow resistance is increased, a slow, deep breathing pattern may occur. These factors of ventilatory mechanics are important to consider when a patient is ventilator dependent. The adopted breathing pattern of the patient must be considered when setting the ventilator controls (for example, in the assist ventilation mode or in the intermittent mandatory ventilation mode). Understanding a patient's adaptive pattern of breathing resulting from changes in ventilatory mechanics is important in respiratory care. It is also important to note that the performance of work requires increased oxygen consumption. If the work of breathing is increased by a change in ventilatory mechanics, oxygen consumption with breathing may be significantly elevated. This oxygen consumption factor must be considered when planning the care of a patient who has increased work of breathing. The practitioner should include physical rest and education in the techniques of energy conservation and efficient breathing patterns to decrease ventilatory requirements in these patients.

There are many differences between the pulmonary system of the infant and that of the adult. However, in comparing the general state of maturity and function, the breathing apparatus of the neonate is as adequate as that of the adult. At birth, lung compliance is very low. It takes a large amount of pressure to cause a small inspiration during the first breath in the newborn because of the air-liquid contact in the alveoli, the viscosity of the lung fluid, and the tissue resistance. Lung compliance increases after the first few breaths. The chest wall of the neonate has almost infinite compliance capacity, with the rib cage and intercostal muscles offering little elastic resistance to expansion. Because of the narrower airways, airway resistance is much greater in the neonate. However, the energy expenditure against elastic and resistive forces relative to average ventilation in an infant is nearly equal to that in an adult.

The interrelationship of the elastic and resistive forces of the neonatal ventilatory system is best illustrated by breathing frequency. The breathing frequency of the neonate is nearly twice that of the adult. An explanation of this increased rate is that the sum of the work needed to overcome elastic and resistive forces is minimized at a rate of about 35 to 40 breaths per minute in the neonate. Therefore breathing frequency is controlled to a rate that allows the maximal amount of ventilation at the minimal energy cost.

Lung perfusion

Blood flow or perfusion is the second major process in the physiology of the respiratory system. The pulmonary capillary bed forms a dense network in the alveolar unit, which makes an exceedingly efficient arrangement for gas exchange. The pulmonary capillaries are offered little support from the epithelial lining of the alveoli; therefore they are subject to collapse or distension, depending on the pressures within or around them. These pressures may become clinically significant in problems such as pulmonary edema, positive pressure ventilation, and fluctuations in cardiac output.

The lung has a dual blood supply: it receives deoxygenated blood via the pulmonary artery and oxygenated blood through the bronchial circulation. In the neonate, pulmonary circula-

tion is a changing process from fetal circulation to neonatal circulation. Disruption of the normal progression to a complete neonatal circulation may cause changes in neonatal pulmonary perfusion. An example of this is in persistent fetal circulation in which the ductus arteriosus does not close. Therefore blood is shunted from the pulmonary artery to the aorta without oxygenation occurring. This causes a lowering of the Pao_2 because of the mixing of blood that has passed through the lungs for gas exchange with the blood that has not (venous admixture).

The pulmonary capillary bed is a low-pressure circuit containing approximately 50 to 60 ml of blood in the adult. There are about 6 billion capillaries in the lung of a human adult, but only 25% to 35% of these capillaries are being perfused under resting conditions.[28] Because it is a very distensible circuit, the capillary system can accommodate a large increase in blood flow by means of *recruitment* and *dilation*. Recruitment means the opening of capillaries which are not open during resting blood flow. Dilation refers to the distensibility of the currently open capillaries to accommodate the increased perfusion. Therefore, in the normal lung when cardiac output is increased (for example, during exercise), pulmonary vascular resistance is decreased, and the pressures in the pulmonary vasculature remain essentially unchanged.

Positioning and the effects of gravity play important roles in the perfusion of different areas of the lung. As with ventilation, the distribution of perfusion in the lungs is not equal at the apex and the base. In the upright position, a majority of the pulmonary blood flow goes to the lung base rather than the apex. When a patient is in the supine position, a majority of blood flow is distributed to the dependent or posterior segments of the lung. When a patient is in the side-lying position, perfusion is increased to the dependent lung. Perfusion may be changed in different zones of the lung by either an increase or decrease in pulmonary artery pressure or alveolar pressure. Some factors that may also alter the distribution of perfusion are intermittent positive-pressure breathing, positive end-expiratory pressure, continuous positive-pressure breathing, exercise, or a change in the cardiac output.

Diffusion

In a discussion of ventilation and perfusion of the lung, the process of diffusion cannot be forgotten. Diffusion refers to the passive transfer of gases to and across the blood-gas barrier or alveolar capillary membrane. Diffusion is a passive process, because no extra energy is required for the transfer of gas to occur. Movement of gas is from an area of higher partial pressure to an area of lower partial pressure. The rate at which the gas diffuses depends on the steepness of the concentration gradient and the diffusing properties of the gas. The diffusing properties of the gas are determined by the solubility and molecular weight of the substance.

Factors that may influence the total quantity of gas crossing the membrane include (1) pressure difference between the alveolar gas and capillary blood, (2) total surface area of the alveolar-capillary membrane, (3) membrane thickness, and (4) the membrane diffusion coefficient.[26] The diffusion partial pressure gradient is a major determinant of the rate of diffusion. The larger the gradient, the more easily the gas will diffuse across the membrane. The surface area of the membrane is important in diffusion because it is a variable that can easily be altered during a disease process. Factors affecting the surface area for diffusion include changes in lung volume, changes in pulmonary capillary perfusion, or loss of lung tissue. The thickness of the membrane must also be considered, since increasing the thickness of the membrane will impair diffusion of gases. Clinical examples of this include interstitial edema or fibrotic thickening of the membrane. The membrane diffusion coefficient depends on the solubility and density of the gas. Carbon dioxide diffuses approximately 20 times more rapidly than does oxygen because of the solubility of carbon dioxide. Thus clinical problems with CO_2 diffusion at the alveolar-

capillary level are seen much less frequently than are problems with O_2 diffusion across the barrier.

In describing the diffusion of O_2 and CO_2 at the alveolar-capillary level, one must first discuss the alveolar-capillary membrane. The thickness of the alveolar-capillary membrane is only about 0.2 to 0.5 μm.[26] Since this membrane is quite thin, it provides little resistance to the movement of gases across it. Oxygen moves through the alveolar-capillary membrane, where it combines chemically with hemoglobin or remains dissolved in the plasma. The membrane contains several layers that the gas must traverse. Oxygen must diffuse through the following layers: (1) pulmonary surfactant, (2) alveolar epithelium, (3) interstitium, (4) capillary endothelium, and (5) into the erythrocyte or into the plasma. When a person is breathing room air, the partial pressure of alveolar oxygen (PAo_2) is about 105 mmHg, whereas the partial pressures of mixed venous blood oxygen ($P\bar{v}o_2$) is 40 mmHg. Thus there is a diffusion gradient of 65 mmHg (105-40) between the alveolar gas and venous blood. The rate at which oxygen moves into the blood depends not only on the diffusion properties of the alveolar-capillary membrane but also on the rate of chemical combination of oxygen with hemoglobin in the blood. Under typical resting conditions, equilibrium between alveolar air and blood is reached in about 0.3 seconds. Blood passing through the lung is only in the pulmonary capillary for about 0.75 seconds. Therefore at a normal alveolar O_2 and cardiac output, the hemoglobin becomes nearly saturated with oxygen as it passes through the pulmonary capillary bed.

Carbon dioxide moves across the alveolar-capillary membrane in the opposite direction from that of oxygen. The diffusion pressure gradient for carbon dioxide is only about 6 mmHg ($P\bar{v}co_2$ = 46; $PAco_2$ = 40). Carbon dioxide diffuses much more easily across the membrane because of its solubility coefficient. Therefore a high diffusion pressure gradient is not necessary for this gas. Equilibrium across the alveolar-capillary membrane takes about 0.3 seconds, the same as for oxygen. Because of the high diffusing capacity of carbon dioxide, the alveolar CO_2, which is very difficult to measure directly, can be reasonably estimated to be equal to the arterial CO_2.

Ventilation/perfusion matching

It is imperative that the alveolar gas and the pulmonary blood flow come into contact with one another. Overall in the normal lung, the ventilation to perfusion ($\dot{V}/\dot{Q}$) ratio is approximately 0.8.[43] This means that there is slightly more perfusion than ventilation in the lung as a whole. This ratio changes throughout different areas of the lung. If either perfusion or ventilation is altered, interference with normal gas exchange will result. This is referred to as a $\dot{V}/\dot{Q}$ *imbalance* or mismatch. Often in the critical care patient a $\dot{V}/\dot{Q}$ mismatch will be apparent. For instance, ventilation can be decreased by any clinical condition that results in airway closure or narrowing. Therefore these areas are still being perfused but are not adequately ventilated. This results in a $\dot{V}/\dot{Q}$ ratio of less than 0.8. Examples of causes of decreased ventilation to areas of the lung include atelectasis, pneumonia, pulmonary edema, and mucous plugging. On the other hand, perfusion may be impaired to certain areas of the lung, resulting in an increased $\dot{V}/\dot{Q}$ ratio (greater than 0.8). This results in wasted ventilation. Clinical examples of this are pulmonary emboli and loss of capillary bed, such as seen in emphysema.

Problems with $\dot{V}/\dot{Q}$ matching may be related to the *percent of pulmonary shunt,* which is defined as that portion of the cardiac output (pulmonary blood flow) that is perfusing nonventilated alveoli or not participating in gas exchange. Measuring the shunt allows one to quantitiate the percentage of cardiac output that returns to the left side of the heart unoxygenated. In the normal person, this shunt is in the range of 3% to 5%. However, in the critically ill patient a shunt of greater than 15% is not uncommon.

A qualitative estimate of the pulmonary shunt can be obtained by allowing the patient to breathe 100% oxygen for 20 to 30 minutes. After this 30-minute period, an arterial blood gas reading is obtained to measure the Pa_{O_2}. If there is a greater than normal amount of unaerated blood being added to the aerated blood, the Pa_{O_2} will not reach the expected value of greater than 500 mmHg. In summary, this means that much of the cardiac output is not participating in gas exchange and is being returned to the left side of the heart unoxygenated.

Gas transport
Oxygen

Oxygen is transported in the blood in two ways. It can be carried in the blood in combination with hemoglobin in the red blood cells or in solution dissolved in the plasma. The mechanisms for O_2 transport are shown in Fig. 3-6. Transport of the O_2 by either method (in solution or attached to hemoglobin) depends on the partial pressure (P) of O_2 in the arterial blood (Pa_{O_2}).

The amount of O_2 dissolved in the plasma is quite small compared to the amount carried by the hemoglobin. Dissolved O_2 in the plasma accounts for approximately 1.5% of the total amount of O_2 actually transported in the blood. At a temperature of 37° C (98.6° F), normal arterial blood with a Po_2 of 100 mmHg contains only about 0.003 ml of oxygen per milliliter of blood or 0.3 ml of oxygen per 100 ml of blood. The blood O_2 content is expressed in milliliters of O_2 per 100 ml of blood, which is referred to as *volumes percent.*

Under normal conditions (normal F_IO_2 and barometric pressure), O_2 in the plasma is insufficient to satisfy the resting body requirement for O_2, which is approximately 250 ml O_2/min. In fact, if this were the only mechanism for transport of O_2, then a cardiac output of 83 L/min. would be required to satisfy the body's resting O_2 needs.

Recent years have seen the development of a new technique in which dissolved O_2 can play a significant role in the total O_2 delivery to the body. This technique is called *hyperbaric oxygen therapy*. During this therapy the patient's body is enclosed in a sealed chamber filled with 100% O_2 at up to three times normal atmospheric pressure. The effect is to raise the PaO_2 to as high as 2000 mmHg. Of course, at a PaO_2 above 150 mmHg, all hemoglobin is essentially saturated with O_2. However, under these conditions a significant amount of O_2 can be physically dissolved in the plasma. In fact, it is possible in the hyperbaric oxygen environment for a patient to exist without hemoglobin for O_2 transport. Of course, these chambers are not used for continuous, long-term therapy. The usual length of therapeutic treatment is no longer than 2 hours. Hyperbaric oxygen therapy is finding increasing acceptance as an adjunct to the treatment of ischemic injuries, crush injuries, compromised skin grafts, thermal burns, and carbon monoxide poisonings.[11] In these cases the beneficial effects of hyperbaric oxygen therapy are mediated almost entirely through the carriage of O_2 dissolved in the plasma. This is one of the only known conditions in which dissolved O_2 transport is of clinical importance.

Hemoglobin accounts for over 98% of the total amount of O_2 carried in the blood. Each gram of hemoglobin can combine with 1.34 ml of O_2 at 37° C (98.6° F). Normal adult hemoglobin is known as *hemoglobin A. Hemoglobin F* (fetal) makes up part of the hemoglobin of the newborn infant and is gradually replaced over the first year of postnatal life. Hemoglobin that is combined with O_2 is called *oxyhemoglobin,* whereas unoxygenated hemoglobin is referred to as *deoxyhemoglobin* or reduced hemoglobin. In a normal person with a hemoglobin of 15 gm/100 ml of blood, this results in an O_2 carrying capacity of approximately 20 ml of O_2/100 ml of blood (20 volumes percent).

In discussing O_2 transport, one must fully understand the terms used to describe the transport. Three terms used are similar, but have unique differences. The *content* of O_2 per 100 ml of blood is the sum of the actual amount of O_2 carried in solution (dissolved) and the amount in combination with hemoglobin. Oxygen transport *capacity* refers to the maximal amount of O_2 that could be transported by hemoglobin if the hemoglobin were 100% saturated. The *percent saturation* is the relationship between the actual

Fig. 3-6. Oxygen transport. (1) Oxygen transported in the dissolved form. (2) Oxygen transported in combination with hemoglobin.

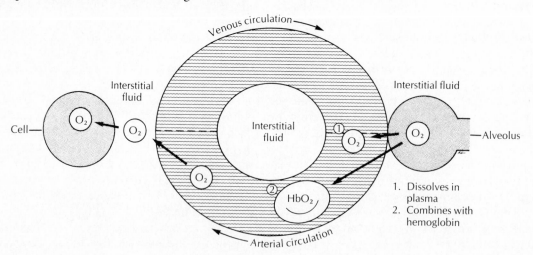

amount of O_2 being carried with hemoglobin, compared to the potential amount that could be carried or transported. It is expressed as follows:

$$\text{Saturation} = \text{Actual/Capacity} \times 100$$

The actual amount of O_2 that is combined with the hemoglobin depends on the partial pressure of O_2 dissolved in the blood.

Although the amount of O_2 carried in physical solution is a linear relationship, the amount of O_2 carried with hemoglobin is a nonlinear relationship. The relationship of the amount of O_2 combined with hemoglobin is described by the oxyhemoglobin dissociation curve. This curve shows the relationship of the Pa_{O_2} and the percent saturation of the hemoglobin. A comparison of the neonatal and adult oxyhemoglobin dissociation curves is shown in Fig. 3-7.

As one can see, the Pa_{O_2} and O_2 saturation of hemoglobin are related to each other in a definite fashion. This curve is derived by plotting the amount of O_2 in combination with hemoglobin (percent saturation) versus incremental Pa_{O_2}s. The sigmoidal shape of this curve has many physiological advantages. The flat upper portion demonstrates that if the Pa_{O_2} drops from 100 mmHg to 70 mmHg in the adult, the saturation only falls to 90%. Therefore adequate amounts of O_2 will be combined with the hemoglobin and carried to the tissues even in the presence of a reduced Pa_{O_2}.

Another significant characteristic of the dissociation curve is the steep midportion. Below a Pa_{O_2} of approximately 60 mmHg in the adult, slight reductions of Pa_{O_2} will produce contrastingly large reductions in the saturation of hemoglobin with O_2. Therefore, in the lower ranges of Pa_{O_2} (30 to 60 mmHg), a small change in the Pa_{O_2} will have a dramatic effect on hemoglobin saturation.

The position of the oxyhemoglobin dissociation curve is not fixed; it may be affected by many factors. An increase in temperature, increased amounts of 2,3-diphosphoglycerate (2,3-DPG), increased Pa_{CO_2}, and decreased pH all shift the oxyhemoglobin dissociation curve to the right. This means that oxygen is unloaded rapidly by hemoglobin at the tissue level. Therefore, if the tissue temperature increases or the patient's body fluids become more acidotic, then the hemoglobin will have a decreased affinity for O_2 and more O_2 will be unloaded from the hemoglobin at the tissue level. A shift of the dissociation curve to the left is produced by the opposite change in the variables just mentioned. When discussing shifts to the left, neonatal respiratory care is important. The neonatal dissociation curve is normally shifted slightly to the left of the adult curve. Large quantities of fetal hemoglobin will shift the dissociation curve even farther to the left. The increased O_2 affinity of fetal hemoglobin is important for oxygen delivery to the fetal tissues. For effective O_2 transport from the placenta to the fetus to occur, fetal hemoglobin must be loading O_2 at the same Pa_{O_2} at which the maternal hemoglobin is unloading oxygen. With the shift to the left, the fetus is able to load larger amounts of O_2 with hemoglobin at lower Pa_{O_2}s. Also, the O_2 and hemoglobin have a greater affinity for each other. The fetal hemoglobin provides an es-

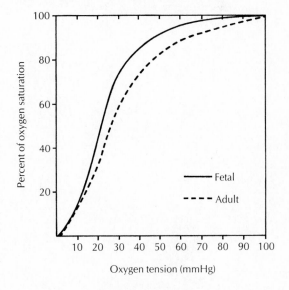

Fig. 3-7. Oxyhemoglobin dissociation curve.

sential advantage to the fetus in the low-oxygen environment of the womb, but these same properties are a disadvantage to the neonate breathing air from the external environment.

Since the standard oxyhemoglobin dissociation curve applies only to normal conditions, the critical care practitioner must relate all the patient factors that may change the position of the curve. The amount of O_2 that leaves the blood will depend on local needs and conditions in the tissue being perfused. The need for adequate oxygenation is of prime importance when caring for a critically ill patient. Arterial hypoxemia (lowered Pa_{O_2}) in either a right or left shift situation will cause an impairment in O_2 delivery compared to when the curve is in a normal position.

Carbon dioxide

Carbon dioxide (CO_2) is the major end product of cellular metabolism and is continuously produced by all cells in all tissues. The average person produces CO_2 at a rate of approximately 200 ml of CO_2 per minute. Carbon dioxide is carried in the blood in three forms: (1) 5% to 10% is physically dissolved in the blood, (2) 5% to 10% is transported as carbamino compounds, and (3) 70% to 90% is carried in the form of bicarbonate (HCO_3^-).[28] These three forms are shown in Fig. 3-8. At 37° C (98.6° F), about 0.0006 ml of CO_2 per mmHg of Pco_2 will dissolve in 1 ml of plasma. Therefore, in 100 ml of plasma or whole blood at a Pco_2 of 40 mmHg, there is about 2.4 ml of CO_2 in physical solution. The total CO_2 content of whole blood is about 48 ml of CO_2 per 100 ml of blood.[28] Therefore approximately 5% of the CO_2 carried in the arterial blood is in physical solution. Carbon dioxide can also be transported in blood proteins, forming carbamino compounds. Because hemoglobin is the protein found in the greatest concentration in the blood, most of the CO_2 transported by this method is bound with hemoglobin.

As stated earlier, the majority of CO_2 in the body is transported in the form of HCO_3^-. The CO_2 is produced metabolically in the tissues and is physically dissolved in the plasma. While in the plasma, the CO_2 enters the red blood cell

Fig. 3-8. Carbon dioxide transport. (1) In the dissolved form. (2) In combination with hemoglobin. (3) In the form of HCO_3^-.

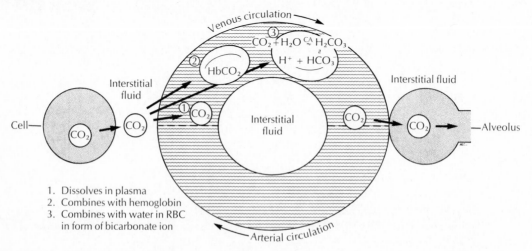

1. Dissolves in plasma
2. Combines with hemoglobin
3. Combines with water in RBC in form of bicarbonate ion

and under the influence of carbonic anhydrase forms carbonic acid (H_2CO_3). This H_2CO_3 can in turn dissociate to form H^+ and HCO_3^- in a reversible equation:

$$CO_2 + H_2O \overset{CA}{\rightleftharpoons} H_2CO_3 \rightleftharpoons H^+ + HCO_3^-$$

Carbonic anhydrase is an enzyme present in high concentrations in the red blood cell, and it makes this reaction occur very quickly. As H^+ and HCO_3^- are formed, an accumulation of HCO_3^- occurs within the red blood cell. Some HCO_3^- diffuses into the plasma where it is carried in this form. To maintain electron neutrality, as HCO_3^- diffuses into the plasma, chloride anions move into the red blood cell. This movement to maintain electric neutrality is termed the *chloride shift*.

For the lungs, the equation reverses. The H^+ combined with hemoglobin are released. They combine with HCO_3^- to form H_2CO_3. The H_2CO_3 then dissociates into CO_2 and H_2O. Simultaneously CO_2 is released from the carbamino compounds. The CO_2 then diffuses out of the red blood cells and plasma into the alveoli. The chloride shift once again occurs, this time into the plasma, to maintain electron neutrality.

The amount of CO_2 carried in the blood is related to the partial pressure of CO_2. The CO_2 dissociation curve, which shows the relationship between CO_2 partial pressure to CO_2 content, is essentially linear. The linearity of this CO_2 curve allows for the maintenance of an essentially normal Pa_{CO_2}. Hyperventilation in one lung zone compensates for hypoventilation in another, with the resulting maintenance of a normal Pa_{CO_2}. Therefore mixing of shunted blood with blood from a well-ventilated area of the lung does not significantly raise the Pa_{CO_2}.

The unloading of O_2 and CO_2 at the tissue level are mutually helpful processes. The relationship exists in such a way that at the tissue level an increased Pa_{CO_2} aids in the unloading of O_2 and a decreased Pa_{O_2} aids in the loading of CO_2. At the lung level, the reverse occurs.

Therefore it must be noted that there is a firm relationship between the degree of hemoglobin oxygenation and the effect of the CO_2 dissociation curve.

Acid-base balance

Traditionally the acid-base status of the body has been characterized by the acid-base status of the blood. Since the blood does come into contact with all organs of the body, the acid-base balance of the blood reflects the acid-base balance of the body. Arterial blood gas (ABG) analysis is a way of measuring the acid-base status of the body. The parameters provide valuable information to the practitioner caring for the critically ill patient. The clinical interpretation of the ABG analysis requires not only knowledge of some basic chemistry but also a foundation in basic physiology. This section on acid-base evaluation will present some basic concepts and the physiological background. The interpretation of ABG results is further discussed in the assessment section, under "Laboratory Data" (p. 204).

First, one must look at the basic definitions of acid-base balance. By definition, pH stands for the negative logarithm of the hydrogen ion (H^+) concentration (pH = $-\log H^+$). Therefore the pH is inversely proportional to the H^+ concentration. One of the most important factors in the cellular environment is H^+ activity. Acids are defined as substances that tend to donate H^+, whereas bases are substances that remove or accept H^+ from solution. Chemical buffers are substances that act to minimize changes in the pH of a solution when acids or bases are added. A buffer system is composed of a weak acid and its conjugate base, called an *acid-base buffer pair*.

Hydrogen ion activity

In clinical medicine, emphasis is placed on the H^+ concentration (pH). The Henderson-Hasselbalch equation is a mathematical statement of the pH and is as follows:

$$pH = pK' + \log \left(\frac{base}{acid} \right)$$

We can apply the Henderson-Hasselbalch equation to the bicarbonate buffer system, which is the most powerful buffering system in the body. The pK of the bicarbonate-carbonic acid buffer system under physiologic conditions is 6.1. This value varies for each acid-base system and is also dependent on temperature. In this equation the base is HCO_3^-, and the acid is carbonic acid (H_2CO_3). Since carbonic acid is not normally reported in the ABG results, we replace the carbonic acid in the equation with the term ($Paco_2 \times 0.03$) which is approximately equivalent. Thus the equation would be as follows:

$$pH = 6.1 + \log \left(\frac{HCO_3^-}{Paco_2 \times 0.03} \right)$$

One can then substitute the normal values for HCO_3^- at 24 mEq/L and arterial $Paco_2$ of 40 mmHg into this equation. The equation can once again be rewritten as follows:

$$pH = 6.1 + \log \left(\frac{24}{40 \times 0.03} \right)$$

$$pH = 6.1 + \log \left(\frac{24}{1.2} \right)$$

$$pH = 6.1 + \log \left(\frac{20}{1} \right)$$

$$pH = 6.1 + 1.3$$

In solving the equation, one finds the pH to be 7.4. Humans are able to maintain a fairly stable extracellular H^+ concentration at a pH of 7.4. The maintenance of this normal arterial pH of

Fig. 3-9. Henderson-Hasselbalch equation.

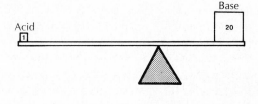

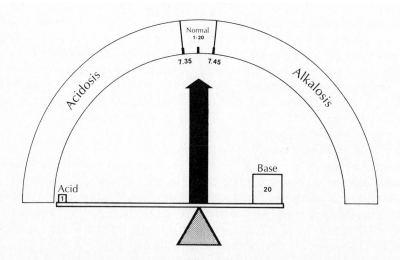

7.4 depends on a multicomponent buffering system that prevents significant changes in extracellular pH. An important point is that the body exercises acid-base homeostasis by controlling arterial Pa_{CO_2} and HCO_3^- levels to maintain this 20:1 ratio and a pH of 7.4 (Fig. 3-9). Therefore the Henderson-Hasselbalch equation can be functionally expressed as follows:

$$pH = 6.1 + log\left(\frac{HCO_3^- \text{ (regulated by kidneys)}}{Pa_{CO_2} \text{ (regulated by lungs)}}\right)$$

Acid-base regulation

When we speak of the regulation of acid-base balance, it actually means regulation of H^+ concentration of the body fluids (Fig. 3-10). Slight changes in H^+ concentration from the normal value can cause significant alterations in the rates of chemical reactions in the cells. Some reactions are depressed, whereas others are accelerated in light of acid-base disturbances. Therefore the regulation of H^+ concentration is the most important aspect of homeostasis of the system. Three mechanisms exist that resist pH change in response to an excessive acid or base load in the system: (1) buffering mechanisms, (2) lung regulation, and (3) kidney regulation.

Buffer systems. Knowledge of the buffering systems of the body is important in understanding the total body response to changes in the parameters of the acid-base system. Buffers do not prevent changes in pH when strong acids or strong bases are added to solutions; they simply minimize these changes. There are three principle buffer systems in the body's fluids: (1) bicarbonate, (2) phosphate, and (3) protein. These buffering systems respond immediately to any change in H^+ concentration.

Bicarbonate. The bicarbonate (HCO_3^-) buffer system plays an important role in the acid-base balance of the body. It is the major buffer system. Because the concentration of HCO_3^- in the blood is not great, the HCO_3^- buffer system derives its power from the fact that it is an open-ended system; that is, the individual components of the system can be regulated. The lung and the kidney can both act to adjust the concentration of the components of the HCO_3^- buffer system.

From the Henderson-Hasselbalch equation one can see that an increase in the HCO_3^- concentration or a fall in the Pa_{CO_2} causes the pH to rise or become alkaline. Conversely, an increase in the Pa_{CO_2} or a fall in the concentration of HCO_3^- decreases the pH or shifts it toward an acidotic state. The respiratory system can change the concentration of CO_2 by increasing or decreasing the rate and depth of ventilation. On the other hand, the kidneys can increase or decrease the concentration of HCO_3^- in the body by retaining or excreting the ions.

Bicarbonate is formed in the blood in the following sequence:

$$CO_2 + H_2O \overset{CA}{\rightleftharpoons} H_2CO_3 \rightleftharpoons H^+ + HCO_3^-$$

The addition of water (H_2O) to CO_2 to form carbonic acid (H_2CO_3) is a very slow reaction in the extracellular fluid and the plasma. However, in the red blood cell, the reaction occurs rapidly because of the presence of carbonic anhydrase (13,000 times faster).[28] It reaches complete equilibrium within fractions of a second. As the concentrations of these ions rise within the red blood cell, HCO_3^- quickly diffuses out into the plasma, but the H^+ cannot, because of the impermeability of the cell membrane to cations. Therefore, to maintain electron neutrality, chloride ions diffuse into the cell from the plasma.

Some of the liberated H^+ is bound to the hemoglobin. Keeping in mind the equation for the HCO_3^- buffer system, consider the following example. Acid or H^+ is added to the blood. This H^+ combines with HCO_3^- to form H_2CO_3, which in the presence of carbonic anydrase dissociates into CO_2 and H_2O. This CO_2 is then excreted by the lungs. The higher the level of HCO_3^-, the greater the acid load the system can handle. Remember that the pH changes in a buffered system in response to an acid or base, but the magnitude of the change is much less than if there were no buffer. By reviewing the sequence of HCO_3^- formation, one can see that the reaction can shift to the left or right to maintain a balance in the system.

Phosphate. The phosphate buffer system acts in a way similar to the HCO_3^- system but is composed of a buffer pair of two phosphate ions, monohydrogen phosphate (HPO_4^{2-}) and dihydrogen phosphate ($H_2PO_4^-$). The pK of the phosphate buffer system is 6.8 and therefore it acts as a strong buffer. Remember that the maxi-

mum buffering power is achieved when pK = pH. Although it is a strong buffer system, the concentration of phosphate buffer is only approximately one sixth that of the HCO_3^- buffer system.

The phosphate buffer system is especially important in the kidney, where H^+ can combine with the phosphate buffer pair in the distal tubular lumen, thus providing an additional means of

Fig. 3-10. Alterations in acid-base balance (changes in the Henderson-Hasselbalch equation and the resulting changes in pH).

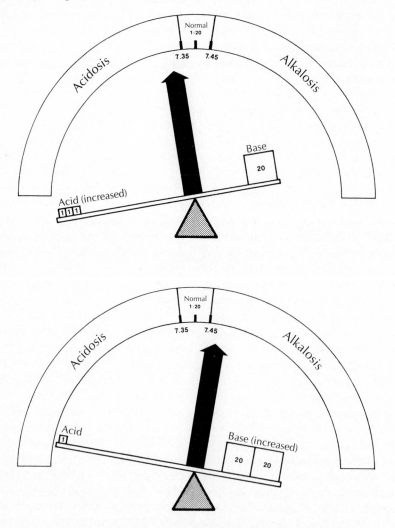

H^+ loss and HCO_3^- preservation. This process also allows for retention of sodium ions because sodium is returned to the blood along with HCO_3^-.

Protein. The most plentiful buffers in the body are the proteins of the cells and plasma. A protein is composed of amino acids bound together by peptide linkages. Some of these amino acids act as H^+ donors and some act as H^+ acceptors. Each protein molecule will therefore have some portions that act as an acid and some portions that act as a base. In the blood, most of the buffering of H_2CO_3 is performed by the protein hemoglobin. The presence of large amounts of hemoglobin allows the H^+ in transit from systemic capillaries to pulmonary capillaries to be buffered effectively by the red blood cell. Reduced hemoglobin has a greater affinity for H^+ than does oxyhemoglobin.

All of the body's buffer systems function in harmony to maintain acid-base homeostasis. Addition or removal of H^+ from the body fluids affects all of the buffer system simultaneously.

Respiratory regulation of pH. The respiratory system plays an important role in acid-base balance by controlling the CO_2 tension of arterial blood. As shown with the reaction previously discussed with HCO_3^- buffering, Pa_{CO_2} also influences H^+ concentration of body fluids. An increase in CO_2 tension will push the reaction to the right, resulting in an increase in the H^+ concentration, decreasing the pH. Three effects occur if alveolar ventilation is decreased: (1) CO_2 will accumulate in the blood, (2) carbonic acid concentration will increase, and (3) the blood pH will fall.

A decrease in CO_2 tension will shift the reaction to the left, resulting in a fall in the free H^+ concentration, causing a more alkaline pH. If ventilation increases and CO_2 elimination exceeds CO_2 production, the blood CO_2 concentration will fall, leading to an increased pH. It can readily be seen that any change in alveolar ventilation may profoundly influence pH. Alveolar ventilation is normally controlled so that blood pH changes are kept to a minimum.

Changes in arterial CO_2 concentrations are sensed within minutes by the chemoreceptors in the medulla, causing changes in ventilation.

Renal regulation of pH. The renal system helps to regulate acid-base balance by controlling H^+ concentration and electrolytes (see Unit 5 for a more detailed discussion). This is accomplished by (1) increasing urinary excretion of H^+ and conservation of HCO_3^- when the blood is too acidic, and (2) increasing urinary excretion of HCO_3^- and conservation of H^+ when the blood is too alkaline. The renal control mechanism has a slower response time than the respiratory system in regulating pH. It may take 24 to 48 hours for the renal system to return the pH to a near-normal range.[25] The compensatory mechanisms of both the lungs and the kidneys are used to minimize pH changes. Neither system overcompensates to correct a problem with the pH.

Renal control of acid-base balance involves four different processes. First, reabsorption of filtered HCO_3^- occurs. This process consumes most of the H^+ secreted by the kidney tubule cells. Through the exchange across the cell membrane to maintain neutrality, sodium ions associate with the HCO_3^- to return sodium bicarbonate to the blood. Second, the renal system is able to help maintain acid-base balance by the formation of titratable acid. Titratable acid is the amount of H^+ present in the urine that is combined with other buffers that will be excreted. Phosphate is the major filtered buffer that functions in this capacity. For each H^+ ion excreted in this form, a new HCO_3^- ion is generated by the kidney and returned to the body. The third process of renal regulation of pH is the control of the excretion of ammonia (NH_3). Ammonia, a urine buffer, is produced within the kidney tubule cells from amino acids brought to the kidneys by the blood. This NH_3 diffuses into the tubular urine, where it reacts with H^+ to yield ammonium (NH_4^+).[24] Ammonium becomes trapped in the urine because of its high solubility. For each H^+ ion excreted in this fashion, an equivalent amount of $NaHCO_3^-$ is added to the blood. Fourth, the potassium ion (K^+) that is regulated by the renal tubular cells has an important role in acid-base balance. There is an inverse relationship between K^+ and H^+ excretion. As H^+ excretion increases, K^+ is conserved. Conversely, when K^+ excretion increases, H^+ is conserved.[5] The exchange of H^+ and K^+ also occurs between the tissue cells and extracellular fluid. An example is when H^+ concentration increases, as with an acute acidemia, K^+ moves out of the tissue cells and into the extracellular fluid in exchange for H^+. The opposite occurs in an acute alkalemia as K^+ moves into the cells in exchange for H^+ ions.

It can be readily seen that the renal system plays an important role in the homeostasis of acid-base balance in the body. In the critically ill patient, problems with acid-base balance are frequently seen. Therefore it is important that the practitioner be aware of the normal mechanisms of acid-base regulation to extrapolate this knowledge for problems in the clinical setting.

ASSESSMENT

An overall assessment of the critically ill patient provides the practitioner with vital information regarding the planning and implementation of care. The critical care practitioner is responsible for making clinical assessments and judgments based on utilization of these skills.

The respiratory history

Although it may be difficult to obtain the critical care patient's respiratory history on admission to the unit, it remains an important part of the assessment process. The patient may not be able to answer pertinent historical questions, but a family member, friend, or the patient's previous hospital record may be able to provide the practitioner with these facts. First, the patient's pulmonary history should be obtained. It should be ascertained whether the patient had an acute or chronic pulmonary problem before admission. The pulmonary history should focus on key pulmonary symptomatology: breathlessness,

cough, sputum production, hemoptysis, chest pain, wheezing, ankle edema, and frequency of chest infections. With an infant or pediatric patient, pertinent facts relevant to respiratory problems at birth may be of importance.

Breathlessness (shortness of breath)

Breathlessness is a subjective sensation experienced by the patient and can be defined as a heightened awareness of difficulty in breathing.[7] The practitioner must first assess the patient's past history of this symptom. Included in the assessment of breathlessness is the mode of onset, its severity, and its duration. As the practitioner assesses this symptom, the minimal amount of activity associated with it must be determined.[7] It is important to establish whether the breathlessness occurs at rest, with exertion, during sleep, in relation to body position, or with emotional upset.

Cough

Cough may also be a symptom of historical importance experienced by the patient with pulmonary problems. As with the symptom of breathlessness, the practitioner should establish certain characteristics about the cough, such as onset and duration, frequency during the day and night, whether there are paroxysms of cough, productivity, and any accompanying symptoms (nausea, vomiting, chest pain, dizziness). It is often helpful to ask family members about the symptoms of cough, because they may have a more heightened awareness of this symptom than does the patient.

It is important to distinguish characteristics of the sputum if the patient has a productive cough. Sputum may be expectorated or swallowed by the patient. Often the infant or pediatric patient will swallow the sputum. This should be assessed by questioning the patient or family. Questions regarding sputum production that should be asked by the practitioner should include the following areas:

1. Amount—best described by the patient in simple terms (for example, teaspoon,

half a cup, number of tissues used per day)

2. Color—clear, white, green, yellow, reddish tinged
3. Character and consistency—thin, thick, particulate matter, odor
4. Associated symptoms

It may also be helpful for the practitioner to ask patients whether they have ever had their sputum "checked" by a physician or have ever been on antibiotics for a respiratory infection.

Coughing up of blood

Hemoptysis is the coughing of blood from the lung. It must be established whether the patient is expectorating blood from the lung, vomiting blood from the gastrointestinal system (hemataemesis), or experiencing a posterior nosebleed. The practitioner should establish the onset and duration of the blood expectoration along with the amount of blood. Often the patient tends to exaggerate the amount of blood expectorated. The practitioner should ask in-depth questions about the amount in simple terms for the patient, as was done with the amount of sputum production. It should also be noted whether the patient is concomitantly having symptoms of an acute respiratory infection. The color and characteristics of the expectorated material should also be ascertained—blood-tinged, fresh blood, clotted blood. The practitioner should ask whether the patient has taken any inhaled medications. Some inhaled medications may cause a discoloration of the sputum.

Chest pain

Chest pain is a very nonspecific symptom that must be reviewed in detail. Diseases of the lungs may produce chest pain or discomfort. It is often hard to distinguish the origin of the chest pain. Only by obtaining an in-depth history of this symptom is one able to determine its cause. The following characteristics of the chest pain should be determined:

1. Onset, location
2. Duration, frequency

3. Characteristics or quality of the pain
4. Pain in relationship to food, swallowing, rest, exertion, position, inspiration, or cough
5. Relieving factors
6. Associated symptoms—cough, breathlessness, hemoptysis

Wheezing

Wheezing or noisy breathing is both a sign and symptom of airway obstruction. The patient may describe wheezing or "whistling" from their lungs associated with breathlessness. The practitioner should establish the following facts about the patient's wheezing episodes: localized or diffuse, duration and frequency, association with an allergen, rest, exertion, cough, sputum production or breathlessness. It should also be noted whether the wheezing is on both inspiration and expiration and how relief is obtained.

Swelling (edema)

Edema may also be a sign of pulmonary dysfunction. There are many causes of edema, which will be further discussed later in the chapter. The practitioner should determine the following about the patient's edema:

1. Onset, duration, frequency
2. Part of body affected
3. Effect of body positioning
4. Precipitating or relieving factors
5. Associated symptoms—breathlessness, chest pain, cough

Past history

The complete respiratory history also includes a discussion of the patient's past problems and hospitalizations. The frequency and duration of respiratory infections should be determined by the practitioner. A respiratory infection may exhibit many or all of the symptoms previously described. In addition, fever and chills, weight loss, or fatigue may also accompany an infection. The examiner should ask the patient whether he has recently been treated by the doctor for an infection and the type of medication that was prescribed.

Establishment of the patient's past and present medication history is also important. It should be ascertained whether the patient is allergic to any medications. If possible, the practitioner should determine the last time that any medications were taken before admission. This would include regularly prescribed or over-the-counter medications, illicit drugs, or medications given by the physician (flu vaccines, antibiotics).

Finally, the practitioner should determine the patient's smoking history, along with any occupational exposure that may be relevant to the patient's present pulmonary symptomatology. It may also be helpful to ask whether the patient has any history of tuberculosis or has ever had a skin test for the disease. Although many other questions should be asked in order to formulate a comprehensive historical assessment of the patient, the ones which have been mentioned are those which may be most helpful to the critical care practitioner in planning care for the patient.

Physical examination

The four methods used to examine the respiratory system are inspection, palpation, percussion, and auscultation. A systematic approach in assessing the patient helps to prevent oversight of any important aspect of the examination. Although the critical care practitioner may not do a complete physical assessment each time the patient is examined, it is imperative that one remember the importance of each method and integrate these facts when doing a complete assessment. In addition to the initial physical examination of a patient entering a critical care unit, it is essential to consider pertinent laboratory data and the patient's history. The historical perspectives of the problem may often illuminate findings in the physical examination that may then be considered more significant.

In preparation for the examination, the patient should be in a sitting position if possible. In a critical care area, it may be necessary to have the patient in a supine position with good body alignment. Good lighting should be available. The examination should occur in a quiet setting, although this is difficult in most critical care units. The patient should have his chest bared so that a proper examination can be done, although the patient's privacy must always be considered.

Inspection

General appearance. Inspection or observation of the patient is perhaps the most underrated facet of respiratory assessment. Often the practitioner rushes through the process, missing vital information that can be obtained only by using a thorough inspection technique. First, the examiner should observe the general nutritional status and musculoskeletal development of the patient. Patients with chronic obstructive lung disease sometimes have increased development of the accessory muscles in the neck and shoulder region. The color and condition of the skin should also be noted. In general, the skin of the thorax reflects the overall character and coloration of the skin elsewhere on the body.[35]

Next, the extremities should be examined for signs of cyanosis, edema, or clubbing. Peripheral cyanosis is seen in the extremities as a result of cooling of the area, lack of circulation, or hypoxia of the tissues. Central cyanosis is most important in the pulmonary examination and is best seen in the lips or buccal mucosa. The bluish discoloration of central cyanosis occurs secondary to unoxygenated hemoglobin (reduced hemoglobin) in the capillaries. Central cyanosis is not perceptible until there are at least 5 gm of reduced hemoglobin per 100 ml of blood[6]; thus it is a late sign of hypoxemia. In the infant, cyanosis may not be apparent with lung disease until the child becomes extremely hypoxemic. Factors that may alter the observation of cyanosis include the practitioner's color perception, the lighting conditions, and the patient's skin pigmentation. In assessing for cyanosis, the patient's hemoglobin level must be taken into consideration.[7] Extremely high or low levels of hemoglobin in the body will alter the patient's presentation of cyanosis. Other signs of hypoxemia must also be assessed to evaluate the patient's oxygenation status.

Edema is an excessive accumulation of interstitial fluid, which is commonly associated with congestive heart failure. It may also be secondary to hypoxemia and subsequently pulmonary hypertension or cor pulmonale. Edema resulting from pulmonary dysfunction is most often seen in the ankles or in the presacral area of the supine patient. Usually the more dependent areas of the body are most affected by the edema. Edema is best appreciated by the examiner pressing his thumb or fingers into the area that is preferably against a bony structure. The edema is usually described as 1+, 2+ or 3+ (pitting edema). A fluid accumulation of 10 pounds must result before pitting edema is noted.

The extremities must also be inspected for clubbing. Clubbing is defined as a bulbous enlargement of the fingernails or toenails (Fig. 3-11). The earliest sign of clubbing is sponginess or mobility of the fixed end of the nail plate. As clubbing enters advanced stages, the nail becomes thickened, ridged, and curved.[7] The exact cause of clubbing is unknown; it is associated with several serious disorders. One explanation of the cause is that tissue hypoxia causes an increase in the number of arteriovenous anastomoses in the digit.[7]

Head and neck region. After observing the general appearance of the patient, the practitioner should next examine the head and neck region. It should be noted whether the patient is breathing primarily through the nose or the mouth. An abnormality that may be observed is flaring of the nares, which may be indicative of respiratory distress in the infant. Also, one may observe the use of pursed-lip breathing in the patient with chronic obstructive lung disease. This technique is thought to help prolong the expiratory phase of ventilation, which helps lessen resistance to airflow and reduce the work of breathing. Therefore the patient can increase the amount of air exhaled with each breath. This helps to decrease air-trapping in the patient with chronic obstructive lung disease.

Often forgotten as important parts of the respiratory system are the nose and throat, which should also be inspected. It should be noted whether the nasal mucosa is inflamed or whether nasal polyps are present. The mouth and throat should be inspected for any signs of inflammation or problems with the tongue or teeth that might cause airway obstruction.

The neck should be inspected for signs of venous distention while the patient is in the supine position or sitting up at a 45-degree angle (see Fig. 2-21). Next, the practitioner must observe the trachea for its normal, midline position. A shift in the position of the trachea is often suggestive of a pneumothorax in a critically ill patient. Finally, it should be noted whether the patient is using the accessory muscles of the neck and shoulders to assist in breathing. Use of these accessory muscles is indicative of increased work of breathing.

Thorax. Before proceeding with the inspection of the thorax, it is important that the practitioner be familiar with the topographic anatomy

Fig. 3-11. A, Normal angle of nail. **B,** Slight clubbing. **C,** Severe clubbing.

From Abels, L.F.: Mosby's manual of critical care, St. Louis, 1979, The C.V. Mosby Co.

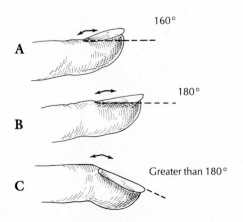

used to describe the findings. The examiner must know the location of the underlying structures and position of any abnormalities detected on the anterior, lateral, and posterior surfaces of the thorax. Diagrams of these important landmarks are shown in Fig. 3-12. It is also of utmost importance that the examiner describe the physical assessment observations in relation to the topographic landmarks. This provides better documentation of the findings and more descriptive information for the other members of the health care team.

In beginning the inspection of the thorax it-self, the chest wall excursion should be noted. The two sides of the chest should move synchronously and expand equally. Next, the practitioner should note the anteroposterior diameter of the thorax. The anteroposterior and transverse diameters of the thorax are nearly equal in the newborn (1:1). Over time there is a greater increase in the transverse diameter. Therefore by the time the child reaches puberty, the chest contour has adult proportions (1:2). The thorax in the normal adult is more elliptic, whereas in the infant it is more cylindrical in shape.

The overall configuration of the thoracic

Fig. 3-12. Landmarks for physical examination. **A,** Anterior landmarks. **B,** Lateral landmarks. **C,** Posterior landmarks.

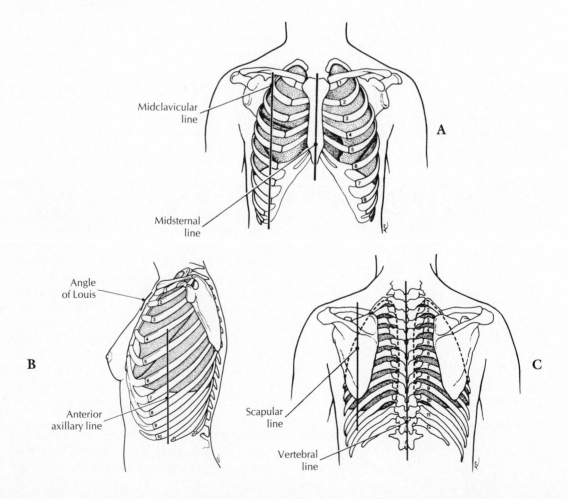

cage should be noted. Alterations in the shape of the thorax may include the following:

1. Barrel chest—an increase in the anterior-posterior diameter found frequently in patients with chronic obstructive pulmonary disease. This may also be seen in the normal process of aging.
2. Funnel chest (pectus excavatum)—a depression of part or all of the sternum.
3. Chicken or pigeon breast (pectus carinatum)—an anterior protrusion of the sternum with a series of vertical depressions along the costochondral junctions.
4. Harrison's groove—a horizontal groove or indentation located at the level of the diaphragm, with some flaring of the rib cage below the groove.
5. Scoliosis—a lateral curvature of the spine.
6. Kyphosis—a forward curvature of the spine.

In an infant, *pectus excavatum* may be seen in early infancy, with significant midline substernal

Fig. 3-13. Abnormal chest configurations. **A,** Barrel chest. **B,** Funnel chest. **C,** Pigeon chest. **D,** Harrison's grooves.

From Abels, L.F.: Mosby's manual of critical care, St. Louis, 1979, The C.V. Mosby Co.

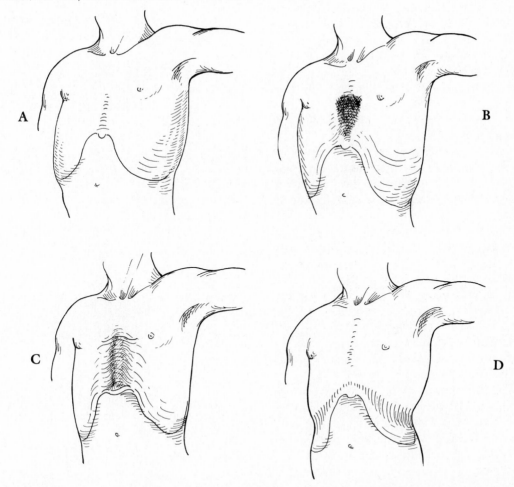

retractions during normal respiration (Fig. 3-13). Other deformities, such as *pectus carinatum,* may not become evident until early childhood. Often the chest deformities listed above do not inhibit the patient's gas exchange mechanism but may inhibit chest wall excursion.

The slope of the ribs should also be noted. Normally the ribs are situated at about a 45-degree angle to the spine. It is best to have the patient in a sitting or supine position when observing the rib angle, because a side-lying position may impair the movement of the rib cage.

Assessment of the patient's work of breathing is accomplished by inspection. Bulging or retraction of the interspaces should be noted. Because the increased compliance in the infant's chest wall, it is often easy to observe the bulging or retractions of the interspaces. These may be described as suprasternal, intercostal, or subcostal. Retraction of the interspaces, which is usually noted on inspiration, indicates obstruction to inspiratory air flow. Bulging of the interspaces may occur with massive pleural effusion or tension pneumothorax and is usually seen during expiration.

Other observations of respiratory effort should be made by the practitioner. The type, rate, depth, and quality of the respirations should be noted. Areas to be assessed include the following:

1. Type of respirations
2. Rate (with or without ventilator assistance)
3. Inspiratory/expiratory ratio
4. Estimated depth of respirations (shallow versus deep)
5. Use of accessory muscles
6. Symmetry of movement
7. Abdominal versus upper thoracic movement

The patient's respiratory rate should first be determined. Observation of the rate should be done for 30 seconds, then multiplied by 2. If there is an abnormal pattern, the rate should be assessed for a full minute. Normal rates are listed as follows:

Neonate 30-50
Infant   6 mo to 2 yr, 20-30
         2 yr to adolescence, 12-20
Adult   16-20

If the patient is on a ventilator and has some spontaneous ventilations, the patient's own res-

Fig. 3-14. Patterns of respiration.

Normal

Bradypnea

Tachypnea

Hyperventilation

Sighing

Cheyne-Stokes

Kussmaul

Biot's

Ataxic

piratory rate along with the ventilator rate should be noted.

There are several respiratory patterns with which the practitioner should be familiar. These patterns of respiration are briefly described and diagrammed in Fig. 3-14.

An additional pattern the practitioner must observe for is a discoordinated or asynchronous chest wall movement. Two types of asynchronous breathing patterns may be noted. In the *flail chest* pattern, usually two or more ribs are broken on one side of the chest wall, which results in a distortion of the structural aspect of the thoracic cage. The affected side of the thorax will move asynchronously with inspiration and expiration. On inspiration, the affected area will move inward, and on expiration it will bulge outward. Another type of asynchronous breathing is seen when the respiratory muscles become discoordinated because of fatigue. In this breathing pattern the intercostal muscles and diaphragm do not contract simultaneously. They appear to contract in sequence and tend to oppose each other.[40]

Palpation

The thorax should next be examined by palpation. Palpation is used to confirm observed findings and to obtain supplemental information. It may be used to assess the structural integrity of the chest wall, check the position of the trachea, or further investigate areas of inflammation or tenderness. Many times thoracic excursion or expansion can be better appreciated by palpation than by simple observation. The anterolateral and posterolateral aspects of the rib cage should be palpated during both quiet and deep breathing. The practitioner's hands should be placed over the lower anterolateral area of the chest wall with the thumbs along the costal margin, each pointing toward the xiphoid process. The palms and fingers should then be extended over the anterolateral wall. The expansion should also be palpated over the posterolateral chest wall in the same manner. As the patient's chest expands with inspiration, the practitioner's

hands should separate simultaneously and should be equidistant from the vertebral column at end-inspiration. Disorders that interfere with lung expansion, such as pneumothorax or pneumonia, can cause asymmetrical chest movement, as can diaphragm disorders or phrenic nerve injuries. In the critically ill patient, the respiratory excursion may be difficult to determine with this method, but palpation and measurement may prove beneficial. The symmetry of movement of the chest wall is important to note, along with any differences in excursion.

In addition to palpation, the practitioner must also consider assessing the presence and quality of vocal fremitus. *Fremitus* simply means vibration. Vocal or tactile fremitus is the sensation of sound vibrations produced in the airways when the patient speaks. The vibrations may be perceived through the thoracic wall by the palm of the hand or the fingertips. In eliciting vocal fremitus the patient is instructed to count "1, 2, 3" or to say "99" or the letter "e." The patient should speak in a normal voice so as not to increase or decrease the intensity of the fremitus. Each side of the chest wall should be compared for symmetry of fremitus. Normal variations of tactile fremitus are determined by the intensity and pitch of the voice, along with the relationship of the bronchi to the chest wall. Although the infant cannot be instructed to say words, tactile fremitus can be felt easily during crying episodes. In general, tactile or vocal fremitus is more prominent in areas where the large airways are closest to the thoracic wall. Alterations of vocal or tactile fremitus include increased, decreased, or absent fremitus. In reviewing some of the basic principles of physics, it can be recalled that a solid medium of uniform structure conducts vibrations better than does a porous structure of solid and air. With any additional medium through which the fremitus or vibrations must pass (air, fluid, solid), the sounds may be distorted. Increased vocal or tactile fremitus may be caused by consolidated tissue, atelectasis or a mass in the lung. Decreased or absent fremitus may be caused by a pleural

Table 3-2. Classification of percussion notes

Sound	Characteristics	Cause	Representative site or condition
Resonant	Moderately loud, low-pitched, long, hollow sound	Normal ratio of air-containing tissue to solid tissue under area of percussion	Normal lung
Hyperresonant	Very loud, low-pitched, long, booming type of sound	Increased ratio of air-containing tissue to solid tissue	Emphysema Pneumothorax Conditions with "air trapping" in the lung
Tympanic	Loud, high-pitched, moderately long, drumlike sound	Air under pressure	Tension pneumothorax Gastric air bubble
Dull (hyporesonant)	Moderately soft, high-pitched, long, thudding sound	Decreased ratio of air-containing tissue to solid tissue	Atelectasis Consolidation Liver
Flat	Soft, high-pitched, short, flat sound	Greatly decreased ratio of air-containing tissue to solid tissue	Muscle Bone

effusion, pneumothorax, or blockage of the airways.

Crepitations or subcutaneous emphysema may be palpated when the subcutaneous tissue contains air. This condition is caused by an escape of air from the lung into the subcutaneous tissue. Crepitus or a crackling sensation can be felt by compression of the affected tissues. Often the crepitations are the result of thoracic trauma or leaking of air into the tissues around a chest tube or tracheostomy tube.

Percussion

After the thorax has been palpated, the practitioner must percuss the chest wall. Percussion is the art of tapping the chest wall in a systematic way to elicit a sound. Over the lungs, sonorous percussion is usually performed to evaluate the density of underlying tissues. It has been shown that the sounds produced by percussion probably do not penetrate more than about 4 to 5 cm below the chest wall surface.[35] Percussion helps to determine whether the underlying tissues are air filled, fluid filled, or solid.

Percussion is difficult to master and takes a great deal of practice, as do some of the other processes of physical examination. The most common type of percussion used is called *mediate percussion*. This technique includes the practice of the following key points. First, the middle pleximeter finger of the left or right hand is hyperextended and placed firmly on the surface to be percussed. It is important to avoid contact by any other part of the hand on the chest wall, because this will dampen the vibrations produced. Next, the opposite hand should be placed near the hand that is placed on the chest wall. The middle finger of the "striking" hand should be poised partially flexed, but relaxed wrist above the hand on the chest wall. With a sharp but relaxed motion, the pleximeter finger is struck on the chest wall with the right middle finger of the opposite hand.[35] Use of the finger tip and not the finger pad will produce the most distinct percussion note. The motion should be done smoothly and quickly so as not to dampen the percussion note. Percussion should be done on all aspects of the chest wall. The sound produced should be noted and compared with the sounds from the contralateral side.

Percussion is performed above the clavicles in the supraclavicular spaces, followed by percussion of the interspaces, always comparing both sides for symmetry. The examiner should proceed down the posterior thoracic wall. The pleximeter finger should always be parallel to the ribs—never across them—because this may dampen the sound produced. The lateral and anterior surfaces should also be examined in the same manner.

Sounds produced by percussion are influenced by the character of the immediate underlying structures of the thoracic wall. The examiner must learn to distinguish certain notes that are characteristic of percussion so that abnormalities may be detected along with the location of normal underlying structures. The sounds of percussion have four characteristics: intensity, pitch, quality, and duration.[35] The classification of percussion notes or sounds is shown in Table 3-2.

Positioning of the patient may affect the percussion note obtained. The anterior and anterolateral wall of the chest may be satisfactorily examined in the supine position. If the patient is in the lateral recumbent position, the following factors may cause changes in sound: the surface of the bed may act to dampen the percussion sounds. The hemidiaphragm on the side next to the bed may be elevated because pressure from the abdominal contents. On the "down" side, there may be some widening of the interspaces as compared to the "up" side. This results from the slight curvature of the spine in the side-lying position. This curvature can be minimized if the body alignment is improved by removal of the pillow under the patient's head.[35] These changes are shown in Fig. 3-15.

Auscultation

The final step of the physical assessment of the thorax includes auscultation of the chest. Auscultation is the art of listening to the sounds produced within the lungs with a stethoscope; the examiner listens for three different sounds in the chest: normal breath sounds, adventitious breath sounds, and voice sounds.

The stethoscope is an important tool of physical examination of the thorax. When listening to the chest, the diaphragm of the stethoscope is used to listen to the higher pitched sounds. If only an adult-size diaphragm is avail-

Fig. 3-15. Effect of lateral recumbent position on percussion note. *A,* Zone of relative dullness next to bed. *B,* Zone of dullness caused by pressure of viscera. *C,* Area of dullness at approximately the tip of the scapula.

From Prior, J.A.: Silberstein, J.S., and Stang, J.M.: Physical diagnosis: the history and examination of the patient, ed. 6, St. Louis, 1981, The C.V. Mosby Co.

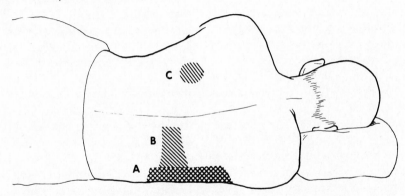

Table 3-3. Descriptive review of normal breath sounds

Sound	Normal location	Abnormal location	Duration	Characteristics
Bronchial or tracheal	Over trachea and large airways	Over small airways (in periphery of lung)	$E > I$	Loud, tubular, harsh sounds; have a "blowing" quality
Vesicular	Over all areas of lung except where large airways are close to surface	—	$I > E$	Soft, low pitched rustling sound

able when listening to a small chest wall, the bell of the stethoscope should be used, because a smaller area is covered and auscultative perception can be more precise. When using the bell of the stethoscope, it should be lightly placed on the chest wall above an intercostal space for the best transmission of sounds.

Breath sounds result from air moving through the tracheobronchial tree: the sounds are produced by turbulence in the airways. Analysis of breath sounds includes four areas: pitch, intensity, quality, and duration. Auscultation should be done systematically, starting at the apical areas of the lung and listening to both sides of the chest for comparison. The examiner should move down the chest wall, being sure to include the anterior, posterior, and lateral aspects. It is best to perform auscultation with the patient sitting erect with the shoulders slightly forward, but this may be difficult in a critical care setting. If the patient is supine, he should be rolled first on one side while the examiner listens to the anterior, posterior, and lateral sounds of the "up" side. Then the patient should be rolled to the opposite side-lying position for comparison of sounds. Putting the patient in the side-lying position helps to minimize compression of the lungs on the "up" side, thus decreasing the chance of misinterpretation of sounds.

There are some factors that may alter the auscultative findings in the critical care patient. If the patient has a nasogastric tube attached to a suction apparatus, the sounds from the suction may interfere with the auscultative process. If possible, the nasogastric tube should be clamped while the practitioner auscultates the lung. A ventilator may also change the characteristics of breath sounds. Although mechanically ventilating the lungs does not produce adventitious breath sounds, it may amplify the breath sounds. If the patient can tolerate being taken off the ventilator for a short time receiving ventilation with a positive pressure inflation bag, the examiner should do so. If the patient is ventilator dependent, this should be taken into account when noting the characteristics of the sounds. If the patient is on a high-flow oxygen system, the sound of the oxygen appliance may interfere with the auscultative process. Also water accumulation in the oxygen appliance or ventilator tubing may interfere with listening to the chest sounds. Finally, a chest tube may produce a pleural friction rub in the areas adjacent to the insertion site.

When beginning the auscultative examination of the lungs, the examiner must understand that there are sounds of the tracheobronchial system that are considered normal. There are two types of normal sounds that are distinguishable in the chest: bronchial or tracheal and vesicular breath sounds.[29] The characteristics of these sounds are reviewed in Table 3-3. A third type of sound, bronchovesicular, may be referred to in some textbooks, but it has been dropped from the American Thoracic Society nomenclature.[29] It is of prime importance to note the location and intensity of the normal breath sounds. If a normal sound is heard

Table 3-4. Descriptive review of abnormal or adventitious breath sounds

Sound	Characteristics	Cause	Example of disease process where sound may be heard
Wheeze	High pitched continuous sound heard primarily on expiration	Narrowing of airways in periphery of lung	Asthma
Rhonchus	Low-pitched, continuous sound heard primarily on expiration; a "snoring" sound	Narrowing of large airways; may be associated with accumulation of sputum in large airways	Sputum accumulation in large airways; loss of muscle tone in upper airway
Fine crackle	Discontinuous, explosive type of sound heard primarily on inspiration	Sudden opening of small airways and alveoli Air moving through fluid in the airway	Pulmonary fibrosis; atelectasis; early stages of pneumonia Early stages of congestive heart failure; pulmonary edema
Coarse crackle	Discontinuous, low-pitched, bubbling sound heard primarily on inspiration but may be heard on both inspiration and expiration	Rupture of fluid films or bubbles in the airways	Pulmonary edema; resolution of pneumonia

somewhere other than in its usual location, this would be considered abnormal. An example of this would be a bronchial breath sound found in an area where vesicular breath sounds should be heard. This is a typical finding over an area of consolidation or atelectasis.

Adventitious or abnormal breath sounds are those sounds other than the bronchial, tracheal, or vesicular sounds. According to the recommended American Thoracic Society nomenclature, the four types of abnormal breath sounds are coarse crackle, fine crackle, wheeze, and rhonchus.[29] The pleural friction rub is also considered to be an abnormal breath sound. It is easiest to identify the characteristics of the abnormal sounds as (1) continuous or intermittent, and (2) inspiratory or expiratory. Shown in Table 3-4 are the primary characteristics of the adventitious sounds.

Before attempting to summarize auscultatory findings in specific pulmonary conditions, it is helpful to discuss the general associations of the adventitious sounds mentioned previously. Continuous sounds usually reflect abnormalities

of the airways, whereas discontinuous or intermittent sound reflect abnormalities of the parenchyma and/or airways. High-pitched continuous sounds (wheezes) are associated with narrowing of central airways. Wheezes may be caused by bronchospasm, edema of the airway lining, mucous plugging and foreign bodies, or tumors. When a high-pitched continuous sound is confined to inspiration or is accentuated during inspiration, it is called *stridor*. Stridor is commonly associated with extrathoracic obstruction. Lower pitched continuous sounds (rhonchi) are usually associated with secretions of the large, central airways. These rhonchi often change significantly after cough and expectoration. Intermittent sounds (crackles) are usually heard on inspiration and reflect abnormality in the peripheral airways and lung parenchyma. They are sometimes referred to as *rales*. Crackles are explosive sounds caused by vibrations from the sudden release of energy stored in the elastic or surface forces in the lung.[29] The coarse crackles of pulmonary edema or other conditions with fluid accumulation in the airways are thought to be caused by rupture of fluid films or bubbles.[29] These crackles often occur during both inspiration and expiration and may change after a cough or a change in position.

Compared to the coarse crackles of pulmonary edema, the fine crackles heard in pulmonary fibrosis or early congestive heart failure are not a result of fluid in the airways; these fine crackles are thought to be caused by the delayed opening of airways during inspiration that have closed at the end of the previous expiration.[29] These fine crackles are heard primarily on inspiration.

Finally, the pleural friction rub is a discontinuous, grating type of sound that is heard on both inspiration and expiration. It indicates distortion of the normal anatomy of the pleural surface, usually from inflammation.

Voice sounds may also be evaluated in the auscultative process. The vibrations produced by a whispered or spoken voice can be heard with a stethoscope. Changes in these sounds are helpful in detecting consolidation and atelectasis.

There are some differences noted between auscultation of the child and adult. Breath sounds in small children and infants are more harsh and sound louder than do the breath sounds in adults. This results from the thin chest wall and the proximity of the airways to the chest wall. The child's head should be in a central forward position when auscultating the chest. The types of breath sound heard in the child are similar to those of the adult. In the infant, fine inspiratory crackles may be heard immediately after birth. This probably results from the initial opening of unexpanded airways and alveoli.[7] These are similar to the fine crackles heard in the adult with pulmonary fibrosis or early congestive heart failure.

In summary, the respiratory physical assessment of the neonate, pediatric, or adult patient is a comprehensive process that involves inspection, palpation, percussion, and auscultation. By integrating all of this data and considering the patient's clinical condition, the practitioner is better able to provide comprehensive care to the critically ill patient. Although the complete re-

spiratory physical assessment may be time consuming and involved, the practitioner should be skilled in all facets and be able to selectively apply these skills in the clinical setting.

Laboratory data

Several different laboratory examinations are necessary to thoroughly evaluate the patient's respiratory status. It is necessary for the critical care practitioner to be knowledgeable about the tests and results as applicable to a specific patient and his condition. Most often in a critical care setting comparative findings in laboratory data are valuable in assessing patient status. The practitioner must understand the significance of changes or trends in the data obtained on a patient.

Arterial blood gas analysis

When assessing a patient's respiratory status, one often thinks of the arterial blood gas (ABG) measurement. It is an important tool in assessing the patient for problems with ventilation, oxygenation, metabolic disorders, and effects of treatment. Unfortunately, the interpretation of the ABG is often a difficult task for the beginning practitioner. If the analysis is approached in a logical manner with a sound knowledge of the basics of acid-base balance and the mechanisms of hypoxemia, the ABG interpretation can provide valuable information plus a broadened clinical assessment of the patient.

One must always remember that laboratory findings may be incorrect; the practitioner must be able to recognize values that are questionable. In interpreting ABG results, the practitioner must review and compare the patient's physical condition and the laboratory findings. As with any laboratory values, there are "normal" ABG values. It is important to point out that a patient who had pulmonary dysfunction before entering the critical care unit may not have "normal" values as a baseline even in his optimal pulmonary status. Thus one should be aware of previous underlying pulmonary problems when interpreting these values. The normal arterial

Table 3-5. Normal arterial and venous blood gas values

Value	Arterial	Venous
pH (negative logarithm of H^+ ion concentration)	7.35 to 7.45	7.31 to 7.41
P_{CO_2} (partial pressure of CO_2)	35 to 45 mmHg	41 to 51
P_{CO_2} (partial pressure of O_2)	80 to 100 mmHg	35 to 40
HCO_3^- (bicarbonate ion concentration)	22 to 26 mEq/L	22 to 26
O_2 saturation (extent to which Hgb is saturated with O_2)	95% or greater	70 to 75%
Base excess (total buffering capacity in solution)	−2 to +2	−2 to +2

and venous blood gas values are shown in Table 3-5.

Venous blood gases may be used to determine the extraction of oxygen at the tissue level. Since the metabolic rate can differ in the various areas of the body, the O_2 and CO_2 content of venous blood in these areas can also differ. Therefore for most purposes it is important to secure a mixed venous blood sample. These venous blood samples are usually obtained from a catheter placed in the pulmonary artery (Swan-Ganz catheter). A fiberoptic pulmonary artery catheter can also be used to assess tissue oxygenation. By attaching this catheter to an oximeter, continuous monitoring of the saturation of venous blood ($S\bar{v}O_2$) is possible. Thus one can measure the $S\bar{v}O_2$, along with the usual measurements of pulmonary vascular pressures and thermodilution cardiac output. Fiberoptic pulmonary artery catheters can provide early warning of deterioration in cardiopulmonary function. The practitioner can use the continuous monitoring of $S\bar{v}O_2$ to determine the effects of certain procedures (suctioning, turning) on tissue oxygenation and to guide patient care.

pH. As stated earlier in the chapter, pH level describes the patient's general acid-base status. An arterial pH of less than 7.35 indicates acidemia, whereas an arterial pH of greater than 7.45 indicates alkalemia. An acid-base abnormality can be judged as being respiratory, metabolic, or a combination of the two. When using the Henderson-Hasselbalch equation, primary disturbances involving the HCO_3^- (the numerator) are metabolic, and those involving the

CO_2 (the denominator) are respiratory in nature.

Pa_{CO_2}. The respiratory parameter of the ABG is the Pa_{CO_2} or partial pressure of arterial carbon dioxide. This parameter allows determination of the adequacy of alveolar ventilation. The Pa_{CO_2} is inversely related to the alveolar ventilation. This parameter is affected by the alveolar ventilation and the production of CO_2 through metabolism in the cells. An increased Pa_{CO_2} indicates hypoventilation at the alveolar level, whereas a decreased Pa_{CO_2} indicates hyperventilation at the alveolar level. If the amount of alveolar ventilation is too small for the level of CO_2 production, there will be an elevated Pa_{CO_2} in the blood and the condition of hypercapnia or hypercarbia will exist. Similarly, if the level of alveolar ventilation is too high as compared with the CO_2 production of the body, the Pa_{CO_2} will be decreased and the condition of hypocapnia (hypocarbia) will exist. It must also be noted that increased or decreased values of Pa_{CO_2} may also signify compensation for metabolic disturbances as well as primary respiratory imbalances.

As previously stated, the Pa_{CO_2} has a direct relationship to the pH, as shown in the Henderson-Hasselbalch equation. If one assumes that the HCO_3^- stays stable or normal, a direct relationship between pH and CO_2 results. This relationship is inverse and is nearly linear. For every increase of 10 mmHg in Pa_{CO_2}, the pH will decrease by 0.08 units. These changes occur if this is an acute situation in the patient. In the patient with a chronic pulmonary problem, the kidneys

Table 3-6. Causes of metabolic acidosis with an increased and normal anion gap

Normal anion gap	Increased anion gap
Renal tubular acidosis	Lactic acidosis
Diarrhea or GI fluid loss of HCO_3^-	Renal failure
Administration of ammonium chloride, carbonic anhydrase inhibitors (Diamox)	Poisonings (salicylate, paraldehyde, ethylene glycol, methyl alcohol)

Anion gap = Serum $Na^+ - (HCO_3^- + Cl^-)$
Normal anion gap < 15 mEq/L

will act to increase reabsorption of HCO_3^-. This increased HCO_3^- will add to the buffering mechanism of the blood so that an increase of 10 mmHg in the Pa_{CO_2} will only cause a decrease of 0.03 pH units.[10]

One must pay particularly close attention to the Pa_{CO_2} in the critically ill patient. Understanding the basis of fluctuation in Pa_{CO_2} through changes in the patient's condition or alterations in therapy are important in understanding and instituting patient care.

HCO_3^-. Bicarbonate is the metabolic parameter of ABG analysis. Regulation of HCO_3^- is primarily a function of the kidneys. Since the kidneys are the prime regulators of HCO_3^-, changes in the parameter are slow (24 to 48 hours), compared to the changes in Pa_{CO_2}, which occur within minutes.[25] However, HCO_3^- changes can be manipulated quickly by artificial administration of sodium bicarbonate or ammonium chloride to the patient.

The HCO_3^- represents the primary blood base. Strictly speaking, an increase in HCO_3^- causes metabolic alkalosis, whereas a decrease causes metabolic acidosis. One must also consider the parameter of Pa_{CO_2} before an interpretation of the ABG can be made. Metabolic alkalosis can occur as a result of H^+ loss or bicarbonate gain. Metabolic acidosis in the critically ill patient is often caused by decreased tissue perfusion. It can also occur as a result of an increase in measurable or unmeasurable anions. To determine whether metabolic acidosis has resulted from an increase in measurable or unmeasurable anions, the following formula can be used:

Anion gap = Serum $Na^+ - (HCO_3^- + Cl^-)$

If the difference is greater than 15 mEq/L, there is an increase in unmeasurable anions. Table 3-6 shows causes of metabolic acidosis with an increased and normal anion gap.

Pa_{O_2}. Normal Pa_{O_2} is dependent on age, position, and altitude. Therefore hypoxemia is defined as a Pa_{O_2} that is less than predicted. There are five basic causes of hypoxemia: (1) ventilation/perfusion imbalance or mismatch, (2) anatomical right to left shunt, (3) ambient hypoxemia (altitude), (4) absolute hypoventilation, and (5) diffusion abnormality. The Pa_{O_2} of ABG analysis is used to guide the O_2 and ventilatory management of the patient. Although the Pa_{O_2} is often labeled the most vital parameter of the ABG, it actually provides little information about the acid-base status of the patient. It, along with other parameters, provides information about the patient's oxygenation status. In the critical care patient the practitioner must look at the Pa_{O_2}, saturation of hemoglobin, hemoglobin value, and fraction of inspired O_2 (F_IO_2) to determine the patient's oxygenation status.

Often in the critically ill patient the mixed venous partial pressure of O_2 ($P\bar{v}_{O_2}$) will also be obtained. The $P\bar{v}_{O_2}$ reflects the amount of O_2 that has been removed or extracted during passage through the body. A normal $P\bar{v}_{O_2}$ is 40 mmHg (patient breathing room air). Thus a $P\bar{v}_{O_2}$ greater than 40 signifies decreased O_2 extraction at the tissue level while a $P\bar{v}_{O_2}$ less than 40 indicates an increased O_2 extraction at the tissue level. The $P\bar{v}_{O_2}$ may be affected by either the oxygenation component (lung), the tissue perfusion component (heart, circulation), or both.[5] Thus if a patient has an abnormal $P\bar{v}O_2$, the practitioner must further differentiate the cause.

In the critical care area, the alveolar-arterial gradient of O_2 (A-a O_2 gradient) is often a useful measurement. This value signifies the gradient between the alveolar and arterial partial pressure of O_2. It is used to assess the ventilation and perfusion matching in the lungs and the amount of venous admixture. A normal A-a O_2 gradient is less than 20 mm Hg. A simplified equation that may be used to easily assess the A-a O_2 gradient is:

$$\text{A-a } O_2 \text{ Gradient} = PA_{O_2} - Pa_{O_2}$$

where $\quad Pa_{O_2}$ = Arterial blood gas value (example, Pa_{O_2} = 90 mmHg)

PA_{O_2} = [(Barometric pressure − 47) × F_IO_2] − (Pa_{CO_2} × 1.2)

EXAMPLE: $\quad PA_{O_2} \quad = [(760 - 47) \times 0.21] - (40 \times 1.2)$

$PA_{O_2} \quad = 150 - 48$

$PA_{O_2} \quad = 102$

$PA_{O_2} - Pa_{O_2} = 102 - 90$

A-a O_2 Gradient $= 12$ mmHg

O_2 saturation. Oxygen saturation is equal to the actual amount of O_2 carried with hemoglobin divided by the O_2 capacity. Usually an O_2 saturation equal to or greater than 90% is considered acceptable. This minimum saturation (90%) corresponds approximately to a Pa_{O_2} of 60 mmHg. It is important to remember that if the hemoglobin value is lower than normal, then the amount of O_2 that can be transported per liter of blood is decreased.

Base excess. Base excess is defined as the total amount of buffering or base in solution. The base excess is expressed in mEq/L above or below the normal buffer base range (normal $O \pm 2$ mEq/L). The base excess serves as an index of metabolic acidosis, and it can be used both diagnostically and therapeutically. A negative base excess is considered along with the pH in determining the administration of sodium bicar-

bonate to the patient for correction of metabolic acidosis.

In analyzing the acid-base status of the patient, it is imperative that the practitioner understand the importance and meaning of each parameter. Only by understanding the cause and effect relationship of each parameter can one properly interpret the results. To describe the acid-base condition of a patient, the correct terminology must be used. Some basic definitions are as follows:

acidemia Acid condition of the blood of a pH less than 7.35.
alkalemia Alkaline condition of the blood of a pH greater than 7.45.
acidosis Process causing acidemia.
alkalosis Process causing alkalemia.

The pH is the measurement used to determine the body's H^+ concentration. Thus in analyzing ABG results, one must first determine whether the blood is acidemic (pH less than 7.35) or alkalemic (pH greater than 7.45). Second, the practitioner must identify the cause of the pH abnormality. It may be a respiratory process, a metabolic process, or a combination of these two causing the abnormality. Once the primary cause or process has been determined, the practitioner must determine whether compensation is occurring. An important point to remember is that the body never overcompensates when attempting to correct acid-base balance. Third, the practitioner must determine the severity of the disturbance. There are four primary processes that the practitioner must consider in analyzing the acid-base data: respiratory acidosis, respiratory alkalosis, metabolic acidosis, or metabolic alkalosis. It must be noted, however, that a combination of these primary processes may occur, especially in the critically ill patient. The box on p. 209 shows causes of the four acid-base disturbances; the changes that are seen in the ABG values are shown in Table 3-7.

Respiratory acidosis. Respiratory acidosis results from retention of CO_2 with an increase in the Pa_{CO_2} and carbonic acid. The cause of the

Table 3-7. Alterations in arterial blood gas values

Condition	pH	$PaCO_2$	HCO_3^-
Normal ABG values	7.35-7.45	35-45	22-26
Acute respiratory acidosis	↓	↑	↔
Compensated respiratory acidosis	↔ or slight ↓	↑	↑
Acute respiratory alkalosis	↑	↓	↔
Compensated respiratory alkalosis	↔ or slight ↑	↓	↓
Metabolic acidosis*	↓	↓	↓
Metabolic alkalosis*	↑	slight ↑	↑

*Respiratory compensation for metabolic disorders occurs very quickly, but this compensation is usually incomplete.

respiratory acidosis is alveolar hypoventilation or failure to eliminate adequate CO_2 from the lungs. In acute respiratory acidosis, the $PaCO_2$ is higher than normal, the pH is acidemic, and the HCO_3^- is within the normal range. If the respiratory acidosis is a chronic problem, with compensation the $PaCO_2$ will be higher than normal, the HCO_3^- will be increased, and the pH will be in the acidotic range or near normal. Most often the diagnosis of acute respiratory acidosis is established by an increase in arterial $PaCO_2$ and a fall in pH as determined by the analysis of the ABG.

Treatment of respiratory acidosis is aimed at improving alveolar ventilation. This may require the use of assisted ventilation or changes in the ventilator settings if the patient's lungs are already being mechanically ventilated. It is important to attempt to locate and treat the cause of the patient's hypoventilation, whether it is an obstruction of the airway, an increase in anatomical or physiological dead space, or one of the other causes listed.

Respiratory alkalosis. Respiratory alkalosis results from hyperventilation of the alveoli, causing a decreased $PaCO_2$ with a resulting increase in pH. Respiratory alkalosis is very common in the critically ill adult patient, resulting from a variety of problems. First, hyperventilation occurs in many hypermetabolic states such as fever, a response to pain, or stress. Prolonged hyperventilation and respiratory alkalosis may characterize the early stages of acute respiratory failure. Overventilation of a ventilator-dependent patient is a common problem in the critical care setting. This can be caused by a large tidal volume, a ventilatory rate which is too fast or a combination of the two. It must be noted, however, that the use of a high volume or rate may be necessary for adequate oxygenation even at the expense of hyperventilating the patient.

Excessive respiratory alkalosis is undesirable in a number of critically ill patients. Those patients with heart disease and especially those receiving digitalis are subject to increased arrhythmias under alkalotic conditions. The cerebral blood flow may also be affected by decreased levels of CO_2 in the blood. Patients with increased cerebral pressure sometimes receive hyperventilation therapy to reduce the cerebral edema and pressure. One must note, however, that when the $PaCO_2$ falls below 20 mmHg, the cerebral blood flow falls by almost one third. Thus very low $PaCO_2$ levels may cause brain damage as a result of lack of perfusion.

As with respiratory acidosis, the underlying cause must be treated. It is probably best to attempt to keep the $PaCO_2$ above 30 mmHg so as not to introduce other problems in the patient. Correction of respiratory alkalosis of the patient on the ventilator is often simply accomplished. If the minute ventilation and tidal volume cannot be reduced because of the need for adequate oxygenation, some type of deadspace or rebreathing apparatus may be added to help increase the $PaCO_2$ level. In this instance, the F_IO_2 may need to be increased to maintain adequate oxygenation while increasing the $PaCO_2$.

Metabolic acidosis. Metabolic acidosis is defined as an increase in nonvolatile or fixed acid or a loss of base in the acid-base system. The clinical problems involving this process can be divided into two categories: (1) conditions in

---

CAUSES OF ACID-BASE DISTURBANCES

Causes of respiratory acidosis ($\uparrow$ Paco$_2$)
(hypoventilation)

Obstructive lung disease
Oversedation
Neuromuscular disorders
Hypoventilation with mechanical ventilation

Causes of respiratory alkalosis ($\downarrow$ Paco$_2$)
(hyperventilation)

Hypoxia
Nervousness and anxiety
Brain injury
Pulmonary embolus
Pulmonary fibrosis
Pregnancy
Hyperventilation with mechanical ventilation
Gram-negative septicemia
Fever

Causes of metabolic acidosis ($\downarrow$ HCO$_3^-$)

Diabetic ketoacidosis
Lactic acidosis
Renal failure
Diarrhea
Drainage of pancreatic juice
Ureterosigmoidostomy
Poisonings—salicylate, ethylene glycol,
   methyl alcohol, paraldehyde
Treatment with acetazolamide
Dilutional acidosis

Causes of metabolic alkalosis ($\uparrow$ HCO$_3^-$)

Vomiting, N-G tube drainage
Overusage of diuretics
Rapid correction of chronic hypercapnia
Treatment with corticosteroids
Hyperaldosteronism
Severe potassium depletion
Treatment with alkaline substances

---

which loss of base represents the primary mechanism, or (2) conditions in which acidic compounds accumulate in the extracellular fluid. Diagnosis of metabolic acidosis is seen as a decrease in pH and HCO$_3^-$ levels in the blood. Although the Paco$_2$ may also be decreased, the HCO$_3^-$ parameter is significantly decreased.

The first priority of treatment of metabolic acidosis lies in treating the underlying cause. Under some conditions it may be necessary to first treat the acidosis itself with administration of sodium bicarbonate. This correction should be done slowly and should not be done to completely correct the metabolic acidosis. There are problems that may occur in reversal of an acidosis with the administration of sodium bicarbonate. Serum potassium will be elevated in the presence of acidosis as a result of the potassium

moving into the extracellular fluid. With rapid correction of acidosis, the potassium again moves back into the cell and a significant deficit in serum potassium may occur. In addition it must be noted that ultimately HCO$_3^-$ added to the body will be converted into CO$_2$. Unless the lungs are able to eliminate this acid load, a respiratory acidosis will occur.

Metabolic alkalosis. Metabolic alkalosis is characterized by an increase in HCO$_3^-$ in the extracellular fluid or a loss of acid from the extracellular fluid. Various factors may cause a metabolic alkalosis. As with the other processes, treatment is aimed at the underlying cause of the metabolic alkalosis. Often volume depletion of the patient is associated with metabolic alkalosis. Replacement with a saline solution is indicated, along with careful monitoring of the serum potassium levels. Parenteral administration of an acid is usually not indicated in the treatment of metabolic alkalosis.

Combined or mixed acid-base disturbances. Often the acid-base abnormality is a complex situation, with multiple processes causing the disturbance. Clinically it is very common to see mixed respiratory and metabolic problems. The disturbances are particularly severe if the processes are in the same direction (for example, respiratory and metabolic acidosis). In this case the pH is severely acidotic and there is little question regarding the possibility of compensation occurring. The practitioner must analyze each parameter of the ABG individually to determine its contribution as a primary or secondary cause of the disturbance. Often in mixed disturbances the dominant disorder is reflected by the status of the pH, but the clinical evaluation of the patient may serve as the guide to the major problem. The practitioner must not only evaluate the ABG results but must also assess the patient's clinical status to gain a total perspective of the patient's condition.

Compensatory mechanisms. The compensatory mechanisms of the body are never complete, so that despite respiratory or renal compensation the pH remains slightly abnormal in the direction of the primary disturbance. Overcorrection is possible in the critical care setting, since changes in the ventilator settings may provide abrupt changes in the Pa_{CO_2} levels and intravenous medications can cause significant changes in the acid-base status. Further information on compensation was discussed in the acid-base regulation section of this chapter, pp. 189-192.

Complete blood count

A complete blood count (CBC) may play a role in evaluating the patient's pulmonary status. Symptoms, along with an increased white blood cell count, may provide information indicating an acute respiratory infection. Hemoglobin and hematocrit values are also important in evaluating the patient. Since hemoglobin is the major carrier of O_2 in the blood, evaluation of this parameter is important in assessing a possible cause of hypoxemia. The hematocrit is also an important parameter to evaluate in the critically ill patient. As a compensatory mechanism, the chronically hypoxemic patient may have an increased hemoglobin concentration in the body's attempt to provide greater O_2 carrying capacity. Thus the hematocrit level is evaluated. Usually an elevated hematocrit is seen as a chronic or long-term compensatory mechanism.

Electrolytes

Serum electrolytes are also valuable in assessing the respiratory patient. The HCO_3^- level, which is regulated by the kidney, represents the main indicator of primary metabolic acidosis or alkalosis. An increased HCO_3^- level may also indicate compensation for chronic respiratory acidosis. Development of respiratory acidosis is also associated with a shift of potassium out of the cells. This results in increased renal excretion and depletion of body potassium stores despite relatively normal or even high serum potassium levels. With the correction of the acidosis, potassium reenters the cells, and a low serum potassium level may result. Diuretics may also play a part in potassium depletion. Thus the practitioner must be aware of these changes and closely monitor the serum electrolytes in the critically ill patient.

Electrocardiogram

In the critical care setting, the electrocardiogram (ECG) may demonstrate changes resulting from pulmonary problems. Hypoxemia is frequently associated with supraventricular and sometimes ventricular arrhythmias.[7] Suggestive findings on the ECG may be found in the patient with chronic obstructive lung disease. These findings include evidence of right ventricular hypertrophy, right atrial enlargement (P-pulmonale), and poor R-wave progression in leads V_1 to V_3 along with low voltage. Although these changes are not specifically diagnostic, they may help in assessing the previous and present pulmonary status of the patient.

Chest roentgenogram

Also of importance in assessing the respiratory status of the patient is the chest roentgenogram (chest X-ray). In the critical care setting, chest roentgenograms are frequently taken to assess changes in pathologic conditions of the lung, to check for correct placement of an artificial airway, to look for abnormalities in the pleural space (pleural effusion, pneumothorax), or to check for correct placement of catheters. Although it may not be practical for the practitioner to have in-depth expertise in reading chest roentgenograms, it is necessary for the practitioner to recognize normal patterns and gross abnormalities that may appear during the patient's critical care course.

Different structures in the chest appear as different densities on the roentgenographic film. The four types of densities (blackness) seen on a chest film are air or gas, water, fat, and metal. Gas is the least dense and absorbs little of the X rays; thus such air-filled structures as the lungs appear blackest on the film. Water density is seen with soft tissue, muscle, and blood; therefore these structures are lighter in appearance. The lightest structures seen on the roentgenogram are the fat and bony structures (metal density).

Most frequently a posterior-anterior (PA) and lateral chest roentgenogram are taken. In the critical care setting, however, an anterior-posterior (AP) film is most commonly done because the patient is either supine or in the sitting position. One must note that there is some difference in the magnitude and size of structures in comparing a PA and AP chest film. Thus this point must be considered when attempting to compare films using these two different techniques.

In assessing a chest roentgenogram the practitioner should first review the normal structures in a systematic fashion. Too often an inexperienced practitioner will quickly identify the gross abnormalities and will miss smaller, less discrete problems. The following is a list of structures that should be inspected:

1. Bony structures—sternum, ribs, clavicles
2. Hemidiaphragms—normally the right hemidiaphragm is slightly higher than the left
3. Left and right heart borders
4. Tracheal air shadow and mainstem bronchi
5. Lung fields—density of lung fields, vascular markings to the periphery

Many abnormalities may occur on a chest roentgenogram of the critically ill patient. Some of the more frequent abnormalities seen in this setting are listed below:

1. Incorrect placement of an artificial airway—the distal tip of the tube should be two inches above the carina
2. Silhouette sign—obliteration of the borders of the heart, aorta, or diaphragm by a condition producing of water density; normally these borders can be distinguished
3. Consolidation—areas of increased density (whiteness) on a roentgenogram; this may be caused by atelectasis, pneumonia, or any process causing alveolar filling
4. Airspace bronchogram—normally, the bronchi cannot be seen because they are air-filled structures; when the lung tissue around the bronchi becomes a water density (lighter in color), the air-filled bronchi become outlined on the roentgenogram; this process may be caused by pneumonia, pulmonary edema, pulmonary infarctions, etc.
5. Pneumothorax—seen as increased radiopacity of the collapsed lung tissue, and the vascular markings do not extend to the periphery of the lung; there may be tracheal or mediastinal shift away from the affected side

The practitioner must be knowledgeable about the "normal" landmarks on the chest roentgenogram, along with the roentgenographic placement of the various catheters and tubes used in the critical care setting. One must be able to identify basic changes and correlate

Table 3-8. Diagnostic studies for evaluation of respiratory disorders

Test	Description	Indication
Theophylline level	Determines blood theophylline level; therapeutic level in pediatric and adult patients is 10-20 μg/ml	Used in monitoring blood level of methylxanthine bronchodilator medications; indication is the need to maintain a therapeutic level without the occurrence of centrally mediated side effects
Pulmonary function tests*		
Vital capacity (VC)	Volume of gas that can be expired from the lung after a maximal inspiration	May be used as criterion for ventilator discontinuation; patient should be able to generate 15 ml/kg
Forced expiratory volume in one second ($FEV_{1.0}$)	Volume of gas that can be expired as forcefully and rapidly as possible in 1 second after a maximal inspiration	May be used as criterion for ventilator discontinuation; patient should have a $FEV_{1.0}$ greater than 10 ml/kg
Minute ventilation ($\dot{V}_E$)	Total volume of gas either inspired or expired in 1 minute	May be used as criterion for ventilator discontinuation; should be less than 10 L/min
Maximum voluntary ventilation (MVV)	Maximum minute ventilation achieved over 15 seconds and multiplied times four	May be used as a criterion for ventilator discontinuation; gives an estimate of ventilatory reserve; MVV should be greater than two times the $\dot{V}_E$
Maximal inspiratory force (MIF) or inspiratory effort (IE)	Generation of negative pressure against an occluded airway; unlike the VC, $FEV_{1.0}$ and MVV, the MIF can be measured without the patient's cooperation	May be used as a criterion for ventilator discontinuation; gives an estimate of respiratory muscle strength; should be greater than -20 cm H_2O pressure.
Deadspace (V_D/V_T)	Measurement of physiologic dead space to tidal volume ratio; physiologic dead space = anatomic dead space + alveolar dead space $$V_D/V_T = (Pa_{CO_2} - Pe_{CO_2})/Pa_{CO_2}$$	Used to assess the percentage of tidal volume that does not participate in effective gas exchange; normal ratio is 0.3 or less
Effective dynamic compliance (C_{dyn})	Comparison of patient's tidal volume with the peak airway pressure on the ventilator $$C_{dyn} = \frac{Volume}{Peak\ pressure - PEEP\ (if\ any)}$$	Used to quickly assess compliance and airway resistance characteristics of the lungs; least accurate compliance measurement, because it is not measured under static conditions and does not factor out the effects of airway resistance

*Many other pulmonary function tests are available, but these are the ones most often used in the critical care setting.

Table 3-8. Diagnostic studies for evaluation of respiratory disorders—cont'd

Test	Description	Indication
Effective static compliance (C_{st})	Comparison of patient's tidal volume to the plateau airway pressure on the ventilator; made under conditions of no airflow; an estimate of true effective static compliance of the lung $$C_{st} = \frac{Volume}{Plateau\ pressure - PEEP}$$ (if any)	Used to assess the compliance characteristics of the lungs under conditions of no flow; because peak pressures reflect both compliance and airway resistance pressures, and plateau pressures reflect the compliance, the difference between these measurements provides an estimate of the magnitude of airflow resistance at that tidal volume
Sputum specimen	Collection and evaluation of sputum sample	Used to detect infectious organisms, cellular debris, and abnormal cells; may also be used in antibiotic susceptibility testing
Bronchoscopy	Visual examination of the tracheobronchial tree using a bronchoscope	Used to examine the tracheobronchial tree for abnormalities, collect brushed cell samples, and biopsies may be performed; may also be used to aspirate retained secretions
Pleural fluid examination	Pleural fluid obtained by thoracentesis	Used to evaluate pleural effusion fluid for content and color
Pulmonary angiography	Radiopaque dye is injected into the pulmonary circulation; allows visualization of the pulmonary circulation	Used in the diagnosis of massive pulmonary embolism and also in the investigation of pulmonary hypertension
Radioisotope lung scanning	Radioisotope injection or inhalation to assess perfusion and/or ventilation abnormalities	Perfusion scans are valuable in detecting thromboembolic disease, and ventilation scans are valuable in a variety of bronchopulmonary disorders
Tomography	Provides films of sections of the intrathoracic structures at different levels	Used to more clearly define lesions, masses, cavities, or shadows seen on a normal chest roentgenogram; may also be used to assess tracheal or mainstem bronchi narrowing
Transthoracic needle biopsy	Under fluoroscopic control, a biopsy of a suspected lesion is obtained with a narrow-gauge cutting needle passed through the chest wall	Used to obtain an etiologic diagnosis of a pulmonary lesion when other measures have failed and when it is desirable to avoid a thoracotomy

these findings with the patient's presentation and the physical assessment. To increase one's expertise in interpreting chest films, one must continue to review both normal and abnormal films on an ongoing basis.

Table 3-8 gives a brief description of other pulmonary tests used in the critical care setting.

ALTERATIONS—A PATHOPHYSIOLOGIC EXPLANATION

Many alterations or clinically significant symptoms may occur in the critically ill patient. Some of the symptoms may be attributed to several systems in the body. The pathophysiology of alterations associated with pulmonary problems is reviewed in this section.

Shortness of breath (dyspnea)

Dyspnea is a subjective sensation experienced by the patient. It has been described as uncomfortable, disordered, or difficult breathing. The patient becomes increasingly aware of her breathing pattern. Although it is usually not painful, dyspnea may illicit an uncomfortable or fearful response by the patient.

Once it is established that the patient does have dyspnea, it is important for the practitioner to define the circumstances in which it occurs and to assess associated symptoms. To quantitate or grade the dyspnea, the practitioner should examine the level of activity needed to precipitate the dyspnea. Some patterns of dyspnea are not related to physical exertion. These episodes should be fully described regarding the position of the patient, onset of dyspnea and precipitating factors.

Possible physiologic mechanisms causing dyspnea have been described by many. In fact, the actual mechanisms of dyspnea have not as yet been truly defined. It is known that dyspnea occurs whenever the work of breathing is excessive. Some part of the respiratory system becomes overstressed, resulting in disruption of the homeostatic properties, leading to an increased workload. In all likelihood a number of different mechanisms operate to different de-

grees to evoke dyspnea in a patient. It has been proposed that dyspnea may be partly caused by stimulation of the type J receptors located in the interstitium of the lung. There may also be receptors that originate in the upper respiratory tract, airways, and respiratory muscles, or a combination of these structures. In general, there is a reasonably good correlation between the severity of dyspnea and the disturbances of pulmonary or cardiac function that are responsible.

Determining the possible relationship of dyspnea to pulmonary problems may be difficult for the practitioner. A dyspneic episode with an acute onset may be caused by an extrathoracic or intrathoracic obstruction of the airways. Acute upper airway obstruction (extrathoracic) may be caused by aspiration of a foreign body or inflammation of a structure in the airway (for example, epiglottitis). Chronic forms of upper airway obstruction may be seen with tumors or fibrotic stenosis of the trachea. Whether the extrathoracic obstruction is acute or chronic, the cardinal symptom is dyspnea. Associated physical findings may include stridor and retraction of the supraclavicular fossa with inspiration.

Obstruction of intrathoracic airways may be acute, chronic, or intermittent. Most episodes of intrathoracic obstruction will generate some degree of dyspnea in the patient. An acute asthma attack causes narrowing of the airways, airway inflammation, and increased mucus production. This airway obstruction causes an increased work of breathing, leading to dyspnea. Intermittent airway obstruction may be seen in the critical care patient as a result of increased mucus production and plugging of airways. Usually this obstruction can be removed by cough, chest physical therapy, and suctioning of the airway. Many years of exertional dyspnea that slowly progresses to dyspnea at rest may characterize the patient with chronic obstructive lung disease. Chronic obstruction of the peripheral airways leads to increasing degrees of dyspnea.

Dyspnea may be experienced in a variety of other clinical problems. Pulmonary vascular occlusive disease, such as pulmonary emboli, may cause an acute onset of dyspnea as a result of the sudden decrease or cessation of blood flow to an area of the lung. Restrictive lung disease, diseases of the chest wall or respiratory muscle insufficiency may also cause dyspnea as a result of the increased work of breathing. It may be difficult for the practitioner to differentiate the cause-response relationship of the anxiety and dyspnea. Certain clues may be helpful in distinguishing the psychogenic cause of dyspnea. In anxiety-induced dyspnea, frequent, sighing respirations, along with an irregular breathing pattern, may be seen.[12] Usually the respiratory pattern returns to normal during sleep.

Positional breathing problems

Orthopnea is defined as difficulty in breathing experienced by the patient while in the recumbent position. It is characteristic of those forms of heart failure associated with elevation of pulmonary venous and capillary pressures. Orthopnea is associated with the redistribution of blood in the recumbent position, along with the increase of intrathoracic blood volumes. In this position the diaphragmatic excursion may also be impaired. The combination of increased pulmonary blood volume, along with decreased lung volume, may result in significant alterations of gas exchange. These alterations in the processes of ventilation, diffusion, and perfusion lead to the development of orthopnea. Patients with chronic obstructive lung disease may often complain of orthopnea. This orthopnea results in part from heart failure but also includes the instability of the accessory muscles in the supine position. Therefore in the supine position the patient must use excess energy to move the accessory respiratory muscles, along with the major muscles of respiration.

Some patients with unilateral lung diseases may have difficulty breathing while lying in certain positions. Examples of persons with unilateral lung problems may include postoperative thoracic surgery patients or patients with unilateral infiltrates. The practitioner must assess the patient's difficulty in breathing and assist the patient in assuming the most comfortable position in bed.

Cough

Cough must be considered an alteration of normal respiratory function. It is a defense mechanism of the respiratory system that provides a means of clearing the tracheobronchial tree of secretions and foreign bodies. It should be noted that a chronic cough is not considered normal. Cough may be evoked by a reflex stimulation of inflammatory, mechanical, chemical, or thermal stimuli in the respiratory system.[6]

The practitioner may evaluate the cause of the cough by many methods. First, a thorough history of the course of the cough may offer valuable clues as to its cause. Often cough may be associated with other problems, such as excessive mucus production or dyspnea. Second, physical examination may reveal further information regarding the source of the cough. Auscultatory findings, such as stridor, wheezes, or crackles, may suggest the site of the pulmonary problem. Thirdly, a chest roentgenogram may disclose a possible cause of a cough, such as an intrapulmonary lesion or a process that may cause alveolar filling with an exudate. Screening pulmonary functions may contribute additional information regarding a type of pulmonary disease process that may be associated with cough. Finally, sputum examination may be used to determine the nature of sputum being produced by the patient. Gram stain and culture of a deeply-coughed specimen may reveal specific bacterial, fungal, or mycoplasmal causation of a cough. A cytologic examination of the sputum may also be done to determine the possibility of a pulmonary neoplasm.

In children, cough may be attributed to a variety of causes. Respiratory infections are probably the primary cause of cough in this age group.[12] Cystic fibrosis is a diagnostic consideration in infants who have a persistent cough or frequent respiratory infections. Allergic airway disease (asthma) may also be a source of cough in the young, as well as mechanical obstruction of the airways. Foreign bodies, copious secretions, an isolated tracheoesophageal fistula, or an extrinsic tumor or abscess may all produce obstruction of the airways, which in turn may cause a cough.[23]

In adults, a respiratory infection of some type is usually the major cause of cough. It must be remembered that cough is so common in the smoker that it is often ignored or minimized. A "smoker's cough" should be evaluated carefully. It is often the first sign of a disease process, such as chronic bronchitis or carcinoma. Acute bronchospasm, such as asthma, may also illicit a cough. As in children, an intrinsic or extrinsic airway obstruction may evoke a cough in an adult.

Severe coughing episodes may precipitate complications in a patient. Paroxysms of cough may cause syncope and nausea, while strenuous coughing may produce rupture of an emphysematous bleb or rib fractures.

Hemoptysis

Hemoptysis is described as the production of blood from the respiratory tract. It is important to establish that the blood is coming from the respiratory tract and not the nasopharynx or gastrointestinal tract. The practitioner must first establish the history of the hemoptysis, which may provide valuable information as to its cause. The amount of blood coughed from the respiratory tract can range from small amounts of blood-streaked sputum to large volumes of expectorated blood (frank hemoptysis). Physical examination may also help to differentiate the origin of the hemoptysis in the respiratory tract. Finally, the chest roentgenogram may be helpful in locating an abnormality in the chest. Bronchoscopy may be used to visualize the origin of the bleeding, to obtain a biopsy of the tissue, or to obtain bronchial washings for further examination.

In children, hemoptysis may be caused by several disease processes. Massive pulmonary hemorrhage may occur in low-birth-weight newborn infants who have been hypoxemic. An acute or chronic pulmonary infection may prompt an episode of hemoptysis or a foreign body in the respiratory tract may irritate the tissues and cause bleeding. Also, any hemorrhagic disorders or friable lesions in the respiratory tract may potentiate an episode of hemoptysis in the young. In young adults, hemoptysis may be seen as a complication of cystic fibrosis.

Adults have many of the same causes of hemoptysis as children. The causes of hemoptysis in adults may be classified as inflammatory, neoplastic, vascular, traumatic, or hemorrhagic.[12] Respiratory infections of an acute or chronic nature may cause hemoptysis. Examples of these infections are tuberculosis, bronchiectasis, lung abcess, pneumonia, or bronchitis. A neoplastic lesion itself may be vascular and may also be a source of bleeding. Second, a neoplastic lesion may erode into vascular tissues and cause hemoptysis. Other vascular causes of hemoptysis should also be considered. Left ventricular failure, mitral stenosis, pulmonary thromboembolism, and pulmonary hypertension can all precipitate bleeding from the respiratory tract. A foreign body or lung contusion may be considered traumatic causes of hemoptysis. Finally, such hemorrhagic disorders as excessive anticoagulant therapy must also be considered as a cause of bleeding.

Cyanosis

Cyanosis refers to a bluish discoloration of the skin and mucous membranes resulting from increased amounts of reduced or unoxygenated hemoglobin in the blood. It is usually most notable in the lips, nailbeds, ears, and buccal membranes. The degree of cyanosis may be modified by the quality of cutaneous pigment, the color of the blood plasma, the thickness of the skin, the state of the cutaneous capillaries, and the perception of the examiner. In deeply pigmented persons, cyanosis may be apparent only in the tongue and mucous membranes.

Frequently the detection of the presence and degree of cyanosis is difficult. In general, cyanosis becomes apparent when the mean capillary concentration of reduced hemoglobin exceeds 5 g/100 ml.[6] It must be remembered that the degree of cyanosis is determined by the reduction of the total amount of hemoglobin available for saturation with the O_2 molecules. Cyanosis may also be observed when nonfunctional hemoglobin is present in the blood.

Cyanosis may be subdivided into central and peripheral categories. In central cyanosis there is a large amount of desaturated or unsaturated hemoglobin in the blood throughout the body. Peripheral cyanosis is caused by a slowing of blood flow to a peripheral area, such as the fingertips, resulting in increased extraction of O_2 from the hemoglobin into those tissues. Peripheral cyanosis may result from vasoconstriction and decreased blood flow to an area. Peripheral and central cyanosis differ in that the patient with central cyanosis suffers from a lowered hemoglobin saturation of all the blood in the body, whereas the patient with peripheral cyanosis has decreased oxygen saturation only in the affected peripheral areas.

In newborn infants, central cyanosis may be noted in the tongue and mucous membranes with only 3 g of reduced hemoglobin and an arterial O_2 saturation of 75% to 88%. Because of the high affinity of fetal hemoglobin for O_2 and the large amount of such hemoglobin in the newborn, dangerous degrees of hypoxemia may be present in the absence of cyanosis. Cyanosis may be attributed to abnormal forms of hemoglobin in the blood. Another general cause of cyanosis is decreased alveolar ventilation, which may be attributed to many things. The hemoglobin is thus unable to become fully oxygenated during the diffusion process. Cyanosis may also be caused from hemoglobin passing in reduced form through unaerated, venoarterial shunts from the heart's right side to the arterial blood in the lungs or through the foramen ovale or ductus arteriosus. This is called *pulmonary shunting*.

In adult patients, many of the same causes of cyanosis can be cited. Central cyanosis may be caused by decreased arterial O_2 saturation from (1) decreased atmospheric pressures, (2) impaired pulmonary function, (3) anatomic shunts, or (4) hemoglobin with a low affinity for O_2. Hemoglobin abnormalities, such as methemoglobinemia or carboxyhemoglobinemia, may also cause central cyanosis. Peripheral cyanosis may be caused by reduced cardiac output, exposure to cold, redistribution of blood flow from the extremities, or vascular obstruction.

Chest pain

As with any type of pain, chest pain must be precisely described so that the cause may be identified. The most important point in evaluating chest pain includes a complete history, along with a definitive physical examination. Chest pain may be a fairly common complaint for both pediatric and adult patients with respiratory problems.

Chest pain may be musculoskeletal in origin and may develop as a result of muscle or ligament strains brought on by unaccustomed exercise, cough or trauma. It may be felt in the costochondral or chondrosternal junctions or in the anterior chest wall muscles. Usually chest pain resulting from chest wall problems is sharply localized and exhibits point tenderness. It may be made worse by tensing the muscles, coughing, or sneezing. Rib fractures will also cause chest pain. This type of chest pain also exhibits point tenderness and may be caused by trauma to the ribs or severe paroxysms of coughing.

Pleuritic pain may also be identified by the patient as chest pain. It results from stretching of inflamed parietal pleura. The visceral pleura is not pain sensitive. Pain receptors lie close to the endothoracic fascia and superficial to the parietal pleura. Pleuritic pain is usually found in the lateral aspects of the chest wall and is usually sharply localized. Diaphragmatic pleural pain is often referred to the shoulder. This chest pain is of sudden onset and may be aggravated by deep breathing, coughing, and positioning. On physical examination a pleural friction rub may be heard over the area of inflammation.

Dysfunction of an intrathoracic structure

may result in the symptom of chest pain. Conditions causing a lowered arterial O_2 tension or a disease impairing the transport of O_2 by the red blood cell may cause or aggravate angina. Similar to angina, chest pain may be caused by pulmonary artery hypertension secondary to hypoxemia. Usually chest pain resulting from pulmonary hypertension is of a crushng or gripping quality and is felt in the center of the chest. It is retrosternal and felt deeply in the chest but does not radiate to the jaw or down the arms. Usually this type of chest pain will develop before the symptom of dyspnea.

A pulmonary embolus or emboli may also cause chest pain. Massive pulmonary emboli may cause severe, persistent, substernal stabbing pain, presumably caused by the distention of the pulmonary artery. This pain may last from a few minutes to hours. For the diagnosis of pulmonary embolus to be made, several examinations may be done. The patient's history is important, along with distinguishing risk factors that may make the patient subject to this problem. Arterial blood gases may show a decreased Pao_2, while a chest roentgenogram may exhibit an area that lacks pulmonary vascular shadows. A wedge-shaped infiltrate may indicate an area of pulmonary infarction. However, the chest roentgenogram is frequently of little diagnostic value, since it is usually difficult to obtain technically good films in these very ill patients and the changes are rarely detected with portable roentgenographic equipment. Lung perfusion scans may be used to assess the problem of pulmonary embolus, along with pulmonary arteriograms.

There are many other causes of chest pain. Pneumothorax may cause chest pain that is of the pleuritic type and is associated with dyspnea. The severity of chest pain the patient experiences is not a guide to the size of the pneumothorax. Some disease processes, such as acute tracheobronchitis, may also cause a mild chest pain perceived as soreness or burning high in the retrosternal area. Lung lesions may affect any thoracic structure. Tumors or other infiltrative processes may involve the bony skeleton or tissue structures in the lung, leading to chest pain.

Finally, chest pain may be associated with O_2 toxicity. Administration of high O_2 concentration ($F_IO_2 > 0.60$ for a period of 72 hours or greater) may result in changes in the pulmonary pathology.[3] Initially the lung responds to high levels of O_2 with changes in the alveolar-capillary endothelial cells. Interstitial and alveolar edema, alveolar hemorrhage, and alveolar epithelial damage may occur. This is followed by thickening of the alveolar-capillary membrane.[31] These changes in pulmonary pathology may cause retrosternal burning and chest pain.

Swelling (edema)

Edema is an alteration that may be caused by a problem in the respiratory system. It is defined as an increase in the extravascular component of the extracellular fluid volume. Edema associated with pulmonary problems is most commonly caused by congestive heart failure. In left-sided heart failure, there may be formation of edema in the lungs that impairs gas exchange and may induce hypoxemia. With right-sided heart failure, edema is also seen. This edema is usually dependent, occurring in the legs, particularly in the ankles and feet of ambulatory patients and in the sacral region of bedridden individuals.

In patients who experience chronic hypoxemia and subsequent pulmonary hypertension, cor pulmonale is often seen. Cor pulmonale denotes altered function and enlargement of the right ventricle secondary to lung dysfunction. Cor pulmonale is often precipitated by ventilatory failure because of the increased pulmonary hypertension induced by hypoxemia. Fluid retention in the dependent areas of the body is often observed in the patient with this diagnosis.

Confusion, restlessness, and fatigue

Confusion, restlessness, and fatigue can be considered together when discussing the patient with respiratory insufficiency. All of these symptoms may result from hypoxemia or hypercapnia. Tissue hypoxia, whether acute or chronic, is associated with problems in neuro-psychologic function. Hypoxemia may produce dysfunction in visual integration and perception, thus causing confusion for the patient. The type of alteration manifested in the patient depends on the degree of hypoxemia and whether it is acute or chronic in nature. Respiratory acidosis may further potentiate the symptoms seen with hypoxemia.

INTERVENTION
Ventilation
Airway establishment

In any patient, the establishment and maintenance of a patent airway is of prime importance in the practitioner's planning and management of care. The airway may be maintained in a variety of ways ranging from correct positioning of the patient to more sophisticated artificial modes. In attempting to establish an airway, the practitioner should begin with the most basic techniques. More complex maneuvers and equipment should be used only as the patient's condition warrants.

Positioning of the airway. The most simple method of establishing an airway is by positioning the patient's head and neck so that the upper airway is patent. The most basic causes of airway obstruction are foreign bodies and relaxation of the oropharyngeal muscles, leading to airway closure. According to the American Heart Association's Standards for Basic Life Support in the infant or child, the method of opening the airway is the head tilt—chin lift method.[1] The practitioner should first tip the child's head backward with gentle pressure on the forehead. One must be careful not to hyperextend the neck because this may cause tracheal collapse or cervical spine injury.[1] Next, the extension on the head is maintained by pressure on the forehead. The tips of the fingers of the opposite hand are used to lift the bony portion of the jaw near the chin in a forward motion.

In the adult, the head tilt is the initial and most important step in opening the airway. This simple procedure may be assisted by the chin lift method. The head tilt method is accomplished by placing the hand on the patient's forehead and applying firm backward pressure with the palm of the hand. This will maximally tip the patient's head backward. Even though the head is tilted back and the neck extended, the lower jaw may need support to adequately lift the tongue and open the airway. The head tilt–chin lift method is accomplished first by tilting the head backward as described earlier. Next, the tips of the fingers of one hand are placed under the lower jaw on the bony part near the chin, bringing the chin forward.[1]

Airway assistance devices. If the patient is unable to maintain a patent airway, then artificial means of airway establishment must be considered by the practitioner. The most elementary way to assist in the maintenance of the airway is by inserting an oropharyngeal or nasopharyngeal airway. The advantage of the nasopharyngeal airway over the oropharyngeal airway is that it is much better tolerated by the semicomatose or awake patient. These mechanical aids may be useful in the restoration and maintenance of a patent airway. These two types of airways may be inserted in the upper airway but will not guarantee the maintenance of patency. Frequently even with a airway assistance device, the head must be tilted back or the mandible supported to ensure an open airway. The oropharyngeal airway may also serve as a bite block when used with an endotracheal tube.

Artificial ventilation

If the establishment of a patent airway fails to produce chest movement in the patient, then artificial ventilation must be initiated to ensure adequate oxygenation. Various means may be used to ventilate the patient's lungs. In the adult, mouth-to-mouth ventilation may be the easiest method if a resuscitator bag and mask are not readily available. With the patient's head tilted and his airway clear, the patient's nose is then pinched. The resuscitator takes a deep breath and then obtains a tight seal around the patient's mouth with his mouth. The rescuer then forcefully exhales into the patient's lungs. He removes his mouth to allow passive exhalation by the patient.

Mouth-to-nose ventilation may be the method of choice if the rescuer is unable to obtain a tight seal around the patient's mouth. First, the rescuer tilts the patient's head to open the airway. The rescuer closes the patient's lips by lifting the lower jaw. Once again, the rescuer makes a tight seal around the patient's nose and forcefully exhales. The rescuer removes his mouth to allow passive expiration by the patient. To facilitate exhalation by the patient it may be helpful to open the patient's lips if the soft palate causes nasopharyngeal obstruction. In infants and small children, both the mouth and the nose are closed by the rescuer's mouth. Gentle puffs of air are used in ventilating infants to avoid trauma to the lungs.

If a patient has had a laryngectomy, mouth-to-stoma ventilation must be initiated. This technique does not require the head to be tilted back, since the upper airway is essentially nonfunctional. The rescuer's mouth is placed over the stoma, and artificial ventilation proceeds as with the other techniques described.

In a critical care setting, a manual positive pressure inflation bag of some sort should always be available at the bedside to artificially ventilate a patient's lungs. Artificially ventilating the lungs with this type of bag is a relatively simple procedure, but it must be done properly to ensure effective ventilation. A frequent misconception is that all resuscitator bags connected to a source of O_2 will deliver a 100% O_2 concentration. Depending on the type of bag used and adaptive equipment, the fraction of inspired O_2 delivered will vary. Often an adapter or reservoir is used to facilitate the delivery of higher concentrations of O_2. The practitioner must be aware of the concentration of O_2 needed to adequately oxygenate the patient. Use of concentrations higher than needed may result in a dangerous situation for the patient. The size of the bag should also be appropriate to the ventilatory needs of the patient.

It is important to review the technique of manually providing pressure ventilation to a patient. Manual positive pressure inflation bags can be used with a mask or directly attached to an artificial airway such as an endotracheal tube or tracheostomy tube. When using a bag and mask, a tight, leakproof seal must be created with the mask on the patient's face. The practitioner must hold the mask firmly in place with one hand and squeeze the resuscitator bag with the other until the chest rises. The bag should be abruptly released to allow exhalation. When manually ventilating a patient's lungs, it is important to note the resistance of the lungs to positive pressure ventilation. This is a direct result of the patency of the airway and compliance of the lungs. The rate at which the lungs should be ventilated is also important. Overventilation or underventilation by artificial means may lead to dangerous changes in the ABGs. A neonates lungs should be ventilated rather rapidly with an infant or pediatric resuscitator bag at a rate of 30 to 50 times per minute; infants to small children should have a rate of 20 to 30 ventilations per minute. Adults should receive artificial ventilation at a rate of 12 to 20 times per minute. The inflations of the chest should be rhythmic. If the patient is spontaneously attempting to ventilate, the resuscitator should attempt to coordinate the positive ventilations with the patient's spontaneous respirations.

Manual positive pressure inflation bags are sometimes equipped with a valve that releases air from the bag at a preset pressure. When approximately 40 cm H_2O of inspiratory pressure is obtained, the one-way valve opens and the pressure is vented away from the patient's airway. These bags with a pressure pop-off valve are frequently used with infants or pediatric patients to avoid subjecting the patient's lungs to high inflating pressures. It may be necessary to use a resuscitator bag without a pressure-relief valve if the patient's lungs are difficult to ventilate. To facilitate adequate ventilation it may be necessary to generate higher pressures to deliver an adequate volume of gas to the patient, especially in a patient with noncompliant or stiff lungs.

Manual artificial ventilation is useful only

when one can establish or maintain an adequate airway. When controlled or prolonged ventilatory assistance becomes necessary, mechanical ventilation may be the mode of therapy chosen. Mechanical ventilation will be discussed later in the chapter.

Artificial airways

When the simple maneuvers mentioned in the preceding pages are not adequate for establishment of a patent airway, the use of an artificial airway must be contemplated. An artificial airway will provide a patent airway, protect the lower airway from foreign body aspiration, and provide an accessible route for artificial ventilation and tracheal suctioning.

There are significant hazards involved with the establishment and maintenance of artificial airways. Although many of the complications depend on the type of artificial airway and the appropriateness of care during its maintenance, there are several universal problems that must always be considered by the practitioner caring for the patient. The establishment of an artificial airway bypasses the normal defense mechanisms that protect the lower airway from bacterial contamination. Second, the artificial airway reduces the effectiveness of the cough maneuver because the vocal cords are rendered nonfunctional. An endotracheal tube prevents the cords from approximating, whereas a tracheostomy tube bypasses the cords. Third, an artificial airway removes the patient's ability to communicate vocally.

The severity of complications from artificial airways depends on numerous circumstances. Trauma during the intubation may predispose the patient to further complications. Such factors as the type of airway used, length of intubation, patient complications and airway care must all be considered when discussing problems of the artificial airway.

Intubation. Intubation of a patient with an artificial airway requires special skills and should not be undertaken by a practitioner who is unfamiliar with the technique. Before intubating the trachea, it is important to have all necessary equipment at the bedside so that there is no delay once the procedure has started. The correct type and size of laryngoscope blade and endotracheal tube should be chosen according to the size and age of the patient.

Before intubation, the practitioner must ensure appropriate positioning of the patient's head, neck, and shoulders. It is essential to have as straight a line as possible between the open mouth and glottis to facilitate intubation of the larynx. In both infants and adults, the neck should be slightly flexed and the head extended in what is frequently described as a "sniffing" position (Fig. 3-16). It may be helpful to have a folded towel under the head or shoulders to assist in optimal positioning during the procedure. The most common mistake made in positioning is to overextend the neck and head. When opening the airway of an infant or an adult, the practitioner must carefully consider any facial or cervical spine injuries experienced by the patient. These types of injuries may drastically alter the method used in establishing and maintaining the airway.

The appropriate equipment must be used for the intubation procedure. This equipment includes appropriate size endotracheal tubes, suction catheters, suction apparatus, a stylet, and a laryngoscope. A stylet may be helpful in providing rigidity and appropriate curvature to the endotracheal tube during intubation. The stylet must be used with care so as not to damage the airway. Laryngoscopes are divided into two groups: those with straight blades and those with curved blades. During intubation, a straight blade tip will lie posterior to the epiglottis, while a curved blade tip will lie in the vallecula, anterior to the epiglottis. A straight blade is sometimes recommended in the intubation of infants and small children, since the epiglottis may obscure one's view of the glottis unless it is elevated with the tip of the blade.[2]

The practitioner should stand at the head of the bed in direct line with the patient. After properly positioning the patient, the laryngoscope handle is held in the left hand for right-handed individuals and the moistened or lubricated tip of the blade is inserted into the right side of the patient's mouth. The tongue should be moved to the left side of the mouth as the blade is brought to midline. The procedure is reversed in people who are left-handed. Care should be taken to avoid trauma to the lips and teeth. Anatomic landmarks should be identified as the laryngoscope blade is advanced. These landmarks include the base of the tongue, uvula, epiglottis, and vocal cords. Once the vocal cords are adequately visualized, the lubricated endotracheal tube is passed with the curve facing forward into the right side of the mouth, using the laryngoscope blade as a guide.[2] The tube should be slowly passed between the vocal cords. In infants, the endotracheal tube is inserted 2 to 5 cm beyond the vocal cords. In adults, the cuff of the endotracheal tube should be advanced beyond the vocal cords to avoid trauma to the cords during inflation of the cuff.

Fig. 3-16. Head and neck position for intubation. **A,** Use of the curved blade laryngoscope and its position (anterior) in relation to the epiglottis. **B,** Use of the straight blade laryngoscope and its position (posterior) in relation to the epiglottis.

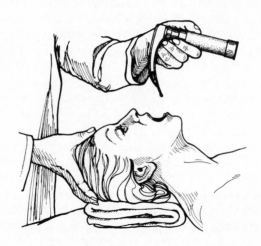

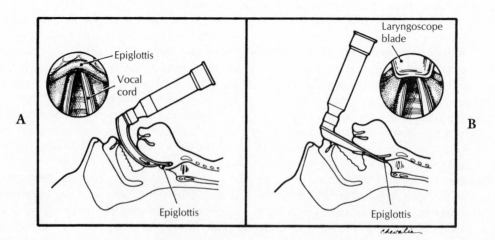

Table 3-9. Guide to size and length of endotracheal tubes in children

Age	Weight		Interior diameter of tube (in mm)	Exterior diameter (French)	Tracheal length (cord to carina, cm)	Length of tube (cm)
	kg	lb				
Neonate	1.5-3.5	3-7	2.5-3.5	11-16	4.0	10-12
1-6 mo	3.5-6.5	7-14	4.0-4.5	16-18	4.0-4.2	12-14
6-12 mo	6.5-9.5	14-20	4.5-5.0	18-20	4.2-4.3	14-16
2-3 yr	12.5-14.0	27-31	5.0-5.5	20-22	4.5-5.3	16-18
4-6 yr	16.0-22.5	35-50	5.5-6.5	24-26	5.4-5.7	18-20
7-10 yr	24.0-36.5	55-80	6.5-7.0	26-28		20-22
10-14 yr	45.0-50.0	100-120	7.0-7.5	28-30		22-24

From Cullen, S.C., and Larson, C.P.: Essentials of anesthetic practice, Copyright © 1974 by Year Book Medical Publishers, Inc., Chicago. Used by permission.

On placement of the endotracheal tube, its position should be checked. Auscultation of the chest should reveal bilateral breath sounds. In addition, a chest roentgenogram should be performed to verify the tube's location. Improper advancement of the endotracheal tube will usually result in intubation of the right mainstem bronchus rather than the trachea. The right mainsteam bronchus has a greater diameter and branches off the trachea at an angle less than that of the left. Thus if the tube is advanced too far or accidently slip down further into the airway, one can predict that it will be displaced into the right mainstem bronchus.

As stated earlier, because intubation is a complex and potentially dangerous procedure, the inexperienced practitioner should obtain more complete training in this procedure along with clinical experience under direct supervision. An inappropriately placed or nonfunctioning endotracheal tube can cause more problems than the patient's own poorly functioning airway.

Endotracheal tubes. Endotracheal tubes vary greatly in size and design. Factors that must be taken into consideration when choosing a tube are (1) age of the patient, (2) size of the trachea, and (3) the need for positive pressure ventilation. Most endotracheal tubes are disposable and are made of polyvinyl chloride, silicone, or nylon. The tube may or may not have a cuff, depending on how the tube will be used. Oral intubation is preferred for emergency situations, but for prolonged intubation, a nasotracheal tube should be considered because its placement is easier to maintain. The nasotracheal tube is easier to stabilize in the airway and is better tolerated by the patient. However, one must consider that the diameter of the nasotracheal tube is limited by the size of the nostrils and turbinates.

Endotracheal tubes used in neonates and small children may or may not have a cuff because of the size of the trachea. An airtight seal is achieved by selecting a tube that fits snugly in the cricoid ring without causing trauma to the mucosa. A tube that is too large will be traumatic, whereas one that is too small will create excessive airway resistance. A formula that assists the practitioner is choosing the correct size in children adds the age in years plus 18 to identify the appropriate size in the French scale. (See Table 3-9 for further information.)

Tracheostomy. A tracheostomy is indicated in patients requiring prolonged tracheal intubation, mechanical ventilation, and in patients whose upper airways are obstructed. As with endotracheal tubes, tracheostomy tubes are either cuffed or uncuffed. In infants and small children an uncuffed tube may be used. In adults, a cuffed tube is usually used in the critical care setting. A variety of sizes and types of tracheostomy tubes is available, including single cannula, double cannulae, fenestrated tubes and speaking tubes. All tracheostomy tubes should have a matching obturator taped to the head of the bed. It is used to reinsert the tube if it should become dislodged or removed.

A tracheostomy may be performed in an operating room setting under controlled conditions or electively at the bedside in the critical care setting. After insertion of the tube, the practitioner should assess bilateral expansion of the chest along with the presence of equal breath sounds. A chest roentgenogram should also be obtained to ensure proper placement. Also, if the tube is cuffed the practitioner should ascertain that the proper amount of air has been used to inflate the cuff. An extra tracheostomy tube of the same size should always be kept at the patient's bedside for emergency use.

Cuff inflation. Adult-sized and larger-sized pediatric nasotracheal, orotracheal and tracheostomy tubes used for mechanical ventilation all use an inflatable cuff to seal the tube within the trachea. The presence of a cuff permits the administration of positive pressure ventilation and decreases the likelihood of aspiration of gastrointestinal and nasopharyngeal contents into the lungs. The cuff should be inflated during positive pressure ventilation, if the patient is unable to defend his airway, in the presence of nausea and vomiting, and both during and 30 minutes after bolus tube feeding of the patient. If the patient is receiving intermittent or continuous nasogastric feedings, it may be wise to keep the cuff inflated continuously and keep the head of the bed slightly elevated.

For a number of years, the cuff used was a low-volume, low-compliance structure that often required 100 cm H_2O pressure or more to inflate it. Frequently that pressure was transmitted directly to the tracheal wall, occluding capillary blood flow and resulting in tissue damage and necrosis. More recently, high-volume, high-compliance cuffs that seal the trachea with 10 to 15 cm H_2O pressure or less have been introduced. These cuffs allow capillary blood flow to be maintained and are associated with a much lower degree of tracheal injury. A variety of cuffs and other devices have been developed to provide controlled positive ventilation with the minimum of tracheal injury.

The most effective way of preventing tracheal injury is to use a large residual volume, large-diameter, low-pressure cuff. This type of cuff occludes the lumen of the trachea by conforming to the configuration of the tracheal wall. A danger of the low-pressure cuff is overinflation. Cuffs should be inflated only to a point where a seal is obtained at peak airway pressure. If more air is inserted than necessary, the cuff pressure and cuff tracheal pressure will increase markedly, defeating the purpose of the soft, low-pressure cuff. Underinflation of the cuff will not provide an airway seal for controlled ventilation and may permit aspiration. Additionally, if there is an inadequate seal of the cuff on the airway wall, this allows a slight movement of the tube with each positive pressure ventilation. This movement and friction can cause additional tissue damage.

The careful filling of the low-pressure cuff with air to the no-leak or minimal leak point is the simplest method of preventing overinflation. One technique used to place the correct amount of air into the cuff is called the "minimal occlusive volume" technique. It is based on the assumption that during positive pressure ventilation, the tracheal diameter is maximal at the time of inspiration. With this technique, the practitioner first deflates the cuff. A stethoscope is then placed on the anterolateral portion of the neck adjacent to the trachea. At this point, harsh bronchial or tracheal breath sounds should be heard. During inspiration only, the practitioner slowly injects air into the cuff. As more volume is placed in the cuff, the tracheal breath sounds decrease. When tracheal breath sounds are no longer heard, cuff inflation should cease. The minimal occlusive volume has been reached in the artificial airway cuff. Therefore, if the cuff barely occludes the trachea during each positive pressure ventilation, there will be the least possible pressure on the tracheal mucosa during the expiratory phase. Another technique used is called the "minimal leak" technique. Using this technique, air is added to the cuff until the minimal occlusive volume is achieved. Then a small amount of air (0.5 to 1.0 cc) is withdrawn from the cuff. With this method, the practitioner should be able to hear a small leak over the trachea during the inspiratory and expiratory phase of ventilation.

Some practitioners find it helpful to monitor the cuff pressure. Cuff measurements of over 25 cm H_2O may occlude the capillary blood supply in the tracheal tissue. If continued high pressures are needed to obtain a minimal occlusive volume or minimal leak technique, then two possibilities must be considered: (1) the endotracheal tube and cuff are too small for the patient and should be replaced; or (2) the pressure of the cuff is producing a structural change in the tracheal wall—thus higher pressures and volumes are required.

Care of the artificial airway. Maintenance of an artificial airway involves many aspects of care. First the endotracheal tube should be taped securely to ensure stabilization without putting tension on the tube, tongue, or nares. Artificial airway ties and stabilizers are available commercially for use in the critical care setting. These products provide such features as Velcro fasteners and padding for the neck and face. With orotracheal intubation, a bite block may be used to prevent pressure on the tube by the teeth or gums. If the patient has an orotracheal tube, it may be helpful to move the tube from side to side every 8 to 12 hours to prevent pressure necrosis on the sides of the mouth. The practitioner may also mark the placement of the endotracheal tube. A small piece of tape should be placed at that point where the tube exits the mouth or nose. In this fashion, the practitioner can tell at a glance whether the tube has slipped further down into the trachea or has become dislodged.

When caring for the patient with a tracheostomy tube, meticulous care by the practitioner can prevent most complications. Infection at the tracheostomy site may occur if improper wound care and proper suctioning techniques are not used. Tracheostomy care includes changing the dressing as needed and cleansing the area. Good skin care is important to prevent skin breakdown at the stoma site. The tracheostomy ties should be secured so as not to allow excessive movement of the tracheostomy tube, but the practitioner should be able to comfortably place one finger between the ties and the neck. If the tracheostomy tube has an inner cannula, it should be removed and cleansed as often as necessary. Excessive secretions in the tube may cause increased airway resistance and respiratory distress for the patient.

Along with the direct care given to the artificial airway, the practitioner should frequently assess the patency of the airway. Observation of chest movement and respiratory rate along with frequent auscultation of breath sounds are mandatory. The frequency of suctioning required should be assessed by the practitioner. The practitioner should also check to see that proper humidification is being delivered to keep the secretions thinned and mobile. Mouth care is very important in a patient with an artificial airway, and oral secretions should be frequently suctioned. The patient with an artificial airway also needs psychologic support from the staff. Reassurance and explanation of the need for the artificial airway and associated procedures helps to allay apprehension and encourage cooperation by the patient. Communication becomes a major problem for the patient with an artificial airway. The patient should be provided with some alternate means of communicating, whether by written method or by a call-bell device of some type. A fenestrated tracheostomy tube may enable the patient to verbally communicate to some degree, as will a "talking" tracheostomy tube.

Extubation. Before removing an endotracheal or tracheostomy tube, the airway should be adequately cleared of secretions. Failure to do so may lead to respiratory distress after extubation. Extubation should only be performed when the patient is able to breathe on her own, is sufficiently alert to protect her own airway, and has oxygen requirements that can be met without the use of positive pressure ventilation.

A greater degree of flexibility and variability in extubating techniques exists with a tracheostomy than with the endotracheal tube. A fenestrated tracheostomy tube is a tube in which a "window" or fenestration has been cut in the posterior wall of the outer cannula. It is possible to have the patient breathe around the tube and through the fenestration without actually removing the tube. This is accomplished by removing the inner cannula, deflating the cuff, and placing a cork or button in the opening of the outer cannula. This procedure will enable the patient to breathe through the upper airway in a normal fashion and clear secretions through the mouth. Once the tracheostomy is removed, the stoma edges are approximated and the stoma is covered with a sterile dressing to permit healing. Another method that may be used in removal of a tracheostomy tube is a tracheostomy "button." With this method, the tracheostomy tube is removed and a tracheostomy "button" is placed in the stoma site. This allows the patient to have the tube removed, but the stoma and track are kept open for easy access to the trachea if needed. Humidification may be used after extubation to soothe the airway and keep the secretions thinned. Postintubation sequelae include pharyngitis, laryngitis, and/or tracheitis secondary to edema or infection. Tracheal stenosis and granuloma formation may also occur as a side effect of prolonged intubation.

Airway maintenance

In addition to the establishment of a patent airway, adequate ventilation, and specific care of the artificial airway, other measures must be considered when caring for a patient with respiratory problems. Such measures as positioning, cough, breathing exercises, suctioning, chest physical therapy, and patient monitoring are vital in the care of this type of patient.

Positioning. Positioning or turning the body is frequently overlooked as an important measure for the patient with respiratory problems. As discussed earlier in the chapter, changes in body position affect both ventilation and perfusion distribution in the lung. Positioning facilitates bilateral chest expansion and mobilizes secretions for expectoration. Although side-to-side positioning is very important, the semiprone position is often overlooked.[15] This position is helpful in mobilizing secretions in the posterior areas of the lungs. It can be safely accomplished with the use of strategically placed pillows for bridging techniques and careful observation of the patient's intravenous lines, oxygen therapy, and response to the positioning.

A device that assists the practitioner in continuously repositioning the patient is the rotokinetic bed. This bed is being used more frequently in critical care because it provides continuous side-to-side rotation of the patient. The continuous positioning of the patient not only assists in the prevention of pressure sores but also has an effect on the ventilation and perfusion of the lung. Another proposed benefit of this bed is that it provides continuous bronchial drainage of the airways.

When positioning patients, it is important that the practitioner monitor changes in the patient's ventilatory status. The ventilatory rate and effort should be monitored, along with changes in skin color. If ventilatory monitoring equipment of any type is being used, it should be closely watched for changes that occur with positioning of the patient.

Cough. If the patient is able to cough effectively, it is important that he be taught to maximally protect his own airway. The effectiveness of a cough is determined by the velocity of expiratory flow. Since a cough is only effective out to approximately the fifth branching of the airways, it is imperative that other methods be used to help mobilize the secretions in the periphery of the lung. To enhance the effectiveness of the cough, the patient should be in a comfortable position with his abdominal muscles relaxed. The effectiveness of the cough cannot be judged only by the aspect of sputum production. A nonproductive cough may be useful in moving secretions into the larger airways for later expectoration or removal via suctioning. It must be noted that coughing may be very tiring for the patient. The practitioner must assess the patient's cough technique and assist the patient in developing a more effective method. A good review of alternative cough tehniques is provided by Traver.[40]

Other means may be used to initiate a cough in a patient. Manual pressure applied lightly over the suprasternal notch causes an obstruction that may trigger an involuntary cough reflex. It is important to note that the intubated patient has a depressed cough reflex and cannot exert a large intrathoracic pressure against a closed glottis. The patient with an artificial airway may use a "huffing" maneuver to force secretions out of the airway. Suctioning may also stimulate a cough reflex in a patient. If the patient has an artificial airway, instillation of small amounts of normal saline into the airway during inspiration usually initiates a cough reflex. If this method is used to initiate a cough, the practitioner must suction the patient to help remove both the normal saline and secretions.

A third method used to initiate a cough is a cough tube or "tickle" tube. With this method, a small catheter is inserted into the trachea through the cricothyroid membrane and is securely taped in place. Small amounts of normal saline can be instilled during inspiration into the trachea to stimulate a cough. It is important to note that both methods of instilling normal saline into the trachea can be very frightening experiences for the patient. In an alert patient, it may provoke a choking, suffocating sensation. By far, it is best to attempt to instruct the patient to effectively cough without using the instillation of normal saline. Normal saline instillation may also be used for other purposes. It may be used to loosen thick, tenacious secretions for easier expectoration. With this technique, normal saline may be very useful in removing secretions and maintaining airway patency.

Breathing exercises or techniques. Breathing exercises or techniques may be helpful in the removal of pulmonary secretions and improvement in the ventilation of the lungs. The most important factor when developing new breathing patterns is patient relaxation. The practitioner must carefully instruct the patient and give continuous feedback regarding his efforts. Unnecessary muscular activity must be minimized to improve ventilation, decrease the body's O_2 needs, and decrease the work of breathing. Much has been written regarding the use of breathing exercises to alter the distribution of ventilation in the lungs. In the critical care patient, this is often a difficult task. With these patients, decreasing the respiratory rate and the work of breathing are probably the most important reasons for using breathing exercises.

In any patient in whom there is an abnormal breathing pattern, breathing exercises or retraining may be an aid. The abnormal breathing pattern may result from pathophysiologic causes, pain, apprehension, bronchospasm, airway obstruction, or a variety of other reasons. Use of the tactile sense is very important when instructing a patient in a more efficient breathing pattern. The practitioner's hands should be placed over the areas where muscular and rib cage movement are desired. The patient is encouraged to concentrate on expanding that part of the rib cage under the practitioner's hands. The practitioner may assist in slowing the breathing pattern of a patient who is tachypnic by using gentle pressure with his or her hands on the chest wall to prolong expiration. This technique for slowing respirations should be done very slowly and gently with much verbal encouragement from the practitioner. As stated earlier, relaxation and concentration by the patient are essential in changing his breathing pattern.

Various respiratory maneuvers have been designed to increase transpulmonary pressure, to prevent reduction of lung volumes, and to induce maximal inspiration in patients. These deep-breathing maneuvers attempt to increase the inspiratory lung capacity to volumes that will possibly prevent alveolar closure or cause reexpansion of those alveoli that are collapsed. It is proposed that the optimal deep-breathing maneuver is a deep breath with a 3- to 5-second sustained maximal inspiration (inspiratory hold). This deep-breathing maneuver should be done at intervals throughout the day. During the past few years various products have been marketed to assist the patient in periodic deep-breathing exercises. These devices are called *incentive spirometers* or deep breathing exercisers. These devices have become very popular because the visual feedback they provide for the patient.

Suctioning. Suctioning is yet another way of helping the patient to maintain a patent airway. It is the practitioner's responsibility to determine the frequency at which tracheal aspiration should be carried out. The best way to detect secretions in the airways is to auscultate the chest. After determining the need for suctioning, the correct size and type of suction catheter should be obtained. If the patient has an artificial airway, ideally the catheter should be half the diameter of the tube. It is not necessary to deflate an artificial airway cuff before the suctioning procedure.

Meticulous suctioning technique should be followed so as not to induce infection or tracheal damage during the procedure. In the neonate without an artificial airway, suctioning can be performed with a bulb syringe or a suction catheter that is attached to a DeLee trap or to mechanical suction. Suctioning in the adult without an artificial airway is done by the nasopharyngeal or oropharyngeal method.

If the patient has an artificial airway, a lubricated catheter is placed into the tube and the suctioning procedure is accomplished via this route. In the adult, the catheter should be introduced into the trachea without suction applied until resistance is felt. In the neonate, care must be taken to insert the catheter only 1 to 2 cm beyond the carina. After the catheter has been inserted to the desired level, the catheter should be slowly withdrawn from the tube, using intermittent suction and a gentle twisting motion of the catheter. The length of each suctioning procedure should not exceed 10 to 15 seconds. Several suction adapters are available to assist in suctioning the airways of a patient receiving mechanical ventilation. These adapters allow the practitioner to suction the patient's airways as mechanical ventilation continues. In patients who require positive end expiratory pressure, an adapter is available to maintain positive airway pressure during the suction procedure.

It is important that the correct negative pressure be used when suctioning a patient. The recommended negative pressures are: adults, -100 to -120 cm H_2O pressure; children, -80 to -100 cm H_2O pressure; and infants, -60 to -80 cm H_2O pressure. The use of excessive negative pressures may cause damage to airway mucosa. On some equipment it is possible to preset a maximal suction negative pressure so that airway damage can be minimized. It must be remembered, however, that many factors may be responsible for the negative pressure being induced in the airway during suctioning: the size of catheter, the amount of negative pressure used, and the length of time that the suction is applied.

When suctioning a patient's airway, the practitioner may find that it is often difficult to place the catheter into the left mainstem bronchus because of its anatomic size and placement in relation to the right mainstem bronchus. Because of this difficulty with left mainstem bronchus suctioning, there is a reportedly high incidence of left lower lobe abnormalities in intubated patients who require suctioning to remove the tracheobronchial secretions.

Several procedures have been studied to evaluate their effectiveness in left mainstem bronchus suctioning. The most recent areas studied are head position, body position, and type of intubation.[18,22] One method that has been suggested to improve the likelihood that a suction catheter will enter the left bronchus is to turn the patient's head to the right. Another suggestion is to turn the patient to his left side so that gravity will assist in catheter placement. These studies were inconclusive regarding the use of different head and body positioning for selective left mainstem suctioning. Studies have indicated that the type of intubation may make a difference in the success rate of left bronchus entrance by a catheter, with greater probability of success in patients with tracheostomy tubes.[22] Many studies have investigated different types of catheters. Curved-tip catheters enter the left mainstem more frequently than straight-tip catheters, although the chance of entering the left side remains less than optimal. Another variable that may make a difference in successful entry into the left bronchus is the type of packaging of the catheter. It is important for the practitioner to take into account all these ideas when attempting to selectively suction the left bronchus.

As a patient is suctioned, oxygen is removed along with the secretions. To minimize this possible suction-induced hypoxemia, presuction and postsuction hyperinflations should be used. The patient's lungs should be hyperinflated with three to five breaths of 100% O_2 before and after suctioning. These hyperinflations may be given with a resuscitation bag attached to an O_2 source or by the mechanical ventilator. In some patients, however, a high concentration of O_2 may be contraindicated. In these patients, the hyperinflation should be done with a lower oxygen concentration.

Besides hypoxemia, other complications may occur as a result of suctioning. These include patient anxiety, tissue trauma, bradycardia, atelectasis, increased intracranial pressure, and ventricular ectopy.[13] It is important that the practitioner closely monitor the patient during and after the suctioning procedure. Although suctioning is routinely performed and is often taken for granted, it is commonly traumatic to the patient and may have serious side effects.

Chest physical therapy. The technique of chest physical therapy is a method used to maintain a patent airway in a patient. It is composed of three basic maneuvers: positioning, percussion, and vibration. Positioning or postural

drainage uses gravity to drain secretions from segments of the lungs into the larger bronchi and trachea, where they can be expectorated or aspirated. Obviously postural drainage must be based on a firm knowledge of the tracheobronchial anatomy. There are 12 postural drainage positions employed to drain individual lung segments in the adult; Fig. 3-17 illustrates these positions. In the critical care setting, these positions are often modified and individualized to meet the needs of the patient.

Percussion is a manual cupping or clapping of the chest wall, which loosens and dislodges mucus and secretions from the airways. It is often used in conjunction with postural drainage. The object is to maintain a cupped-shaped hand and "clap" the chest wall. This clapping traps air between the hand and the chest wall. The sudden compression of air produces a vibration that is transmitted through the chest wall to the lung tissue. The procedure is performed by rhythmically and alternately striking the chest wall with the cupped hands. Bony prominences, such as the sternum and spinal column, along with the female breast tissue should be avoided. Percussion is more difficult to perform with an infant, since the adult is usually much larger than the infant's thorax. In many cases, a small plastic medicine cup or a small infant mask may provide effective percussion with a cupping-like action. Depending on the amount of secretions in the airways, percussion should be done for 2 to 3 minutes in each postural drainage position. As with other procedures, the practitioner must individualize the treatment for each patient. This may include focusing the percussion on a problem area of the lung or integrating the treatment into patient care throughout the day.

Vibrations applied to the chest wall during exhalation are transmitted to the airways in the underlying segments of the lungs. This helps to promote loosening and movement of secretions "downstream" (toward the mouth). With the fingertips or palm of the hand, three to five vibrations are usually done at the end of each percussion maneuver in each postural drainage po-

Fig. 3-17. Positions for postural drainage. **A,** Lower lobes in apical segment are drained by placing patient in prone position with pillow under abdomen. **B,** Lower lobes in anterior basal segment are drained by placing patient in supine position with pillow under knees and foot of bed elevated 14 to 16 inches. **C,** Lower lobe in lateral basal segment is drained by placing patient on unaffected side with pillow under hips and foot of bed elevated 14 to 16 inches. **D,** Lower lobes in posterior basal segment are drained by placing patient in prone position with pillow under hips and foot of bed elevated 14 to 16 inches. **E,** Right middle lobe in medial or lateral segment is drained by placing patient on back, turned to 45-degree tilt toward left, and elevating foot of bed 12 inches. **F,** Left lingula in left lingular segment is drained by placing patient on back, turned to 45-degree tilt toward right, and elevating foot of bed 12 inches. **G,** Upper lobes in anterior segment are drained by placing patient in supine position with pillow under knees to facilitate relaxation. **H,** Upper lobes in posterior segment are drained by placing patient on left side at 45-degree tilt forward. **I,** Upper lobes in posterior segment are drained by placing patient on right side at 45-degree tilt forward. Shoulders should be elevated approximately 12 inches.

From Abels, L.F.: Mosby's manual of critical care, St. Louis, 1979, The C.V. Mosby Co.

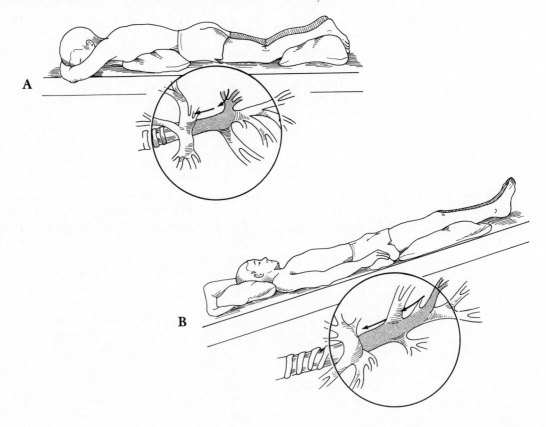

Fig. 3-17, cont'd. For legend see opposite page.

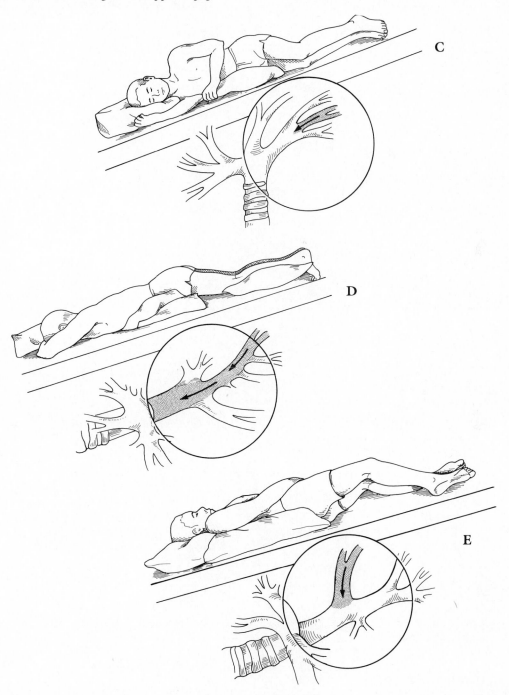

Continued.

Fig. 3-17, cont'd. For legend see p. 230.

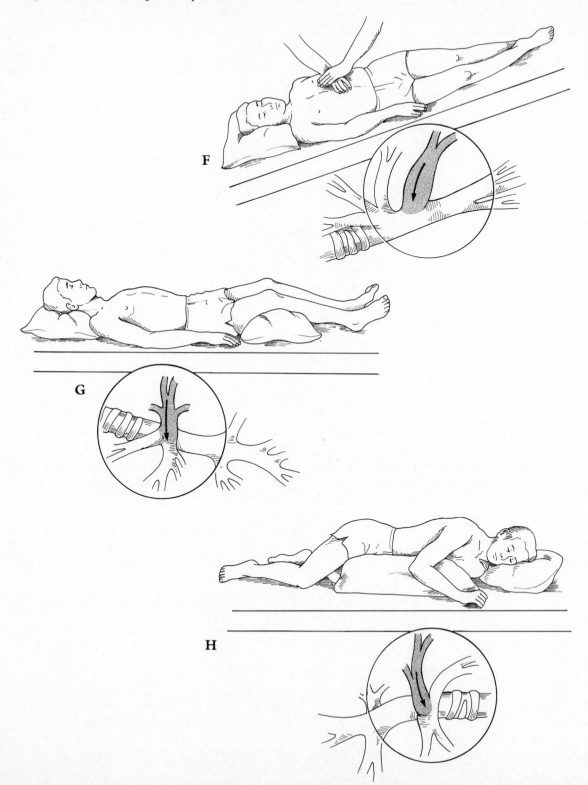

Fig. 3-17, cont'd. For legend see p. 230.

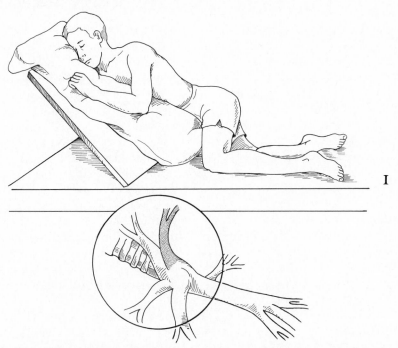

I

sition. In infants, it may be helpful to use an electric or battery powered toothbrush to perform vibrations. Only the handle or motorized mechanism without the toothbrush attached should be used. This must be wrapped in a cloth or gauze so as to not irritate the infant's skin. Vibrations with the electric toothbrush can be used instead of manual percussion of the segments of the lungs. One should be careful to avoid the hazards of using electric equipment such as this around O_2 devices.

Chest physical therapy is a very helpful technique in maintaining a patent airway in the critically ill patient. For some patients, this may be a fatiguing procedure. A routine should be instituted whereby chest physical therapy is worked into the basic care of the patient. Chest physical therapy treatment may be integrated with the turning schedule of the patient. Practitioner responsibilities during chest physical therapy include observing and monitoring the patient for signs of cardiorespiratory distress. A position change (especially the Trendelenburg position)

may cause significant stress on the cardiopulmonary system. Also, the head-down position may diminish venous return from the head and result in increased intracranial pressure. Certain patients may not be able to tolerate the percussion and vibration techniques. The potential benefit of the treatment versus the potential risk and discomfort must be assessed for each patient. In the final analysis, the decision should be based on the practitioner's and physician's clinical evaluation. There are rotokinetic beds available that offer an alternative for this type of patient. These beds are electrically controlled and gently produce a continuous side to side rocking movement for the patient. This slow rocking movement provides continuous bronchial drainage for some segments of the lung.

The chest physical therapy procedure must include deep-breathing exercises by the patient both during and after the treatment. It must be stressed that the patient should be able to clear his airways of these mobilized secretions. If the patient is unable to cough, then suctioning must be employed to remove the secretions. In some instances a bronchodilator medication may be administered via a nebulizer to the airways before a chest physical therapy treatment. This is done in an attempt to maximally dilate the airways before the mobilization of secretions. If the chest physical therapy treatment causes bronchospasm in a patient, it may be helpful to divide the dose of nebulized bronchodilator so that the patient receives half before the treatment and the remaining dose of medication after the therapy is complete.

Oxygen therapy

There are three goals that may be accomplished with proper O_2 therapy: (1) to treat hypoxemia, (2) to decrease the work of breathing, and (3) to decrease the myocardial workload. There are many different O_2 delivery systems available for use in patients of all ages. The practitioner should be aware of the therapeutic goal of the O_2 therapy and should assess the patient carefully to ensure that this goal is being met. When determining which type of O_2 therapy is appropriate for a patient, several parameters must be assessed. First, the fraction or concentration of inspired oxygen (F_IO_2) must be determined. An ABG analysis should be done to determine the patient's oxygenation status and predicted needs. In some cases a noninvasive estimate of oxygenation, such as ear oximetry or transcutaneous O_2 monitoring, can be used. Secondly, it should be determined which type of appliance would be best tolerated by the patient, taking into account his condition and physical and psychological status.

By first establishing the cardiopulmonary system's need for increased oxygenation, one may more effectively choose an O_2 system most beneficial to the patient. The use of higher concentrations of O_2 than is physiologically necessary can be hazardous to the patient, especially the neonate. High concentrations of O_2 at atmospheric pressure can affect the stability of the red blood cell membrane and possibly alter the neonatal brain. Obvious effects of O_2 toxicity have been observed in the retinal vessels and the lungs of premature neonates, especially if the arterial Po_2 rises above 150 mmHg to 200 mmHg.[25] For the sick infant, the general practice is to maintain the Pao_2 between 60 to 80 mmHg. For the healthy but small premature infant, a Pao_2 of 40 to 60 mmHg may be adequate. If these O_2 tensions cannot be maintained with a F_IO_2 of below 0.40, a different type of O_2 and ventilatory support system may be required.

In infants, pulmonary O_2 toxicity or bronchopulmonary dysplasia (BPD) may also result from using assisted ventilation with high concentrations of O_2 over a prolonged period of time. This usually occurs in patients whose lungs have been mechanically ventilated with FIO_2s greater than 0.60 for longer than 5 to 6 days. In adults, O_2 toxicity may also be a problem. Subjecting a patient to FIO_2s greater than 0.60 for prolonged periods of time may cause alveolar cell dysfunction. The relationship of the duration of therapy and the concentraton of O_2 in causing physiologic changes in the lung is not known. Studies in both animals and humans have associated O_2 toxicity with a number of findings, including destruction of type I alveolar lining cells, alveolar and interstitial edema, alveolar hemorrhaging, capillary endothelial damage, and alveolar membrane thickening.[3,20,33]

Another effect of high O_2 concentrations is the development of absorption atelectasis, which occurs when high O_2 concentrations wash out nitrogen in the lungs. If the alveoli then become partially obstructed, the O_2 in the alveoli will diffuse into the pulmonary circulation faster than it can be replaced. This results in the alveoli shrinking in size and collapsing. Absorption atelectasis is more likely to occur at low lung volumes or at normal lung volumes in the absence of coughing or sighing.

Excessive administration of O_2 to some patients may suppress the respiratory drive. This occurs in patients who are stimulated to breathe by a "hypoxic" drive rather than the normal "hypercarbic" drive. An example of this would be the patient with severe chronic lung disease

Table 3-10. Appliances used for oxygen administration

Type	Description	Oxygen delivery	
Nasal cannula	Cannulas or prongs that are inserted into nostrils; patient may breathe through the mouth or nose; is available for both adults and children; F_IO_2 depends on liter flow, respiratory rate, and tidal volume.	22%-40%	1-6 L/min
Simple face mask	No valve or reservoir bag; exhaled air is vented through holes in body of mask; air is drawn through exhalation ports and around oxygen mask if oxygen supply is interrupted; sizes available for infants through adults.	34%-45% 45%-55% 55%-65%	6-8 L/min 8-10 L/min 10-12 L/min
Partial rebreathing mask	Combined face mask and reservoir bag; reservoir bag conserves oxygen, enabling the patient to rebreathe one third of expired air from reservoir bag, which is still high in oxygen; exhalation ports are provided so that carbon dioxide levels remain negligible if flow rate remains above 4 L/min.	60%-90%	6-10 L/min
Nonrebreathing mask	Tight-fitting mask with reservoir bag and one-way valve system that eliminates rebreathing of expired air; allows oxygen to be inspired from the bag and expired air to be discharged through exhalation valve; provides high concentrations of oxygen.	90%-95%	10 L/min or greater
Venturi mask	Delivers a variety of oxygen concentrations; principle is called *high-airflow*, and precisely controlled concentrations can be delivered; entrained air combines with oxygen to deliver variable concentrations.	24%-50%	Liter flow depends on company recommendations

or the patient who is under the influence of large amounts of respiratory depressant drugs.

Adequate humidification must also be delivered along with the O_2 therapy to prevent the drying effect of the gas. The administration of moist inspired gas is essential to prevent the accumulation of dry secretions with consequent obstruction of the airways.

The oxygen hood or the nasal catheter are two common methods used to deliver an oxygen-enriched atmosphere to a spontaneously breathing infant. With the oxygen hood, air and oxygen proportional controllers allow for the delivery of O_2 (21% to 100%) through a cascade humidifier to the hood. The air-oxygen mixture must be humidified and warmed to the same temperature as that of the incubator air.

In older children and adults, O_2 may be administered in a variety of ways, depending on the individual needs of the patient. In most institutions, this equipment is provided and maintained by the respiratory therapy department, but every practitioner should be familiar with the equipment used, including its operation, benefits, and limitations. It is not within the scope of this book to fully describe every O_2 device available. Table 3-10 describes some of the the more commonly used pieces of equipment.

Carbon dioxide therapy

It is sometimes necessary to increase the CO_2 tension in the blood. The simplest way of increasing the CO_2 level is to allow the patient to rebreathe part of his own exhaled air. In the critical care setting, this may be accomplished by adding mechanical "dead" space to the ventilator tubing. The addition of this tubing is done by placing a small length (usually 12 to 15 cm) of tubing between the artificial airway and the "Y" piece of the ventilatory tubing for the adult. This "extension" of the trachea allows for partial rebreathing of the patient's own exhaled gas. The use of deadspace tubing for increasing the carbon dioxide tension is a reliable and predictable method with the controlled mode of ventilation.

Another method that may be used to increase the CO_2 tension in the blood is by decreasing the rate of ventilator-controlled breaths or decreasing the tidal volume delivered to the patient. This method allows for retention of some CO_2, although it may also have a deleterious effect on oxygenation. No matter what method of increasing the CO_2 tension is used, it is important to monitor the ABG parameters frequently to avoid possible complications from hypercarbia or hypoxemia.

Ventilator therapy

The conservative approach to maintaining adequate ventilation should always be the first method of choice. If the patient needs added ventilatory support, then mechanical ventilation may be indicated. The purpose of a mechanical ventilator is simply to provide mechanical work to inflate the lung in a physiologic fashion. Four clinical indications for mechanical ventilation that have universal application are (1) apnea, (2) acute ventilatory failure, (3) impending ventilatory failure, and (4) inadequate oxygenation. Practitioners are often frightened or frustrated by their lack of knowledge concerning the capabilities of the ventilator and its effects on the patient. Understanding the concepts of mechanical ventilation is a key factor in the provision of optimum care for the patient. Several types of ventilators are available on today's market. The basic concepts of ventilation are applicable to all types of machinery in any critical care setting.

Ventilators differ according to their primary control of cycling mechanism. The four main types are (1) volume cycled, (2) pressure cycled, (3) time cycled, and (4) flow cycled. The volume cycled ventilator is most commonly used in adult critical care. With this type of ventilator, a preset volume of gas is delivered to the patient with each breath. These machines are effective in that even when lung compliance is decreased or airway resistance is increased, the patient will continue to receive a consistent tidal volume. A pressure cycled ventilator delivers gas to the patient until a preset pressure is obtained on each breath. A disadvantage with this type of ventilator is that lung compliance and airway resistance will alter the volume delivered to the patient. With a time cycled ventilator, inspiration and expiration are terminated by a preset cycle duration. Many of the infant ventilators used are time cycled ventilators. Primary time cycled ventilators deliver a tidal volume in the time allotted for inspiration. These machines have a wide range of available flow rates, thus they can accommodate changes in lung compliance and airway resistance. The last type of ventilator, flow cycled, is cycled from inspiration to expiration by a drop of pressure to a preset level. These ventilators are not frequently used in critical care.

Negative pressure ventilation may also be employed in critical care. In this type of ventilation, a negative pressure is applied to the chest wall during inspiration. This creates a negative pressure in the airways themselves and air is pulled into the lungs. This type of ventilator is more frequently called an "iron lung" or a cuirass ventilator. Adaptations have been made to this concept of ventilation in its use today. A fiberglass shell is used that fits tightly over the anterolateral chest wall. In this way, the negative pressure concept can be applied without having to use a total body chamber. Although not frequently used in the critical care setting, it is used for long-term or nighttime ventilatory support of some patients.

Ventilatory modes. Most ventilators offer different modes of handling the expiratory/inspiratory changeover. These modes of therapy are shown in Fig. 3-18. The practitioner must be aware of the mode in which a patient is being mechanically ventilated and his response to the type of ventilation. If the patient is on a *controlled ventilation* mode, the ventilator cycles automatically at a rate determined by the operator, regardless of the patient's need or desire for a breath. The patient takes no active role in the ventilatory cycle. This mode is frequently used in critically ill patients, because the machine can provide the total work of breathing. Controlled mechanical ventilation may be employed in several circumstances: (1) when apnea is present, either because of primary central nervous system dysfunction or excessive sedation; (2) as a back-up for assisted ventilation should the patient fail

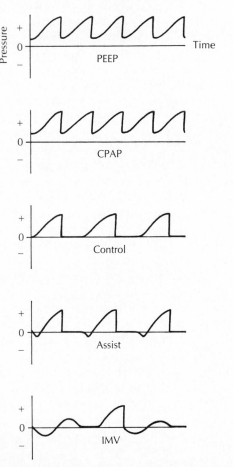

Fig. 3-18. Modes of mechanical ventilation. The pressure changes with the modes of therapy are shown. Zero (o) is atmospheric pressure.

to sustain spontaneous ventilatory activity; (3) under conditions when spontaneous ventilatory effort may be felt to be deleterious, such as flail chest; and (4) if the therapy involved, such as high-level positive end-expiratory pressure (PEEP) makes other modes ineffective or unreliable. Patients receiving controlled ventilation may attempt to take more breaths than the ventilator will provide. This leads to considerable anxiety and may increase the work of breathing. Sedation, muscle relaxants, and paralyzing medications can be used to manage the patient who becomes agitated on controlled ventilation. Extreme caution must be taken by the practitioner caring for this type of patient. With this mode of ventilation, the patient becomes totally dependent on the ventilator and the staff to meet his physiologic and psychologic needs.

In the *assisted ventilation* mode, the machine begins inspiration when the patient creates a subatmospheric pressure in the airway. The respiratory rate is determined by the patient, although a minimum ventilator rate is frequently set. Thus the ventilator will continue to provide an adequate minute ventilation if the patient becomes apneic. On the ventilator, the amount of subatmospheric pressure needed for the patient to "trigger" the ventilator is referred to as "sensitivity." Some proposed benefits of this mode of ventilaton are (1) subatmospheric pressure before each inspiration will increase venous return, (2) a more "normal" pH and Pa_{CO_2} are attained because the patient determines his own rate of ventilation, and (3) the psychologic benefit of the patient having control over his ventilation. These proposed benefits of assisted ventilation may not be clinically significant. First, the subatmospheric pressure generated with each inspiration may have little effect on venous return. Also, if the sensitivity is not set at an optimal level, the machine may "autocycle" or be difficult for the patient to trigger. These situations may agitate the patient, cause an increase in the work of breathing, and precipitate dramatic changes in the ABGs.

Intermittent mandatory ventilation (IMV) allows the patient to breathe on his own, determining his own rate and tidal volume. A mandatory breath is supplied by the machine at a predetermined volume and frequency without regard to the patient's demand. There are several advantages of this mode. First, the patient is responsible for regulating his own ventilatory pattern, which may provide more "normal" ABG values and provide more psychologic satisfaction. Second, the mean intrathoracic pressure is lower and venous return is less impeded than with controlled ventilation. Finally, atrophy of the muscles of ventilation is prevented because of their continued normal functioning. The IMV mode of mechanical ventilation is frequently used in the weaning process. Using IMV, weaning can be accomplished in a way that appears more physiologically sound than the older, conventional method of trial periods off the ventilator. Intermittent mandatory ventilation allows a smooth transition from controlled to spontaneous ventilation by gradually decreasing the ventilator rate as the patient assumes an increasing percentage of the total work of breathing. Two disadvantages of this mode must be mentioned. If the patient becomes apneic during the IMV mode of ventilation, adequate ventilation may not be delivered by the ventilator. Second, the patient's own breath and the machine-delivered breath may occur simultaneously. Thus the patient receives a larger breath than normal. This is regarded as a "sigh" or hyperinflation and is usually not thought to be a problem.

A modification of the IMV ventilator mode is the *synchronized intermittent mandatory ventilation (SIMV)* or *intermittent demand ventilation (IDV)*. This mode is very similar to the IMV mode in that the patient is allowed to breathe spontaneously. At intervals predetermined by the operator the machine "assists" the patient's next spontaneous breath. This alleviates the problem of a spontaneous patient breath and ventilator-delivered breath occurring concurrently. An excellent review of the IMV mode of therapy is provided by Weisman et al.[41]

Yet another technique of ventilation is *positive end-expiratory pressure (PEEP)*. In the previously mentioned modes of ventilation, positive airway pressure is applied during inspiration. At the onset of expiration, airway pressure is allowed to return to atmospheric pressure. With the PEEP mode of mechanical ventilation, a positive plateau pressure is maintained at end expiration. Most of the newer ventilators have PEEP as a feature on the ventilator. This is accomplished by pressurizing the expiratory valve during expiration. Positive end-expiratory pressure has been proven to be valuable in counteracting airway collapse, which may produce profound arterial hypoxemia, and reduced lung compliance. It increases the volume of air left in the lung at end-expiration (functional residual capacity) and alveoli are stabilized above their closing volume (the volume at which they would normally close). With the improved alveolar expansion, intrapulmonary shunting is reduced and the Pao_2 is improved. This improvement in Pao_2 may allow for a reduction in the F_IO_2.

Usually PEEP is started at 2 to 4 cm H_2O in the neonate and 5 to 10 cm H_2O in the adult patient. The PEEP along with the F_IO_2 can be titrated to achieve optimal oxygenation at the lowest F_IO_2. A potential hazard of PEEP therapy is a reduction in cardiac output. Three factors are thought to contribute to this decrease in cardiac output: (1) decreased venous return, (2) increased right venticular afterload, and (3) decreased left ventricular distensibility.[34] An excellent review of the PEEP mode of therapy is provided by Shapiro et al.[37]

Ventilation can also be assisted by expansion of the lungs with *continuous positive airway pressure (CPAP)*. Continuous positive airway pressure is similar to the technique of PEEP, but the patient is breathing spontaneously. It is particularly useful for infants but may also be used in adults. The constant positive pressure in the airways during both inspiration and expiration helped to counteract the tendency for alveoli to collapse; thus gas exchange is improved. As with PEEP, the major goals of CPAP therapy are to reexpand collapsed alveoli, increase the functional residual capacity, and reduce the work of breathing.[19]

As with PEEP therapy, CPAP therapy also has undesirable side effects. The most frequent complications are pulmonary air leak, inspissated secretions, pressure necrosis, and reduction in cardiac output. A pulmonary air leak may initially be seen as an interstitial emphysema, pneumothorax, or pneumomediastinum. Inspissated secretions may result from inadequate humidification of the inspired gas. Pressure necrosis of the nares, face, or neck may occur, depending on the method of CPAP administration. Finally, CPAP may also cause a reduction of cardiac output, which may occur for the same reason as was mentioned with the PEEP mode of therapy.

To conclude this section on ventilatory modes, a new technique must be mentioned. This ventilatory technique uses very small tidal volumes (less than the anatomic dead space) delivered at respiratory frequencies ranging from 60 to 100 cycles per minute.[38] The generic name for this mode of ventilation is *high-frequency positive pressure ventilation (HFPPV)*. Since its development, modifications of HFPPV have occurred to provide even higher rates of ventilation. These modifications are known as high-frequency jet ventilation or high-frequency oscillation. Some applications for this mode of ventilation include tracheal surgery, emergency and pediatric ventilation, and ventilatory support and weaning of patients with respiratory distress syndrome and bronchopleural fistulas.

In comparison to standard tidal volume ventilation, this new technique offers several potential advantages, including reduction of tidal fluctuations in alveolar pressure. Thus the risk of hemodynamic compromise and the likelihood of pulmonary air leak may be reduced. Although initial clinical reports have been promising, the use of HFPPV has been limited by two major problems. The first is that in many HFPPV circuits the tidal volume actually delivered to the patient differs substantially from the tidal volume generated by the ventilator. Thus a consistent data base describing the frequency and tidal volume dependence of gas exchange is not available. Second, optimal ventilatory settings must be determined empirically for each patient. The trial and error method used to determine optimal settings is a time-consuming and potentially dangerous process that consists of several trials of various combinations of tidal volume and frequency.

Although HFPPV is being used in some clinical settings, there are many issues that remain to be resolved before this technique can be generally applied as an accepted mode of mechanical ventilation. From a technical standpoint many questions remain unanswered along with a need for controlled clinical trials to distinguish which patients will benefit most from this type of ventilation.

Complications of mechanical ventilation

Airway complications. Complications resulting from problems with an artificial airway are the most common in mechanical ventilation. A complete discussion of the establishment and maintenance of an artificial airway is found earlier in the chapter. It must be reinforced, however, that the practitioner must monitor the cuff care and proper inflation technique to prevent tracheal necrosis. Care must also be taken to prevent kinking of the ventilator tubing. This may be prevented by making sure there is no tension on the artificial airway and ventilator tubing when the patient is in various positions. One may use swivel adapters and tubing support devices to prevent this problem.

Infections. Patients receiving mechanical ventilation are extremely susceptible to nosocomial infections. These patients are usually critically ill, and their resistance to infection is low. Most importantly, the normal defense mechanisms of the respiratory system are inhibited by the artificial airway. The use of antibiotics for other purposes may predispose the patient to the development of superimposed infections. Often these superimposed infections are highly resistant to antibiotic therapy.

Three areas that may contribute to the spread and growth of infectious organisms are the care of the artificial airway, suctioning technique, and cleaning of the respiratory therapy equipment. First, the artificial airway and its surrounding area are excellent mediums for bacterial growth. Secretions plus a warm, moist environment play a major part in the growth of organisms. Meticulous care of the artificial airway is an essential part of infection control. Included in the care of the artificial airway is the use of proper suctioning technique. The manual pressure inflation bag, another source of bacterial growth, should also be changed routinely and more frequently if the patient has copious amounts of secretions.

In addition, one must also consider possible contamination when the patient is disconnected from the ventilator or oxygen appliance. The ventilator tubing should be placed upright so as not to contaminate the connector site. If possible, the connector should be placed on a clean towel and not on the patient's bedclothes or linen. The practitioner should be sure that the proper care and cleaning of equipment takes place by the responsible personnel. In many institutions, culture and sensitivity tests are done routinely on respiratory therapy equipment to check for bacterial growth. It is also important for the practitioner to assess the patient for signs of respiratory infection. These include fever, change in the color of sputum, increased respiratory difficulty, or a change in laboratory values.

Cardiovascular impairment. Mean intrathoracic pressure is increased during mechanical ventilation because of the positive pressure inspiratory phase. The high pressures produced during mechanical ventilation may be transmitted to the heart and large vessels. This causes a decrease in venous return to the heart and a drop in cardiac output. In return, a drop in blood pressure may ensue. Factors that may predispose a patient to cardiovascular complications include high intrathoracic pressures, preexisting left ventricular problems, hypovolemia, vasodilation, and highly compliant lungs.

Previously the diminished cardiac output observed with PEEP therapy was attributed only to the impedance of venous return to the heart. There is now evidence that a variety of mechanisms are involved in this process.[34,37] Even under conditions of adequate fluid therapy, in most patients there is a PEEP level at which cardiac output diminishment becomes detrimental to the patient. Thus it is important to weigh the effectiveness of the PEEP therapy (improved oxygenation) against the deleterious effects on cardiac function.[37]

The IMV mode of therapy, along with the PEEP therapy, may help to lessen the intrathoracic pressures being generated. Spontaneous ventilations assist in reestablishing normal intrathoracic pressure relationships.

Pulmonary complications. As discussed earlier in the chapter, *oxygen toxicity* may also be a problem in the ventilator-dependent patient. Oxygen can produce toxicity when given in a large dosage for extended periods of time. Microscopic pulmonary changes occur with prolonged ventilation with increased O_2 tensions (F_IO_2 greater than 0.60).[3,31] In order to prevent this complication, the lowest possible F_IO_2 that will produce adequate oxygenation should be used. After O_2 toxicity occurs, no specific therapy is yet available to counteract the effects. On a trial basis, PEEP therapy may be instituted to assess if the F_IO_2 can be reduced while maintaining adequate oxygenation.

Barotrauma refers to the consequences of alveolar overdistention, which results from excessively high intrathoracic pressures being generated by positive pressure ventilation. This complication can be avoided if the ventilation is carefully monitored to provide adequate oxygenation and ventilation while minimizing the positive pressure being transmitted to the lungs. This is one reason the practitioner should monitor proximal airway pressure on the ventilator.

Fluctuations in H^+ concentrations may also occur in mechanical ventilation of a patient. The ventilator is a powerful instrument that may cause as well as correct acid-base derangements.

When support is initiated, special care should be exercised not to reverse acidosis too quickly or to cause significant respiratory alkalosis and the concomitant electrolyte changes. In the assist mode, marked fluctuations in pH and $PaCO_2$ can occur in patients who excessively trigger the ventilator. It is important to understand the interdependence between changes in the tidal volume and the ventilator rate and their relationship to changes in H^+ concentration.

Weakening or discoordination of respiratory muscles may occur as the burden of the timing and pattern of breathing are controlled by the machine for prolonged periods. Good nutritional support and use of the IMV mode of mechanical ventilation will allow the patient to continue to use her respiratory muscles. Thus muscle loss or weakness can be prevented or minimized. Other measures that will assist the patient in strengthening her muscles of respiration are early ambulation and breathing exercises.

Aspiration pneumonia may occur before, during, or after intubation and placement on a mechanical ventilator. Once aspiration occurs, the extent of pulmonary damage depends on the acidity and volume of the aspirated material. In addition to the effect of the acid, the composition of the aspirate affects the degree of pulmonary insult. Aspiration may occur even if the cuff of the artificial airway is seemingly properly inflated. Use of positive pressure mechanical ventilation necessitates the need for cuff inflation, thus helping to minimize the occurrence of aspiration. If a cuffless artificial airway is being used (for example, in infants and small children), the practitioner must take every precaution to minimize the possibility of aspiration.

Fluid retention. Continuous positive pressure ventilation of any type may result in a decrease in urine output and water retention. The exact cause of this fluid retention and antidiuresis is not known, but factors that may contribute to the problem include increased circulating levels of antidiuretic hormone (ADH), fluid overload, unrecognized cardiac failure, and changes in in-

trarenal blood flow. It is important for the practitioner to closely monitor the fluid status of the patient by observing for edema, to accurately measure intake and output and body weight, and to monitor cardiovascular function and changes in chest roentgenograms (increased intravascular markings).

Gastric problems. Gastric dilation may occur if the positive pressure gas is allowed to enter the stomach. This may occur if there is a small leak around the endotracheal or tracheostomy tube. A practitioner should routinely check for bowel sounds and the circumference of the abdomen at regular intervals. Insertion of a nasogastric tube will help to prevent or correct the situation.

Stress ulcers may occur in the ventilator-dependent patient. Some possible causes of stress ulcers are gastric acid hypersecretion and disruption of the gastric mucosal barrier. Antacid therapy as well as H_2 blocker medications seem to reduce the occurrence of stress ulcers in the critically ill patient. Care to prevent this occurrence includes proper administration of the medications and tube feedings, along with encouraging normal intake of foods when this is possible. It is also advisable for the practitioner to check periodically for occult stool in the ventilator-dependent patient.

Psychologic complications. The patient who is receiving mechanical ventilation therapy is under constant stress, both physically and from the environment. Usually the critical care milieu is one of continuous, excessive sensory stimulation for the patient. An attitude by the practitioner of confidence and knowledge of the equipment will help allay the patient's fears of safety. Communication becomes an almost intolerable problem for the patient receiving mechanical ventilation therapy. The patient must have some means of communication to relay his needs and feelings to his family and the health care team.

Regression, dependency, and anger are all emotions that may surface in the ventilator-dependent patient. Regression is fostered by an environment that is very structured and does not allow the patient to make decisions. Ventilator dependency may occur psychologically as well as physiologically. A patient may become fixated on his dependence on the mechanical ventilator because he realizes this is a life-supporting device. Perhaps having experienced feelings of suffocation and fear in respiratory distress, the patient feels very secure and comfortable while receiving mechanical ventilation. Patient dependence also occurs with the caregivers and family, physically and psychologically. The patient should be encouraged to participate in his care as much as possible and to develop a sense of independence. Continuity of caregivers who are compatible and accustomed to the patient is also important in fostering the sense of independence and control.

A trusting relationship must develop between the patient and his caregivers. This relationship is needed if behavior modification techniques are used with the patient, most importantly when the ventilator weaning process is begun. Only with a calm, motivated, and secure patient and staff will the weaning process be incident free and successful.

Weaning from ventilator support. Weaning is the staged withdrawal of ventilator support from those patients who will not tolerate sudden, complete cessation. For the patient and the caregivers, the weaning process can be a difficult and slow task. This is especially true of patients who have been on prolonged ventilation therapy and those patients with underlying chronic lung disease. The weaning period is critical to the patient's needs.

The method of weaning chosen for a patient should be individualized to his needs. The practitioner plays a valuable role in the weaning process. Psychologic preparation for weaning should begin with the initiation of mechanical ventilation and be maintained throughout by frequent references to the temporary nature of the treatment. The practitioner should be in constant attendance during the initiation of the weaning process. Psychologic support, along with motivation and positive feedback to the pa-

tient, are necessary for a successful transition from the ventilator to spontaneous breathing.

During the weaning period, the practitioner should assess the patient for any signs of respiratory distress, such as increased respiratory rate, increased heart rate, increased anxiety, excessive use of the accessory muscles, asynchronous breathing pattern, arrhythmias, or a significant change in the patient's overall physical status. If respiratory distress occurs, the patient should be reconnected to the ventilator or the IMV rate should be increased. It is important for the practitioner to offer emotional support to the patient after an unsuccessful attempt at weaning so that the patient will not be frightened of future attempts. Weaning of the patient from the ventilator must be conducted in a controlled atmosphere with the patient and caregiver knowing exactly what to expect. Each patient will need an individualized plan devised for the weaning process. In essence, the plan for weaning a patient from the ventilator should begin immediately after mechanical ventilation has been initiated.

The inability to discontinue mechanical support often results from failure to correct one or more of the factors that adversely effect the patient: strength and nutrition, coping abilities, ventilatory requirements, gas exchange, or lung mechanics. Before beginning the weaning process the patient should have good electrolyte, acid-base, and fluid balance. Infection, arrhythmias, and heart failure should all be under control. The airways should be optimally bronchodilated and cleared of secretions. In addition, the patient should be rested and mentally prepared for the weaning process.

Nutrition is a vital need that is often overlooked during mechanical ventilation.[16] Gastric feedings or intravenous hyperalimentation are necessary if the patient is unable to orally ingest fluids or foods. Weaning a patient from mechanical ventilation puts an added load on the patient's energy and O_2 requirements. When the patient begins to spontaneously ventilate, the work of breathing increases along with the energy requirements of the respiratory musculature.

Thus poor nutrition may be a cause of unsuccessful weaning of a patient from a ventilator.

There are also several suggested ventilatory parameters that aid in the assessment of ventilatory strength or reserve relative to requirements. Almost all parameters depend on patient cooperation.

The following are some parameters in common use:

1. Vital capacity > 10 to 15 ml/kg
2. Forced expiratory volume in 1 second > 10 ml/kg
3. Maximal inspiratory effort > −25 cm H_2O
4. Minute ventilation < 20 L/min
5. Maximal volume ventilation > minute ventilation × 2
6. Pa_{O_2} > 60 mmHg on 40% O_2

The vital capacity and inspiratory effort may suffice in most clinical situations.[40] Good parameters provide data supportive of ventilator discontinuation, but poor ones do not preclude a T-piece trial or an attempt to wean if clinical judgment suggests a favorable outcome.

Initially a T-piece trial is a brief but stringent test of the patient's ability to sustain spontaneous ventilation. Passing of this trial justifies discontinuing the ventilator abruptly, whereas failing the trial indicates that weaning is necessary. The weaning process should be started in the morning when the patient is well rested and an adequate number of staff members is available. The optimally prepared patient is placed in a comfortable semi-Fowler's position, the airway is suctioned, and vital signs are measured before the weaning process begins.

Basically, two methods are available for weaning a patient from a mechanical ventilator. First, a Briggs adapter or T-piece may be used. This allows the patient to be disconnected from the ventilator and to breathe spontaneously while heated humidified gas is delivered to the patient via widebore corrugated tubing. With this method, the patient must be closely monitored by the practitioner for signs of fatigue and respiratory difficulty. The patient is alternately put on the T-piece for short periods of time and then reconnected to the ventilator. This allows the patient time to rest. As the weaning process progresses, the patient is left on the T-piece for increasing periods of time until he is able to tolerate the T-piece continuously. If the patient is able to tolerate the T-piece for long periods at a time with no evidence of deterioration, extubation should be considered.

The second method of weaning from the mechanical ventilator is via the IMV ventilator mode. It allows the ventilator-delivered respiratory rate to be slowly decreased and provides a method for gradually transferring the work of breathing from the machine to the patient. It is a potentially advantageous method for patients who cannot withstand sudden increments in venous return or the burden of total unaided ventilation. Furthermore, IMV provides periodic controlled ventilations and allows the patient to retrain and strengthen his ventilatory muscles.

The IMV method of weaning is not without some disadvantages. It may increase the work of breathing and unnecessarily prolong the weaning process. Unlike the T-piece method, IMV requires that the tube cuff remain inflated, thus increasing resistance in the airway. Finally, one of the greatest dangers of the IMV method is that the patient will not be monitored closely for signs of deterioration because the patient is "on the ventilator."

Monitoring devices

Several methods are available for monitoring the respiratory status of patients in the critical care setting. Equipment is available to monitor respiratory activity, ventilation, and the oxygenation and perfusion status of the patient. Although many types of monitors are available, any type of monitoring equipment should be used to supplement the practitioner's care, not replace it.

In the newborn or pediatric critical care setting, respiratory monitors are frequently used to monitor ventilation. The most common apnea monitors use the technique of impedance pneumography to register respiratory activity by sensing the resistive changes to the movement of air into and out of the lungs. Other types of apnea monitoring equipment available are the air mattress monitor and sensor pad monitor.

Apnea monitors are infrequently used in the adult critical care setting. Because of the sensing mechanisms, it is difficult to adapt this system to the adult. If the adult is receiving ventilatory therapy, these machines are equipped with numerous alarms to check for both patient distress and machine failure.

Other types of noninvasive monitors are available to monitor respiratory status. Transcutaneous monitors use the phenomenon that gases diffuse through the skin, making possible second-by-second recording of these gas levels. Transcutaneous monitoring is available for both O_2 and CO_2. Several companies have developed a single skin electrode that measures both of these gases. The transcutaneous skin P_{CO_2} is thought to measure arterial P_{CO_2} to an accuracy of $3 \pm$ mmHg.[17,36] The skin P_{O_2} measurement, however, is not as accurate in measuring arterial P_{O_2}. Factors that may affect the skin P_{O_2} measurement are skin perfusion, skin preparation, and choice of skin site.[36] Transcutaneous O_2 and CO_2 measurements are important tools in respiratory care. These monitors are most helpful in continuously assessing the patient and his responses to ventilatory changes and such activities as turning and suctioning.

Use of the ear oximeter is another noninvasive method to continuously monitor the patient's respiratory status. The ear oximeter measures oxygen saturation by optical methods: the system uses a fiberoptic cable to pass light from the instrument to the headpiece or earpiece, which is attached to the pinna of the ear. It can be used in both pediatric and adult patients. The O_2 saturation obtained by this method may be more accurate than that from an arterial blood gas analysis, which is calculated from the O_2 tension. The continuous monitoring of the O_2 saturation is helpful in determining transient or long-term periods of desaturation resulting from

changes in therapy or response to various procedures.

Either the transcutaneous O_2 monitor or the ear oximeter will faithfully record changes in the O_2 status of the patient. It is important, though, to correlate the reading obtained by the noninvasive device with an ABG at the start of the period. Currently all noninvasive devices that monitor O_2 status depend on skin perfusion for this correlation between noninvasive and invasive O_2 monitoring techniques.

Measurement of end-tidal capnography (CO_2) via an infrared analyzer allows the practitioner to continuously monitor CO_2 levels in the patient. Because CO_2 is so easily diffusable, the end-tidal CO_2 is a good estimate of the arterial CO_2 level. This analyzer connects to the end of the artificial airway, between the airway and the ventilator tubing. This type of monitoring is of value because continuous monitoring of the patient can occur and it lessens the need for frequent ABG measurements.

A newer, invasive respiratory monitoring device was mentioned previously in the text. The fiberoptic pulmonary artery catheter can be used to continuously monitor the oxygen saturation of venous blood. The practitioner can use this continuous monitoring to determine the effect of certain procedures on tissue oxygenation and to guide patient care.

Pharmacologic interventions

There are numerous sites for drug actions to occur in the lungs. First, several receptors lie in the smooth muscle of the airways. The alpha-receptors act on the smooth muscle to cause vasoconstriction and contraction. Beta-2 receptors are also found in the smooth muscle. The response of the beta-2 receptor is relaxation or bronchodilation. Cholinergic receptors in the airway's smooth muscle have a bronchoconstrictive response. A second site for drug action to occur is during cellular metabolism. Certain respiratory drugs have an effect on the production and breakdown of cyclic adenosine monophosphate (AMP). Cyclic AMP is one of the intermediaries of cellular metabolism in the sequence of energy production. Another site where drug action may occur is in the mast cell in the airways. Certain drugs stabilize the mast cell, preventing the extrusion of histamine and other reactive agents that cause bronchoconstriction during an allergic response. The drugs used most commonly in the critical care setting will be discussed in this section.

Bronchodilators. Bronchodilators are of major importance when discussing pharmacologic intervention in respiratory care. The two classifications of bronchodilators are the methylxanthines and the sympathomimetics.

The methylxanthine drugs work as bronchodilators by increasing levels of cyclic AMP through inactivating phosphodiesterase, a substance that normally breaks down cyclic AMP. Theophylline is the foremost methylxanthine for use in the treatment of bronchospasm. Other effects of theophylline include inhibition of mast cell degranulation and subsequent mediator release and an increase in mucociliary transport rates.[27] Theophylline not only acts on the airways but also effects the cardiovascular system, central nervous system, and kidney.[27] Although it is primarily used in pulmonary care, it does have other uses.

In the critical care setting, an intravenous infusion of aminophylline is most often used. Aminophylline is another name for theophylline ethylenediamine. The ethylenediamine is a solvent in which theophylline is 20 times more soluble than in water. As a result, aminophylline can be given intravenously, whereas theophylline cannot. The dosage of the methylxanthines is calculated by the patient's weight in kilograms and other factors that potentiate or decrease the action of the drug. With intravenous administration of aminophylline, frequently a loading dose will be given, followed by a maintenance dosage via continuous infusion. Side effects of the methylxanthine group includes nausea and vomiting, nervousness, arrhythmias, and seizures. Theophylline serum levels are drawn at frequent intervals to monitor the level of drug in the body. The usual therapeutic range for a theophylline level is 10 to 20 μg/ml. Toxic levels of the drug may occur in the blood very quickly with continuous infusion. Thus the practitioner must be alert to the side effects of the drug, factors that may potentiate or decrease the action of the drugs, and the serum levels of theophylline.

Usually the methylxanthines and sympathomimetic drugs are used together to offer a synergistic effect. Therefore maximal bronchodilation is achieved. As stated earlier, the most common methylxanthine used in the critical care setting is intravenous aminophylline. Numerous combination preparations of theophylline and its derivatives are available in tablet and liquid forms. These preparations are used when the severe bronchospasm is relieved and intravenous infusion is no longer required. For any given preparation containing theophylline, the exact amount (milligrams and/or percentage) of anhydrous theophylline base in the preparation must be determined to appropriately calculate a specific patient dosage.

A sympathomimetic drug is one that stimulates the action of the sympathetic nervous system. Adenylate cyclase, the beta-2 receptor, is an enzyme that is stimulated in the presence of the sympathomimetic drugs. Increasing adenylate cyclase catalyzes the conversion of adenosine 5'-triphosphate (ATP) to cyclic AMP, thus providing smooth muscle relaxation in the airways.

There are several sympathomimetic drugs used to control bronchospasm. These drugs all have side effects similar to the methylxanthines. Nausea, nervousness, palpitations, headache, and tremor may be seen with increased dosages of the drug. Some commonly used sympathomimetic agents used are isoetharine (Bronkosol), terbutaline (Brethine, Bricanyl), metaproterenol (Alupent, Metaprel), and albuterol (Proventil, Ventolin). Epinephrine is a powerful bronchodilator; however, because of its increased action on the beta-1 receptors in the myocardium, it is used less frequently. Isoproterenol (Isuprel) also has powerful beta-2 stimulation properties and therefore relaxes smooth muscle in the bronchial tree. Because of its strong beta-1 activity on the myocardium and the side effects, this may not be the bronchodilator of choice, since more selective beta-2 drugs are available.

It is the practitioner's responsibility to administer the bronchodilator drugs correctly and to be alert for any side effects. Awareness of dosages and length of action, along with potential drug interactions, is also of importance. The sympathomimetics may have potential interactions with propranolol and other sympathomimetic agents. Intravenous administration of aminophylline may be complicated by incompatibilities in the intravenous solution with many drugs, including penicillins, insulin, morphine sulfate, phenytoin sodium, epinephrine, tetracyclines, and vitamins. Because there are many other drug incompatibilities, the practitioner must closely monitor all infusions of aminophylline.

Corticosteroids. Corticosteroids may be used to treat pulmonary problems. There are several proposed mechanisms of the action of corticosteroids on lung tissue. First, corticosteroids may be used in an effort to halt inflammation and restore the integrity of cell membranes in the lung. Some other beneficial actions of these drugs are (1) inhibition of antibody formation, (2) inhibition of formation of messenger agents, such as histamine, which are involved in the asthmatic response, and (3) inhibition of various cellular mechanisms involved in bronchoconstriction.[27]

The corticosteroids in general usage are the glucocorticoids. These are steroidal agents possessing antiinflammatory and gluconeogenic properties. As with any corticosteroid medication, many side effects may occur with the drug. With prolonged large dosages of the drug, the following may occur: hyperglycemia, depletion of bone potassium, impairment of the immunologic response, reduction of the inflammatory response, elevation of blood pressure, and problems with the clotting mechanisms of blood.

Usually, once the patient's bronchocongestion and bronchospasm are stabilized, the patient is changed to an oral steroidal preparation. The lowest dosage of corticosteroids that can maintain the desired clinical response is always preferred. This helps to prevent or minimize side effects. For long-term care, an inhaled steroid, beclomethasone dipropionate, may also be used. The inhaled preparation has a topical effect on the airways while maintaining low systemic activity. This type of inhaled preparation is not used in the critical care setting but is used for maintenance therapy in the inpatient and outpatient setting.

Although not approved by the Food and Drug Administration, triamcinolone acetonide (Aristocort, Kenalog) is sometimes used in an aerosol form to decrease airway mucosal inflammation. As with the advantage of beclomethasone dipropionate, this drug has a topical effect while minimizing systemic activity. Side effects from aerosolized triamcinolone include hoarseness, voice weakness, and oropharyngeal candidosis.[27]

In the critical care setting, an intravenous corticosteroid will probably be used. Because of the numerous and dangerous side effects of these preparations, the practitioner should administer these drugs with caution.

Mucokinetic agents. Mucokinetic agents may be used to facilitate airway clearance and thus ventilation. These drugs are administered in an aerosolized or systemic form. They tend to lower the surface tension and viscosity of the mucus, which helps to enhance airway clearance. Some commonly used mucolytic agents are normal saline, water, N-acetylcysteine, and propylene glycol. The practitioner must be aware that these drugs may promote airway blockage and bronchospasm as a result of the mobilization of secretions. Thus if the patient is unable to voluntarily cough, suctioning of the tracheobronchial tree must be done by the practitioner.

Antimicrobial agents. Infection is often a predisposing factor in the cause of respiratory failure, especially in those patients with chronic lung disease. In a critically ill patient, infection may be the cause of the patient's illness or may result from treatments, procedures, or care given to the patient. Bacteria can enter the body from several sources: artificial airways, contaminated equipment, intravenous or arterial cannula sites, a urinary catheter, or improper clean or sterile technique used by the practitioner.

The antimicrobial of choice will depend on isolation of the organism by culture and sensitivity. Antimicrobials produce their effects by interfering with cell structure or function. They can be given via several routes. Most commonly in the critical care setting they will be given intravenously. Aerosolization of certain liquid antimicrobials can also be used to treat respiratory infections. When used, they should be combined with appropriate systemic antimicrobials. Aerosolized antimicrobials are used sometimes in special situations, for example, patients with cystic fibrosis and in some patients with fungal infections.

Some commonly used antimicrobials are the penicillins and cephalosporins, which act on the cell wall synthesis; polymyxin, which acts on the cell membrane function; aminoglycosides, chloramphenicol, and the tetracyclines, which inhibit protein synthesis; and sulfonamides, which act on bacterial metabolism.[27] Most antimicrobials are capable of producing various side effects. The practitioner should be familiar with the possible side effects and observe for them.

Analeptic drugs. Analeptic drugs are those that increase primarily the depth of respirations, but also the rate. Doxapram hydrochloride (Dopram) is an analeptic drug that may be used to stimulate the respiratory center. Its site of action is thought to be direct stimulation of the carotid bodies. It may be useful in severe respiratory depression caused by hypnotic and sedative-hypnotic agents. Doxapram hydrochloride may also be used to stimulate breathing in postanesthetic patients. Some practitioners feel, however, that direct supportive measures such as mechanical ventilation and maintenance of cardiovascular function are more useful. The drug

has several side effects indicative of central and autonomic nervous system stimulation. Some side effects of this drug are tachycardia, arrhythmias, sneezing, vomiting, itching, tremors, and muscle rigidity. The practitioner should be aware that this drug may also cause a rise in blood pressure and produce bronchospasm and laryngospasm in patients with asthma.

Narcotic antagonists. Narcotic antagonists are drugs that may be used in patients being treated for narcotic overdoses or to reverse respiratory depression caused by therapeutic doses of narcotics. The narcotic antagonist drugs are given intravenously. Naloxone (Narcan) is an agent frequently used because it is a pure narcotic antagonist. In the absence of narcotic drugs it exhibits no pharmacologic effect. Levallorphan tartrate (Lorfan) is also a narcotic antagonist. Compared to naloxone, this drug may have a depressant effect on respirations in the absence of narcotic drugs. Physostigmine salicylate, an anticholinesterase agent, may be useful in reversing the central anticholinergic syndrome produced by overdosage of such drugs as phenothiazines, antihistamines, tricyclic antidepressants, and diazepam.

Sodium bicarbonate

Sodium bicarbonate is an agent that functions physiologically as an inorganic buffer. It may be used to increase the level of bicarbonate in the blood in the correction of metabolic acidosis. With the administration of sodium bicarbonate, the bicarbonate level increases, which is then available to combine with the excess H^+. The result of this reaction is carbonic acid, which then becomes dehydrated to form CO_2 and H_2O. The CO_2 is then excreted by way of the lungs.

Careful monitoring of the ABG pH is important in guiding the administration of this drug. Large amounts of sodium bicarbonate may be necessary to correct metabolic acidemia caused by the accumulation of lactic acid during cardiac arrest. The practitioner should remember that the goal of sodium bicarbonate therapy may not be to fully correct the metabolic acidemia, since other acid-base buffering mechanisms will act to correct the condition simultaneously. The effects of these other buffering systems may not be seen for hours. In addition, one should remember that sodium bicarbonate will lower serum potassium. Therefore one must also pay close attention to these levels when administering large amounts of sodium bicarbonate.

Tris(hydroxymethyl)aminomethane (THAM). THAM is a buffer that has been used in neonates in the treatment of acute respiratory acidosis. It combines with CO_2 to form bicarbonate and thus restore pH. Some problems with the use of this drug have been cited. As with sodium bicarbonate, the rapid injection of THAM may be associated with a rapid change in serum osmolarity. With this brisk change in serum osmolarity, many other parameters may be altered. The rapid infusion of a hypertonic solution produces a sudden rise in cerebrospinal fluid pressure and venous pressure. This is followed by a steep drop in cerebrospinal fluid pressure. Profound effects on the brain may occur, including depressed respiration and apnea. Because of its potential side effects, the administration of this drug should be closely monitored by the practitioner.

Acetazolamide (Diamox). Acetazolamide may be used to potentiate the excretion of excess bicarbonate from the patient. Thus this drug may be used to partially correct metabolic alkalosis. It inhibits the action of carbonic anhydrase, which results in slowing the CO_2 uptake from the tissues and CO_2 unloading in the lungs. With this, ventilation is usually improved, accompanied by improved oxygenation in the blood. The practitioner must remember that the action of this drug is slow and may persist for days.

Perfusion

Procedural intervention

Several procedural interventions are used to improve perfusion of the lungs. Many of these techniques have been alluded to in earlier parts of this chapter. These interventions range from simple techniques to very complex ones that are infrequently used in the critical care setting. For instance, a very simple technique to enhance lung perfusion is frequent repositioning of the patient. This improves perfusion as well as ventilation of the lung. Fluids and blood may also be administered to increase blood volume and increase the blood hemoglobin level, thus improving oxygen-carrying capacity. Improvement of the cardiovascular status of the patient is yet another method that improves perfusion of the lung. Finally, control of the acid-base status and oxygenation of the patient also play an important role in improving the perfusion of the lungs. More complex measures such as extracorporeal membrane oxygenation (ECMO) are available as a measure to artificially maintain perfusion in a patient in a critical situation.

One must note that along with the benefits of procedural interventions for perfusion and also ventilation, some deleterious effects may also be caused in the attempt to improve perfusion of the lung. Two of the areas of procedural interventions, positive pressure ventilation and continuous positive pressure to the airways (PEEP, CPAP) have already been discussed earlier in the chapter.

ECMO is a method of artificially maintaining perfusion in a patient. With ECMO, the patient's blood is passed through artificial lungs in a manner similar to that for hemodialysis. Certain patients in acute, reversible, respiratory failure, despite maximum efforts of conventional ventilatory care, are unable to maintain adequate arterial oxygenation. Thus ECMO has been used in an attempt to maintain perfusion. Use of ECMO may allow for more time and the institution of specific therapy to allow for restoration of the lung function. Few centers have the resources to initiate ECMO in the critical care setting, and although it may be helpful as an emergency measure, there are no data to show that it is effective in long-term usage.[44] The significant hazards of ECMO are bleeding, infection, and mechanical failure.

The practitioner is responsible for monitoring the patient in regard to problems with ECMO therapy, poor oxygenation, and lowered cardiac output. Maintenance of a patent airway by positioning, chest physical therapy, and suctioning are all necessary to promote healing of the lungs. Weaning a patient from ECMO therapy presents many problems. The effect on arterial oxygenation of reduction of flow rates through the oxygenator provides a means of determining whether a patient can be weaned from the oxygenator or not. Usually, if the patient can maintain a PaO_2 of 50 mmHg or greater for a number of hours, mechanical perfusion can probably be stopped.

Pharmacologic intervention

Diuretics. Diuretics are indicated to promote loss of salt and water in fluid-retaining states and for control of blood pressure. The primary use of diuretics in respiratory patients is to treat fluid overload and congestive heart failure, which may be secondary to their pulmonary disease. There are several types of diuretics available. Their mode and duration of action vary. The type of diuretic ordered will depend on the severity of fluid overload and the estimated duration of therapy.

Furosemide (Lasix) and ethacrynic acid (Sodium Edecrin). Furosemide and ethacrynic acid are the most potent diuretics available. Both drugs exert their major effect by blocking reabsorption of sodium along the entire ascending limb of the loop of Henle and possibly along the proximal and distal convoluted tubules. After intravenous administration of one of these drugs, profound diuresis occurs within 30 minutes and reaches a maximum in 60 to 90 minutes. Both drugs are excreted from the liver and kidney. The prompt beneficial effect of these drugs in relieving pulmonary congestion and acute pulmonary edema frequently precedes any diuresis and results from a decrease in left ventricular filling pressures. Serum electrolytes should be closely monitored during and after the administration of these drugs. Some side effects are alkalemia, electrolyte depletion, weakness, dizziness, lethargy, and postural hypotension. The practitioner should closely observe fluid balance when either of these drugs is being given.

Thiazides. Thiazides are excellent oral diuretics because of their potency, repetitive effectiveness, and relative lack of side effects and toxicity. They act by inhibiting sodium reabsorption in the ascending limb of the loop of Henle and also exhibit properties of carbonic anhydrase inhibition. A large number of thiazide preparations is available. They differ in dosage, degree, and duration of action. All of these drugs cause a loss of potassium. Serum potassium should be monitored, and the use of a potassium supplement may be necessary. Some side effects of the thiazide preparations are skin rashes, gastric irritation, nausea, weakness, fatigue, and anorexia.

Other diuretic preparations. Other diuretic preparations exist that are potentially potassium sparing. Although usually not as strong as the thiazide preparations, they may be used in conjunction with other types of preparations for an adequate diuretic effect.

Thrombolytic/anticoagulant agents. Following an embolic episode, therapy is directed at two goals. First, supportive therapy is used to maintain cardiopulmonary function and relieve breathlessness, pain, and hypoxemia until the thrombi begin to lyse. The second goal is the lysis and prevention of further venous thrombosis and embolization to the lungs by thrombolytic agents and anticoagulants. Surgical intervention may be used, depending on the size and area of the embolism.

Thrombolytic agents (urokinase, streptokinase). These drugs promote dissolution of thrombi by stimulating the conversion of endogenous plasminogen to plasmin. Two other actions of these drugs are to decrease the viscosity of the blood and decrease the erythrocyte aggregation tendency. Treatment with these drugs should be started as soon as possible after the objective diagnosis of pulmonary embolism has been made. They are given for 12 to 24 hours, then the patient is switched to anticoagulant therapy. Not all patients are candidates for this therapy. A clinical decision whether to use these agents is based on the total assessment of the patient and the size, severity, and recurrence of the thromboembolism.

Thrombolytic drugs may produce profound changes in hemostasis and a greater degree of bleeding than heparin or oral coumarin anticoagulation therapy. The bleeding that may occur with this therapy is often more severe and difficult to manage. Concurrent use of other anticoagulants with a thrombolytic agent may be dangerous. During thrombolytic treatment, coagulation tests do not correlate with the drug's effects or side effects. Observing the patient for bleeding (at needle punctures, chest tubes, catheters, etc.) and taking care to avoid unnecessary trauma are more important than quantitative tests.

Heparin. The prevention of further venous thrombi is accomplished by anticoagulation. This is initiated with heparin rather than an oral anticoagulant because of heparin's rapid action. Heparin acts to alter the configuration of antithrombin, which in turn inhibits thrombin, preventing clot formation. It is given intravenously either intermittently or by continuous infusion to the patient. The patient is monitored daily with coagulation tests. Intravenous heparin is usually administered for 5 to 10 days, at which time the patient is switched to a deep subcutaneous heparin injection or oral anticoagulant therapy. The practitioner must be aware of the patient's coagulation laboratory values, along with any signs of blood dyscrasias and bleeding disorders that may occur with anticoagulation therapy.

Nutritional intervention

As stated earlier in this chapter, adequate nutrition is of utmost importance in the overall management of the critically ill patient. If a ventilator-dependent patient has a poor nutritional status, this may contribute to a difficult weaning process even when other aspects of his lung disease have been resolved. Later it is possible to successfully wean these patients from mechanical ventilation after they have improved their nutritional status. For the patient who is spontaneously breathing and making slow progress, adequate nutrition is necessary to provide sufficient energy for the patient to begin sitting up in the chair and begin ambulating. Improved nutrition and progressive ambulation both play intricate roles in improvement of lung perfusion and ventilation. All aspects of the patient's care and their independence must be taken into account by the practitioner to provide a comprehensive pulmonary care plan.

Nutritional intake may be provided by a variety of methods. Nutrition must be carefully evaluated for each patient. The presence of a tracheostomy tube is not necessarily a contraindication to oral feedings. Once gastrointestinal system function has been established, oral feedings may be attempted. As stated earlier, aspiration into the lungs may be a problem with oral feedings. This may be prevented by the slow progression of fluids and foods to the tracheostomized patient and meticulous cuff and oral care. Usually the patient with a tracheostomy tube will be able to eat only a soft diet, since the inflated tracheostomy cuff often produces some difficulty in swallowing. If the patient is unable to maintain an adequate oral intake of foods, then another method of alimentation must be used.

Hydration is important to facilitate the removal of secretions from the tracheobronchial tree. Unless it is contraindicated, a patient receiving oral intake should receive large amounts of water or fluids (1500 to 2000 ml) daily. Proper hydration is also important to minimize hypovolemia, which in turn may result in decreased cardiac output in the patient receiving mechanical ventilation therapy. Humidification and nebulization are necessary to avoid drying and encrusting of secretions.

However, the benefits of humidification and hydration are sometimes offset by the potential for generalized fluid overload. Under most circumstances the fluid requirements of a patient receiving mechanical ventilation therapy are less than those of a patient breathing spontaneously. Ventilators prevent respiratory water loss that normally occurs with spontaneous breathing. In addition, patients on ventilators who are in a state of negative nitrogen balance may develop protein depletion, cell destruction, and generalized edema. It is the practitioner's responsibility to monitor fluid intake and prevent overload by careful daily measurements of intake, output, and body weight and examination of the serum electrolytes. If fluid overload does occur, diuretics may be administered and a restricted amount of fluid intake may be ordered to reestablish fluid balance.

A low-sodium diet is indicated in patients who are subject to fluid retention and weight gain. Minimizing sodium intake of a patient will reduce the possibility of sodium and fluid retention, which in turn may put an added burden on both the heart and lungs.

Finally, one must take into consideration any medications the patient is receiving that promote fluid retention. An example of a medication that does promote fluid retention is the corticosteroids.

REHABILITATION

Rehabilitation is an important aspect of care for the critically ill respiratory patient. Rehabilitation in the critical care setting simply means restoring the patient to the fullest physical and emotional potential of which he or she is capable. Depending on the degree of pulmonary problems the patient has, the goals of rehabilitation will vary. Rehabilitative measures should be initiated on the patient's admission to the critical care unit and should extend beyond hospital discharge to the home setting. The process of rehabilitation is multifaceted, involving many disciplines of the health care team. The patient, family, and practitioner all play active roles in the process of rehabilitation.

Education

Education of the patient and family is an important aspect of the rehabilitation process. It is an ongoing process that should be continued throughout the patient's stay in the hospital. Cooperation by the patient and his family may be increased when simple explanations about procedures and treatments are given. Increased knowledge and understanding also helps to alleviate fear and apprehension experienced by the patient and his family. Once the patients' condition improves, education regarding his disease process, medications, bronchial hygiene, and preventitive measures of respiratory disease should all be included in the teaching process.

Physical therapy

In the critical care setting, physical therapy is a vital discipline for the pulmonary patient. Implementation of relaxation and breathing techniques are important to facilitate improved ventilation (see "Airway Establishment," p. 219). The patient should be taught to use more efficient breathing patterns. It is important for the patient to use these relaxation and breathing techniques during the weaning process from mechanical ventilation.

Once the patient is able, his cough effectiveness should be evaluated. Often a patient must be taught to cough effectively while using the least amount of energy. In the critical care setting, cough is very important once the patient's artificial airway has been removed. Protection of his airway is important to prevent aspiration and facilitate airway clearance.

Conditioning exercises by the physical therapist can be started in the critical care setting. As stated earlier, prolonged ventilatory assistance leads to respiratory muscle weakness and markedly interferes with the patient's ability to breathe spontaneously. Breathing exercises or changes in the patient's breathing pattern will help to condition the respiratory muscles by two methods. First, muscle strengthening can be accomplished. Second, with a more efficient breathing pattern, the work of breathing will be lessened. Thus the patient uses O_2 more efficiently.

The patient should be repositioned frequently in bed to facilitate ventilation and perfusion. As soon as possible, the patient should sit in a chair, if only for brief periods of time. This may also improve the ventilation and perfusion of the lungs. Early ambulation is very important in the critical care setting. Although this process may be time consuming for the practitioner, the eventual benefits far outweigh the problems. Ambulation helps the patient's ventilatory, circulatory, and psychologic status. If the patient is completely bedridden, the physical therapist or practitioner must initiate passive or active range of motion exercises for the joints and limbs. This helps to prevent venous stasis, loss of joint motion, and muscle deconditioning.

Whether it is the physical therapist or the practitioner who is responsible for these rehabilitative techniques, they should be continued on discharge from the critical care unit and the hospital. Continuity of these physical therapies yields the best results for the patient.

Occupational therapy

Occupational therapy is another aspect of the rehabilitative process. It involves teaching the patient and his family how to use the least amount of energy when performing activities. If energy conservation is increased, then the patient's O_2 demands are decreased. In the critical care setting, energy conservation techniques may be employed when getting the patient into a chair or when ambulating the patient. Performance of such daily activities as grooming and eating all have areas of energy use that may be improved. Through occupational therapy, the patient should be able to continue and improve on these techniques once he is transferred from the critical care setting.

Diversional activities may be an aspect of occupational therapy in the critical care setting. Diversional activities may help to relax an alert patient, thus improving his ventilatory status and work of breathing.

All aspects of occupational therapy rehabilitation are individualized, depending on the patient's status and needs. If part of the therapy is initiated and fails during the initial care of the patient in the critical care setting, it should not be forgotten. Often, once the patient improves and becomes more involved in his care, these same techniques may become very helpful.

REFERENCES

1. American Heart Association: Student manual for basic life support, Dallas, Tx, 1981, The Association.
2. American Heart Association: Textbook of advanced cardiac life support, Dallas, Tx, 1981, The Association.
3. Arey, L.B.: Developmental anatomy, ed. 7, Philadelphia, 1974, W.B. Saunders Co.
4. Block, E., and Ryerson, G.: Safe use of oxygen therapy, Part 1, Respiratory Therapy 13(1):17, 1983.
5. Brody, J.: Lung development, growth, and repair. In Fishman, A.P., editor: Assessment of pulmonary function, New York, 1980, McGraw-Hill Book Co.
6. Broughton, J.O.: Understanding blood gases, Madison, OH, 1979, Medical Product Reprint Library.
7. Burrows, B., et al.: Respiratory disorders: a pathophysiologic approach, Chicago, 1983, Year Book Medical Publishers, Inc.
8. Cherniack, R., and Cherniack, L.: Respiration in health and disease, Philadelphia, 1983, W.B. Saunders Book Co.
9. Chow, M.P., et al.: Handbook of pediatric primary care, New York, 1979, John Wiley and Sons.
10. Coates, J.E.: Lung function: assessment and application in medicine, Oxford, 1979, Blackwell Scientific Publications.
11. Davis, J.C., and Hunt, T.K.: Hyperbaric oxygen therapy, Gaithersburg, MD, 1977, Impressions, Ltd.
12. DeGowin, E., and DeGowin, R.: Bedside diagnostic examination, New York, 1981, Macmillan Publishing Co.
13. Demers, R.: Complications of endotracheal suctioning procedures, Respiratory Care, 17(4):453, 1982.
14. Dorinsky, P., and Whitcomb, M.: The effect of PEEP on cardiac output, Chest 84(2):210, 1983.
15. Douglas, W., et al.: Improved oxygenation in patients with acute respiratory failure: the prone position, Am. Rev. Respiratory Disease 115:559, 1977.
16. Driver, A.G., and LeBrun, M.L.: Iatrogenic malnutrition in patients receiving ventilatory support, JAMA 244:2195, 1980.
17. Eberhard, P., et al.: Methodologic aspects of cutaneous Pco_2 monitoring, Crit. Care Med. 7:249, 1981.
18. Fewell, J., et al.: The effect of head position and angle of tracheal bifurcation on bronchus catheterization in the intubated neonate, Pediatrics 64(3):318, 1979.
19. Finer, N., and Kelly, M.: Optimal ventilation for the neonate. Part 1, CPAP, Respiratory Therapy 13:43, 1983.
20. Fisher, A.B.: Oxygen therapy: side effects and toxicity, Am. Rev. Respiratory Disease 122:61, 1980.

21. Fishman, A.P.: Assessment of pulmonary function, New York, 1980, McGraw Hill Book Co.

22. Freedman, A., and Goodman, L.: Suctioning the left bronchial tree in the intubated adult, Crit. Care Med. 10(1):43, 1982.

23. Green, M.: Pediatric diagnostic interpretation of symptoms and signs in differential age periods, Philadelphia, 1980, W.B. Saunders Co.

24. Huber, G.L.: Current concepts: arterial blood gas and acid-base physiology, The Upjohn Company Monographs, 1978.

25. Kendig, E., and Chernick, V.: Disorders of the respiratory tract in children, Philadelphia, 1983, W.B. Saunders Co.

26. Klocke, R.A.: Diffusing capacity. In Fishman, A.P., editor: Assessment of pulmonary function, New York, 1980, McGraw Hill Book Co.

27. Lehnert, B.E., and Schachter, E.N.: The pharmacology of respiratory care, St. Louis, 1980, The C.V. Mosby Co.

28. Levitzky, M.G.: Pulmonary physiology, New York, 1982, McGraw-Hill Book Co.

29. Murphy, R.L., and Halford, S.K.: Lung sounds, basics of RD, New York, 1980, American Lung Association.

30. Murray, J.F.: The normal lung, Philadelphia, 1976, W.B. Saunders Book Co.

31. Newman, T.: Pulmonary oxygen toxicity. In Bordow, R., et al., editors: Manual of clinical problems in pulmonary medicine, Boston, 1980, Little, Brown & Co.

32. Ng, L., and McCormick, K.: Position changes and their physiological consequences, Adv. Nurs. Sci. 4:13, 1982.

33. Phibbs, R.H.: Oxygen therapy: a continuing hazard to the premature infant, Anesthesiology 47:486, 1977.

34. Pick, R., et al.: The cardiovascular effects of PEEP, Chest 82(3):345, 1982.

35. Prior, J., et al.: Physical diagnosis: the history and examination of the patient, ed. 6, St. Louis, 1981, The C.V. Mosby Co.

36. Severinghaus, J.W.: Transcutaneous blood gas analysis, Respiratory Care 27:152, 1982.

37. Shapiro, B., et al.: PEEP therapy in adults with special reference to acute lung injury: a review of the literature and suggested clinical correlations, Crit. Care Med. 12(2):127, 1984.

38. Sjostrand, U.: High frequency positive pressure ventilation: a review, Crit. Care Med. 8(3):345, 1980.

39. Slonim, N.B. and Hamilton, L.H.: Respiratory physiology, ed. 4, St. Louis, 1981, The C.V. Mosby Co.

40. Traver, G.S.: Respiratory nursing: the science and the art, New York, 1982, Wiley Medical Publications.

41. U.S. Department of Health, Education and Welfare: Chronic bronchitis and emphysema (Ch. 8) and Magnitude of the problem (Ch. 2). In Epidemiology of respiratory diseases, Task Force Report, NIH Publication No. 81-2019, 1980.

42. Weisman, I.M., et al.: Intermittent mandatory ventilation, Am. Rev. Respiratory Disease 127:641, 1983.

43. West, J.B.: Respiratory physiology, Baltimore, MD, 1974, Williams & Wilkins Co.

44. West, J.B.: Ventilation/blood flow and gas exchange, Oxford, 1977, Blackwell Scientific Publications.

45. Zapol, W.M., et al.: Extracorporeal membrane oxygenation in severe acute respiratory failure: a randomized prospective study, JAMA 242:2193, 1979.

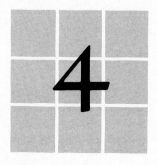

4 The Nervous System

LINDA ABELS
ANN BELCHER
BARBARA L. RUSSO

The myriad of symptoms resulting from alterations in the function of the nervous system presents a challenge for the critical care practitioner. Anatomically and physiologically, the nervous system is perhaps the most complex of the body's systems. Because the nervous system is the body's main regulatory system, disease and trauma to it often cause, contribute to, or are a consequence of other multisystem problems. In the critical care setting, the potential for rapid deterioration and nonreversible damage makes survival and quality of life after recovery very dependent on skilled nursing care.

Concepts of neurologic disease have been changed by our expanding knowledge of brain chemistry, functions, and pathology, and of the physiology and pathology of the peripheral and autonomic nervous systems. Research has revealed new information about neurotransmitters and neuromodulators. In the past decade, the major advances of computerized axial tomography and transaxial tomography have revolutionized diagnosis of cerebral and spinal disorders. Recent advances in microscopic techniques during neurosurgical procedures have greatly reduced morbidity and mortality statistics.

These advances in the knowledge of diseases of the nervous system have required a thorough understanding of neuroanatomy, physiology, and pathophysiology. The critical care practitioner must be educated to make definite judgments so as to ensure quality care.

EMBRYOLOGY

No other organ in the body can equal the specificity and complexity of interrelationships or the heterogeneity of form and physiologic properties acquired by the cells of the developing nervous system.

Central nervous system tissue develops from the outer layer of cells in the developing embryo, the ectoderm. Neuroectoderm thickens by the process of invagination (growth of cells by the depositing of particles between those cells already existing); the neuroectoderm forms the neural tube from single cells of the neural plate (Fig. 4-1). The first indication of brain formation is the enlargement of the neural folds (of each side) of the neural groove of the neural tube (Table 4-1). The neural tube has three distinct layers: (1) the ependymal (inner) layer, (2) the mantle (middle) layer, and (3) the marginal (outer) layer. The spinal cord neurons and macroglial cells that make up the supportive tissues of the brain and spinal cord are derived from the ependymal layer. The marginal layer of axions and glial cells eventually becomes the white matter in the spinal cord as it receives the axons from the brain, the dorsal root ganglia, and the cell bodies of the neurons in the mantle layer. The neuroblasts in the mantle layer become neurons.

Differentiation of glial cells occurs at the same time as that of the neurons. (The astrocyte is a major type of glial cell that appears in the third month of embryologic development; see Table 4-1.) Cytoplasmic material from astrocytes surrounds blood vessels that penetrate the nervous system; this phenomenon may help to explain the physiologic basis of the blood-brain barrier. The presence of cytoplasmic material surrounding the blood vessels results in no extracellular collagen-containing space around small vessels of the brain and spinal cord.[7]

As cells proliferate in the neural tube, the lateral walls thicken. Different rates of thickening result in the bilateral formation of a longitudinal groove, the sulcus limitans. The sulcus limitans divides the ependymal and mantle layers into two laminae, the basal (ventral) plate and the alar (dorsal) plate (Fig. 4-2). Key components of the nervous system can be catego-rized, with few exceptions, by functional variation in relation to their origin from the alar or basal plate. Overall, neuronal cells of the alar plate develop into sensory and internuncial cells, and those of the basal plate develop into motor cells. Separate areas of the nervous system, including the spinal cord, medulla, brainstem, cerebellum, and cerebrum, show some degree of this three-layer cellular pattern and the derivation of motor cells from the basal plate and sensory cells from the alar plate.

Myelination of the central and peripheral nervous systems occurs during most of the second and third trimesters of fetal formation and continues during infancy. Myelination contributes significantly to brain weight. At 12 years, the brain weighs four times more than at birth.[7]

Brain development

Around day 26 of embryonic development, the rostral end of the neural tube differentiates into three primary cerebral vesicles or dilations:

Fig. 4-1. Horizontal section through embryo at about 20 days of gestation. Neuroectodermal cells (shaded areas) remain at periphery to form neural crests after neural tube has fused. Neural crest will become neural folds and can be fused at midline by twenty-fourth day of gestation.

From Conway B.L.: Carini and Owens' neurological and neurosurgical nursing, St. Louis, 1978, The C.V. Mosby Co.

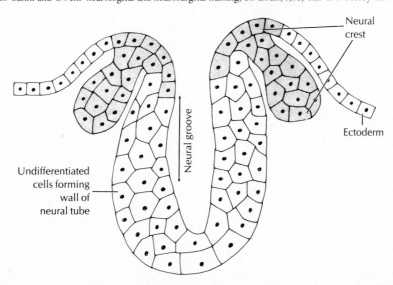

Table 4-1. Development of human nervous system

Age in weeks	Size (crown-rump) in mm	Nervous system	Age in weeks	Size (crown-rump) in mm	Nervous system
2.5	1.5	Neural groove indicated	8	23.0	Cerebral cortex begins to to acquire typical cells
3.5	2.5	Neural groove prominent; rapidly closing			Olfactory lobes visible
		Neural crest a continuous band			Dura and pia-arachnoid distinct
4	5.0	Neural tube closed			Chromaffin bodies appearing
		Three primary vesicles of brain represented	10	40.0	Spinal cord attains definitive internal structure
		Nerves and ganglia forming	12	56.0	Brain attains its general structural features
		Ependymal mantle and marginal layers present			Cord shows cervical and lumbar enlargement
5	8.0	Five brain vesicles			
		Cerebral hemispheres bulging			Cauda equina and filum terminale appearing
		Nerves and ganglia better represented			Neuroglial types begin to differentiate
		(Suprarenal cortex accumulating)			
6	12.0	Three primary flexures of brain represented	16	112.0	Hemispheres conceal much of brain
		Diencephalon large			Cerebral lobes delimited
		Nerve plexuses present			Corpora quadrigemina appear
		Epiphysis recognizable			Cerebellum assumes some prominence
		Sympathetic ganglia forming segmental masses	20-40 (5-10 mo)	160.0- 350.0	Commissures completed (5 mo)
		Meninges indicated			Myelinization of cord begins (5 mo)
7	17.0	Cerebral hemispheres becoming large			Cerebral cortex layered typically (6 mo)
		Corpus striatum and thalamus prominent			Cerebral fissures and convolutions appearing rapidly (7 mo)
		Infundibulum and Rathke's pouch in contact			Myelinization of brain begins (10 mo)
		Chorioid plexuses appearing			
		Suprarenal medulla begins invading cortex			

Modified from Arey, L.B.: Developmental anatomy, a textbook and laboratory manual of embryology, ed. 7, Philadelphia, 1974, W.B. Saunders Co. Reprinted with permission.

(1) the proencephalon or forebrain, (2) the mesencephalon or midbrain (located behind the proencephalon), and (3) the rhomencephalon or hindbrain (Fig. 4-3).

Adult brain structures derived from the proencephalon are the preoptic region and the paired cerebral hemispheres from the telencephalon, a division of the proencephalon. The other division, the diencephalon, is the basis for the hypothalamus and thalamus. Further development of the mesencephalon forms the mentencephalon and the myelencephalon. These structures give rise, respectively, to the pons, the cerebellum, and the medulla oblongata, and both give rise to part of the fourth ventricle. As the proencephalon divides, two precursors for the lateral ventricles evolve. The third ventricle is formed between the lateral ventricles.

Spinal cord development

The spinal cord develops from the caudal portion of the neural tube. Around the second month of fetal development, the earliest tracts of nerve fibers appear. The third month brings the appearance of long association tracts, with pyramidal tracts forming in the fifth month. Nerve fiber myelination of the spinal cord starts in the middle of fetal life and is not completed in some tracts for 20 years. Table 4-1 reviews the embryology of the human nervous system.

Development of special sense organs

Because of the complex, elaborate nature of special sense organs, we will not attempt to describe the embryonic development of these structures. Table 4-2 presents the major landmarks in the development of special senses.

PHYSIOLOGY
General physiologic properties of neuronal cells[1,16,39,41]

Structure

The functional conductive cell of the nervous system is the neuron. The neuron consists of a cell body, the *soma,* containing a nucleus and cytoplasm with intracytoplasmic organelles including Nissl substance, Golgi bodies, and mitochrondria. One or more dendrites and one axon project from the neuron body (Fig. 4-4). The dendrites receive information that is projected to the soma. The axon then transmits away from the soma.

Neurons may be classified as afferent, internuncial, or efferent. Afferent fibers are sensory or receptor neurons and receive incoming stimuli, projecting information into the brain or spinal cord. Internuncial neurons, also called *interneurons* or *association neurons,* transmit incoming information to efferent neurons. Efferent fibers, also called *motor neurons,* communicate with effector organs, conveying impulses away from the spinal cord or brain.

Many peripheral nerve fibers are enclosed in a myelin sheath and a neurolemma that covers the myelin. Small gaps (nodes of Ranvier) occur at regular intervals in the myelinated fibers to facilitate impulse conduction. Other nerve fibers have no myelin sheath and are referred to as unmyelinated.

Neurons are supported by nonexcitable cells that help to insulate, separate, and protect them. These cells, which may also be of value

Fig. 4-2. Basal and alar plates: key to functional variation.

From Conway B.L.: Pediatric neurological nursing, St. Louis, 1977, The C.V. Mosby Co.

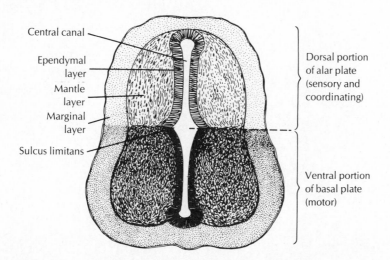

Central canal
Ependymal layer
Mantle layer
Marginal layer
Sulcus limitans
Dorsal portion of alar plate (sensory and coordinating)
Ventral portion of basal plate (motor)

Fig. 4-3. Five stages in early development of brain and cranial nerves of young human embryos. **A,** At 20 somites—approximately 3½ weeks fertilization age; **B,** At 4 mm—probably 4 weeks fertilization age; **C,** At 8 mm—fertilization age a little over 5 weeks; **D,** At 17 mm—fertilization age about 7 weeks; **E,** At 50-60 mm—fertilization age of about 11 weeks. Cranial nerves are indicated by the appropriate Roman numerals. (Hy = hyoid arch; Md = mandibular arch; V Mand = mandibular branch of trigeminal nerve; V Max = maxillary branch; V Ophth = ophthalmic branch.

Redrawn from Patten, B.M.: Human embryology, ed. 2, New York, 1968, McGraw-Hill Book Co.

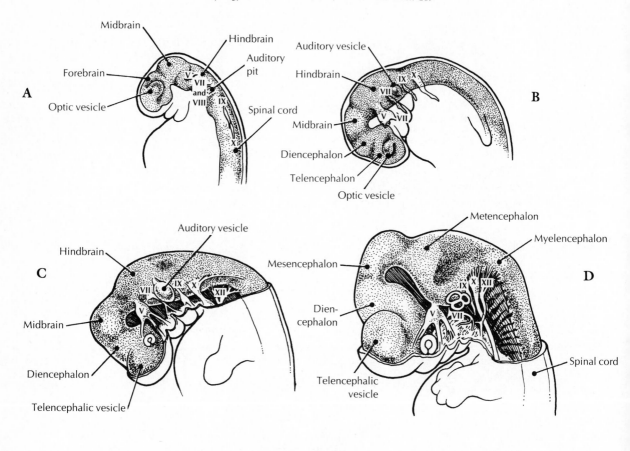

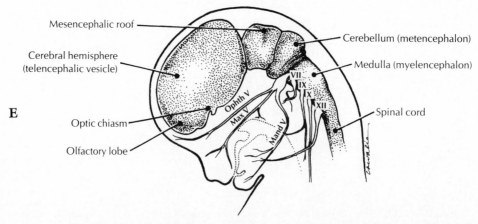

Table 4-2. Development of human sense organs

Age in weeks	Length (crown-rump) in mm	Sense organs	Age in weeks	Length (crown-rump) in mm	Sense organs
2.5	1.5	—	8	23.0	Eyes converging rapidly; exterior, middle, and interior ear assuming final form; taste buds indicated; exterior nares plugged
3.5	2.5	Optic vesicle, auditory placode present; acoustic ganglia appearing			
4	5.0	Optic cup and lens pit forming; auditory pit becomes closed, detached otocyst; olfactory placodes arise and their nerve cells differentiate	10	40.0	Iris, ciliary body organizing; lids fused; lacrimal glands budding; spiral organ begins to differentiate
5	8.0	Choroid fissure prominent; lens vesicle free; vitreous anlage appearing; endolymphatic duct budding from elongated otocyst	12	56.0	Characteristic organization of eye attained; retina becoming layered; fusions of nasal septum, palate completed
6	12.0	Optic cup shows nervous and pigment layers; nasolacrimal duct; modeling of exterior, middle, and interior ear under way	16	112.0	Eye, ear, nose grossly approach normal appearance; organs of general sensation differentiating
7	17.0	Choroid fissure closes around central retinal artery; nerve fibers invade optic stalk; Lids, fibrous and vascular coats of eye forming; olfactory sacs open into mouth cavity	20-40 (5-10 mo)	160-350	Nose and ear ossify (5 mo); retinal layers completed, light-perceptive (7 mo); sense of taste present (8 mo); eyelids reopen (7-8 mo); mastoid cells unformed (10 mo)

Modified from Arey, L.B.: Developmental anatomy, a textbook and laboratory manual of embryology, ed. 7, Philadelphia, 1974, W.B. Saunders Co. Reprinted with permission.

metabolically, respond to injury by phagocytizing debris and forming scar tissue. They are called *glial cells* in the central nervous system (CNS) and *Schwann cells* in the peripheral nervous system (PNS).

There are four kinds of glial cells: astrocytes (astroglia), oligodendrocytes (oligodendroglia); microglia, and ependymocytes. Astrocytes respond to injury by forming gliofilaments that fill the lesion, adding strength to necrotic and damaged areas. Oligodendroglia produce and maintain axonal myelin sheaths in the CNS. Microglia phagocytize in response to injury, removing debris in the CNS. Ependymocytes, which line

the ventricular system, are thought to assist in the exchange of metabolites between the cerebrospinal fluid and the extracellular spaces of the brain and spinal cord.[7]

Supporting cells in the PNS are called Schwann cells. They separate, insulate, and myelinate axons. Schwann cells also phagocytize debris in responding to degenerative processes such as demyelination.[31]

Central nervous system

The central nervous system (CNS) processes conscious and unconscious sensory information from the external and internal environment and compares and coordinates suitable motor responses that are elicited in effectors. Consisting of the spinal cord and brain (Fig. 4-5), it is made up of both gray matter and white matter. Gray matter contains cell bodies of neurons; each cell body contains a nucleus embedded in a neuropil, a dense network of cytoplasmic processes of nerve cells and dendrites. White matter contains axonal processes surrounded by myelin sheaths, which give it its characteristic white color. In some areas of the CNS, there are regions that are an admixture of gray and white matter.

Spinal cord. The spinal cord represents the lowest level of integration of activity within the central nervous system. The spinal cord forms a continuous structure with the brainstem, serving as a link between the brain and the periphery (Fig. 4-6). It extends from the foramen magnum at the base of the skull to the body of the second lumbar vertebra, where it terminates in a fibrous band attached to the coccyx. In infants, it ends in the sacral region. The cord consists of 31 segments, each with a spinal nerve for both sides of the body. There are 8 cervical, 12 thoracic, 5 lumbar, and 5 sacral segments, and 1 coccygeal segment. Sensory and motor nerves leave the vertebral column separately. Sensory nerves project into the dorsal root of the cord; motor fibers exit ventrally. The sensory and motor fibers converge outside the vertebral column to form the spinal nerve.

Autonomic fibers are added to the spinal nerve to form the peripheral nerve (Fig. 4-7). Each spinal nerve innervates a segmental field of skin called a *dermatome* (Fig. 4-8). Such exten-

Fig. 4-4. Cell body of a neuron.

From Conway B.L.: Pediatric neurological nursing, St. Louis, 1977, The C.V. Mosby Co.

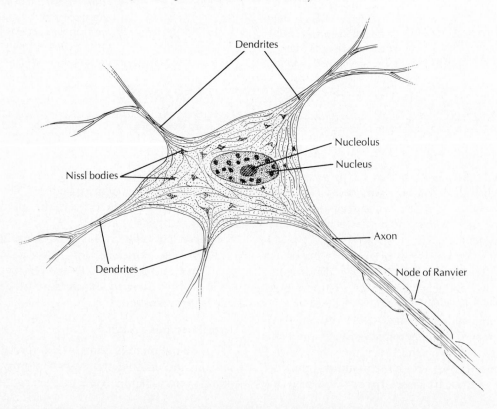

sive overlapping minimizes the loss of sensory or motor function that might be incurred with the interruption of a single spinal nerve. Knowledge of the dermatomes is necessary for localizing disorders of the spinal cord.

Brainstem. The brainstem controls most of the subconscious activities of the body. Consisting of the medulla oblongata, the pons, the mesencephalon, and the diencephalon, it controls numerous autonomic functions. The brainstem regulates some motor movement, supports the body against gravity, and gives rise to 10 of the 12 pairs of cranial nerves. Table 4-3 outlines the functional physiology of the anatomic divisions of the brainstem.

Medulla oblongata. The medulla oblongata is the most caudal portion of the brainstem. Forming a structure that is continuous with the spinal cord, it extends upward to the lower border of the pons. The rostral part of the medulla forms the floor of the fourth ventricle.

Different autonomic functions are controlled by the medullary vasomotor center. Cardiovascular centers regulate blood pressure and heart rate. The lateral portion of this center is tonically active, firing continuously at a slow rate to maintain a partial state of contraction in the blood vessels (vasomotor tone). This vasoconstrictor effect can be inhibited by impulses from the medial region of the vasomotor center, allowing dilation of the blood vessels.

The vasomotor center simultaneously regulates heart rate and controls the degree of vascular constriction. Excitatory impulses that increase heart rate are transmitted from lateral portions of the vasomotor center via sympathetic

Fig. 4-5. Sagittal section through midline of the brain.

From Anthony, C.P., and Thibodeau, G.A.: Textbook of anatomy and physiology, ed. 11, St. Louis, 1983, The C.V. Mosby Co.

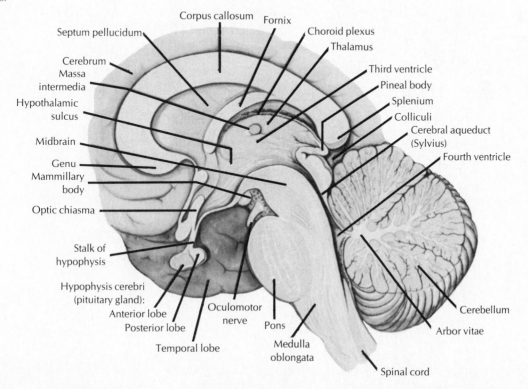

Fig. 4-6. A, Posterior view of brainstem and spinal cord in situ with spinal nerves and plexuses. **B,** Anterior view of brainstem and spinal cord. **C,** Lateral view of brainstem and spinal cord illustrates relationship of spinal cord to vertebrae.

From Mettler, F.A.: Neuroanatomy, ed. 2, St. Louis, 1948, The C.V. Mosby Co.

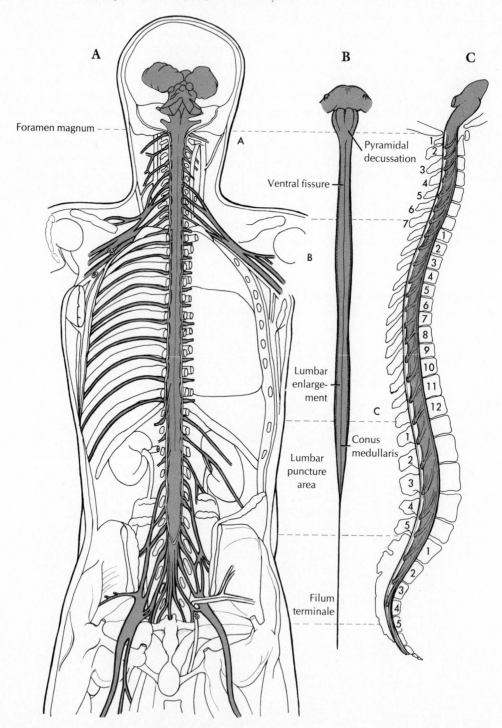

fibers to the heart, while the medial portion transmits impulses through parasympathetic vagal fibers to slow the heart rate.

Medullary respiratory centers regulate the involuntary act of breathing, establishing the basic rhythm of respiration. Inspiratory and expiratory neurons transmit excitatory or inhibitory impulses in a rhythmic fashion to coordinate the rhythm of inspiration and expiration.

Pons. The pons is situated above the medulla. It gives rise to four cranial nerve nuclei. It also houses the accessory respiratory centers, the apneustic and pneumotaxic centers. The apneustic center remains tonically active, continually

exciting the medullary inspiratory neurons, while the pneumotaxic center inhibits inspiratory activity either via inhibition of the apneustic center or by acting directly on the inspiratory neurons of the medullary center.

Mesencephalon. The mesencephalon (midbrain) is a short segment located between the pons and the diencephalon. It gives rise to the nuclei of the third and fourth cranial nerves. This region functions as a relay center for visual and auditory reflexes. It also serves as a center for postural reflexes and for the righting reflex, responsible for maintaining the head in an upright position in relation to the environment.

Fig. 4-7. Cross sectional diagram of vertebral column and spinal cord.

From Schottelius, B.A., and Schottelius, D.D.: Textbook of physiology, ed. 18, St. Louis, 1978, The C.V. Mosby Co.

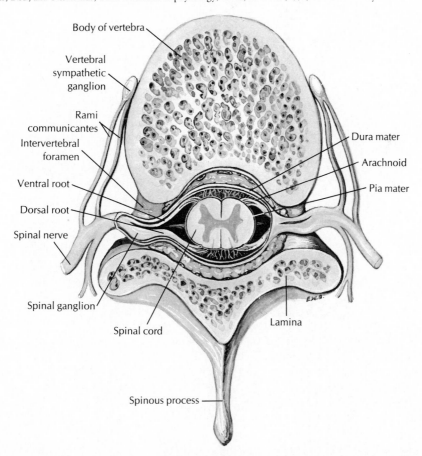

Diencephalon. The diencephalon, a direct continuation of the brainstem, is bounded by the mammillary bodies caudally, the anterior commissure, and lamina terminales at the upper end of the third ventricle just above the optic chiasm. It consists of the thalamus, hypothalamus, and epithalamus (pineal body). The subthalamus is also part of the diencephalon but is more often considered an accessory nucleus with the basal ganglia. Referred to as the *interbrain,* the diencephalon is involved with sleep, emotions, thermoregulation, hormonal homeostatic mechanisms, and autonomic activities.

THALAMUS. The thalamus, which forms part of the lateral wall of the third ventricle, can be found between the hypothalamus and the epithalamus. It is the largest part of the diencephalon and is divided into two parts (medial and lateral) by the internal medullary lamina, a sheet of myelinated fibers. Each of these parts contains nuclei that have specific functions. In general, the thalamus is involved in the relay of all somatic and special sensory impulses—with the sole exception of olfactory stimuli—into the cortex via thalamocortical pathways. It also serves as an integrating center for motor func-

Fig. 4-8. The dermatomes.

From Conway-Rutkowski, B.O.: Carini and Owens' neurological and neurosurgical nursing, ed. 8, 1982, St. Louis, The C.V. Mosby Co.

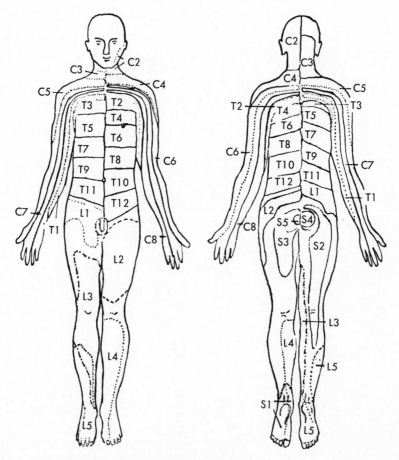

Table 4-3. Functional physiology of the brainstem

Medulla oblongata	Pons	Mesencephalon	Diencephalon
Origin of cranial nerves 9, 10, 11, and 12 nuclei	Origin of cranial nerves 5, 6, 7, and 8 nuclei of accessory respiratory centers that modify medullary activity: apneustic center—excites medullary inspiratory neurons facilitating inspiration; pneumotaxic center—inhibits inspiratory activity either via the apneustic center or by direct action on medulla	Origin of cranial nerves 3 and 4	Thalamic tracts relay all somatic and special sensory impulses except olfaction
Cardiac centers responsible for control of heart rate and force of contraction*		Relay center for visual and auditory reflexes	Thalamic nuclei involved in synchronization and desynchronization of cerebral cortical activity
Vasomotor centers that regulate blood pressure and the distribution of blood flow		Center for postural reflexes (static and labyrinthine reflexes)	Thalamic nuclei process, store, and modify incoming signals
Primary respiratory centers responsible for genesis of inspiration and expiration		Center for righting reflex that maintains the head in an upright position in relation to environment	Hypothalamic centers regulate anterior and posterior pituitary output
			Hypothalamic centers regulate body temperature
			Hypothalamic centers involved in expressive emotions
			Hypothalamic centers integrate autonomic output
			Hypothalamic appetite centers control satiety

*Not responsible for the genesis of the heartbeat.

tions, since some thalamic nuclei receive the principal efferent projections from the cerebellum and corpus striatum. Parts of the thalamus play a dominant role in the maintenance and regulation of the state of consciousness, alertness, and attention through their influence on the cerebral cortex. These nuclei are concerned with both general and specific types of awareness as well as with the emotional connotations that accompany sensory experiences. Thus the thalamus transmits sensory information and is intimately involved with input and output tuning, synchronization and desynchronization of cerebral cortical activity, processing of information, and storing and modification of signals.[76]

HYPOTHALAMUS. The most ventral part of the diencephalon is the hypothalamus. It is situated beneath the thalamus and above the hypophysis (pituitary gland) and forms the floor and part of the lateral wall of the third ventricle. It is bound by the optic chiasm (anteriorly) and the mammillary bodies (posteriorly). The hypothalamus can be subdivided into several regions. Located in the medial zone of the hypothalamus is the preoptic area. The supraoptic region, also in the medial zone, is somewhat adjacent to the preoptic area. It contains the supraoptic nucleus, the paraventricular nucleus, and the anterior hypothalamic and lateral hypothalamic areas. Within the tuberal region in the medial zone are many small nuclei such as the dorsomedial nu-

Table 4-4. Hypothalamic hormones influencing the adenohypophysis

Hypothalamic hormone		Anterior pituitary tropic hormone	Target tissue	Physiologic function
Releasing	Inhibiting			
Growth hormone–releasing hormone, somatotropin (GHRH)	Growth hormone–inhibiting hormone, somatostatin (GHIH)	Growth hormone	Many	Protein synthesis
Thyrotropin-releasing hormone (TRH)		Thyroid-stimulating hormone, thyrotropin (TSH)	Thyroid gland	T₃ and T₄ production and release
Corticotropin-releasing hormone (CRH)		Adrenocorticotrophic hormone, corticotropin (ACTH)	Adrenal cortex	Corticosteroid synthesis and release
Lutienizing hormone–releasing hormone (LHRH)		Luteinizing hormone, interstitial cell–stimulating hormone (LH or ICSH)	Female, follicle Male, testes	Ovulation, formation of luteum, and progesterone secretion Testosterone secretion
Follicle stimulating hormone-releasing hormone		Follicle-stimulating hormone (FSH)	Female, follicle Male, testes	Maturation of follicle Spermatogenesis
	Prolactin hormone-inhibiting hormone	Prolactin	Mammary gland	Milk production
Melanotropin-releasing hormone	Melanotropin-inhibiting hormone	Melanocyte stimulating hormone, melanotropin	Melanocytes	Pigmentation

cleus, the ventromedial nucleus, and the arcuate nucleus. The mammillary region, also found in the medial zone, consists of mammillary nuclei and the posterior nucleus. Major nuclear groups derive their names from their location in relation to these regions. Basically, the hypothalamus, which is the chief subcortical center, plays an integral role in the regulation of metabolic activities and in the control of the autonomic nervous system. It is also involved in the behavioral responses to emotional states. Parts of the hypothalamus are involved in the regulation of pituitary hormone output, the control of body temperature, drinking, eating, sleeping, and wakefulness. The hypothalamic regulatory mechanisms are mediated by both neuronal and humoral connections.

Hypothalamic supraoptic and paraventricular nuclei exhibit an intimate relationship with the endocrine system. Neurohypophysial hormones–vasopressin (ADH) and oxytocin–are synthesized in the hypothalamus and released by neurosecretory cells into the bloodstream to the neurohypophysis (posterior pituitary), where they exert their primary effect. Vasopressin acts as an antidiuretic* (see Unit 5) and a vasoconstrictor, although the latter role is of little importance physiologically. Oxytocin stimulates smooth muscle contractions in the uterus and the breast.

Additional nuclei from widespread regions of the hypothalamus release hormonal releasing factors and inhibiting factors that are transported to the adenohypophysis (anterior pituitary) via the hypophyseal portal blood system. These releasing factors either stimulate or inhibit the release of anterior pituitary hormones. Table 4-4 describes the hypothalamic hormones and their relationship to the adenohypophysis.

The hypothalamus plays an integrative or regulative role in both the sympathetic and parasympathetic nervous systems. Control of sympathetic activities is located in the lateral and posterior hypothalamic regions. Stimulation of these areas, especially the posterior region, activates thoracolumbar outflow. As a result, there is an increase in metabolic and somatic activities associated with emotional stress: pupillary dilation, increased heart rate, blood pressure elevation, increased rate and depth of respiration, sweating, hyperglycemia, and cessation of gastrointestinal motility. Parasympathetic responses are controlled in the anterior and medial hypothalamic areas and include a decrease in heart rate, peripheral vasodilation, and an increase in the tone and motility of the gastrointestinal tract and vesical walls.

Thermoregulation is accomplished by nuclei in both the anterior and posterior hypothalamus (see Unit 8). These areas coordinate sympathetic and parasympathetic responses to produce heat (shivering, vasoconstriction, activation of the thyroid and adrenal glands) or to promote heat loss (vasodilatation and sweating).

The role of the hypothalamus in the expression of emotional states is related to the integration of activity from the cortical centers. Thus, the hypothalamus controls the expressive or motor aspects of emotion.

Portions of the hypothalamus regulate food and water intake. Apparently, separate but interconnected areas control the many aspects of eating and drinking. Anterior regions of the hypothalamus seem to be associated with thirst, resulting, on stimulation, in the consumption of large amounts of water. Osmotic receptors close to the cells of the supraoptic nuclei also influence water intake. The lateral hypothalamus has been identified as a feeding center, and the medial hypothalamic area has been labeled the satiety center.

Evidence suggests that there is no single sleep center in the hypothalamus. However, sleep and sleeplike states can be produced with hypothalamic stimulation. Further study is necessary to determine the exact role of the hypothalamus in the sleep-wakefulness cycle.

---

*The supraoptic nucleus functions as an osmoreceptor, responding to changes in the osmolarity of the blood flowing through this area.

EPITHALAMUS. The *epithalamus* collectively includes the pineal body, habenula, habenula commissure, and striae medullares. All of these structures are situated superiorly, caudally, and medially in relation to other divisions of the diencephalon. Little is known about the exact physiologic function of the pineal body, which is the most important of these epithalamic structures in humans. Pineal secretions include serotonin, norepinephrine, and melatonin. The gland also contains concentrations of thyrotropin-releasing factor, luteinizing hormone-releasing factor, and somatostatin. Pineal secretions may alter hypothalamic functions after entering the general circulation.[15]

Reticular formation. There exists in the brain-stem a diffuse network of neurons collectively called the *reticular formation*. This area, which helps to regulate the brain's level of awareness, begins at the upper end of the spinal cord and extends upward through the central portion of the thalamus into the hypothalamus and into other areas adjacent to the hypothalamus. Both motor and sensory neurons are found in the reticular formation. It contains nuclei that serve the extrapyramidal motor control system and is also the site of the reticular activating system (RAS), a system that controls the overall degree of CNS activity and regulates, in part, the ability to direct attention toward specific areas of the conscious mind.

Cerebellum. The cerebellum is a collection of

Fig. 4-9. Left lateral view of the human brain illustrating division of cerebral hemisphere into four lobes: frontal, parietal, temporal, and occipital.

From Schottelius, B.A., and Schottelius, D.D.: Textbook of physiology, ed. 18, St. Louis, The C.V. Mosby Co.

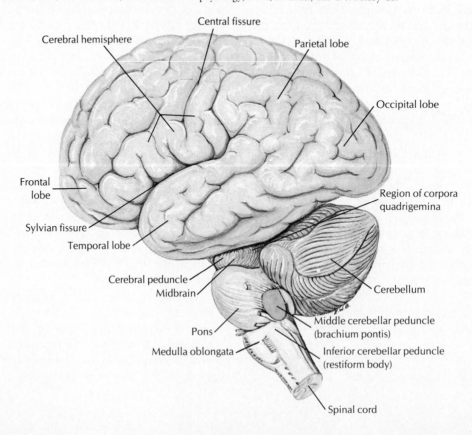

neurons located above the pons and medulla that is connected with the brainstem by three bundles of nerve fibers: the inferior, middle, and superior cerebellar peduncles. Cerebellar activities regulate the reflex tonus of skeletal musculature and are involved in the control of voluntary activity and in the maintenance of equilibrium. The cerebellum integrates sensory and motor input to smooth and coordinate muscle activity through connections with cells of upper motor neuron systems. This input, which travels via sensory cerebellar circuits through one of the cerebellar peduncles, informs the cerebellum of the position and state of contraction of the muscles and the tension on the tendons throughout the body, the position of the head in space, and the general activity of total body sensation. Each side of the cerebellum receives information from the ipsilateral side. Once this information is integrated, cerebellar output provides control over upper motor neuron systems only. It influences lower motor neurons indirectly through the upper motor neuron pathways.

Telencephalon. The telencephalon consists of

the cerebral cortex or cerebrum, the corpus striatum, the limbic system, and the medullary center.

Cerebrum. The cerebrum is the largest part of the CNS. It functions to integrate afferent information from the contralateral side of the body into complex perceptual images and refines control over all efferent systems. The cerebrum consists of two similar halves (hemispheres), one of which is functionally more dominant than the other.* The left hemisphere is dominant for the function of speech in 90% of the population, regardless of handedness.

Each hemisphere is divided into four lobes: frontal, parietal, temporal, and occipital (Fig. 4-9). Fissures identify the boundaries between the various lobes. The fissure of Rolando (central fissure) separates the frontal and parietal lobes. The parietooccipital fissure divides the parietal lobe from the occipital lobe. The temporal lobe is separated from the frontal and parietal lobes

---

*At birth, both hemispheres have the same capability of developing. With growth and speech, the interpretative functions of one hemisphere become highly developed.

Fig. 4-10. Lateral view of cerebral hemisphere showing localization of cortical motor and sensory functions.

From Schottelius, B.A., and Schottelius, D.D.: Textbook of physiology, ed. 18, St. Louis, 1978, The C.V. Mosby Co.

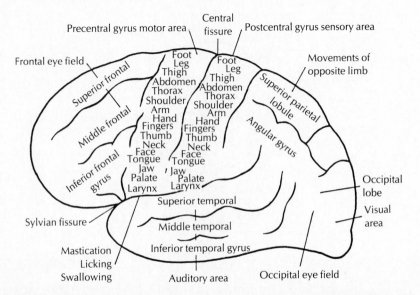

by the sylvian fissure (lateral fissure). Fig. 4-10 illustrates cortical motor and sensory functions.

Corpus striatum. The corpus striatum is made up of a large mass of gray matter and is found at the base of each cerebral hemisphere. It consists of caudate and lentiform nuclei, the latter being further divided into the putamen and globus pallidus. This structure, together with the claustrum and the amygdaloid body, is often labeled as the basal ganglia, although clinically the term *basal ganglia* refers to the corpus striatum, the subthalamic nucleus, and the substantia nigra. The three areas have motor functions. They are often described as being involved with the maintenance and programming of stereotyped repetitive and routine motor behavior,[31] and they appear to suppress unwanted movements.

Limbic system. Emotional responsiveness and expression, and short-term memory, are controlled by the limbic system. This area also controls the responsiveness of the visceral and endocrine hypothalamus. It plays a minor role in olfaction in humans.

Medullary center. Bounded by the cortex, lateral ventricle, and corpus striatum, the medullary center, which is made up of white matter, accommodates the numerous fibers running to and from all parts of the cortex.

Vascular and ventricular systems

Blood supply. Blood is supplied to the brain by the carotid arteries lying anteriorly, and by the vertebral arteries lying posteriorly (Fig. 4-11). The carotid and vertebral arteries anastomose intracranially by means of the circle of Willis, which lies at the base of the brain. Before anastomosing with the circle of Willis, the vertebral arteries, which lie lateral to the medulla, unite to form the basilar artery, which lies in front of the brainstem as it travels superiorly.

Fig. 4-11. Diagram of principal arteries and circle of Willis.

From Conway-Rutkowski, B.L.: Carini and Owens' neurological and neurosurgical nursing, ed. 8, St. Louis, 1982, The C.V. Mosby Co.

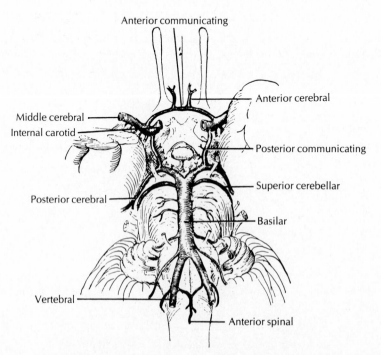

The basilar artery terminates by dividing into the posterior cerebral arteries.

The carotid arteries enter the intracranial cavity through the carotid canals in the base of the skull. They then travel through the cavernous sinus on either side of the pituitary fossa and divide into their two terminal branches, the anterior and middle cerebral arteries. Before terminating, the internal carotid artery gives off a posterior communicating artery that joins the anterior and posterior components of the circle of Willis. The middle cerebral artery travels up the sylvian fissure between the frontal lobe above and the temporal lobe below. The anterior cerebral arteries run along the midline and communicate by means of the anterior communicating artery, completing the anterior loop of the circle of Willis.

Posteriorly, the basilar artery divides into the posterior cerebral arteries, which join with posterior communicating arteries, completing the posterior loop of the circle of Willis. The circle of Willis is a very important anastomosis that allows perfusion of the brain, even though one or more of the carotid or vertebral arteries may be occluded. Besides the circle of Willis, other sources of vascular anastomosis include communication between branches of the external carotid with the ophthalmic artery, a branch of the internal carotid; by retrograde flow through the external carotid to supply the internal carotid after occlusion of the common carotid proximally; and by meningeal branches of the external carotid with cortical branches of the internal carotid—the rete mirabile.

The terminal branches of the carotid arteries and the vertebral arteries course over the brain surface, supplying the cortex, and also send deep perforating branches to supply the white matter and subcortical brain matter. The anterior cerebral runs up over the corpus callosum anteriorly and superiorly to supply the medial cortex of the frontal lobe and the frontoparietal region. Consequently it supplies the cortex responsible for motor function of the leg on the opposite side. The middle cerebral artery runs up the syl-vian fissure between the frontal lobe and the temporal lobe, supplying much of the lateral aspect of the cerebral hemisphere as well as much of the basal ganglia. The cortex supplied by the middle cerebral artery innervates the motor function of the opposite face and arm. The middle cerebrals also irrigate the parietal cortex, which is responsible for speech on the dominant side and for cortical sensory function, and anastomose with the posterior cerebral artery to contribute to the occipital cortex, which is responsible for vision. The posterior cerebral arteries supply the lateral, medial, and inferior occipital cortex, responsible for vision. The vertebral and basilar arteries supply both the brainstem and cerebellum by circumferential arteries such as the superior cerebellar, by the anterior inferior cerebellar, and by the posterior inferior cerebellar, and also supply the brainstem by means of midline perforating branches. Fig. 4-12 summarizes the anatomic distribution of the cerebral arteries.

Venous blood drains through superficial and deep veins into the venous sinuses, which eventually empty into the internal jugular veins (Fig. 4-13).

Regulation of cerebral blood flow (CBF). The human brain is an extremely complex organ that can only function with aerobic metabolism. Because the CNS requires a constant supply of oxygen and glucose to function normally, neurologic dysfunction will generally occur within a few minutes of cessation of cerebral blood flow. For normal function, the brain requires 50 to 60 ml of blood/100 g of tissue per minute or approximately 700 to 800 ml for the total brain per minute in the adult. When perfusion drops below 30 ml/100 g per minute, neurologic dysfunction resulting from ischemia will occur. To maintain adequate perfusion of the brain, a vascular regulatory system has developed that allows constant cerebral blood flow despite changes in systemic blood pressure. This is known as cerebral autoregulation. Cerebral autoregulation will allow adequate perfusion to the brain despite changes in the systemic systolic blood pressures from 70 to 200 mmHg. This autoregulation is possible as the cerebral blood vessels alter their resistance independent of the systemic blood vessels. This is possible because the cerebral blood vessels do not receive much sympathetic innervation, unlike the systemic vessels. The cerebral vessels instead alter their resistance depending on intraluminal pressure and also on changes in the carbon dioxide, oxygen, and hydrogen ion concentrations. When systemic blood pressure falls, cerebral resistance vessels dilate rapidly, decreasing resistance and increasing brain perfusion. Below a systemic pressure level of 50 to 70 mmHg, cerebral perfusion falls as the vessels are maximally dilated. With increased systemic blood pressure, the cerebral vessels constrict until the systemic systolic pressure reaches 200 mmHg. At this point, cerebral

Fig. 4-12. Diagram of areas of distribution of anterior, middle, and posterior cerebral arteries.

From Mettler, F.A.: Neuroanatomy, ed. 2, St. Louis, 1948, The C.V. Mosby Co.

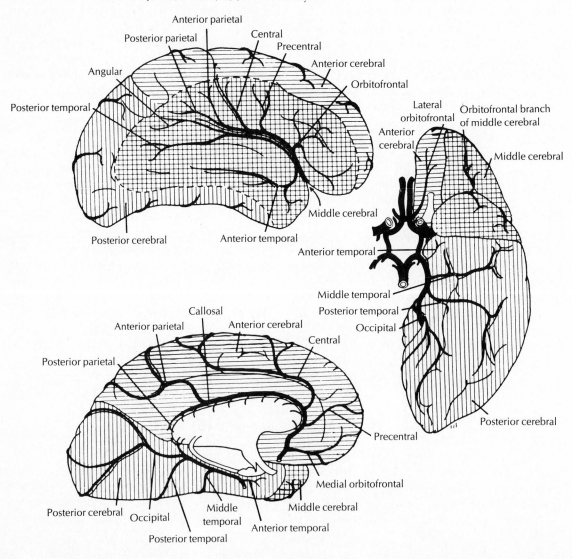

vessels lose their ability to regulate and dilate.

In addition to autoregulation of cerebral perfusion by pressure-sensitive changes, cerebral resistance also responds to changes in Pco_2, Po_2, and pH. Increases in carbon dioxide levels result in dilation of the cerebral vascular vessels, with decreased cerebral vascular resistance and increased perfusion of the brain. This compensatory increase in cerebral blood flow, or CBF, dilutes and removes excess CO_2 in an effort to increase the pH, since acidosis can depress neuronal activity. CBF increases approximately 2 ml/100 g of tissue for each mmHg increase in Pco_2, an increase of approximately 4%. Cerebral blood volume changes 0.04 ml per 100 g/mmHg change in Pco_2, or about 9 ml when Pco_2 drops from 40 mm to 25 mm.

Pco_2 works through changes in the extravascular cerebrospinal fluid (CSF) pH. Hydrogen ions (H^+) freely cross the blood-brain barrier (BBB). The set point for normal is adjusted in patients with chronic increased intracranial pressure (ICP). In aging and in cerebral vascular disease, this vasodilator response of CO_2 is diminished. In areas surrounding infarction, the vessels also lose response to Pco_2 and become maximally dilated, resulting in a shunting of blood away from the infarcted and ischemic area—the luxury perfusion syndrome. Changes in the oxygen level also change cerebral vascular resistance and consequently cerebral perfusion. These effects are somewhat less pronounced than those resulting from changes to the Pco_2. Increased oxygen levels result in cerebral constriction and reduction of CBF. Decreased oxygen level, conversely, results in vasodilation. Changes in pH may also change cerebral perfusion independently of the Pco_2 level, with acidemia resulting in an increase in cerebral perfusion.

Other influences may also alter cerebral perfusion, however, including systemic arterial pressure, central venous pressure (CVP), and ICP.

Extracranial mean arterial blood pressure (MABP). The brain has a vascular autoregulatory system that will allow adequate perfusion despite decrease in systemic blood pressure to 70 mmHg. Adequate cardiac output is also essential

---

Fig. 4-13. Diagram of intracranial veins and drainage pathways.

From Conway-Rutkowski, B.L.: Carini and Owens' neurological and neurosurgical nursing, ed. 8, St. Louis, 1982, The C.V. Mosby Co.

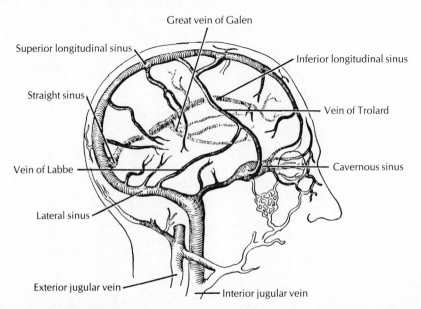

in maintaining adequate cerebral perfusion. Often the earliest clinical sign of shock is agitation and confusion.[41]

Extracranial venous return. The actual cerebral perfusion blood pressure is the pressure derived from subtracting the CVP and ICP from the MABP. Cerebral blood flow (CBF) can be decreased by factors that increase cerebral venous pressures. These include increased central venous pressure secondary to heart failure or fluid overload, jugular venous obstruction from IVs, trauma, or head position, and increased intrathoracic pressure from positive pressure ventilation and positive end-expiratory pressure (PEEP).[41]

The effect of increased venous pressure can easily be negated in most patients by elevating the head of the patient's bed. A CVP of 15 cm of water can be changed to zero simply by holding the patient's head 15 cm higher than his heart.[41]

Intracranial pressure. Cerebral perfusion pressure (CPP) was previously mentioned as MABP − (CVP + ICP). Because the normal MABP is 100 mmHg, normal CVP is zero, and normal ICP is approximately 15, the normal CPP is 85 mmHg. Ischemia is seen with CPP of less than 35 mmHg. Increases in ICP can cause symptoms due to regional ischemia by increasing vascular resistance and by vascular compression due to shifts of brain substance.[41]

Blood-brain barrier. The blood-brain barrier is a complex network of structures that help to maintain a stable environment in the CNS by regulating the movement of chemical substances between the plasma, cerebrospinal fluid, and brain. Certain substances are prevented from passing into central nervous system tissue. These substances, which ordinarily have access to nonnervous tissues, remain bound to plasma protein molecules that are unable to leave cerebral blood vessels. This phenomenon is thought to result from tight junctions that exist between endothelial cells and special properties in their internal plasma membranes.[6] The highly selective permeability of the blood-brain barrier maintains precise qualitative and quantitative limits. It breaks down in infected or irradiated areas or at the locus of tumors. Clinically it is important

Fig. 4-14. Diagram of ventricular system illustrating its relationships to various parts of the brain.

From Conway-Rutkowski, B.L.: Carini and Owens' neurological and neurosurgical nursing, ed. 8, 1982, St. Louis, The C.V. Mosby Co.

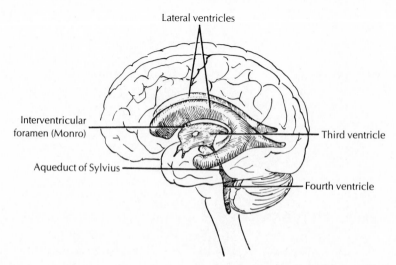

Lateral ventricles

Interventricular foramen (Monro)

Aqueduct of Sylvius

Third ventricle

Fourth ventricle

Table 4-5. Cranial nerves

Nerve	Mode	Function	
		Sensory	Motor
I Olfactory	Sensory	Relays chemical information from nasal receptors	—
II Optic	Sensory	Conveys visual information to thalamus and midbrain	—
III Oculomotor	Mixed	Pupil diameter; accommodation	Controls extrinsic eye muscles (4 of 6)
IV Trochlear	Motor	—	Controls extrinsic eye muscles (1 of 6)
V Trigeminal	Mixed	Somatic sensation of face (that is, pain, touch, and pressure)	Supplies muscles of mastication
VI Abducent	Motor	—	Controls extrinsic eye muscles (1 of 6)
VII Facial	Mixed	Taste; facial proprioceptive information	Controls facial muscles of expression
VIII Vestibulocochlear	Sensory	Vestibular—information from equilibrium apparatus; cochlear—hearing	—
IX Glossopharyngeal	Mixed	Pharyngeal sensory activities	Salivary secretion; swallowing, speech
X Vagus	Mixed	Pharyngeal sensory activities	Swallowing
XI Spinal accessory	Motor	—	Supplies sternocleidomastoid and trapezius muscle
XII Hypoglossal	Motor	—	Controls tongue movement

From Pflanzer, R.: Personal communication, Nov., 1984.

to understand what drugs can permeate this barrier.

Ventricular systems. An ultrafiltrate of blood, cerebrospinal fluid (CSF), is found in both the subarachnoid space and the ventricles within the brain. CSF is produced by the choroid plexus from arterial blood and by leakage of extracellular fluid (ECF) into the ventricles. It serves a protective function by cushioning the brain from contact with the skull. It may also provide a channel of communication for CSF-borne substances that affect neurons (Fig. 4-14).

Peripheral nervous system

The peripheral nervous system (PNS) includes all neural structures that lie outside the spinal cord and brain. It contains cranial (Table 4-5) and spinal nerves associated, respectively, with the brain and spinal cord. Peripheral nerves convey neural messages from the sense organs and sensory receptors to the CNS and transmit neural impulses from the CNS as motor output to the muscles and glands of the body. The PNS also communicates sensory stimuli from the viscera to the CNS for processing and transfers the appropriate responses to the involuntary (smooth) and cardiac musculature and glands of the viscera.

The PNS can be subdivided into somatic and autonomic components.

Somatic division

The somatic component of the PNS has both sensory and motor functions. It conveys and processes conscious and unconscious afferent information from the head, body wall, and extremities, and is involved with motor control of the voluntary (striated) muscles.

Sensory receptors. Somatic sensory receptors can be classified into three types, which differ physiologically: (1) mechanoreceptors, (2) thermoreceptors, and (3) pain receptors. Since some of these cutaneous receptors are exterior, they are often referred to as exteroreceptors. They respond to touch, pressure, heat, cold, and pain. Other deep receptors are named proprioceptors, whereas those on the viscera are referred to as interoceptors. Receptors may respond to epicritic modalities such as fine discriminative touch, vibration, two-point discrimination, stereognosis, and proprioception, or protopathic modalities including pain, temperature, and light moving touch.

Mechanoreceptors respond to mechanical deformation of the receptor or of cells adjacent to the receptors. There are many different mechanoreceptors known. Those located within the epidermis and dermis include free nerve endings, expanded tip endings (Ruffini's end or-gans, Merkel's discs), encapsulated endings (Meissner's corpuscles, Krause's corpuscles, and pacinian corpuscles), and hair-end organs. Others are found in deep body tissues where they detect stretch, deep pressure, and any other type of tissue deformation. They consist of free nerve endings, expanded tip endings (Ruffini's end organs), encapsulated endings (pacinian corpuscles), and specialized endings (muscle spindles and Golgi tendon receptors).

Temperature changes are detected by thermoreceptors located in subepithelial tissues. Warm receptors fire at temperatures from 20° to 45° C; cold receptors are sensitive to temperatures between 10° and 41° C. Warm receptors stop firing at temperatures greater than 45° C. At such extremes, cold receptors surprisingly begin firing simultaneously with pain receptors.

Pain receptors are found in practically every body tissue. Since pain perception has a large subjective component, painful sensations are often protective, as opposed to other sensory modalities that are informative. Different types of pain are recognized depending on their source. Cutaneous pain is superficial and localized on body surfaces. Deep pain emanates from muscles, tendons, joints, and fascia. Visceral pain occurs in response to the appropriate stimulation of visceral organs. Cutaneous and deep pain are labeled as somatic pain. Stimulation of cutaneous pain receptors is often described as pricking, sharp, or burning. It may be localized or diffuse. Deep visceral pain is usually

---

Fig. 4-15. The action potential of a nerve cell measured with the recording electrode inside the cell. The different phases of the action potential are shown with respect to their time course. The overshoot is the extent to which the potential is reversed. (B = depolarizing after-potential; b = hyperpolarizing after-potential.)

From Strand, F.L.: Physiology: a regulatory systems approach, ed. 2, 1983, New York, Macmillan Publishing Co.

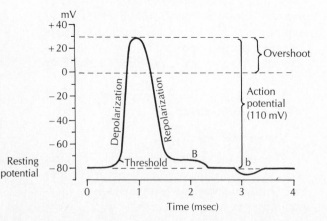

Fig. 4-16. Saltatory conduction along a myelinated axon.

From Guyton, A.C.: Organ physiology structure and function of the nervous system, ed. 2, Philadelphia, 1976, W.B. Saunders Co.

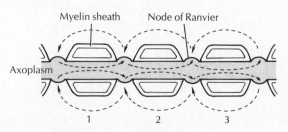

poorly localized (protopathic) and characterized as dull, aching, or throbbing in nature.

Impulse transmission. A local graded response of increasing membrane depolarization is created when a stimulus of at least threshold intensity is delivered to a sensory receptor. Normally, the cell membrane maintains a negative charge of -75 mV, known as the membrane potential, by means of a sodium pump that pumps positively charged sodium ions out into the extracellular fluid. When the local response is sufficiently intense, the membrane becomes permeable to sodium ions, which enter the cell and reduce the membrane potential. As the membrane potential falls to a threshold of -59 mV, an action potential is generated (Fig. 4-15). Depolarization at one point along an axon gives rise to a local response at an adjacent location in the direction of impulse flow. In such a manner, the action potential is transmitted down the dendrite and axon. In cells with myelinated axons, conduction skips down the axon between nodes (nodes of Ranvier) in the myelin. This mechanism is known as saltatory conduction (Fig. 4-16). The impulses reach the axon terminal and are transmitted to other nerve cells, muscle cells, or endocrine cells by release of neurotransmitters from the termination of the axon. These axonal terminations, called boutons, are in close apposition with specialized areas of the surface membrane of the receiving cell, known as the subsynaptic membrane. The axon terminal, the subsynaptic membrane, and the thin extracellular space between the two, known as the synaptic cleft, all form the synapse (Fig. 4-17). Terminal boutons may be excitatory, secreting a substance that excites the neuron, or inhibitory, secreting a substance that inhibits the neuron. They release a neurotransmitter via exocytosis that binds to a receptor molecule on the postsynaptic neuron. The receptor responds to the neurotransmitter in such a way as to increase the membrane permeability to either sodium influx (excitatory transmitter) or potassium efflux (inhibitory transmitter). Thus, release of neurotransmitter by the bouton induces transient postsynaptic voltage changes that may be excitatory (EPSP) or inhibitory (IPSP)* and produce depolarization or hyperpolarization in the receiving cell. Fig. 4-18 illustrates the generation of the EPSP and IPSP. If the membrane potential is

---

*EPSPs and IPSPs can occur in rapid sequence. The synapse can be activated twice in rapid succession, a phenomenon called *temporal summation;* or more than one synapse can be activated simultaneously, a situation known as *spatial summation.*

Fig. 4-18. Generation of EPSP and IPSP in postsynaptic membrane. Action potential spike of presynaptic axon and synaptic delay are shown. Postsynaptic axon action potential is shown after summation of EPSP.

From Schottelius, B.A., and Schottelius, D.D.: Textbook of physiology, ed. 18, St. Louis, 1978, The C.V. Mosby Co.

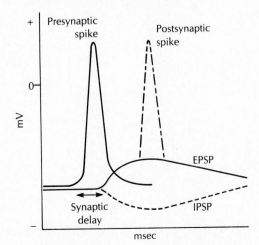

Fig. 4-17. Physiologic anatomy of the neuromuscular synapse.

From Guyton, A.C.: Organ physiology structure and function of the nervous system, ed. 2, Philadelphia, 1976, W.B. Saunders Co.

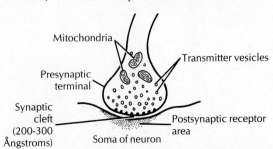

reduced to −59 mV, an action potential is generated in the receiving cell. After release of the neurotransmitter into the synaptic cleft, the transmitter is either biochemically degraded or re-uptaken into the axon bouton and used again. In this manner, an impulse can be transmitted down chains of neurons.

Reflex arc. When an afferent cell has a synaptic arrangement with an efferent cell such that a given stimulus produces a given response, a reflex arc is produced (Fig. 4-19). The elements of a reflex system lie both within and outside of the CNS. In the simplest reflex arc, there are only two neurons in the circuit and there is only one synapse. This reflex is known as a monosynaptic reflex. The best-known monosynaptic reflex is the deep tendon reflex produced by tapping a tendon with a reflex hammer and eliciting a muscle jerk (Fig. 4-20). This is an example of a class of reflexes also called *myotatic* or *stretch reflexes*. The blow stretches the tendon and the stretch receptors in the muscle spindle that serve

as sensory receptors to detect changes in the length of muscle fibers and the rate of change of length. Proprioceptive impulses travel to the cord and return via efferent (motor) fibers to the muscle in which they originate (Fig. 4-21). The flexor muscle is reflexly inhibited by a neuronal mechanism called reciprocal innervation (Fig. 4-22). The ultimate result is the contraction of the extensor muscle and inhibition of the antagonistic flexor. Prolonged contraction is prevented by Golgi tendon organs that are found within the muscle tendons immediately beyond their attachments to the muscle fiber. Stimulated by the degree of tension applied to the tendon by muscle contraction, this apparatus excites inhibitory motor neurons to cause sudden relaxation of the entire muscle. If tension is too little, impulses from the tendon organ cease, removing inhibitions from the motor neuron.

Frequently multiple interneurons are interposed between the afferent and efferent neurons within the NS, producing a polysynaptic reflex.

Fig. 4-19. Reflex arc components. Afferent sensory impulses flow to the spinal cord; efferent motor information leaves the spinal cord. Typical cord segment shows entrance of afferent neuron into posterior root, with exit of efferent fiber from anterior root.

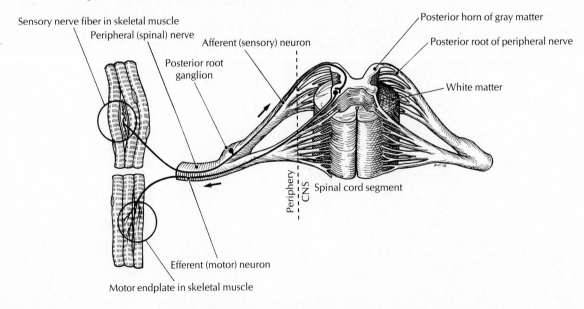

A well-known polysynaptic reflex is the withdrawal of an extremity from a source of pain (Fig. 4-23). In this example, pain impulses are transmitted via afferent fibers to the spinal cord, where the excitatory influence to withdraw a limb from the cause of the pain is mediated through polysynaptic pathways that reach the motor efferent neuron.

Ascending sensory pathways. Afferent information, both conscious and unconscious, is transmitted to the CNS via the posterior columns, the anterolateral spinothalamic, spinoreticular, or spinotectal tracts, the lateral spinothalamic tract, or the spinocerebellar tracts. Fig. 4-24 shows the major ascending pathways, and Table 4-6 outlines the sensory information transmitted by each.

Motor neurons. Axons arising from the ventral root of the spinal cord that provide motor innervation for skeletal muscles are called lower motor neurons. These neurons receive input from afferent impulses that arise in the posterior root and from upper motor neurons that regulate tone, posture, and voluntary movements. Lower motor neurons are divided into two categories: *alpha* and *gamma* motor neurons. The alpha motor neurons, which are under the control of both sensory and supraspinal systems, are

---

Fig. 4-20. Simple reflex arc (knee-jerk reflex). **1,** The *receptor*, the sensory nerve fiber that first picks up the impulse as the hammer strikes the tendon; **2,** the *sensory transmitter*, the afferent neuron that passes the impulse to the spinal cord; **3,** the *motor transmitter*, the efferent neuron that passes the impulse to the effector (muscle); **4,** the *neuroeffector junction*, a specialized endplate of motor nerves; and **5,** the *effector*, a muscle that carries out the actual response (jerking of knee).

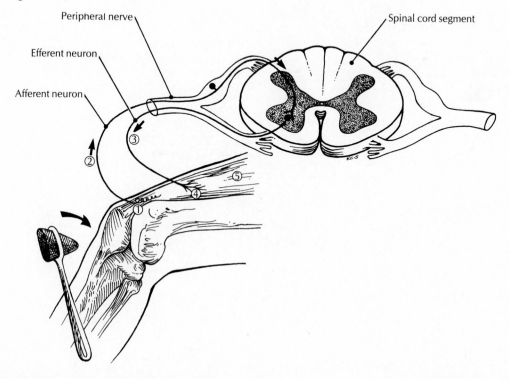

Peripheral nerve

Spinal cord segment

Efferent neuron

Afferent neuron

larger and directly innervate extrafusal striated muscle fibers. Intrafusal fibers, muscle fibers in the muscle spindle, are innervated by the smaller gamma motor neurons that are mainly under the control of supraspinal systems.

Descending motor pathways. Motor neurons are influenced by efferent fibers that descend from the four major regions of the brain. These areas include the cerebral cortex, red nucleus, lateral vestibular nucleus, and central nuclei at the reticular formation. The major descending pathway, the corticospinal (or pyramidal) tract, originates in the frontal and parietal lobes of the cerebrum. Some descending fibers cross to the

Fig. 4-21. Muscle spindle. Neural basis for a stretch reflex illustrating afferent fibers from muscle spindle and tendon organs and efferent fibers to muscle and spindle (gamma fibers). Excitation is indicated by plus signs, inhibition by minus signs. The Renshaw cell is an interneuron that provides recurrent inhibition to the active motorneuron pool. Muscle rigidly fixed at upper end and subject to stretch at lower end in direction of arrow.

From Schottelius, B.A., and Shottelius, D.D.: Textbook of physiology, ed. 18, St. Louis, 1978, The C.V. Mosby Co.

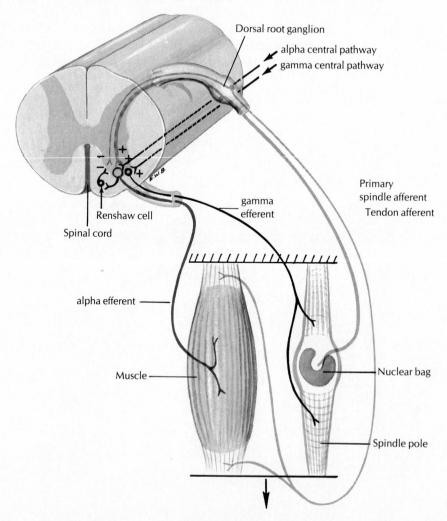

contralateral side at the medulla, continuing as the lateral corticospinal tract. Others continue uncrossed as the anterior corticospinal tract, to cross in the ventral horn through the anterior white commissure of the upper, or cervical, spinal cord to the contralateral side. This pathway regulates fine skilled hand and finger movements and has a dominant influence on flexor lower motor neurons while exerting inhibitory action on extensor muscles.

From the red nucleus of the midbrain arises the rubrospinal tract, a pathway that crosses in the midbrain descending through the ventro-lateral medulla. It regulates fine skilled hand and finger movements, as does the corticospinal tract, but in a more indirect route from the cortex to the cord.

The vestibulospinal tracts originate in the medulla oblongata. Each of these consists of a medial tract with crossed fibers and a lateral tract with uncrossed fibers. The medial tract ends in the cervical spine, and the lateral tracts terminate in the lumbosacral area. These fibers are concerned with the regulation of muscle tone and maintenance of balance, the latter resulting from abundant input from the cerebellum.

Fig. 4-22. Diagram illustrating reciprocal innervation of antagonistic muscles at *a* and *b* and double reciprocal innervation at *c* and *d*. Excitation is indicated by plus signs, inhibition by minus signs.

From Schottelius, B.A., and Schottelius, D.D.: Textbook of physiology, ed. 18, St. Louis, The C.V. Mosby Co.

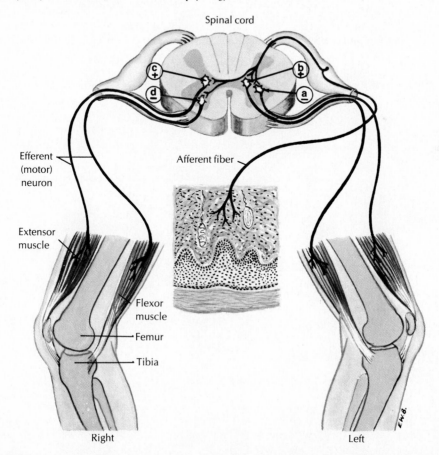

Derived from the portions of the brainstem are the reticulospinal tracts. The pontine or medial reticulospinal tract begins in the reticular activating system of the brainstem, descending uncrossed to the cord. The medullary or lateral reticulospinal tract originates in the medulla and descends to the spinal cord. Most of its fibers are uncrossed, although some do cross in the medulla. These tracts control ordinary activities that require no conscious effort by carrying impulses to the ANS. They also have an effect on motor activities related to posture and muscle tone. The medial tract initiates the extensor reflex while inhibiting the flexor response. The lateral tracts act in the opposite manner.

Neck movement is influenced by the tectospinal tract, which originates in the area of the tectum of the midbrain. Its fibers cross descending to the cervical spinal cord.

Major descending tracts are shown in Figs. 4-25 and 4-26.

Neuromuscular junctions. The neuromuscular junction is the region at the termination of the motor neuron on individual skeletal muscle fibers. When a nerve impulse reaches the neuromuscular junction, a nerve action potential is generated, calcium ions move from the ECF into the membranes of the terminal, and the neurotransmitter acetylcholine is released from synaptic vesicles. In a very short period of time (2 to 3 milliseconds) the acetylcholine, in contact with the muscle fiber, excites it and alters the permeability of the muscle membrane. As a result, there is an increase in the membrane potential in the end plate such that a local end-plate potential is created. Subsequently, the intense local current threshold is reached (approximately −50 mV), and an action potential that spreads in both directions along the muscle fiber is created.

Autonomic division

The autonomic division of the PNS contains fibers that innervate cardiac muscle, smooth

---

Fig. 4-23. Three-neuron reflex arc (flexor withdrawal reflex). Painful stimulus initiates flexor reflexes, which cause withdrawal movements.

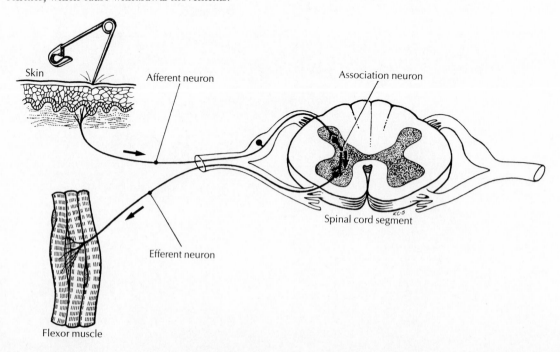

muscle, and glands. Both anatomic and physiologic differences within the autonomic nervous system contribute to its subdivision into the sympathetic and parasympathetic components (Table 4-7). In general, this system can be considered as a two-neuron chain. The cell bodies of the first neuron originate in the CNS. Their myelinated fibers leave at different levels, the sympathetic exiting from the thoracic and lumbar regions of the cord and the parasympathetic exiting from the brain and sacral portions of the spinal cord. Consequently the sympathetic chain is often referred to as the *thoracolumbar division,* and the parasympathetic as the *craniosacral division.*

After leaving the CNS and before arriving at

Fig. 4-24. Major ascending pathways to the thalamus and cerebral cortex.

From Conway-Rutkowski, B.L.: Carini and Owens' neurological and neurosurgical nursing, ed. 8, St. Louis, 1982, The C.V. Mosby Co.

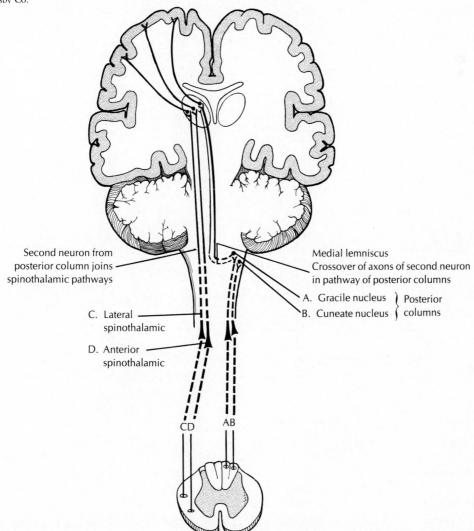

Second neuron from posterior column joins spinothalamic pathways

Medial lemniscus
Crossover of axons of second neuron in pathway of posterior columns

A. Gracile nucleus ⎱ Posterior
B. Cuneate nucleus ⎰ columns

C. Lateral spinothalamic

D. Anterior spinothalamic

CD   AB

Table 4-6. Spinal pathways conveying afferent impulses

Sensation	Course
Pain/thermal impulses	Short posterior root fibers terminate in substantia gelatinosa, which develops into collaterals coursing up and down one or two segments in Lissauer's tract before reaching posterior horn. Fibers of second order decussate and course upward in lateral spinothalamic tract. Medial pain pathways have different route.
Tactile sensations	Fibers enter ipsilateral posterior column, where a few terminate in gracile and cuneate nuclei. Most enter nucleus propius of posterior horn at point of root entry and at higher levels as they ascend in posterior column. Second-order fibers decussate and course upward through anterior spinothalamic tract.
Position sense and kinesthesia	Fibers course through ipsilateral posterior column and upward from there. Alternate route is Morin's tract of ipsilateral lateral column.
Discriminative functions	Fibers course through ipsilateral posterior column and upward from there. Alternate route is Morin's tract.
Vibratory stimuli	Fibers course through ipsilateral posterior column and upward. Possible alternate route is medial portion of ipsilateral lateral column.
Proprioception	Three ipsilateral pathways are used to convey these sensory experiences to cerebellum, including (1) pathways from nucleus dorsalis via dorsal spinocerebellar tract and into inferior cerebellar peduncle, (2) pathways from nucleus of Stilling and postcommissural nucleus through ventral spinocerebellar tract to superior cerebellar peduncle, and (3) pathways from lateral cuneate nucleus through dorsal superficial arcuate fibers and onto inferior cerebellar peduncle.

From Conway-Rutkowski, B.L.: Carini and Owens' neurological and neurosurgical nursing, ed. 8, St. Louis, 1982, The C.V. Mosby Co.

the effector cell, these fibers synapse with unmyelinated fibers of a second neuron in the PNS. These synapses occur in small clusters called *ganglia*. Both subdivisions differ with respect to the location of their ganglia. Some sympathetic ganglia can be found close to the spinal cord, forming paired chains of ganglia called the sympathetic trunk. Others lie halfway between the cord and the innervated organ. All parasympathetic ganglia, in contrast, are located within the walls of the effector organ. Fibers that pass from the CNS to sympathetic or parasympathetic ganglia are *preganglionic autonomic fibers;* those passing from the ganglia to the effector are *postganglionic fibers* (Fig. 4-27).

Neurotransmitters are released at the synapse between preganglionic and postganglionic fibers and between the postganglionic fibers and the effector cell. In both the sympathetic and parasympathetic divisions, acetylcholine is the transmitter at the ganglionic synapse between preganglionic and postganglionic fibers. It is also the neurotransmitter secreted between postganglionic fibers and the effector cell in the parasympathetic nervous system. Fibers that release acetylcholine are said to be cholinergic. The sympathetic postganglionic fibers, however, release norepinephrine and are referred to as adrenergic.

Acetylcholine and norepinephrine stimulate the effector organ by reacting with postsynaptic receptors thought to be located in the cell membrane of the effector cell. There are two mechanisms by which this is postulated to occur. The most likely explanation is that the transmitter substance binds to the membrane receptor, causing a molecular transformation. The structural change that takes place makes the cell membrane more permeable to certain ions, permitting the rapid influx of sodium, chloride, or calcium, or the efflux of potassium. In such a way, an action potential can be generated. In addition, the ions may have a direct effect upon the receptor—such as calcium in the promotion of smooth muscle contraction. The other mechanisms by which receptors can function involve the activation of an enzyme in the cell membrane that can promote a specific chemical reaction.

There are two kinds of acetylcholine receptors: muscarinic and nicotinic. Muscarinic recep-

Fig. 4-25. Pyramidal tracts. Upper motor neurons cross to muscles on opposite side of body. Lateral pyramidal tracts cross high at decussation in medulla oblongata. Ventral tracts cross low.

From Conway-Rutkowski, B.L.: Carini and Owens' neurological and neurosurgical nursing, ed. 8, St. Louis, 1982, The C.V. Mosby Co.

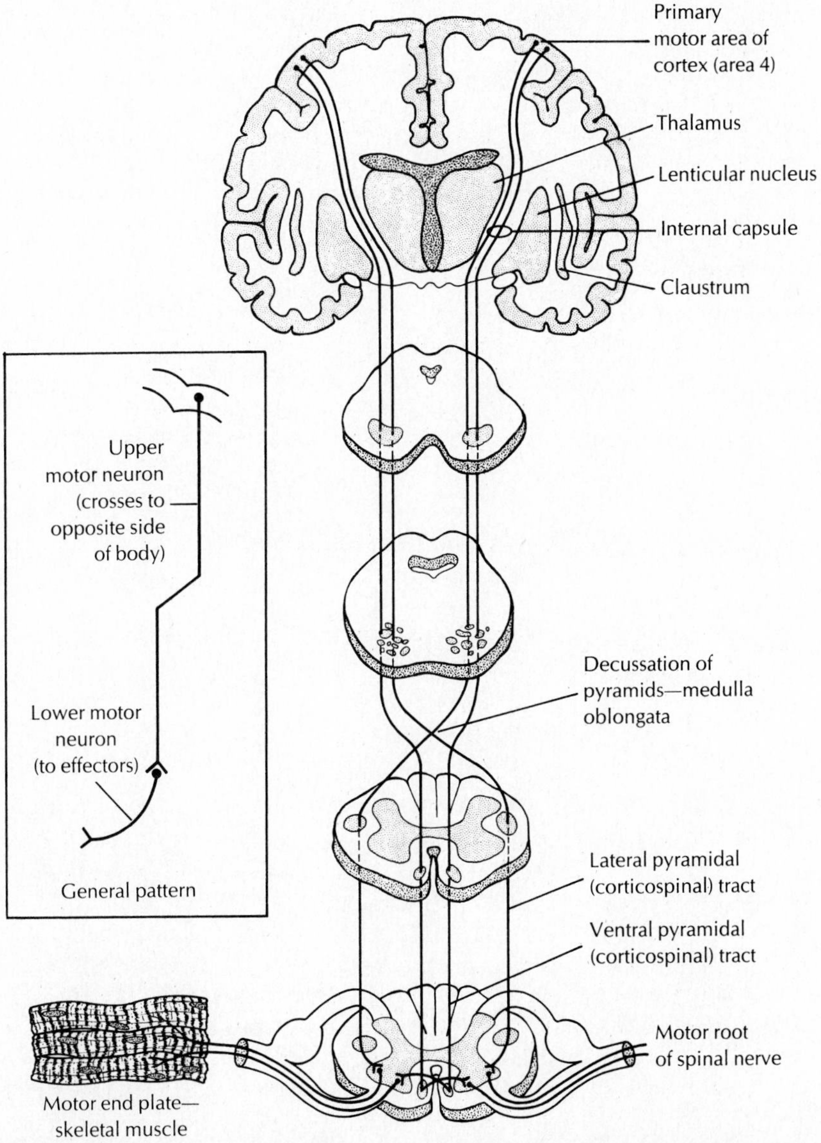

Fig. 4-26. Extrapyramidal descending tracts. Upper motor neurons originate below level of cortex and converge on lower motor neurons along with motor neurons of pyramidal tracts (see Fig. 4-25). *A,* Rubrospinal tract originates in the red nucleus of the midbrain, crosses immediately, and descends contralaterally in opposite cord. *B,* Vestibulospinal tract originates in vestibular nucleus of medulla oblongata and descends ipsilaterally. *C,* Reticulospinal tracts (medial and lateral) originate from reticular activating system of brainstem and descend in general area of *C.* (These are not so well organized as others are.) Interconnections between basal nuclei, midbrain, diencephalon, and cerebellum are extensive.

From Conway-Rutkowski, B.L.: Carini and Owens' neurological and neurosurgical nursing, ed. 18, St. Louis, 1982, The C.V. Mosby Co.

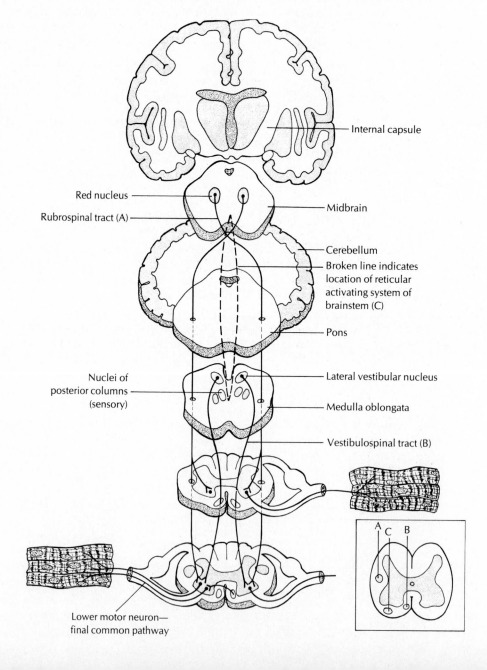

Internal capsule

Red nucleus

Rubrospinal tract (A)

Midbrain

Cerebellum

Broken line indicates location of reticular activating system of brainstem (C)

Pons

Nuclei of posterior columns (sensory)

Lateral vestibular nucleus

Medulla oblongata

Vestibulospinal tract (B)

Lower motor neuron— final common pathway

Table 4-7. Distinguishing characteristics of major divisions of the autonomic nervous system

Parameter	Sympathetic	Parasympathetic
Preganglionic	Leaves via thoracic or lumbar spinal nerves	Leaves via cranial nerves 3, 7, 9, 10 or sacral nerves
Ganglion	Located next to vertebral column (paravertebral) or next to major blood vessels	Located within viscera of area being innervated
Fiber size	Preganglionic and postganglionic fibers about the same size	Preganglionic fibers long; postganglionic fibers short
Neurotransmitter	Preganglionic fibers release acetylcholine; postganglionic fibers release norepinephrine*	Preganglionic and postganglionic fibers release acetylcholine*

From Pflanzer, R.: Personal communication, Nov., 1984.
*A few postganglionic fibers are cholinergic.

tors are located in parasympathetic postganglionic effector cells, as well as those stimulated by sympathetic cholinergic nerve endings.* There are also at least two adrenergic receptors. Currently, they are classified as alpha and beta receptors, but studies have revealed the existence of both alpha and beta 1 and 2 receptors. These receptors are widely distributed and have various effects. Table 4-8 outlines the sites and some of the resultant effects of alpha and/or beta receptor stimulation.

The autonomic nervous system plays a widespread and important role in the maintenance of an internal homeostasis. Its effects are described in Table 4-9. Note that the heart and many glands and muscles are dually innervated.

ASSESSMENT
Neurologic history

The neurologic history frequently provides the most significant data in the overall assessment of the patient with a neurologic deficit. A carefully obtained, appropriately analyzed, detailed account of the patient's symptoms, both past and present, may facilitate the interpretation of the nature and location of the disease process. An accurate history, with a thorough analysis of the chief complaints and course of the

illness, often indicates the probable diagnosis before physical and laboratory examinations are performed.

Since many nervous system dysfunctions are primarily subjective, without outward manifestations, it is important to obtain a good description of the symptoms—the patient's account of the disease. Often it is necessary to encourage the patient to provide a detailed account of his illness in his own words. Little unnecessary interference should be made. However, since a patient's spontaneous narrative is rarely complete, it may behoove the practitioner to intervene in order to exclude obviously irrelevant information, to request amplification of a statement that seems vague or incomplete, or to lead the discussion into directions that will be useful.

Chief complaint

Although the immediate concern must be reported in the patient's own words, it should be recorded in terms that are clearly understood. It is important to have the patient relate the chief concern in detail, because this is the reason for which help is being sought and provides the basis for the objective of treatment.

History of the present illness

Each symptom is described and expanded on in the history of the present illness. The course of the patient's illness must be carefully documented, with an attentive search for the earliest

---

*Nicotinic receptors are found in synapses between pre- and postganglionic fibers in both divisions of the ANS and in the neuromuscular junction in the membranes of skeletal muscle fibers.

Fig. 4-27. Neurotransmitter release from preganglionic and postganglionic fibers in the autonomic nervous system. Sympathetic and parasympathetic preganglionic fibers release acetylcholine and are said to be cholinergic. Postganglionic parasympathetic fibers also secrete acetylcholine. Sympathetic postganglionic fibers release norepinephrine and are referred to as adrenergic.

From Anthony, C.P., and Thibodeau, G.A.: Textbook of anatomy and physiology, ed. 11, St. Louis, 1983, The C.V. Mosby Co.

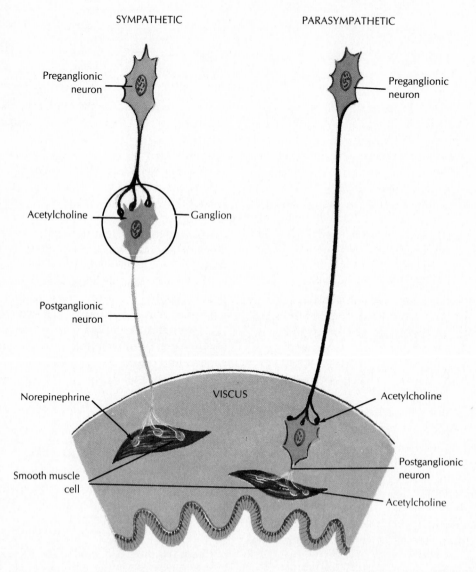

Table 4-8. Response to adrenergic and cholinergic nerve stimulation

Organ or tissue function	Adrenergic receptor	Adrenergic response	Cholinergic response
Heart			
Rate (chronotropic effect)	Beta 1	Increase	Decrease
Contractile force (inotropic effect)	Beta 1	Increase	None
Conduction velocity	Beta 1	Increase	Decrease
Eye			
Pupil size	Alpha	Constriction of radial muscle causing dilation (mydriasis)	Contraction of circular muscle causing constriction (miosis)
Accommodation		No innervation	Contraction of ciliary muscle producing accommodation for near vision
Bronchial smooth muscle	Beta 2	Relaxation	Contraction
Blood vessels (arteries and arterioles)			
Cutaneous	Alpha	Constriction	No innervation
Visceral	Alpha	Constriction	No innervation
Pulmonary	Alpha	Constriction	No innervation
Skeletal muscle	Alpha, beta 2	Constriction*	Dilation‡
Coronary	Alpha, beta 1	Constriction, dilation†	No innervation‖
Cerebral	Alpha	Constriction	
Veins	Alpha	Constriction	No innervation
Gastrointestinal tract (tone, motility, and secretory activity)	Alpha, beta 1	Decrease	Increase
Sphincters	Alpha	Contraction	Relaxation
Splenic capsule	Alpha	Contraction	No innervation
Urinary bladder			
Detrusor muscle	Beta	Relaxation	Contraction
Trigone-sphincter muscle	Alpha	Contraction	Relaxation
Uterus	Alpha, beta 2	Contraction-relaxation	Contraction-relaxation
Glycogenolysis			
Skeletal muscle	Beta	Increase	None
Liver	?	Increase	None
Lipolysis	Beta 1	Increase	None
Renin secretion	Beta 2	Increase	None
Insulin secretion	Alpha	Decrease	Increase

Modified from Craig, C.R., and Stitzel, R.E.: Modern pharmacology, Boston, 1981, Little Brown & Co.
*Low doses of epinephrine of endogenous or exogenous origin plus other beta-receptor agonists dilate these blood vessels.
†Dilation is the dominant in vivo response, owing to indirect effects.
‡Skeletal muscle blood vessels in certain regions of the body receive a sympathetic cholinergic innervation.
‖Exogenously administered cholinergic drugs dilate these blood vessels.

Table 4-9. Systemic effects of autonomic nervous system

Organ	Effect of sympathetic stimulation	Effect of parasympathetic stimulation
Eye		
Pupil	Dilated	Constricted
Ciliary muscle	Slight relaxation	Contracted
Glands		
Nasal	Vasoconstriction and slight	Stimulation of thin, copious
Lacrimal	secretion	secretion (containing many enzymes
Parotid		for enzyme-secreting glands)
Submaxillary		
Gastric		
Pancreatic		
Sweat glands	Copious sweating (cholinergic)	None
Apocrine glands	Thick, odoriferous secretion	None
Heart		
Muscle	Increased rate	Slowed rate
	Increased force of contraction	Decreased force of atrial contraction
Coronaries	Dilated (beta 2); constricted (alpha)	Dilated
Lungs		
Bronchi	Dilated	Constricted
Blood vessels	Mildly constricted	? Dilated
Gut		
Lumen	Decreased peristalsis and tone	Increased peristalsis and tone
Sphincter	Increased tone	Relaxed
Liver	Glucose released	Slight glycogen synthesis
Gallbladder and bile ducts	Relaxed	Contracted
Kidney	Decreased output	None
Bladder		
Detrusor	Relaxed	Excited
Trigone	Excited	Relaxed
Penis	Ejaculation	Erection
Systemic blood vessels		
Abdominal	Constricted	None
Muscle	Constricted (adrenergic alpha)	None
	Dilated (adrenergic beta)	
	Dilated (cholinergic)	
Skin	Constricted	None
Blood		
Coagulation	Increased	None
Glucose	Increased	None
Basal metabolism	Increased up to 100%	None
Adrenal cortical secretion	Increased	None
Mental activity	Increased	None
Piloerector muscles	Excited	None
Skeletal muscle	Increased glycogenolysis	None
	Increased strength	

From Guyton, A.C.: Textbook of medical physiology, ed. 6, Philadelphia, 1981, W.B. Saunders Co.

symptom of neurologic disease. Some neurologic disorders can be present for many years, producing only a few minor symptoms, before help is sought. The exact nature of the symptom, its severity, its body location at onset with any change in pattern over time, and its relationship to other events, should be noted. Also of importance are any related or associated symptoms and a description of what aggravates or alleviates the problem. Previous treatments and effects, and any progress—with descriptions of remissions and exacerbations—should be documented.

Past history

The past medical history should emphasize inquiry into the onset, progression, and resolution of past problems, especially those that influence or predispose the patient to neurologic disorders. Accurate information is important for establishing relationships between past illnesses and current problems (for example, head injury as an adolescent and recurrent headaches as a young adult). Major neurologic complaints that require thorough investigation include headache, dizziness, seizure, seizure-like activity or transient involuntary changes in consciousness or behavior, alterations in consciousness, loss of sensory or motor function, difficulty in speech or expression, and head injury.

Major neurologic concerns

Headaches. With headaches a detailed description may facilitate an accurate diagnosis. Because this symptom is entirely subjective, only the patient can provide the needed information, although family input may be of value in determining whether the headache is incapacitating or whether it interferes with work or sleep. The character of the headache is important. Descriptive terms such as dull, aching, steady, throbbing, burning, gripping, sharp, stabbing, constricting, intermittent, continuous, or paroxysmal are often used. Although it may be difficult to evaluate, the severity or intensity of the headache should be mentioned by the patient or family. A description of how or whether the headache interferes with routine activities may provide the needed answers. An attempt should be made to localize the pain, which may be confined to one area, regional or diffuse, unilateral, bilateral, or bandlike. If the pain is confined to one area, it is necessary to question the patient about whether it is frontal, temporal, occipital, or at the vertex. It is also important to inquire about whether the locus is tender. With headaches, in describing the incidence, onset, duration, and frequency of occurrence, it is significant to note the relationship between the headache and the time of day, month, or season, as well as its connection with food, movement, exercise, position, emotion, stress, or strain. All therapeutic interventions and their results should also be documented. Finally, associated symptoms such as nausea, vomiting, visual disturbances, tenderness, syncope, vertigo, aphasia, alterations in sensorium, or fever must be described.

Dizziness. The difference between dizziness, vertigo, giddiness, and lightheadedness must be established in the history. The nature of these symptoms, together with the mode of onset, duration, frequency, severity, direction, and relationship with any position or postural changes is important. Questions regarding any laterality or the presence of staggering or falling should be asked. Associated phenomena such as nausea, vomiting, tinnitus, deafness, diaphoresis, and prostration also need to be described.

Seizures, seizure-like activity, or transient changes in consciousness or behavior. A complaint of "fits," "convulsions," "spells," or other seizure-like activity must be accompanied by a detailed description of the manifestations of the individual attacks in proper sequence in order to establish a possible etiology. The patient and family should be queried about any precipitating factors or auras that may precede the attacks. The aura may or may not be of localizing value. A descriptive aura that consists of auditory hallucinations, tinnitus, vertigo, visual illusions or hallucinations, an unusual odor or taste, or a recurring thought may help pinpoint the locus of brain disease. The appearance of stuttering, aphasia, and numbness, tingling, or other motor alterations in a specific part of the body before seizure activity is of great localizing value and should be accompanied by a description of the area of onset, mode of extension, severity, and duration. A description of the attack itself is essential. The family, or someone who has observed the activity, must be questioned about the presence of flaccidity or rigidity and akinetic or hyperkinetic movements. Queries about whether movement is focal or generalized are important. Associated motor manifestations must be described—for example, tonic or clonic, bizarre and purposeless or coordinated and purposeful, fighting, or kicking—since such features may facilitate the differentiation between a nonorganic and an organic basis for the attacks. The presence of a cry at the onset or during the attack, flushing, cyanosis, and bladder and/or bowel incontinence all need to be mentioned. Postconvulsion behavior should also be reviewed. The patient should be asked whether he is fatigued, sleepy, confused, or sore after the seizure. He should also be questioned about the existence of any motor weakness, numbness, tingling, nausea, vomiting or headache, and, if present, how long it lasts.

Other historical information that it is important to obtain includes the age of the patient when the first attack was noted, the frequency of seizures and any variation from their normal character, the relationship between the attack and any activity, emotion, or stress, the time of the month at which they occur, the presence of any preexisting illness, infection, or trauma, and the use of any drug therapy. A birth and developmental history may also be of value with some patients.

Alterations in consciousness. The history of the patient with a reduced level of consciousness is often difficult to obtain. A patient may be drowsy, lethargic, apathetic, confused, delirious, semicomatose, stuporous, or comatose. When responses are impaired, the family may be able

to supply the needed information. Questions regarding the patient's preexisting state of health as well as any recent variations in personality or affective responses that may have been noted should be described. A history of head trauma should be noted. If there is a history of traumatic injury, inquiry should be made about any loss of consciousness and its duration; convulsions, amnesia, bleeding from the nose or ears, headaches, memory loss, or personality change. Exposure to industrial hazards, toxins, or the possible abuse of drugs should be explored.

Loss of sensory motor functions. A history of paralysis, atrophy, ataxia, or loss of sensation should include a description of the mode of onset, location, severity, and type, and information about the progression or improvement of the problem. The nature and location, onset, duration, amplitude and frequency, as well as the existence of any exciting factors, should be mentioned in the presence of any hyperkinetic movements. Questions should also be asked about any weakness, fatigue, stiffness, clumsiness, stumbling, staggering, or equilibrium disturbances.

Disturbances in speech. Abnormalities in sound production and word formulation occur frequently in combination with other phenomena. Questions about the individual's ability to comprehend both spoken and written words should be asked. Once again, family members may be the only people able to help.

Head injury. The person who has experienced head trauma may be unable to provide much information of an historical nature. Consequently, individuals who accompany the patient to the hospital should not be permitted to leave until they have been questioned.

Initially, it is important to establish the mechanism of injury. It is also necessary to determine when and where the injury was sustained. Knowing how the injury took place enables one to anticipate what changes in the patient's condition might occur. For example, trauma resulting from the penetration of a sharp object increases the risk of intracranial infection or intracranial hematomas. Or, if trauma occurred secondary to a syncopal episode, one might expect or be prepared for another.

Query must also be made regarding the patient's level of consciousness. A change in the level of consciousness is the most significant factor in the evaluation of a patient who has suffered craniocerebral trauma. The patterns of loss of consciousness are significant. Immediate loss of consciousness followed by a lucid interval and a subsequent progressively stuporous state is suggestive of an epidural hematoma. A lucid interval that is followed by a gradual loss of consciousness may indicate a subdural hematoma. Any history of unconsciousness warrants investigation.

The presence of vomiting and its nature should be described. Although vomiting is not unusual after trauma—because of the emotional and psychological impact of the injury—projectile vomiting may be indicative of increased intracranial pressure.

The position and movement of the patient after head injury should be documented. Life-threatening problems can be anticipated if the patient exhibits decerebrate posturing. If the patient is flaccid, possible neck injury as well as cerebral injury must be considered, and precautions must be taken in turning and positioning the patient to protect against further spinal cord damage.

Questions about the size of the pupils should be asked by the hospital staff of family members or whoever transports the patient to the hospital. Changes in pupil size and reactivity provide valuable data if accurate assessments are recorded over a period of time. Pupillary dilation and inequality may indicate increased pressure and may also facilitate identification of the cerebral hemisphere involved.

Since patients may not be evaluated immediately after experiencing head trauma, families must be questioned about the development of any of the above symptoms.

Review of systems

Because some symptoms may be inadvertently left out by the patient relating his past history, a complete systems review is essential. Particular attention should be given to those problems that may directly or indirectly influence the operation of the nervous system.

Family history

The family history should be obtained in detail since many neurologic conditions have a genetic or familial origin. The ages and/causes of death of parents and siblings must be recorded, together with a description of their physical and mental health during their lifetimes. Direct and collateral lines should be reviewed, with the possibility of consanguinity considered. Questions regarding inherited, familial, and congenital neurologic disorders should be pursued.

Social history

The social history should review the patient's occupational record, with special reference to contact with toxins, industrial hazards, fumes, and so on. Information regarding the duration and nature of employment as well as occupational exposure to physical or mental strain may be of interest. If there is a history of frequent change of employment or absenteeism, questions should be asked in an attempt to discern a cause.

Personal habits also need to be reviewed. Data regarding the use of such items as alcohol, tobacco, drugs, coffee, and tea, or the reasons for abstinence from these substances, are important.

Previous residence in areas where some diseases may be endemic should be documented.

A personality inventory may be of interest, especially when behavior changes have been documented. Reactions, adjustments, and emotional tendencies may assist in establishing a pattern. Some history regarding the patient's cultural and economic background, together with information about race and religion, may explain certain behaviors.

In summary, all of the information elicited becomes part of a permanent record that may not only facilitate a diagnosis but also may be referred to during the improvement or progression of the disease.

Physical examination
Vital signs

Blood pressure, heart rate, and respiratory rate are almost always included in the assessment and observation of the critically ill neurologic patient. Structures responsible for mediating these functions are located in the medulla and brainstem. Therefore, consistent and long-term changes in these functions occur very late in the syndrome of transtentorial herniation. Fluctuating vital signs can reflect changes in intracranial pressure, but relying on vital signs for detection of impending herniation is useless: major vital sign changes will occur too late to prevent irreversible herniation.

Intracranial pressure monitoring[41]

Currently there are three generally used methods of ICP monitoring: intraventricular, subarachnoid, and epidural.

Intraventricular monitoring was used initially by Lundberg. The advantages of intraventricular pressure monitoring include the ability to remove CSF for ICP control or analysis, the ability to measure compliance, and the relatively inexpensive equipment, which is readily available at most neurosurgical centers. Major disadvantages include difficulty cannulating ventricles with high ICP and decreased ventricle size, or with shift in ventricle position secondary to mass effect; increased risk of meningitis; and reliance on pressure transducers, which are susceptible to drift and air bubbles and which tend to become plugged with debris, requiring flushing.

Subarachnoid monitoring is probably the most popular type. A Richmond Screw, simple stopcock or cup catheter is introduced into the subarachnoid space. This method has the advantages of rapid insertion, no brain penetration, the ability to be used for compliance calculations, and inexpensive equipment. Disadvantages include plugging and inaccurate readings, which become more frequent with increased ICP and necessitate frequent flushing; increased risk of meningitis; and dependence on arterial transducers, which tend to drift.

The third method is epidural monitoring. Its advantages include no brain or dural penetration and, therefore, minimal risk of meningitis. Disadvantages with this equipment include its cost and relative unavailability, inaccurate readings if improperly installed, and difficulty with zeroing or detecting drift (depending on model).

Indications for ICP monitoring include trauma, hydrocephalus, encephalopathy, which includes Reye's syndrome, herpes, and postcraniotomy. Monitoring can be continued safely for several days with the intraventricular and subarachnoid methods, and for weeks with the epidural method.

Under normal circumstances, the intracranial pressure is regulated at 5 to 15 mmHg with the patient in a recumbent position. The intracranial contents can be considered to consist of three fluid components—the brain, the cerebral blood volume, and the cerebrospinal fluid—lying within a closed cranial vault. As one of the fluid components increases in volume—for example, enlargement of the brain due to cerebral edema—one or both of the other fluid components must decrease for the intracranial pressure to remain constant. An example is vasoconstriction with decrease in the cerebral blood volume and displacement of CSF from the intracranial to the intraspinal compartments. However, as these compensatory mechanisms are gradually used up—for example, as the ventricles become more compressed with displacement of CSF—the intracranial pressure begins to rise. Finally, when the mechanisms are fully used up, a very small increase in intracranial volume results in a very rapid increase in intracranial pressure. The relationship of changes in intracranial pressure produced by changes in intracranial volume produces a curve known as the cerebral elastance curve.

Before any increase in the baseline intracranial pressure, changes are often seen in the intracranial pressure waves. In patients with normal intracranial pressure, very small pulse waves may be seen which are both arterial and respiratory in origin. The arterial pulsations represent expansion of the cerebral hemispheres during systole. The respiratory waves result from transmission of increased central venous pressure during expiration, with changes in cerebral elastance because of increased volume of the intracranial contents; however, additional intracranial pressure waves are seen that were described by Lundberg originally. Lundberg described A waves, which are large plateau waves reaching pressures of 50 to 90 mmHg and lasting 5 to 20 minutes. They are indicative of a marked decrease in intracranial compliance and are probably the result of transient vasodilation due to loss of autoregulation from ischemia. A waves are a serious indicator suggesting that transtentorial herniation is impending, and they must be treated aggressively. B waves occur at a rate of 0.5 to 4 per minute and peak at 10 to 15 mmHg. They may occur in normal states, but they usually indicate diminished intracranial compliance and often precede development of A waves.

Though increased cerebral volume can be compensated for by changes in cerebral volume and CSF volume, an important mechanism for maintaining intracranial pressure is the blood-brain barrier (BBB). The BBB is the mechanism preventing free passage of many molecules into the brain, and helps to regulate the water content of the brain itself. The BBB is the result of the endothelial cells of the cerebral blood vessels. These endothelial cells are unique in that they have very tight intercellular junctions which block larger molecules from passing from the blood vessel into the brain. This BBB can be reversibly rendered ineffective by arterial perfusion with hyperosmolar agents which dehydrate the endothelial cells, causing them to shrink and opening up the intercellular junctions.

Level of consciousness

Disruption of consciousness, regardless of its cause, is of clinical concern because a disorder in the level of consciousness may produce life-threatening problems such as brain herniation and/or respiratory insufficiency.

To assess level of consciousness most accurately, the practitioner must understand the mechanism of consciousness and its relationship to functional anatomy. Arousal and cognition are the two components of consciousness. Sleep is the only normal form of altered consciousness. Disruptions and altered forms of consciousness are produced by alterations in the functioning of two major brain areas: the reticular activating system (RAS) and the cerebral cortex (see pp. 268-270).

Astute assessment and observation of changing neurological functions assist in detecting early brain variation. In addition, the clinician can determine the remainder of brain still functioning. Once consciousness has been lost, detecting further deterioration depends upon assessing motor function, respiratory patterns, eye movements and pupillary reaction, and vital signs. Anticipating further changes in neurological function will also help to provide protection for the patient to prevent complications resulting from absent gag, cough, swallowing, and corneal reflexes.

One of the most useful assessment measures is the Glasgow coma scale (Table 4-10). This scale evaluates consciousness based on three kinds of response to stimuli: motor activity, verbal performance, and eye-opening ability. If a verbal stimulus does not obtain a measurable response, the assessor administers a painful stimulus. Using assessment data such as respiratory pattern, symmetry and type of motor response, and pupillary reactions and eye movements, this coma scale summarizes progression toward

Table 4-10. Glasgow coma scale*

Score	Eye opening	Talking†	Motor
1	Does not open eyes	Makes no noise	No motor response to pain
2	Opens eyes with painful stimulus	Moans, makes unintelligible sounds	Extensor response (decerebrate)
3	Opens eyes with loud verbal command	Talks, but nonsensical	Flexor response (decorticate)
4	Opens eyes on own	Seems confused, disoriented	Moves part of body but does not remove noxious stimulus
5		Carries on conversation	Pushes away noxious stimulus; localizes pain‡
6		Alert and oriented	Follows simple motor commands

From Jennett, B., & Teasdale, G.: Aspects of coma after severe head injury, Lancet, April 23, 1977, pp. 878-881.
*Features of coma during the first week after severe head injury have been analyzed in 700 patients. Although each step on each part of the scale may not be of equal significance, the method is useful in comparing the overall responsiveness of one patient with another or one series of patients with another. Based on observations of the 700 patients, all combinations that added up to 7 or less were defined as coma. If each response on the scale is given a number (high for normal and low for impaired responses), the responsiveness of the patient can be expressed by summation of the figures. The lowest score is 3; the highest is 15.
†Arouse patient with painful stimulus if necessary.
‡Apply knuckle to sternum, observe arms.

brain herniation and assists in determining the level of brain function.

There are many causes of loss of consciousness which may be related either to actual events in the brain or to conditions imposed by other pathophysiologic mechanisms. The most common of these conditions is metabolic encephalopathy. In this syndrome, loss or impairment of consciousness is a result of disruption in metabolism of the cerebral cortex or spinal cord or both. Certain toxic conditions such as uremia, diabetes, hypoglycemia, alcoholism, drug overdose, and lead poisoning are a few of the etiologic causes in the syndrome of metabolic encephalopathy. When coma results, abnormal motor movements are symmetrical bilaterally. Without drug involvement, pupils are small and reactive bilaterally. If the patient is combative and disoriented, hypoxia or cerebral contusion is suggested. Loss of recent memory or of other more complex intellectual function may suggest an organic dementia. Disordered thinking with hallucinations may suggest psychosis or drug-induced state.

Motor system

In addition to level of consciousness, inspection should also continue with evaluation of the motor system. In the unconscious patient, the symmetry of spontaneous movements should be closely watched. Asymmetrical movement of the extremities should suggest a hemiplegia. In addition, puffing of one of the cheeks during respiration suggests a facial weakness on that side. The presence of any involuntary movements should be noted. Spontaneous movement of the upper extremities but not the lowers might suggest a paraparesis or paraplegia.

In the awake patient, more accurate assessment can be made of strength and tone throughout. Injury to the motor systems acutely will result not only in weakness but also in loss of tone. More long-standing lesions of the motor system result in increased tone and increased deep tendon reflexes known as spasticity. Included in spasticity are flexor and extensor spasms in response to stimuli and also clonus. Cerebral lesions will generally result in weakness of the opposite side of the body or hemiplegia. The hemiplegia may involve the arm or leg to a greater extent, particularly when it is the result of cerebrovascular disease. Involvement of the middle cerebral artery distribution results in ischemia of the lateral cerebral hemisphere and, consequently, greater involvement of the arm and face. Infarction of the anterior cerebral artery distribution results in involvement of the medial cerebral hemisphere and, consequently, greater weakness in the leg than in the arm. Not only is the lower face generally involved in weakness from cerebral lesions, but there also may be weakness of the opposite side of the tongue. In bilateral lesions, there may be a pseudobulbar palsy with consequent dysarthria and dysphasia. If a sensory examination can be performed, there is often noted to be decreased touch sensation and position sense on the same side as the weakness. If the thalamus is also involved, there is pain and temperature loss on the same side as the weakness.

Weakness down one side of the body may also result from injuries with hemisection of the spinal cord. However, in contrast to cerebral lesions, hemisection of the cord will result in pain and temperature loss on the opposite side to the weakness, since the pain and temperature pathways do not cross over until they reach the medulla. This is known as the Brown-Séquard lesion. Generally, however, spinal cord injuries will result in complete or partial weakness below a transverse plane. Injuries to the cervical cord area result in quadriparesis or quadriplegia, and injuries below the cervical level will result in paraparesis or paraplegia of the lower extremities. The diaphragm is innervated from the C3-C4 and C5 levels; consequently, injury at C3 and above will result in partial or complete loss of diaphragm function and resultant apnea. Injuries at this level will also result in complete paralysis of the arms. If there is sparing of the C5 level, then there is function in the deltoids with shoulder abduction. Sparing of C6 will result in function of the biceps, with consequent flexion

at the elbow, and also in some wrist extension on the radial side. With sparing of C7, the tricepts function persists bilaterally, permitting extension of the elbow. With good C7 and some C8 function, the wrist can be flexed and also ulnar wrist extension returns. With good C8 function, finger extension returns, and with T1 function, all hand intrinsics are present. In the lower extremities, the level of bone injury cannot be collated as well with the spinal cord level since the spinal cord ends at the L1-L2 level. Injuries below the L1-L2 level consequently will injure the nerve root and cause a peripheral nerve injury rather than a spinal cord injury. Sparing of the L1-L2 neurologic levels, which come off the spinal cord at about T10-T11, result in preservation of hip flexion. Knee extension results from sparing of L3-L4. Knee flexion comes from sparing of L4-L5. Sparing of L5 will also result in preservation of dorsiflexion of the foot and eversion of the foot; sparing of S1 and S2 will allow plantar flexion and inversion of the foot to be spared. The bowel and bladder are innervated from the S2, S3, and S4 segments.

In addition to assessing for gross strength and tone, the presence of involuntary movements should also be noted. Involuntary movements such as chorea and athetosis may be present, suggesting damage to the basal ganglia, particularly from lesions resulting in cerebral ischemia and infarction.

Reflexes

Reflex examination is often restricted to examination of the deep tendon reflexes and the plantar response or Babinski reflex. Acute central and peripheral nerve injuries will result in loss of both the deep tendon and Babinski responses, but over time, central lesions will demonstrate return of the deep tendon reflexes to an abnormally increased level and also the conversion of the plantar response from plantar flexion to dorsiflexion, otherwise known as a positive Babinski. Clonus and withdrawal spasms may also be noted in these patients.

Senses

Sensory examination is often somewhat limited in severely ill patients but can be of great value in distinguishing cerebral from spinal cord injuries, as mentioned earlier. Assessment of the response to touch, position of the limb, and pain should all be determined. In spinal cord injuries, in particular, there may be preservation of position sense in the lower extremity and also of some pain and temperature in a saddle area around the perineum. This should be specifically examined for in these patients.

Cerebellum

A cerebellar examination often can be made by simply observing the patient. Disorders of cerebellar function will result in ataxia of the extremities or of gait and sometimes of an intension tremor. Ataxia consists of the inability to perform smoothly coordinated movements and also the misjudgment of distance. Consequently, with cerebellar injury, the movements the patient performs are jerky and uncoordinated, and the patient will frequently overshoot while performing a task. These movements are found on the same side as the lesion when the cerebellar hemispheres are involved. When the midline of the cerebellum is involved, there may be marked ataxia of gait, with the patient unable to walk or sit, but no evidence of ataxia in the extremities on testing.

Vision

Examination of the visual system consists of examining the visual acuity, the visual fields, the fundi, and the pupil and its reactivity. Disorders of visual acuity are frequently the result of ocular disease, but damage to the optic nerve tracts or radiation may result in complaints of blurred vision; on examination, there may be a reduction in visual acuity. This can be grossly tested for by having the patient read newsprint. Complete injury to the optic nerve will result in blindness of the eye and loss of the pupillary reaction to light, or in preservation of the consensual light reflex to light applied in the remaining functional eye.

As mentioned earlier, lesions of the optic chiasm will result in bitemporal hemianopsia, and radiation, injury to the optic tracts, and injury to the visual cortex will all result in a homonymous hemianopsia on testing. This can be tested most readily at bedside by confrontation of the patient and having the patient detect the examiner's moving finger. The fundal examination is part of the physician's examination for papilledema, evidence of optic atrophy, and disturbances of the retinal vessels. On pupil examination, note should be made of the size and reactivity of the pupil. Congenital differences in pupil size occur in about 10% to 15% of the population and have little significance. Loss of the response to light may occur with either optic nerve or oculomotor disturbances. With optic nerve injuries, though the direct light response is lost, the consensual response is still present. In oculomotor injuries, such as those seen with transtentorial herniation, both the direct and the consensual reflexes are lost. In lesions farther down the brainstem in the pons, the sympathetic outflow is disrupted but oculomotor function persists. These patients will display pinpoint but reactive pupils.

Laboratory evaluation

Laboratory determinations have gained increasing prominence in the diagnostic evaluation of neurologic diseases. A battery of tests can be used to confirm a clinical impression, to determine the extent and severity of a problem, to rule out a specific diagnosis or disease, as a guide to therapeutic management, or as a prognostic guide.

Many neurologic diagnostic examinations require a trained specialist to perform the procedures and to interpret the results. Proper technique is essential for preventing prelaboratory and laboratory errors.

A carefully performed history and neurologic examination is invaluable in the determination of which part of the nervous system is involved. It is important to establish a clinical impression before laboratory evaluation is begun.

In most cases, the findings of ensuing laboratory tests will confirm this previous impression.

Biochemical analysis

Cerebrospinal fluid examination. A lumbar puncture (LP) is most commonly used to obtain cerebrospinal fluid (CSF) for analysis. The specific site to be used depends on the age of the patient and the presence of any preexisting malformations or abnormalities. Cisternal taps may also be performed, but these require someone experienced in the technique.

Normally CSF is clear and colorless. It is routinely evaluated to measure red and white cell counts, glucose and protein determinations, and a serologic test for syphilis. It may also be used for bacteriologic examination (see Unit 8), to measure pH, and to identify the presence of CSF enzymes in attempts to correlate enzymatic elevations with brain dysfunction.

The presence of blood in the CSF is clearly abnormal. Though usually indicative of an intracranial or intraspinal hemorrhage, it can occur with a traumatic tap. A stat centrifuge test can be performed to determine whether the blood is from a bloody tap or is the result of a preexisting hemorrhage.

A few lymphocytes or monocytes are commonly found in CSF. Generally, a white cell count greater than five is considered pathologic. The presence of one or more polymorphonuclear leukocytes should be investigated further.

Although the exact white cell count is not diagnostic, it tends to fall within a characteristic range that can be correlated with general pathologies. For example, counts between 10 and 100 cells per cubic millimeter are often found in syphilitic CNS disease, encephalitis, encephalomyelitis, and aseptic meningitis. These counts are also characteristic of the early or convalescent phase of diseases caused by pyogenic bacteria. Moderate increases, between 100 and 500 cells per mm³, are common to syphilitic, bacterial, tuberculous, and viral meningitis and are also found in some forms of encephalitis. The highest counts, usually those greater than 1000 cells per mm³, are characteristic of purulent meningitis. A culture or Gram stain in such cases may provide definitive information about the causative infectious agent.

Little protein is normally found in CSF since large protein molecules do not cross the BBB. In most instances, values greater than 45 mg/100 ml of CSF are considered abnormal. An elevation of CSF protein can be traced to a breakdown of the BBB at any level of the neural axis from the cerebral cortex to the nerve roots. The CSF protein elevation is a nonspecific response in a number of varied diseases that may be of an infectious, inflammatory, or neoplastic nature.

The CSF glucose level is approximately two thirds that of the blood glucose level. Thus, a blood sugar should be drawn before—or, with a fasting blood sugar, in conjunction with—the lumbar tap. CSF glucose levels are reduced in both infectious and neoplastic disorders.

Spinal taps are contraindicated in certain situations. A tap performed within 72 hours before myelography or pneumoencephalography may interfere with the introduction of contrast material. In such cases, it is often difficult to introduce contrast into the subarachnoid space without concomitantly injecting dye or air. This procedure is also contraindicated in patients with signs of incipient or ongoing herniation and in the presence of a skin infection in the lumbar region. Patients with increasing intracranial pressure on the basis of a posterior fossa mass are considered high risk, as are persons with suspected brain abscesses, although an LP in the latter group may assist in the identification of the causative agent. Finally, in patients with acute head injuries, an LP is thought to provide little additional information that is of value in their immediate care.

Electroencephalography

The electroencephalograph (EEG) provides a graphic recording of the electrical currents that emanate spontaneously from nerve cells in the cerebral hemispheres. It is performed to localize underlying pathology. The normal EEG apparently is dependent on the interaction of associated cortical projection systems, as well as ascending brainstem pathways. Recently, investigators have suggested that deep midline structures, including the thalamus, may act as a pacemaker to regulate cortical activity.[1] Others emphasize an inherent rhythmicity of electrical discharge characteristic of individual cortical neuronal units.[1]

Ideally, the EEG should be obtained during both waking and sleeping periods, with the patient off all medications. In practice, this is frequently not possible. Patients may be receiving anticonvulsants, sedatives, or a variety of other drugs. Anticonvulsants can alter paroxysmal activity, but they rarely obliterate a seizure pattern completely. Sedatives may help to relax a patient, and the judicious use of some tranquilizers can help suppress involuntary movements that produce artifact—although the latter may concomitantly depress some paroxysmal activity.

Four wave frequencies can be encountered in interpreting the EEG. These include (1) alpha (8 to 13 cycles per second [cps]), (2) beta (greater than 13 cps), (3) theta (4 to 7 cps), and (4) delta (below 4 cps) waves. Although none of these frequencies can be identified as a "normal" or "abnormal" tracing, certain patterns are reviewed as pathologic. Such patterns include (1) spikes with a high voltage potential and a duration of less than 60 milliseconds; (2) sharp waves with a high voltage potential and a duration of greater than 60 milliseconds; and (3) spikes and waves in combination, characterized by single or multiple spikes with slow waves in either an isolated or a synchronous pattern.[32]

The EEG is of value in the diagnosis of seizure disorders, the localization of vascular and neoplastic brain lesions, and the establishment of brain death. Certain metabolic conditions may also be diagnosed by EEG.

Echoencephalography

Echoencephalography (ECHO) is a technique in which pulses of ultra-sonic waves are beamed through the skull from both sides, pro-

ducing echoes from the midline structures of the brain that are reflected back to the receiver and recorded as graphic tracings. These sound waves encounter substances of differing acoustical impedance, yielding characteristic images.

The use of echoencephalography has decreased with the introduction of computerized tomography. However, this procedure is still useful in the screening process of acute head trauma and in the bedside evaluation of infants with suspected intracerebral hemorrhage.

Isotopic scans

The brain scan is the most valuable isotopic study. It was first developed to detect neoplastic growths, but it is also used to evaluate vascular lesions, to determine the extent of trauma, and to identify brain abscesses and other miscellaneous lesions. Isotopic scanning has also been of value in the detection of CSF leakage and low pressure hydrocephalus.

A scanning system is used after the injection of one of a number of radionucleotides. These isotopes accumulate in areas of the brain where there is an altered BBB. The cause of the alteration will determine the pattern and rate of uptake. Blocking agents may be required with certain isotopes that accumulate in target structures outside of the CNS. Specific structures are invariably visible and serve as landmarks in the normal brain scan.

Radiologic studies

Skull films. Roentgenographic films of the skull can be useful in the detection of developmental abnormalities, trauma, and increased intracranial pressure, and in the identification of specific tumors and some infectious disorders. Although portable series may be obtained, they are generally unsatisfactory except in the recognition of obvious pathology. Special views of the skull are often critical, requiring a skilled technician.

Spinal films. Spinal films can be used to review the integrity of the vertebral body, the disk interspace, the lamina, and the pedicles.

Contrast procedures

Arteriography. Arteriography is the most commonly used invasive procedure in the diagnosis of structural lesions involving the CNS above the level of the foramen magnum. It is valuable in the identification of aortocranial and intracranial occlusive vascular disease, cerebral aneurysms, and arteriovenous malformations, and is used to detect alterations in cerebral blood flow characteristic of vascular manifestations, increased intracranial pressure, and tumors.

In this procedure, a contrast agent is injected via one of several approaches. The exact approach is determined by the location of the suspected lesion. Percutaneous puncture of the common carotid artery provides the best visualization of the anterior circulation, including the middle and cerebral arteries on that side. Therefore this approach is favored for frontal, temporal, or anterior parietal lobe suspected pathology. The right retrograde brachial artery approach shows anterior circulation, the basilar artery, and the right and left posterior cerebral arteries. Left brachial arteriography permits visualization of the vertebral-basilar system and both cerebral arteries and is the appropriate choice in the patient with symptoms of a posterior fossa disorder. Less commonly used approaches include bilateral brachial arteriography and direct vertebral puncture. Intravenous angiography has enjoyed only limited use.

The primary contraindication to arteriography is a previous reaction to a contrast agent. Bleeding is also a potential risk, making the procedure of little value for the anticoagulated patient.

Arterial imaging can also be accomplished by the use of an x-ray image intensifier attached to a computer. This is a relatively new procedure referred to as digital-subtraction angiography.

Pneumoencephalography and ventriculography. Pneumoencephalography and ventriculography are used on a limited basis for suspected lesions that touch the ventricular system or alter the flow of CSF. This procedure necessitates the injection of air into the lumbar subarachnoid space. Patients must be in a sitting position so the air rises to outline the cerebral structures and the ventricles. Small amounts of a water-soluble contrast medium may also be used.

Serious complications have been associated with these procedures—which are, in addition, most uncomfortable. Hemiplegia, aphasia related to hypotension, intracerebral hemorrhage, subdural hematoma, cardiac dysrhythmias, and herniation have all been reported.

Myelography. Myelograms are obtained in the presence of suspected degenerative disk disease. An iodinated contrast substance is injected into the lumbar subarachnoid space before films are made.

Computerized transaxial tomography. Computerized transaxial tomography (CT) permits detailed visualization of the normal anatomy of the brain, as well as any structural anomalies, without subjecting the patient to the hazards of an invasive procedure. An X-ray tube rotates axially or coronally around the patient's head, making density measurements. The X-ray source is linked to a computer that is programmed to (1) display the measurements made and (2) translate the information into a picture of the brain. The CT scan is frequently carried out with an iodine dye, which provides better contrast between normal brain structures than when no contrast media is used, as well as outlining abnormal structures when there is an alteration in the BBB. (The test can be performed with or without contrast.)

CT scanning permits the identification of low-grade gliomas that may have been previously unrecognized by both isotopic scans and arteriography. It is also valuable in the diagnosis and management of other tumors and brain abscesses and in the timely detection of intracerebral hemorrhage and nonhemorrhagic vascular insults. The CT scan is useful in head trauma, negating the need for angiography. In addition, degenerative processes and hydrocephalus can be identified and monitored with this procedure. Thus, using radiation approximately equal to that received during conventional skull films, the technique has led to significant advances in the diagnostic evaluation of neoplastic, infectious, vascular, and endocrine abnormalities of the brain.

The patient must be cooperative in order for the technician to obtain a CT scan. The judicious use of sedation may dispel some anxiety or "settle" the restless patient. Since a contrast medium is often used, there is always the risk of an allergic reaction. Patients with a history of allergies or asthma may require antihistamine or steroid therapy before the test.

ALTERATIONS

Pathologic alterations in the nervous system are often divided into three broad classifications: (1) focal lesions that result from a localized disturbance; (2) diffuse or generalized disorders that involve the nervous system and supporting elements; and (3) systemic nervous abnormalities with aberrations that are found in a particular neural tissue, structure, or group of structures. Further subdivision is frequently made on the basis of etiology. Pathologies are described as (1) congenital—stemming from altered development; (2) traumatic—the result of physical or chemical injury; (3) inflammatory (acute, subacute, or chronic)—secondary to infective or allergic processes; (4) neoplastic (benign or malignant, with the latter considered either primary or secondary in origin); (5) degenerative; and (6) metabolic or endocrine.

Clinically, there are literally hundreds of neurologic alterations that can be elicited and interpreted. This variety can be attributed to the complexity of the nervous system itself. Several different diseases may cause the same syndrome, and several syndromes may characteristically occur in any one disease.

In the pages that follow, the pathophysiology of those neurologic syndromes commonly seen by acute care practitioners will be reviewed.

Headache

Headaches are caused by the stimulation of pain-sensitive structures located either within the cranium or outside it, in extracranial tissues in the head and neck. Cranial structures sensitive to mechanical stimulation include (1) the skin, subcutaneous tissue, muscles, arteries, and periosteum of the skull; (2) fine structures of the eyes, ears, and nasal cavity; (3) extracranial and intracranial veins, venous sinuses, and their tributaries; (4) areas of the dura at the base of the brain, together with arteries in the dura mater and pia-arachnoid; and (5) the fifth (trigeminal), ninth (glossopharyngeal), and tenth (vagus) cranial nerves and the first three cervical nerves.[1] The cranial bone, a good portion of the pia-arachnoid and dura, the brain parenchyma, ependymal lining, and the choroid plexus, all lack sensitivity—hence the name pain-insensitive structures.[58]

Headaches may be classified into one of three main groupings to avoid confusion generated from using a system based on a series of disparate headache syndromes. These groups are: vascular, muscle contraction, and traction and inflammatory headaches.

The mechanisms of pain production are as follows:

1. Distention, traction, dilation, and displacement of intracranial or extracranial blood vessels.
2. Compression, traction, or inflammation of sensory, cranial, or spinal nerves.
3. Voluntary or involuntary spasms or interstitial inflammation of cranial and cervical muscles.
4. Irritation and inflammation of the meninges and increased intracranial pressure.[1,58,73]

Vascular headaches include migraines, cluster headaches, toxic vascular, and hypertensive headache. In each situation, pain is thought to be caused by vascular dilation. With some vascular headaches, vasoconstrictive changes may also occur and may be responsible for the painless sensory and motor phenomena that take place. Toxic vascular headaches produced by systemic vasodilation can be traced to fever, alcohol or poison ingestion, retention of carbon dioxide, or the therapeutic use of nitrates. Hypertensive headaches are uncommon and are attributed to the increase in systemic arterial pressure.

Headaches caused by persistent contraction of the muscles of the head, neck, and face are appropriately labeled muscle contraction headaches. These constitute the most common form of headache.

Traction and inflammatory headaches are caused by organic diseases of the skull or its components, including the brain, meninges, arteries, veins, eyes, ears, teeth, nose, and paranasal sinuses. These headaches occur when intracranial lesions or tumors deform, displace, or exert traction on vessels and dural structures at the base of the brain. A traction headache may be evoked by hematomas, abscesses, nonspecific brain edema, and lumbar puncture. It is also a symptom of a brain tumor, especially if the ventricular system is compromised with obstruction of absorption or flow of CSF, causing hydrocephalus.

Although headaches are infrequent with mild to moderate increases in intracranial pressure, they do occur with significant elevations in at least two conditions: acute hydrocephalus and benign intracranial hypertension. The exact mechanism by which pain is produced is poorly understood. It is believed to be related to the traction on pain-sensitive areas that occurs with structural shifts.

Headaches can also be caused by arteritis, phlebitis, and infections. Pain occurs as a result of inflammation of the vessel wall and surrounding perivascular regions. The pain usually coincides with the course of the disorder and abates as the disease is brought under control. Rarely is it recurrent or paroxysmal.

Sensory information from pain-sensitive intracranial structures is transmitted via several cranial nerves. The trigeminal and vagus nerves are considered the principal afferent fibers of the intracranial structures, but the ninth, eleventh, and twelfth cranial nerves and the upper cervical nerves are also involved.[21] Pain emanating from the upper surface of the tentorium and the anterior and middle cranial fossa is communicated by the fifth cranial nerve. Pain from these areas is referred to the eye and forehead on the same side. The upper three cervical nerve roots carry information from the inferior surface of the tentorium and from the posterior fossa.[47] The ninth, tenth, eleventh, and twelfth cranial nerves have also been shown to be sensitive to painful stimulation.[21] This pain is perceived in the back of the head and in the upper part of the neck. Some of the posterior fossa is also supplied by the glossopharyngeal and vagus nerves; consequently, pain may be referred to the ear or throat.[47]

Pain from extracranial arteries is mediated either by the trigeminal nerve or by the upper cervical nerve roots. Painful information from the frontal and superficial temporal arteries is transmitted by the fifth cranial nerve, and that from postauricular and occipital arteries is carried by cervical nerve fibers.[47]

Central pain pathways involve several ascending tracts. Pain fibers from all divisions of the trigeminal nerve are joined by fibers from the glossopharyngeal and vagus nerves in the second cervical segment. After synapsing, second-order neurons cross the midline and ascend through the brainstem to the posteroventromedial nucleus of the thalamus. This is designated the quintothalamic pathway.

Spinothalamic fibers also transmit information to another nucleus, the posteroventrolateral nucleus. Both of these tracts mediate the perception of sharp, localized pain. The apinoreticulothalamic pathway is important in the perception of constant, diffuse pain. This pathway connects with cells in the nucleus reticularis before reaching the medial thalamic nuclei. The affective interpretation of and reaction to pain is mediated by projections from the dorsomedial and anterior thalamic nuclei to the orbital surface of the frontal lobe and limbic system.[48]

Dizziness

Dizziness or vertigo is produced by disorders of the vestibular system. It is characterized by a derangement in equilibrium, manifested as a sensation of rotation of the self or of one's surroundings. Often it is accompanied by unsteadiness, vomiting, pallor, and nystagmus.

Because there are several mechanisms involved in the maintenance of normal posture, different aural and neural pathways must be reviewed to determine the pathophysiology of dizziness or vertigo.

The end organs instrumental in the regulation of vestibular activity are the semicircular canals, which respond to movement and angular momentum, and the otoliths, sense organs of the utricle and saccule responsible for the conveyance of information regarding the position of the head in relation to gravity. Hair cells located within the ampulla of the semicircular canals and in the utricle and saccule, when distorted, transmit impulses to the vestibular nerve. Most of the vestibular nerve fibers end in the vestibular nuclei, situated near the junction of the medulla and pons. Here, these fibers synapse with second-order neurons that ultimately send fibers to the cerebellum, to other areas of the brainstem (particularly the reticular formation), and down the spinal cord via the vestibulospinal and reticulospinal tracts. Other fibers pass without synapsing to the fastigial nuclei and the uvula and flocculonodular nodes of the cerebellum. Signals also pass upward into the brainstem from the vestibular nuclei and cerebellum via the medial longitudinal fasciculus or through reticular tracts to the cerebral cortex, terminating in the cortical equilibrium center located in the parietal lobe. These impulses apprise the mind of the equilibrium status of the body.[35]

Vertigo is caused by an imbalance between vestibular input bilaterally, or by a conflict between visual proprioceptive and vestibular information when one is inappropriate to the other.[48]

Pathologic vertigo may result from infection or vascular disease affecting the labyrinth. The concurrent development of vomiting in children and young adults in the absence of auditory disorders suggests a vestibular neuronitis. This condition, which is severe at the onset but usually subsides gradually, may also involve the cerebellum. In acute cerebellitis, the vertigo is often accompanied by nystagmus, incoordination, and ataxia.[48]

Drugs may also interfere with the vestibular apparatus. There are a number of drugs shown to be ototoxic. Streptomycin and gentamicin primarily produce vestibular impairment. Neomycin, ethacrynic acid, and kanamycin affect both vestibular and cochlear function. Salicylates may also cause mild vestibular disturbances, but these effects appear to be reversible with reduced dosage. Some of these drugs may also be nephrotoxic. In the elderly or in anuric patients, therapeutic doses of many of these agents can destroy labyrinth function.

Transient or persistent vertigo may also be traced to brainstem and cerebellar disorders. Infections and vasocular and neoplastic processes have been cited as etiologic agents. Vertigo has been documented in encephalitis, vertebrobasilar arterial insufficiency, and gliomas.

Vertigo may be seen as a transient symptom in temporal lobe epilepsy. Cortically induced vertigo, however, is not as severe as that originating in the vestibular system or in the brainstem or cerebellum.

Alterations in consciousness

The consciousness system maintains consciousness, alertness, and attention, and regulates the sleep state. A state of wakefulness and alertness is attained by this system through the action of the ascending reticular activating system on the cerebral cortex. The ascending reticular activating system itself is activated by sensory pathways and by fibers from the cerebral cortex.

Consciousness is defined as a state of awareness of one's self and environment. It implies an awake and alert condition in which an individual is able to perceive his internal and external environment and, with an intact motor system, is capable of responding in an appropriate manner to incoming stimuli. There are two components of consciousness: (1) the content of consciousness consisting of cognitive mental functions that reflect the activity of the cerebral cortex, and (2) arousal and wakefulness that are dependent upon the ascending reticular activating system, which is activated via direct stimulation, sensory stimuli, or cortical influences.

Clinically, there are several terms used to describe the states of awareness and responsiveness. These include normal consciousness, inattention, confusion, and clouding of consciousness, delirium, stupor, and coma.

Normal consciousness. Normal consciousness is the state in which an individual who is fully awake is capable of responding to psychologic stimuli, and indicates by his behavior and speech an appropriate awareness of himself and his environment. This condition may fluctuate during a 24-hour period from a state of keen alertness to one of general inattention and drowsiness.

Confusion and clouding of consciousness. Confusion and clouding of consciousness are states characterized by sensorial clouding or imperceptiveness and distractibility of attention. Frequently, the patient fails to take into account all elements of the immediate environment.

The severely confused patient often can do no more than carry out a few simple commands. Thought processes may not be operational. Speech capacity may be limited to a few phrases or may be voluble. These individuals are not aware of much of what goes on around them.

Patients who are moderately confused are easily distracted but can carry on a simple conversation. Often these people think slowly and appear slightly incoherent. They are usually disoriented as to time and place but recognize significant others.

With mild degrees of confusion, the disorder may be so slight as to go unrecognized. The patient may be fairly oriented as to time and place These individuals normally are able to speak freely on almost any subject.

Delirium. Delirium is an agitated state of confusion associated with illusions (false interpretations or misrepresentations of real sensory images), hallucinations (false sensory perceptions that have no external basis), and delusions

(false beliefs or misconceptions uncorrectable by reason). Some regard delirium as a state of confusion with excitement and hyperactivity. The delirious patient normally is unable to sleep and has difficulty responding to events other than those to which he or she is reacting at any one moment in time.

Stupor. The stuporous patient exhibits a moderate amount of spontaneous movement and can be aroused to respond purposefully to afferent stimuli. When sufficiently aroused, these people can give a brief response to questions or simple commands, although mental and physical activity are reduced to a minimum. Tremulous movement, coarse muscular twitching, restless or stereotyped motor activity, and grasping and sucking reflexes may occur.

Coma. Comatose individuals are unreceptive and unresponsive to external stimuli or inner needs. The degree of coma may vary. Semicoma is a lighter stage of coma in which a patient may respond to stimulation with simple withdrawal movements, facial grimaces, or groans. Such an individual may show spontaneous motor activity that includes restless movements, tremors, twitches, or purposeless plucking movements. Although reflexive response varies with the location of the underlying disease, pupillary reflexes, ocular movements, and other brainstem reflexes often can be elicited.

In deep coma, little or no spontaneous movement is evident. Corneal, pupillary, pharyngeal, tendon, and plantar reflexes are all depressed or absent. Extensor rigidity of the limbs and opisthotonos which may or may not be present indicate decerebration if they exist. Breathing is often slow or rapid and may be periodic. Other vital signs may also be altered.

Causes of loss of consciousness

Consciousness may be affected by both (1) physiologic alterations of function that produce a transient loss of consciousness, and (2) structural lesions that result in a loss of consciousness that persists.

A temporary disturbance of consciousness

can occur as a result of a concussion, a generalized seizure, a syncopal episode, metabolic encephalopathy, or drug therapy.

Concussion. A concussion is a momentary loss of consciousness that occurs after a sudden blow to the head. Arousal by vigorous stimuli is usually possible even though the individual is unconscious. Some degree of confusion is common after consciousness returns, and amnesia may persist for a variable period of time. Permanent neurologic complications are rare, although microscopic studies on animals show individual neuronal alterations.

The cause of the transient alteration in consciousness is as yet unproven. Several mechanisms have been postulated. These include (1) a sudden increase in intracranial pressure in the area of neurons critical for maintenance of consciousness, (2) cerebral ischemia, (3) sudden neuronal depolarization or hyperpolarization, and (4) mechanical distortion of neurons or axons that leads to an interference in neuronal activity.

Seizures. The sudden, violent discharge or epilepsy may induce an alteration in consciousness. Rarely does a jacksonian seizure affect consciousness, unless it should happen to spread from one side of the body to the other. A generalized seizure, on the other hand, results in a loss of consciousness because it involves both hemispheres simultaneously or the thalamus and reticular activating system.

Syncope. Syncopal episodes produce a transient loss of consciousness resulting from a decrease in cerebral blood flow and ischemia in the consciousness system. This can be caused by a decrease in the cardiac output, a bradydysrhythmia, or pooling blood in the periphery.

Metabolic encephalopathy. Various systemic disorders produce a metabolic encephalopathy that can cause a temporary alteration in consciousness. Hypoglycemia, hypoxia, hyperosmolar and hypoosmolar states, acidosis, and alkalosis, potassium imbalance, hyperammonemia, and deficiencies of thiamin, nicotinic acid, vitamin B_{12}, pantothenic acid, and pyridoxine are all

examples of conditions that can alter consciousness.

Cerebral blood flow or cerebral metabolism is reduced in all metabolic disorders that lead to coma. In hypoglycemia, the cerebral metabolic rate is reduced while cerebral blood flow remains normal or above normal. This creates a substrate deficiency. With thiamine and vitamin B_{12} deficiency, cerebral blood flow is normal or slightly decreased while the cerebral metabolic rate is low. This is probably a result of insufficient coenzymes. Both cerebral blood flow and cerebral metabolic rate are reduced with significant falls in blood pressure. A drop in the systolic pressure below 70 mmHg deoxygenates neural structures, leading to the described changes in cerebral blood flow and metabolic rate described above. Cerebral metabolic rate is also decreased in the presence of bacterial toxins, although the exact mechanism is unknown. This is the case in diabetic acidosis, uremia, hepatic coma, and the coma of systemic infections. In diabetes there is an accumulation of ketone bodies (acetoacetic acid, beta hydroxybutyric acid, and acetone) or, in the nonketotic form, a lactic acidosis. Phenolic derivatives of the aromatic amoni acids are found in uremia. In both situations, the serum acidosis and dehydration may also be a factor. The serum levels of ammonia are significant in hepatic coma.

Abnormal neuronal activity also affects consciousness. Body temperature extremes—both hyperthermia (temperatures greater than 41° C) and hypothermia (temperatures below 35° C) may induce coma by exerting a nonspecific effect on the metabolic activity of the neuron. Neuronal activity is altered in respiratory and metabolic alkalosis (pH > 7.45) from cardiopulmonary disease, central neurogenic hyperventilation, and alkali ingestion. Membrane excitability is also affected in water intoxication hypoosmolality resulting from hyponatremia and changes in the intracellular potassium.

Coma also occurs in the presence of hypercapnia and hypoxia. Oxygen values of less than 2 ml/100 g of brain tissue per minute are not compatible with an alert state of consciousness.

Alterations resulting from drug therapy. A number of pharmacologic agents exert a depressive effect on the level of consciousness. Barbiturates, bromides, diphenylhydantoin, alcohol, glutethimide, and phenothiazines all have a suppressive effect on neurons in the cerebrum and diencephalon. Others, such as methanol, paraldehyde, and ethylene glycol result in a nonrespiratory acidosis that ultimately affects cerebral blood flow and cerebral metabolic rate. Additional drugs may alter cardiovascular mechanics, causing circulatory collapse that leads to inadequate cerebral blood flow.

Lesions. Coma occurs with lesions that involve the reticular system and its projections or the cerebral hemispheres bilaterally. Infarction, neoplasia, and hemorrhage may depress the consciousness system in the posterior fossa or diencephalon. Diffuse bilateral cerebral lesions such as encephalitis, meningitis, and subarachnoid hemorrhages have a similar effect.

Indirect involvement of the consciousness system can also lead to coma.

Brain lesions such as hemorrhage, tumors, or abscesses occupy space and alter consciousness, either by direct destruction of the midbrain and diencephalon or by producing herniation of the medial part of the temporal lobe through the opening of the tentorium. This either crushes the upper brain against the opposite free edge of the tentorium or causes lateral or downward displacement of the brainstem.

Seizures or seizure-like activity

Seizures represent the sudden, excessive, disorderly discharge of neurons in either a structurally normal or a diseased cortex. The discharge is associated with an almost instantaneous disturbance of sensation, loss of consciousness, and convulsive movement.[73]

There are many classifications of seizures based on their characteristics—pattern, temporal occurrence, etiology, associated behaviors. In 1969, the International League Against Epilepsy recommended a classification system that has been widely used. Three main categories are recognized: partial, generalized, and unilateral. Partial seizures are further subdivided into those with elementary (simple) and those with complex symptomatology. Those with complex symptomatology are considered to originate in areas of higher cerebral organization and to involve a loss of consciousness. It is also acknowledged that partial seizures may secondarily become generalized. Simple partial seizures are divided into motor, sensory, autonomic, and compound forms.

Generalized seizures are also subdivided into primary and secondary types. Primary generalized seizures are generalized from their onset, whereas secondary generalized seizures may be either generalized from the onset or secondarily generalized.

Unilateral seizures are similar to generalized seizures with the exception that they occur principally, if not exclusively, on one side of the body.

This method of classification is summarized in Table 4-11.

The mechanisms by which seizures are produced remains a subject of research. It is believed that synaptic influences upon a cell alter membrane permeability and have a depolarizing action. If a sufficient area of the cell membrane is depolarized, a chain reaction occurs, spreading along the entire cell membrane to adjacent cortical and thalamic brainstem nuclei. Neurotransmitters act postsynaptically to either facilitate or inhibit all discharge. Some chemical transmitters cause hyperpolarization of the cell membrane, increasing cellular stability and decreasing the likelihood of discharge. These transmitters function as anticonvulsants by depressing neuronal discharge.[62,63] Glycine is thought to be an inhibitory transmitter chiefly in the spinal cord, whereas gamma-aminobutyric acid (GABA) serves as an inhibitory transmitter substance in the cerebrum and cerebellum. Substances that block inhibitory neurotransmitters may induce seizure activity. Picrotoxin, used as a CNS stimulant in the treatment of respiratory failure sec-

Text continued on p. 315.

Table 4-11. Clinical and electroencephalographic classification of epileptic seizures*

Clinical seizure type	Electroencephalographic seizure type	Electroencephalographic interictal expression†	Anatomic substrate	Etiology	Age
I. PARTIAL SEIZURES OR SEIZURES BEGINNING LOCALLY Seizures in which the first clinical changes indicate activation of an anatomical and/or functional system of neurones limited to a part of a single hemisphere; in which the inconsistently present electrographic seizure patterns are restricted, at least at their onset, to one region of the scalp (the area corresponding to the cortical representation of the system involved); and in which the initial neuronal discharge usually originates in a narrowly limited or even quite diffuse cortical (the most accessible and vulnerable) part of such a system.					
Elementary or complex symptomatology depending on the discharge of a system localized in one or, sometimes, both hemispheres	Rhythmic discharge of spikes and/or of more or less slow waves more or less localized over one or, sometimes, both hemispheres	Intermittent local discharges, generally over one hemisphere only	Various cortical and/or subcortical regions corresponding with functional representation in one hemisphere	Usually related to a wide variety of local brain lesions (cause known, suspected or unknown). Constitutional factors may be important	Possible at all ages but more frequent with increasing age
PARTIAL SEIZURES WITH ELEMENTARY SYMPTOMATOLOGY					
Generally without impairment of consciousness	Local contralateral discharge starting over the corresponding area of cortical representation (not always recorded on the scalp)	Local contralateral discharges	Usually in the cortical region of one hemisphere corresponding to functional representation	As above	As above
With motor symptoms Focal motor (without march), including localized epileptic myoclonus Jacksonian Versive (generally contraversive) Postural Somatic inhibitory (?) Aphasic Phonatory					

(vocalization and arrest of speech)
With special sensory or somatosensory symptoms
Somatosensory
Visual
Auditory
Olfactory
Gustatory
Vertiginous
With autonomic symptoms
Compound forms‡

PARTIAL SEIZURES WITH COMPLEX SYMPTOMATOLOGY‖

Generally with impairment of consciousness; may sometimes begin with elementary symptomatology	Unilateral or bilateral discharge, diffuse, or focal in temporal or fronto-temporal regions	Unilateral or bilateral, generally asynchronous, focus; usually in the temporal region(s)	Usually cortical and/or subcortical temporal or fronto-temporal regions (including rhinencephalic structures), unilateral or bilateral
With impaired consciousness alone *With cognitive symptomatology* With dysmnesic disturbances (conscious amnesia, "déjà vu," "déjà vécu") With ideational disturbances (including "forced thinking," dreamy state . . .)		As above	As above

---

Recommended by the International League against Epilepsy, the World Federation of Neurology, the World Federation of Neurosurgical Societies and the International Federation of Societies for Electroencephalography and Clinical Neurophysiology.
†The incidence of interictal abnormalities varies; they may be absent.
‡Compound implies a joining together of elementary or (and/or) complex symptoms.
‖Complex versus elementary; implies an organized, high-level cerebral activity.

Continued.

Table 4-11. Clinical and electroencephalographic classification of epileptic seizures—cont'd

Clinical seizure type	Electroencephalographic seizure type	Electroencephalographic interictal expression	Anatomical substrate	Etiology	Age
With affective symptomatology *With "psychosensory" symptomatology* Illusions (for example, macropsia, metamorphopsia) Hallucinations *With "psychomotor" symptomatology* (automatisms) *Compound forms*					
PARTIAL SEIZURES SECONDARILY GENERALIZED					
All forms of partial seizures, with elementary or complex symptomatology, can develop into generalized seizures, sometimes so rapidly that the focal features may be unobservable. These generalized seizures may be symmetrical or asymmetrical, tonic or clonic, but most often tonic-clonic in type	Above discharge becomes secondarily and rapidly generalized			Refer to partial seizures in general	

II. GENERALIZED SEIZURES, BILATERAL SYMMETRICAL SEIZURES OR SEIZURES WITHOUT LOCAL ONSET

Seizures in which the clinical features do not include any sign of symptom referable to an anatomical and/or functional system localized in one hemisphere, and usually consist of initial impairment of consciousness, motor changes which are generalized or at least bilateral and more or less symmetrical and may be accompanied by an "en masse" autonomic discharge; in which the electroencephalographic patterns from the

...start are bilateral, grossly synchronous and symmetrical over the two hemispheres; and in which the responsible neuronal discharge takes place, if not throughout the entire grey matter, then at least in the greater part of it and simultaneously on both sides.

Convulsive or non-convulsive symptomatology, without sign referable to a unilateral system localized in one hemisphere

	Bilateral, essentially synchronous and symmetrical discharge from the start	Bilateral, essentially synchronous and usually symmetrical discharges	Unlocalized (? mesodiencephalon)	No cause found or: All ages (i) Diffuse or multiple bilateral lesions, and/or: (ii) Toxic and/or metabolic disturbances, and/or: (iii) Constitutional, often genetic factors (epileptic predisposition)	
Absences Simple absences, with impairment of consciousness only	With rhythmic 3 c/s spike and wave discharge ("petit mal" or typical absence)	Spike and waves and/or polyspike and wave discharges	As above	As above (organic etiology is unusual)	Especially in children
	Without 3 c/s spike and wave (variant of "petit mal" or atypical absence) Low-voltage fast activity or rhythmic discharge at 10 or more c/s, or More or less rhythmic discharge of sharp and slow waves, sometimes asymmetrical	More or less rhythmic discharges of sharp and slow waves, sometimes asymmetrical	As above	As above (organic etiology is usual; cerebral metabolic disturbances superimposed on previous brain lesion may be important)	Especially in children
Complex absences, with other phenomena associated with impairment of consciousness			As above	As above	As above

Continued.

Table 4-11. Clinical and electroencephalographic classification of epileptic seizures—cont'd

Clinical seizure type	Electroencephalographic seizure type	Electroencephalographic interictal expression	Anatomical substrate	Etiology	Age

Absences—cont'd
  With mild clonic components (myoclonic absences)
  With increase of postural tone (retropulsive absences) with diminution or abolition of postural tone (atonic absences)
  With automatisms (automatic absences)
  With autonomic phenomena (for example, enuretic absences) As mixed forms					

Bilateral massive epileptic myoclonus (myoclonic jerks)	Polyspike and waves or, sometimes, spike and waves or sharp and slow waves	Polyspike and waves or spike and waves, sometimes sharp and slow waves	As above	As above	All ages
Infantile spasms	Flattening of hypsarhythmia during spasm or exceptionally more prominent spikes and slow waves	Hypsarhythmia	As above	As above (cerebral metabolic disturbances superimposed on prior brain lesion may be important)	Infants only

Clonic seizures	Mixture of fast (10 c/s or more) and slow waves with occasional spike and wave patterns	Spike and waves and/or polyspike and wave discharges	As above	As above	Especially in children
Tonic seizures	Low-voltage fast activity or fast rhythm (10 c/s or more) decreasing in frequency and increasing in amplitude	More or less rhythmic discharges of sharp and slow waves, sometimes asymmetrical	As above	As above (organic etiology is usual)	Especially in children
Tonic-clonic seizures ("grand mal" seizures)	Rhythm at 10 or more c/s, decreasing in frequency and increasing in amplitude during the tonic phase, interrupted by slow waves during the clonic phase	Polyspike and waves and/or spike and waves or, sometimes, sharp and slow wave discharges	As above	As above	Less frequent in young children than other forms of generalized seizures; all ages except infancy
Atonic seizures Sometimes associated with myoclonic jerks (myoclonic-atonic seizures)		Polyspike and wave			
Of very brief duration (epileptic drop attacks)	Polyspike and waves (more waves than in the myoclonic polyspike and wave)	Polyspike and waves Polyspoke and wave and/or spike and waves or, sometimes, sharp and slow wave discharges			
Of longer duration (including atonic absences)	rhythmic spike and wave (3 to 1 c/s) or mixture of fast and slow waves with occasional spike and wave patterns				
Akinetic seizures Loss of movement without atonia	Rhythmic spike and wave (3 to 1 c/s) or mixture of fast and slow waves with occasional spike and wave patterns	Polyspike and waves and/or spike and waves or, sometimes, sharp and slow wave discharges	As above	As above	Especially in children

Continued.

Table 4-11. Clinical and electroencephalographic classification of epileptic seizures—cont'd

Clinical seizure type	Electroencephalographic seizure type	Electroencephalographic interictal expression	Anatomical substrate	Etiology	Age
III. UNILATERAL OR PREDOMINANTLY UNILATERAL SEIZURES Seizures in which the clinical and electrographic aspects are analogous to those of the preceding group (II), except that the clinical signs are restricted principally, if not exclusively, to one side of the body and the electrographic discharges are recorded over the contralateral hemisphere. Such seizures apparently depend upon a generalized or at least very diffuse neuronal discharge with predominates in, or is restricted to, a single hemisphere and its subcortical connections.					
Characterized by clonic, tonic, or tonic-clonic convulsions, with or without an impairment of consciousness, expressed only or predominantly in one side. Such seizures sometimes shift from one side to the other but usually do not become symmetrical	Partial discharge very rapidly spreading over only one hemisphere (corresponding with only contralateral seizures), or:	Focal contralateral discharges	Cortical and/or subcortical region in one hemisphere	Wide variety of focal, unilateral lesions, generally in immature brain (constitutional factors may be important)	Almost exclusively in very young children
	Discharges generalized from the start but considerably predominant over one hemisphere, susceptible to change from one side to the other at different moments (corresponding to alternating seizures)	Bilateral and synchronous symmetrical or asymmetrical discharges of spike and waves and/or polyspike and waves	Unlocalized (? mesodiencephalon)	No cause found, or: Diffuse or multiple bilateral lesions, and/or: toxic metabolic perturbations, and/or: constitutional, often genetic factors (epileptic predisposition), generally in immature brain	Almost exclusively in very young children
	Partial discharge, susceptible to change, from time to time, in morphology and topography (from area to area and, sometimes, from one side to the other)	Focal discharges, susceptible to change, from time to time, in morphology and topography	Cortical and/or subcortical region in one or both hemispheres, or unlocalized	Focal or diffuse lesions of diverse etiology or metabolic and/or toxic. Constitutional factors and cerebral immaturity are important	Limited virtually to the newborn

ondary to chronic obstructive disease and in the treatment of depressive drug overdose, decrease synaptic resistance by blocking the effects of GABA.[19] Local application of penicillin to the cortex has the same effect.[19,48]

Other chemical transmitters are excitatory and reduce the potential difference across the cell membrane.[62,63] They increase the efficiency of transmission and have a depolarizing action. Acetylcholine is a proven excitatory transmitter that may be effective in the ascending reticular activating system.[48] Norepinephrine, dopamine, and 5-hydroxytryptamine may mediate transmission in several tracts radiating from the brainstem to the cerebrum and spinal cord. The amino acids L-glutamate and L-aspartate are thought to be transmitters in afferent and efferent central pathways, respectively.[48]

The behaviors exhibited with a convulsion vary depending upon the spread of a seizure discharge from one area of the cortex to another. Motor, sensory, and psychic phenomena may be combined in a number of different sequences.[73] Little is known about what facilitates or inhibits the spread of seizure activity from one part of the brain to another.

It may be difficult to identify the etiology of a convulsive disorder. Both physiologic and psychologic stimuli can evoke a seizure: a flash of light; a series of monotonous or musical tones; touching, rubbing, or hurting a body part; and being subjected to fright or strong emotion have all been described.[73] Numerous disease states may also be accompanied by seizure activity. Febrile disorders associated with significant temperature elevations, bacterial meningitis, uremia, and other disorders such as cardiac arrest, respiratory failure, carbon monoxide poisoning, and NO_2 anesthesia that cause hypoxic encephalopathy may induce seizures. Seizures also occur during withdrawal periods in patients addicted to alcohol or barbiturates. They may also accompany electrolyte imbalance and glucose alterations, and may appear in the terminal phases of many other illnesses.

Numerous physiologic changes are associated with generalized seizure activity. Few systems are immune. Cardiovascular changes include an initial increase in both systolic and diastolic pressure, together with a marked tachycardia that may slow when blood pressure peaks. The arterial hypertension and tachycardia are caused by increased sympathetic stimulation. Late in status epilepticus the blood pressure may fall below normal and hypotension may persist. Cerebral blood flow increases during the early phases of generalized seizure activity either caused by direct neuronally mediated vasodilatation or as a consequence of autonomic discharge related to the seizure activity. Central venous pressure also rises dramatically at the onset and can remain elevated or return to normal.

Respiratory effects are varied and depend on the type of seizure. Tachypnea and transient apnea occur with tonic seizures, and a simple change in respiratory rate is often one of the most obvious signs in petit mal activity. The Pao_2 and $Paco_2$ also may be altered. Initially, oxygen levels may be normal, low, or high; the $Paco_2$ is usually elevated. During the late stages, the Pao_2 is either normal or low, whereas the arterial carbon dioxide level is normal to high. These changes may be a result of the direct effect of cerebral seizure activity on the brainstem respiratory center, the presence of abnormal motor activity that impairs breathing mechanics, or the influence of peripheral autonomic seizure activities that impair gas exchange.

The endocrine consequences of seizure activity are complex. Hyperglycemia follows generalized seizure activity. The blood sugar begins to rise immediately and peaks within 15 to 30 minutes after the onset of the seizure.[62] In some individuals, this is followed by a period of hypoglycemia traceable primarily to the action of insulin, although increased glucose consumption may also play a role.[62]

Generalized seizures also activate the adrenocortical response, resulting in a marked increase in plasma cortisol.[63]

Activation of the autonomic nervous system occurs in generalized tonic seizures.

Metabolic changes occur in the brain both during and as a consequence of seizure activity. Animal studies show an increase in cerebral metabolism.[63] In the presence of an adequate oxygen concentration, the brain is able to increase the rate of oxidative metabolism to produce the high-energy phosphate compounds required for active transport mechanisms.

Impairment in mobility

Impairment in mobility may represent a disorder of the motor system at some point from the cells of the motor cortex to the muscle fiber. It may be manifested as (1) paralysis due to lower motor neuron disease, (2) paralysis secondary to diseases of the upper motor neurons (corticospinal and corticobrainstem), (3) abnormalities of coordination with cerebellar lesions, (4) abnormalities in movement or posture related to disorders in the extrapyramidal motor tract, or (5) apraxic or nonparalytic movements secondary to cerebral involvement.[73]

Paralysis resulting from disease of the lower motor neurons

Damage to the lower motor neuron at some point between the anterior horn cell of the spinal cord and the neuromuscular junction can destroy all voluntary, postural, and reflex movements.[1] The muscle becomes lax and soft or flaccid. Muscle tone is reduced. Ultimately, the denervated muscle atrophies. The muscle stretch reflex is lost. If only a portion of the muscle fibers that supply a muscle is involved, paralysis or paresis ensues, the muscle atrophies less, and the deep reflexes are diminished rather than lost.

The distribution of paralysis depends on the locus of damage. Motor nerve fibers from the anterior roots intermingle with adjacent roots, forming plexuses that innervate muscles segmentally. Whereas each large muscle is supplied by two or more roots, a single peripheral nerve normally provides the complete motor innervation for a muscle or group of muscles. Therefore, paralysis caused by disease of the anterior horn cells differs from that which follows a lesion of a peripheral nerve.[1]

The coexistence of sensory changes usually indicates involvement of mixed motor and sensory nerves or affection of both anterior and posterior roots.[1] In the absence of sensory changes, the lesion may be found in the anterior gray matter of the spinal cord, in the anterior roots, in a motor branch of a peripheral nerve, or in motor axons alone.[1,73]

Paralysis resulting from disease of the upper motor neuron

Paralytic lesions may interrupt the integrity of the corticospinal pathways at many levels. Lesions may be found in the cerebral cortex, subcortical white matter, internal capsule, brainstem, and spinal cord.[1] In only a few documented cases has a pure lesion of the corticospinal system been isolated.[81] Usually, more is involved than just the pyramidal tract.

Although the distribution of paralysis resulting from upper motor neuron disease varies with the locale of the lesion, there are several characteristic features common to all paralytic lesions resulting from upper motor neuron disease. A group of muscles, rather than individual muscles, is always involved. The paralysis never involves all of the muscles on one side of the body, even in severe hemiplegia.[1,73] If volitional movement is possible, the maximum effort is attained, although more slowly than in the normal limb.[73]

Bilateral movements, such as those of the eyes, jaw, pharynx, larynx, neck, thorax, and abdomen are affected minimally, if at all, by lesions in the upper motor neurons.[1,73] Most severely affected are the hand and arm muscles. The leg muscles are next. Of the cranial musculature, only the lower facial and tongue muscles are involved to any significant degree.[73] At lower levels of the cord, lesions may also cause the temporary abolishment of spinal reflexes subserved by segments below the involved area. Referred to as *spinal shock,* this condition is characterized by a period of flaccidity and areflexia followed, after a few days, by a period of hypertonus and spasticity.[1] These changes are not as sharply defined with cerebral lesions as they are with spinal ones. In some instances, both spasticity and paralysis develop together; in others, muscles remain flaccid but reflexes are retained.

Corticospinal lesions are associated with certain involuntary movements known as synkinesias.[73] A paralyzed arm may move suddenly during stretching and yawning. Attempts to flex the arm may result in involuntary pronation. Flexion of the leg may cause plantar dorsiflexion or may cause the foot to evert automatically.

Motor disturbances resulting from cerebellar disease

Diseases of the cerebellum may interfere with balance and coordination. Interruption of the fastigioreticulospinal and dentatorubrothalamocortical fibers blocks cerebellar facilitation. Depressed fusimotor efferent activity in the spinal cord leads to decreased spindle afferent discharge and lessened tonic facilitation of alpha motor neuronal activity.[73] Both of these factors have been used to provide a physiologic explanation for the tremors, ataxia, and hypotonia that develop with cerebellar lesions.

Isolated cerebellar lesions can create grave equilibrium disturbances, which often are manifested when the patient attempts to stand and walk. Involvement of the anterior lobe of the cerebellum results in a disturbance in coordination of volitional movement in the ipsilateral side. This is called ataxia and is characterized by an inappropriate range, rate, and strength of each of the various components of a motor act and by an improper coordination of these components.[73] The lack of coordination is termed asynergia. These defects occur most noticeably in actions that require rapid alternation of movements. Hypotonia is also present and may account for the failure of the antagonistic muscles to come into play at the appropriate time. The patient frequently experiences intention tremors, rhythmic jerks, and oscillations in movements requiring accurate direction.

Lesions of the lateral and inferior cerebellar hemispheres are characterized by ataxia, asynergia, and dysmetria with hypotonia and little intention tremors.[73]

Bilateral lesions cause a severe disturbance in all movements, inhibiting the patient from standing or walking. These are also associated with ocular and speech disorders, including nystagmus and dysmetria, skew deviation of the eyes, and dysarthria.[1,73] Involvement of the cerebellar peduncles results in similar symptomatology.

Movement and posture abnormalities resulting from diseases of the basal ganglia

Motor and postural abnormalities may also be attributed to diseases of the basal ganglia. Lesions can lead to functional deficits or may result in the release or disinhibition of activity of other undamaged portions of the motor nervous system.[1] Because the basal ganglia are involved in the maintenance and programming of stereotyped repetitive and routine motor behavior[31] and appear to suppress unwanted movements, disorders can produce both akinesia and a loss of normal postural reflexes. Akinesia is the absence or disturbance of motion in a muscle without significant diminishment of strength. Involuntary movements (chorea, athetosis, and dystonia) also occur. Choreic movements are arrhythmic, forcible, rapid, and jerky in nature. They may be limited to only one side of the body. Often, these movements are superimposed on voluntary movements and become exaggerated and grotesque. Chorea can be combined with athetosis, a condition characterized by an inability to sustain a body part in one position. Abnormal athetoid movements alternating between extension-pronation, flexion-extension, etc., are common, making discrete voluntary movement difficult. Athetosis may involve all four limbs or may be unilateral. Dystonia refers to an abnormal tonicity of the muscle. Often described as an overextended or overflexed posture, it is closely allied with athetoid movements, differing only in the duration or persistence of the abnormality and the disproportionate involvement of larger axial muscles.[1,73]

Apraxic or nonparalytic movements

Apraxia describes a disorder in motility in which learned sequences of movement are deranged. The apraxic patient has no weakness, is not ataxic, and suffers no other extrapyramidal disorder or loss of the primary modes of sensation. Frequently this individual fails to execute certain acts in the correct context, while retaining the ability to facilitate movements upon which such acts depend.[1]

The cause of apraxic movements can be identified by considering the neural connections in different regions of the cerebral cortex. A lesion that interferes with the connections between the left supramarginal and premotor regions leads to apraxia of both the right and left extremities.[1] Aphasia is also present. Apraxia of the left limbs occurs only with a lesion of the collosal pathway that interrupts the connections between the left and right motor cortex.[73] Normally, this disorder is located at or near the origin of this pathway and includes the Broca's area as well as the left motor cortex. Consequently, a motor speech disorder and a right hemiplegia are apparent, together with apraxia of the nonparalyzed left extremity.[1] Facial apraxia is characteristic, with lesions involving the left supramarginal gyrus or the left motor association cortex. Such lesions may also be associated with apraxia of the limbs. Only the facial musculature will be affected, with lesions restricted to the facial area of the left motor cortex.[1] Apraxic disorders of gait occur with diseases that affect the medial parts of the frontal lobe.[1]

Sensory dysfunction

Although sensory and motor functions are interdependent, loss or impairment of sensory function may occur independently and may be the primary manifestation of neurologic disease.

Somatic sensation depends on impulses excited by the adequate stimulation of receptors that communicate with the CNS via afferent sensory fibers. These receptors are of two types. Exteroceptors are located in the skin and transmit sensory information about temperature, touch, and pain. Proprioceptors, found in the deeper somatic structures, interpret the body's position in space, the force, direction, and range of movements of the joints, and pressure. Cutaneous fibers are carried in sensory fibers or in mixed sensory and motor fibers. Proprioceptive fibers run primarily in motor nerves. The segmental distribution of sensory information is shown in Fig. 4-8. There is considerable overlapping from one segment to another, especially in respect to touch. Sensory information is transmitted to the spinal cord via afferent fibers, into dorsal or posterior roots. Ascending pathways communicate this data to the CNS, where several areas of the cerebral cortex are involved in the perception of sensory stimuli. Fine sensory discrimination involves the sensory cortex.

Sensory dysfunction may be manifested in several ways. Tactile sensation may be completely lost (anesthesia), or an intermediate level of dysfunction may occur in which some sensation is preserved but the ability to discriminate such things as objects and shapes is lost. This phenomenon is explained by the existence of two distinct systems of receptive end organs and conducting neurons: (1) a protopathic system that transmits information about pain and temperature, providing a diffuse, poorly localized impression of the sensation; and (2) an epicritic system that perceives fine variations in touch and temperature.

Other derangements in sensation include dysesthesia, paresthesia, hypesthesia, and hyperesthesia. *Dysesthesia* describes an unpleasant or painful sensory experience induced by a stimulus that ordinarily is painless. A prickling, burning, or tingling sensation, often characterized as feelings of "pins and needles," is called *paresthesia,* whereas a diminution of sensation is called *hypesthesia.* An abnormally increased sensitivity to various stimuli is known as *hyperesthesia.*

Disturbances in sensation can be the result of an interruption of a single peripheral nerve fiber or may be attributable to the involvement of multiple nerves or multiple spinal nerve roots. Dysfunction may also be traced to either complete or partial transection of the spinal cord, lesions of the central gray matter, brainstem, thalamus, or parietal lobe. Also implicated is infarction of the spinal cord.

Disturbances resulting from interruption of a single peripheral nerve

The changes that occur when a single fiber is involved depend on the composition of the affected nerve and whether it is predominantly muscular, cutaneous, or mixed. Because pain fibers overlap, the area of tactile anesthesia is greater with lesions of cutaneous nerves. In addition, because adjacent nerves also overlap, the area of sensory loss after division of a cutaneous nerve is generally less than its anatomic distribution. The sensory defect, when a large area of skin is affected, usually consists of a central portion of anesthesia surrounded by an area of partial loss that becomes less marked as the distance from the center to the periphery increases. The skin along the margin of this zone becomes more sensitive. Deep pressure response and passive movement remain intact, since these modalities are mediated by subcutaneous structures.

Various lesions affect sensory nerve fibers differently. Compression may paralyze larger touch and pressure fibers, leaving smaller pain, thermal, and autonomic fibers untouched.[1] With lesions of the brachial and lumbosacral plexuses, the sensory disturbance is more widespread and is associated with muscle weakness and reflex changes.[73]

Disturbances resulting from involvement of multiple nerves

Sensory dysfunction resulting from polyneuropathy involves all the modalities and is usually symmetric, except in diabetic and periarteritic neuropathy. The loss of sensation is most remarkable over the feet and legs, since the longest and largest fibers tend to be the most affected. The change from normal to impaired sensation is gradual and is associated with varying degrees of motor and reflex loss.

Disturbances resulting from involvement of multiple spinal nerve roots

The division of a single sensory root does not produce complete anesthesia, because there is a good deal of overlap from adjacent roots. Varying degrees of sensory loss occur in a segmental pattern, with loss of pain sensation being greater than loss of the touch sensation. With multiple root involvement, there is an area of complete sensory loss surrounded by a narrow region of partial loss. Tendon and muscular reflexes can also be lost. The involvement of the ventral roots is suggested in the presence of muscle weakness and atrophy.

Disturbances resulting from spinal cord lesions

Complete or partial transection of the spinal cord produces various symptoms, depending on the site of the lesion. With complete transection, all forms of sensation are lost below the level of the lesion. Pain, temperature, and touch anesthesia occur one or two segments below the injury, whereas vibratory and position senses have a less discrete level. Often there is a narrow zone of hyperesthesia along the upper margin of sensory loss. The exact level of the lesion may be difficult to discern, since it may evolve from the periphery to the center of the cord, or vice versa. The former affects the outermost fibers first, producing symptoms accordingly; the latter may involve these modalities in a reverse manner.

Hemisection of the spinal cord results in the loss of pain and temperature sensation on the contralateral side two segments below the lesion. Proprioception is absent on the ipsilateral side. Tactile sensation is unaffected, because fibers that mediate this modality are distributed in the posterior columns and anterior spinothalamic tract.

Disturbances resulting from lesions that involve the posterior roots

Lesions that involve the large proprioceptive fibers and other fibers of the posterior lumbosacral roots result in a loss of vibratory and position sense, primarily in the feet and legs. A loss of superficial or deep pain sense or of touch may occur in severe cases. Bladder atonicity is also noted.

Disturbances resulting from lesions of gray matter

Involvement of the central gray matter leads to the abolition of pain and temperature on one or both sides over several segments (dermatomes). Such lesions have little effect on the sense of touch. Extension to other parts of the gray matter results in differing degrees of segmental amyotrophy and reflex loss. Additional sensory dysfunction may develop if the lesion spreads to the white matter.

Disturbances resulting from brainstem diseases

Brainstem disorders cause a variety of sensory alterations, depending on the exact locus of the lesion. Because the crossed trigemino-thalamic and lateral spinothalamic tracts run together in the upper medulla, pons, and mid-brain, a lesion in these areas results in the loss of pain and thermal sense on the opposite half of the body. A lesion that occupies the upper brainstem causes a loss of all superficial and deep sensation over the contralateral side. This can be attributed to the confluence of the spinothalamic tract and the medial lemniscus in this region. Cranial nerve palsies, cerebellar ataxia, or motor paralysis can also occur. Involvement of other lateral medullary regions often creates sensory disturbances that are crossed. Pain and temperature are lost on one side of the face and on the opposite side of the body. This is caused by the influence of the trigeminal tract or nucleus and the lateral spinothalamic tract on one side of the brainstem.

Disturbances resulting from thalamic lesions

All forms of sensation on the contralateral side of the body are lost or diminished with thalamic lesions. Position sense is frequently af-fected, and deep sensory loss is usually greater than cutaneous sensory loss. Involvement of the posterolateral ventral nucleus of the thalamus may also result in ipsilateral pain or discomfort that can be rather severe. This distress is often accentuated during emotional disturbances. Although persons with this type of lesion tend to "overrespond" to a stimulus, they frequently exhibit an elevated pain threshold.

Disturbances resulting from lesions of the parietal lobe

Parietal lobe lesions interfere with discriminative sensory functions. The face, arm, and leg on the contralateral side are primarily affected. Classically, position sense is lost. Touch and pain stimuli are difficult to localize. Elevation of two-point threshold, astereognosis, and tactile agnosia are common, the latter occurring with a lesion situated in the dominant hemisphere. Sensory extinction or inattention is also characteristic. When symmetric bilateral body parts are tested at the same time, the stimulus may be acknowledged on the sound side or may be improperly localized on the affected side. Appropriate responses are elicited with stimuli applied separately to each side.

Pain, temperature, touch, and vibratory senses may also be impaired with lesions of the parietal cortex. The response to testing is variable, with no sensory dysfunction at all noted on occasion. In other instances, sensory abnormalities have been reported. This type of response has been attributed to hysteria. A circumscribed loss of superficial sensation has also been documented in lesions confirmed to be in the parietal cortex.[1]

Speech and language disorders

Speech and language disorders may be categorized as follows:

1. Cerebral disturbances that result in the loss more or less exclusively of the production or comprehension of spoken speech or written language; this condition is called *aphasia* or *dysphasia*.

2. Defects in articulation that occur in the presence of intact mental functions and normal comprehension and memory of words; can be attributed to a motor disorder of the muscles of articulation and may result from flaccid or spastic paralysis, rigidity, stuttering, or ataxia; called *dysarthria* and *anarthria*

3. Disturbances of speech and language that occur with diseases involving the higher nervous integrations; for example, delirium and dementia; speech is usually not lost but rather deranged

4. Loss of voice secondary to disease of the larynx or its innervation; articulation and inner language are not affected; this is called *aphonia* or *dysphonia*[1,73]

Only the first category will be considered at this time.

Aphasia can be defined as a general impairment of language function resulting from localized pathologic conditions of the cerebrum. There are several varieties of aphasia that can usually be identified with a systematic clinical examination. The most easily recognizable type of aphasia is complete or global aphasia, in which all or almost all speech and language functions are lost. A second major type involves the motor, verbal, and expressive sides of language; this is called *motor* or *Broca's aphasia*. A third variety, *Wernicke's aphasia,* is a receptive form of aphasia with interruption of all language-dependent behaviors. A number of dissociative syndromes exist, such as conduction aphasia, word deafness, word blindness, nominal or amnestic aphasia, pure word mutism, transcortical aphasia, and agraphia.

Complete global aphasia

Global aphasia occurs with a lesion that destroys a large portion of the speech areas of the major cerebral hemispheres. Although it may result from hemorrhage, tumor, or other lesions or may occur as a postictal effect, it is usually caused by an occlusion of the left internal carotid or middle cerebral artery at its origin. The latter blood vessel provides the blood supply to all of the language area of the brain.

Global aphasia affects all aspects of speech and language. Most patients with this form of aphasia cannot read or write and can understand only a few words or phrases. They may be able to perform simple, universally understood gestures. With time, some degree of understanding of spoken speech may be apparent, and they may become able to speak a few words. Clinically, the picture becomes one of expressive aphasia. Rapid improvement is characteristic when the cause is cerebral edema, postconvulsive paralysis, or temporary metabolic disorders that cause old lesions that had affected language areas to worsen. Some deficit may persist with speech loss from a disintegrating embolus of the left middle cerebral artery.

Motor or Broca's aphasia (minor motor aphasia)

Broca's aphasia refers to a primary deficit in language output or speech production. Minor motor aphasia is caused by sharp focal lesions along the anterior and superior sylvian operculum and insula. None of the resulting deficiencies are significant or long lasting. Lesions affect the mechanical elaboration of speech in a circumscribed pattern that depends on the site and extent of the disorder.

There are several forms of focal opercular lesions. Broca's area infarction affects the lower premotor cortex adjacent to the motor cortex for the oropharynx, larynx, and respiratory apparatus. Skilled movements of these muscle groups are damaged. Clinically, the transitions between syllables and words is deranged. In addition, the melodic intonation of phrases is disrupted. Rolandic infarction affects the sensorimotor cortex. It is characterized by poor articulation, lowered volume and pitch of speech, and a nasal quality to the voice. Postcentral anterior parietal infarction leads to errors in the positioning of the oral cavity for individual sounds, syllables, and whole words. All of these types of aphasia may resemble major motor aphasia, except that spoken and written words are understood satisfactorily.

Major motor aphasia is characterized by a failure of the motor aspects of speaking and writing that is accompanied by an agrammatism and a variable deficit in language comprehension. This defect is thought to be caused by a large lesion that affects the cortical and subcortical structures along the frontal and superior sylvian fissure, including the insula. This area is supplied by the upper division of the left middle cerebral artery.

Initially, the entire language mechanism is inactivated. A right hemiparesis and hemisensory syndrome frequently develop and persist. A transient right hemianopia, accompanied by an ipsilateral deviation of the eyes, is also characteristic.

After weeks to years, the disorder of comprehension abates slightly. Speaking and writing deficits remain.

Wernicke's aphasia

Wernicke's aphasia is characterized by impaired comprehension of words and objects, and a general impairment of language-dependent behavior. These deficits reflect involvement of the auditory association areas or their separation from the angular gyrus and the primary auditory cortex of Heschl's transverse gyri.[1]

Wernicke, in his 1874 monograph, theorized that the conduction of sensory impulses to motor patterns was impaired in these individuals;[46] hence the name conduction aphasia.

This defect does not reflect a disturbance in hearing or vision. The speech of Wernicke's aphasia is fluent and paragrammatic; however, it is marked by word substitutions, nonsense words, and poor circumlocution. There is normal intonation but poor comprehension and ability to repeat.

The lesion that causes this speech and language disorder occupies the perisylvian region and usually results from embolic occlusion of the lower division of the left middle cerebral artery. A slit hemorrhage in the subcortex of the tem-

poroparietal region or the presence of a tumor, abscess, or the extension of a small putaminal or thalamic hemorrhage may elicit similar symptoms.[1,73]

Conduction aphasia

Conduction aphasics are relatively fluent, have good comprehension but poor ability to repeat, and a number of phonemic paraphasias. In many features these individuals resemble other aphasics. As in Wernicke's aphasia, speech in fluent. Also, there is paraphasia in self-initiated speech, in repeating what is heard, and in reading out loud. Writing is also impaired. In contrast to Wernicke's aphasia, these aphasics have minimal difficulty in understanding, are aware of their own deficiencies, and attempt to correct them. Since repetition is severely affected, it is this that must be tested specifically to identify conduction aphasics.

The lesion has been found in the cortex and subcortical white matter in the upper bank of the sylvian fissure. It apparently involves the supramarginal gyrus of the inferior parietal lobule and, on occasion, the posterior portion of the superior temporal region.[1,48] The critical structure is the arcuate fasciculus, a fiber tract extending out of the temporal lobe proceeding around the posterior end of the sylvian fissure, where it joins the superior longitudinal fasciculus. From there it proceeds forward through the suprasylvian opercular region to the motor association cortex, including Broca's area.[1,48]

Although the usual cause is an embolus in the ascending parietal or posterior temporal branch of the middle cerebral artery, other types of vascular lesions, neoplasm, or trauma may have a similar effect.[1]

Word deafness

This syndrome is characterized by impaired auditory comprehension and an inability to repeat what is said or to write dictation.[73] Visual comprehension, while not normal, is far better than auditory comprehension.

Pure word deafness, also called auditory verbal agnosia, is an uncommon disorder thought to be caused by a bilateral lesion located in the middle thirds of the superior temporal gyri. Consequently it damages the connections between the primary auditory cortex in the transverse superoposterior portion of the temporal lobe.[1] A few unilateral lesions have been found in part of the dominant temporal lobe.[48] The cause is an occlusive embolus of a small branch of the lower division of the middle cerebral artery.[1]

Word blindness

Word blindness describes a syndrome in which an individual may recognize individual letters but not words. The person can write fluently but cannot read what has been written. Spoken language is easily understood and can be repeated without difficulty. Conversation remains intact. In lesser degrees of severity, reading out loud is possible, but usually a single letter at a time.

This disorder is often discovered accidentally. In modern terminology, it is often referred to as "alexia without agraphia."[46]

Usually the lesion destroys the left visual cortex and underlying white matter, especially the geniculocalcarine tract, as well as the connections of the right visual cortex with the intact language areas of the dominant hemisphere.[1] It has also been found confined to the deep central white matter of the left parietooccipital region, where it interrupts the connections between the angular gyrus and both occipital lobes. In this situation, alexia may be combined with agraphia and with anomic aphasia and elements of Gerstmann syndrome.*

Amnestic aphasia

Amnestic or anomic aphasia encompasses the largest group of aphasics. These persons

have little expressive or receptive difficulty but rather lose the ability to name objects. The anomic aphasic pauses during speech, groping for words. Typically the patient substitutes another word or phrase that will convey the same meaning (circumlocution).

The causative lesion is situated deep in the temporal lobe, where it interrupts connections of sensory speech areas with the hippocampal-parahippocampal regions involved with learning and memory.[73] The lesion may be neoplastic, may be traced to an otogenic abscess, or may be attributable to an occlusion of the temporal branches of the posterior cerebral artery.[1]

Pure word mutism

Also called *subcortical* or *peripheral motor aphasia of Goldstein* or *anarthria of Marie,* pure word mutism occurs as a result of a vascular lesion or some local injury. It is characterized by a complete inability to speak. The ability to write, verbal comprehension, and visual comprehension remain intact.

Although the anatomic basis of the syndrome has yet to be determined, a lesion in the Broca's area has been implicated.

Transcortical aphasia

The destruction of the border zones between anterior, middle, and posterior cerebral arteries results in a disorder characterized by a deficit of auditory and visual word comprehension. Writing and reading are also impossible. Speech is fluent with marked paraphasia, anomia, and empty circumlocution. They may be able to echo word phrases.[1]

Agraphia

Agraphia is a syndrome characterized by the inability to express thoughts in writing. Pure agraphia is rare, although it has been described; it has been associated with a lesion of the posterior perisylvian area.[82] Frequently this disorder is found concurrently with another disturbance such as alexia, constructional apraxia, acalculia, and similar disorders.[46]

---

*Gerstmann syndrome—a disorder caused by a lesion in the angular gyrus of the dominant hemisphere that results in a combination of finger agnosia, right-left disorientation, agraphia, acalculia, and often constrictional apraxia.

INTERVENTIONS

Management of the patient with neurologic dysfunction requires continuous assessment to maintain life at the highest possible level. Problems that develop must be recognized and dealt with to prevent complications through appropriate intervention.

The principles of care are similar, regardless of the cause of the disorder. Because the central nervous system interacts with multiple body systems, circulatory, respiratory, temperature, gastrointestinal, urinary, integumentary, and musculoskeletal functions must be regularly evaluated.

Improved diagnostic studies, coupled with new surgical therapies and a number of intensive care measures, have significantly enhanced the survival rate for many persons with neurologic alterations. Measures including controlled ventilations, continuous ICP monitoring and aggressive control of ICP spikes, as well as institution of barbiturate coma, have contributed greatly to the reduction in mortality.

Surgical therapy[41]

Surgical therapy of neurologic disease is directed at returning the brain and spinal cord to as near normal anatomic location and physiologic function as possible. Surgery for victims of trauma involves removing mass lesions, usually hematomas from the intracranial space, and closure of defects in the normal coverings of the brain, especially the dura and the skin. Defects in the dura are usually closed with grafts of tissue from the pericranium or fascia lata. Surgery for trauma to the spine is infrequent and is aimed at reinstituting normal alignment and stability of the spine as well as removal of material impinging on the spinal cord. Surgery is usually not performed on patients who show evidence of complete anatomic or physiologic transection of the spinal cord.

Operations for brain and spinal cord tumors are aimed at removal of as much of the tumor as possible without increasing the neurologic deficit. The ability to remove the tumor is re-

lated not only to tumor type but also to location and adherence to adjacent vital structures.

Vascular surgery attempts to reconstitute normal cerebral flow or to obliterate anomalies. Intracranial aneurysms are obliterated in several ways. The ideal method is to occlude the aneurysm at its neck with a clip, keeping the parent vessel patent. When clipping is impossible, coating the aneurysm with plastic after wrapping it in gauze is effective. Another method is to occlude the parent vessel on each side of the aneurysm. This depends on adequate collateral flow through the vessels beyond the occlusion. The flow can be asegmented by surgically anastomosing a scalp vessel to the occluded vessel beyond the occlusion. Bypass is also performed for patients with transient ischemic attacks (TIAs) from stenosis or occlusion of the cerebral arteries resulting from atherosclerosis or anomalies. Removal of the offending atheromatous plaque (endarterectomy) can be performed on the carotid artery in the neck.

Increased ICP that is unresponsive to medical therapy can occasionally be lowered by decompressive craniotomy in which a large portion of the skull is removed and the dura mater is opened, thereby increasing intracranial volume.

Medical therapy
Respiratory function

Respiratory medical treatment of neurologic disease is based on (1) maintenance of adequate tissue perfusion and oxygenation and (2) prevention of further deficits. Maintenance of an adequate airway is of paramount importance in maintaining adequate cerebral oxygenation. Obtunded patients are at high risk for aspiration of material into the tracheal bronchial tree and obstruction of their airways. Abnormal respiratory patterns resulting from neurologic disease, such as Cheyne-Stokes respiration and central neurogenic hyperventilation, often lead to problems with acid-base balance and poor oxygenation.

Endotracheal intubation is necessary in most

severely obtunded patients. It is important, however, for the intubation to be rapid and smooth, without prolonged coughing or apnea. Prolonged laryngoscopy with associated hypertension, bucking, or prolonged apnea lead to significantly increased ICP. The increase can be damaging or fatal to the patient with poor cerebral compliance. Sedation with thiopental or inducing paralysis by administration of a muscle relaxant is often necessary. If time permits, giving an osmotic diuretic first will decrease ICP and allow a larger margin of error during the intubation. The goal of intubation should be to maintain normal arterial blood gases and pH. However, as mentioned earlier, decreasing P_{CO_2} is a very effective way of lowering intracranial pressure through decreasing intracranial blood volume. The lower limit to which P_{CO_2} should be lowered is approximately 20 mmHg, or a pH higher than 7.55 to 7.60 as cardiac irritability increases significantly with increasing pH. The most effective way to decrease P_{CO_2} uses controlled ventilation with a tidal volume of 10 to 15 cc/kg and a respiratory rate of 10 to 12. Increasing the rate prevents adequate expansion of the lungs, leading to atelectasis, fever, and inadequate gas exchange.

Adequate ventilation and airway protection are of first priority in comatose patients. If the comatose patient is breathing, ventilation is maintained by mask until cervical spine fracture has been ruled out; then intubation is performed. If ventilation by mask is impossible or the neck is fractured, then nasotracheal intubation is important. Emergency tracheostomy is indicated for some severe facial injuries.

Cardiac function

Cardiovascular stability is of utmost importance. Abnormalities in blood pressure, either hypotension or hypertension, require immediate attention. Systolic hypertension may demonstrate evidence of decompensation resulting from increased intracranial pressure, or hypertension may be a preexisting problem that predisposes the person to a stroke. Regardless of the cause, intervention must be initiated to control the symptom. Monitoring the heart rate and rhythm is also essential in identifying potential life-threatening dysrhythmias.

Urinary function

An indwelling catheter may be needed to manage urinary drainage in the unconscious patient. This also permits monitoring of renal function. Such a patient should receive catheter care at least two times daily to minimize the risk of ascending infection. Continuous bladder irrigations with normal saline and antibiotic solution may also be helpful.

Gastrointestinal function

The nutritional needs of the neurologic patient, especially one who is unconscious, can be complex. Nutrition must be adequate to maintain body function and combat infection. Tube feedings may be necessary for the patient who is unconscious for a long period of time. Unit 6 reviews the principles involved in the enteral feeding.

The regimen for bowel care must also be followed. A drug program that uses stool softeners and laxatives may be instituted to aid in the prevention of constipation and impaction. Enemas are contraindicated in the patient with increased intracranial pressure, since they would initiate a Valsalva-like response that would, in turn, cause further increase in the intracranial pressure.

Integumentary function

Since the skin provides a protective barrier and the first line of defense against infection, its integrity is essential. The thin, bedridden patient is most likely to have bony prominences that are subject to breakdown. Obese patients with folds of skin are also at risk for skin breakdown. A basic plan of care that emphasizes turning and proper positioning, coupled with the use of an alternating-pressure mattress, will minimize the incidence of decubitus development and pulmonary complications.

Musculoskeletal function

Maintenance of muscle tone and prevention of orthopedic disabilities are constant concerns when caring for many patients with neurologic dysfunction. Muscle tone, muscle bulk loss, ankylosis, and contractures can develop quickly in the patient receiving bed rest. These persons who do not bear weight also lose calcium from their bones. This can lead to osteoporosis and renal calculi. A program to prevent functional loss should include frequent repositioning, range-of-motion exercises, and early rehabilitation.

Positioning. The patient should be positioned to prevent deformity. A firm, supportive mattress with a bedboard and alternating-pressure mattress is ideal. A sufficient number of pillows must be available for positioning; trochanter rolls, slings, and sand bags may also be helpful. Frequent repositioning is necessary to maintain good body alignment and may be enhanced by the use of special accessories, such as positioner boots. Placing a pillow in the axillary region will help prevent shoulder adduction. Caution must also be taken to avoid external hip rotation that can prolong the rehabilitation process. Special attention should also be given to paralyzed limbs, which should be slightly elevated to prevent the development of dependent edema, a problem that makes normal range-of-motion exercises difficult. Wrist-palm splints may be required to maintain functional position of the hands. The patient should be turned with enough help to prevent initiation of a Valsalva-like response, which can lead in turn to increased intracranial pressure. Ideally, movement should be coordinated with exhalation. A Trendelenburg position is ordinarily contraindicated.

A Stryker frame is used to change the position of patients with spinal cord injuries. This apparatus permits turning without causing further trauma to the spinal cord by maintaining correct anatomic alignment and immobilization. Independence is fostered with the patient lying on the anterior frame, since whenever possible these patients are encouraged to feed themselves and perform some other activities of daily living or light occupational therapy. The Stryker frame should not be used with cervical cord injuries that are being treated by immobilization and hyperextension without Crutchfield tongs. It is also not appropriate for compression fractures of the thoracic and lumbar spine that are reduced by hyperextension. This equipment is contraindicated for exceptionally tall or obese individuals, for whom it would be unsafe.

Exercises. Exercises may be classified as passive (motion provided to the body by another person without voluntary participation), active (independent voluntary motion to a body joint), or active-assistive (motion to a body joint accomplished by the patient with some outside assistance). Passive exercises do not build strength. They increase blood flow and help prevent the development of deformities. The particular exercise program selected depends on the stage of illness and the neurologic disabilities that exist. During the acute phase of illness, passive exercises are normally performed. As the patient's condition improves, he usually becomes more actively involved in his exercise program and may be taken to an area where more sophisticated equipment is available.

Passive exercises should be performed for all body joints that the patient cannot exercise independently. A regular routine should be carried out four times a day to provide a full range of motion to the joint capsules, muscles, and ligaments. It may be incorporated into other procedures but should be done when the patient is rested and pain free, to gain as much cooperation as possible. Body parts should be moved only to the point of resistance or pain. Under close supervision, body parts can be exercised by a physical therapist to stretch and to increase the range of motion. Although stretching may cause some initial discomfort, there should be no residual pain.

To conduct passive range-of-motion exercises properly, the joint must be supported against gravity or any unwanted movement by placing one hand above the joint. The other hand can be used to move the joint gently with a slow, smooth, regular rhythm.

Muscle strength can be increased by isometric or concentric exercises. Isometric exercises are accomplished by alternately tending and relaxing the muscle without joint movement. Concentric exercises shorten muscles.

Endurance is developed by exercises that consist of low resistance and high repetition. The resistance should range between 15% and 40%. Fatigue will increase progressively with the increase in resistance. Because these exercises must be repeated hundreds of times a day, they may become boring. Variations in approach may help to maintain interest to a limited extent.

Cardiovascular and respiratory function should be monitored throughout any exercise routine implemented to develop strength and endurance. Although maximal safe heart rates have been predicted for endurance exercises, cardiac output decreases with the patient's illness and deconditioning, and the maximal heart rate may increase. Guidelines for monitoring should be provided by the appropriate medical personnel.

Neurorehabilitation

The goal of rehabilitation is to restore an individual to former capacity. Although in some situations this may not be possible, neurorehabilitation strives to assist the disabled patient to achieve an optimal physical, emotional, social, and vocational potential. Independence is encouraged to help the patient maintain dignity and self-respect and improve the quality of life. The objective of care is the maintenance of optimal function and prevention of complications.

Rehabilitative efforts should begin early— when the initial patient contact is made. Rehabilitative potential is determined by the health team based on a thorough assessment of the patient. Both short- and long-term goals must be established, with input from the patient. These goals must be reevaluated frequently to make sure that they are both realistic and attainable. Family members or significant others should be actively involved and should be recognized as a potential support system. Discharge planning ought to be instituted early enough to permit the patient and family to participate in the decision-making process.

Several health care professionals are involved in the development and implementation of a comprehensive rehabilitation program. Although the primary physician assumes the overall responsibility for directing the plan of care, the nurse, psychiatrist, physical therapist, speech therapist, occupational therapist, dietitian, vocational counselor, and social worker may be actively involved.

Comprehensive rehabilitative programs must begin with a consideration of proper positioning, range-of-motion exercises, balance and sitting activities, transfer assistance, ambulation, and accessory equipment to aid in ambulation. Such plans often include exercise protocols aimed at building strength and endurance, bladder and bowel retraining programs, speech therapy, and practices or assistive devices used to foster independence in activities of daily living. Patients and families are taught to cope with a variety of neuromuscular defects in programs individualized for their specific problem.

Thermoregulation

All enzyme systems and therefore metabolic processes and energy requirements are temperature dependent. Fever significantly increases energy expenditure throughout the body and brain. A patient can suffer cell damage if the cerebral metabolic rate is increased in the face of poor perfusion. It is therefore most important to reduce fever rapidly in patients with compromised CNS function. To lower fever rapidly, a cause of the fever must be determined to avoid sequelae in patients with CNS damage. Obtunded patients with multiple catheters in the trachea, bladder, and central and peripheral veins are at risk for septic complications. High-dose steroids and antipyretics will often mask fever or WBC response to infection. Barbiturate coma induces poikilothermia (body assumes room temperature) and further blunts fever response to infection.

Intracranial disease can cause significant fever without infection. Subarachnoid hemorrhage, hypothalamic injury from trauma or tumor, and postoperative aseptic meningitis are all well-known causes of "central" fever. The effect of temperature on energy requirement can be exploited to decrease CNS injury through use of induced hypothermia. The effect of hypothermia on decreasing cerebral metabolic rate and increased ICP was discovered in the early 1960s. Clinical trials found much difficulty as a result of shivering, which significantly increased energy needs, skin burns, and cardiac arrhythmia. Therefore inducing hypothermia fell into disfavor. Moderate induced hypothermia is now being used as an adjunct to barbiturate coma for severely increased ICP. The barbiturates will control shivering. Cardiac arrhythmia can be avoided by maintaining normal electrolytes and not allowing the temperature to drop below 32° C (89.6° F). Hypothermia will cause decreased cardiac output. Hypothermia in conjunction with barbiturates (barbiturate coma) requires additional inotropic support.

Fluid and electrolyte management

Fluid and electrolyte management in the patient with CNS injury is very important and much different from other disciplines.[41] Dehydration is a mainstay of treatment of increased ICP. Furthermore, patients with CNS lesions are very susceptible to the syndrome of inappropriate antidiuretic hormone (SIADH). The goal of dehydration is to remove intracellular fluid and decrease cellular volume. To do this, the osmolality of extracellular fluid is increased. Intracellular water will then leave the cell across the cell membrane down the osmotic gradient. The extracellular osmolality is reflected in the serum osmolality. Osmolality is a measure of particles in the blood—either ions, proteins, or drug molecules. It can be directly measured in most hospital laboratories. It can be accurately estimated by the following formula:

$$2 \times [Na^+] + \frac{[Bun]}{3-5} + \frac{[Glucose]}{18} +$$

$$\frac{[ETOH]}{4.2} + \frac{[Mannitol]}{18}$$

It is important when evaluating a serum osmolality value to determine whether the patient's glucose or BUN is elevated, because either will significantly increase osmolality but they have little contribution to establishing an osmotic gradient as both diffuse fairly freely across the cell membrane. Likewise, patients admitted after having received a head trauma will often have high initial osmolality because of prior alcohol ingestion. Mannitol transiently elevates the serum osmolality but is rapidly excreted, and much of its effect on increasing osmolality results from removal of free water during the resultant diuresis.

Dehydration can either be accomplished rapidly, through use of diuretics to remove water, or gradually through fluid restriction. A normal adult will usually consume approximately 2400 ml in 24 hours. A person needs 50 to 100 mEq Na and approximately 60 mEq K each 24 hours to maintain normal electrolyte balance. Restricting fluids to 30% to 50% of normal will lead to gradual dehydration. The serum osmolality will rise exponentially, however. During the first several days of fluid restriction, there will be almost no change in the serum osmolality. However, once serum osmolality begins to rise, it will increase rapidly if fluid restriction is maintained. This is caused by gradual depletion of excess freewater stores, which will maintain normal osmolality until depleted. Therefore frequent measurement of electrolyte values is necessary throughout the period of fluid restriction and should not be stopped after 2 or 3 days of normal values.

Dehydration as a therapeutic measure in CNS disease, beyond a serum osmolality of 320 to 330, is of little use. Above this limit, there is little further reduction in cell size, and there is much increased incidence of renal failure and hyperosmolar coma.

Pharmacologic therapies[41]

Steroids. The effect of steroids on cerebral edema depends on the type and cause of the edema. The effect is most dramatic in the edema surrounding tumors or abscesses. The effect in ischemic and traumatic edema is controversial. Many early studies showed no effect in steroid doses that were effective in tumors. Several studies in recent years have suggested a possible effect of megadose steroids in ischemic infarction and trauma.

Steroids work predominantly through stabilization of cell membranes and free-radical scavenging. It is theorized that steroids work best in vasogenic edema and minimally in cytotoxic edema. There are multiple steroid preparations; decadron has historically been used for intracranial disease. Its theoretic advantages are less fluid retention and less immunosuppression. Several centers are using medrol for trauma and tumors.

Patients receiving steroid replacement therapy because of pituitary or adrenal insufficiency usually take cortisone acetate each morning and evening.

The use of steroids for cerebral edema is most useful if given before the insult. Therefore preoperative craniotomy or spinal cord patients are given steroids for the 24 hours preceding the operation. For prevention or treatment of cerebral edema from brain tumors a 24-hour equivalent dose of dexamethasome will usually be adequate. For trauma or nontraumatic intracerebral hemorrhage, daily divided doses are given for several days, then tapered over 7 to 10 days. In children, the pharmacologic dose is calibrated according to their weight.

Operations on adrenosuppressed or cortisone-dependent patients can safely be performed by pretreating them with hydrocortisone every 24 hours in the intraoperative and postoperative periods. The patient's medication can be changed to oral cortisone acetate when he is eating, with the dosage tapered over 7 to 10 days. The side effects of corticosteroids are numerous; some can be life threatening. None of the side effects, however, is dose dependent once physiologic levels are exceeded. The side effects are, however, related to duration of treatment. Major side effects are upper gastrointestinal hemorrhage and immunosuppression. Prophylactic use of antacids and cimetidine is recommended, especially since this group of patients is at high risk for stress hemorrhage. Steroids can cause an early leukocytosis, which may mask infection. They also delay and decrease the normal inflammatory response to infection. There must be a high index of suspicion for sepsis. Continuing steroid treatment for longer than 30 days leads to adrenal suppression. Steroid doses are usually tapered because of the "rebound" edema that has been reported with abrupt discontinuation. This will also theoretically allow normal adrenal function to return. Steroid "psychosis" is occasionally seen and will not resolve until steroids are stopped. If the patient displays paranoid ideation, hallucinations, and other symptoms of psychosis, antipsychotic medication may be necessary temporarily. Moonface, osteoporosis, and purple striae are other side effects of long-term steroid administration; however, these are not usually seen in neurosurgical patients.

Hyperosmotic agents. Dehydration is a mainstay of treatment of increased ICP. Agents currently used are mannitol, urea, and Furosemide (Lasix). Mannitol and urea are osmotic diuretics that act to transiently increase the serum osmolality and draw fluid from the extravascular space to the intravascular space. The increased osmolality in the renal tubule also leads to increased excretion of free water. The effect of decreasing ICP is caused by removing intracellular fluid, thereby decreasing cell volume. The diuretics probably remove very little "edema fluid," because often there is associated vascular and cell wall damage. No osmotic gradient can develop, because the mannitol will freely diffuse through the damaged vessel or cell wall. The greatest effect is in dehydration of normal cerebral tissue. Furosemide has been used for many years as a diuretic. It acts at the distal renal tubule to inhibit reabsorption of water. In the past several years, it has been shown to effectively decrease ICP. The effect occurs before any demonstrable change in serum osmolality occurs, and its exact mode of action remains unknown. Mannitol and urea each work within 5 minutes and reach peak effectiveness within 20 minutes of administration. The effect lasts 60 minutes. The onset of action of furosemide is within 20 minutes, peaks at approximately 60 minutes, and lasts up to 4 hours. Frequency of administration is best determined by constant ICP monitoring. There is little further decrease in ICP after the serum osmolality has reached 320. Side effects from all diuretics include depletion of electrolytes, especially potassium, and volume depletion. Potassium and sodium supplementation is usually necessary, as is frequent electrolyte measurement. Urea will cause phlebitis and must be infused through a large vein. Rapid infusion of urea is also reported to cause abnormalities with clotting function and cardiac electrical activity. A temporary volume expansion occurs as fluid is drawn into the intravascular space by mannitol and urea, and transient rebound increases in ICP have been reported. This effect can be decreased by elevating the patient's head.

Barbiturates. The effect of barbiturates on ICP was discovered in the 1920s; however, clinical popularity awaited the introduction of routine monitoring of ICP. The drugs used most commonly are thiopental (Pentothal) and pentobarbital (Nembutal) or secobarbital (Seconal).

Barbiturate coma is induced when ICP control has been unsuccessful with diuresis and hyperventilation therapy. Barbiturate coma necessitates total support of the patient. The minimal monitoring necessary involves constant ICP monitoring, constant arterial pressure measurement, and electrocardiograms. The ability to measure central venous pressure (CVP) or pulmonary capillary wedge pressure (PCWP) and pulmonary artery pressure (PAP) is helpful; measurement of cardiac output is also helpful. Controlled ventilation is necessitated by the significant respiratory depression seen with bar-

biturates. The patients are totally dependent on the monitoring systems, and frequent zeroing and calibration of the monitors is mandatory. Long-term administration of large doses of barbiturates will cause myelosuppression, reflected in decreased platelet count and WBC. Temperature regulation is impaired, and frequent measurement of body temperature is necessary. Abnormalities of electrolytes, liver function, and Ca^{+2} and PO^{-4} have been reported in patients in barbiturate coma, possibly as a result of the associated administration of diuretics and steroids.

Barbiturates cause direct myocardial depression and decreased peripheral resistance. Adequate intravascular volume must be maintained; however, inotropic doses of dopamine are often necessary. To induce barbiturate coma, a loading dose of pentobarbital IV push is usually given over 30 minutes, with constant blood pressure monitoring. A maintenance dose of pentobarbital is given every 1 to 2 hours. Serum levels of barbiturates should be kept between 2.5 and 5.0 mg/100 ml. These levels can be exceeded if necessary, if the patient is not hypotensive. Further doses are based on cerebral perfusion pressure, attempting to keep the CPP greater than 40 mmHg. Barbiturate coma is stopped after normal CPP has been maintained for 24 to 48 hours. The dose is gradually decreased. If CPP falls, then coma is reintroduced for another 24 hours.

Barbiturates decrease ICP through reduction of cerebral blood volume. They cause constriction of small afferent arterioles and arteries. A second important effect of barbiturates is protection of cerebral tissue from hypoxic or ischemic damage. Animals that are treated with barbiturates and then undergo occlusion of a cerebral vessel show significant improvement in survival rates and less neurologic impairment than similar animals not given barbiturates. The exact mechanism of cerebral protection is not known; however, barbiturates are known to decrease cerebral metabolic rate and oxygen and glucose consumption. They are believed to stabilize cell membranes in a method similar to that of steroids. Barbiturates also act as free radical scavengers, and neutralize destructive products of cell breakdown.

Anticonvulsants. Treatment of status epilepticus is a medical emergency. The drug of choice for stopping status epilepticus is intravenous diazepam (Valium).

Diazepam, however, will stop the seizure for only 5 to 10 minutes. During this time, phenytoin (Dilantin) or phenobarbital should additionally be given. Diazepam can be used repeatedly; however, respiratory depression is a frequent complication. A diazepam drip has been used to titrate dosage until adequate levels of anticonvulsants can be obtained.

Phenytoin is one of the oldest anticonvulsants. It acts by preventing propagation of epileptogenic impulses. It should not be used in children because of problems with hirsutism, gingival hyperplasia, and coarse facial features. It is the drug of choice in adults.

A major problem with phenytoin is administration to patients that are NPO. Intramuscular administration is painful and leads to sterile abscess, and absorption is erratic. Rapid intravenous administration will lead to cardiac conduction delay. The cardiac effect is related to age and rate of administration. If administration is kept to a rate less than 50 mg/min, problems are rare, except in elderly persons. Constant cardiac monitoring is recommended. Soluset administration is not recommended by the manufacturer because of precipitation in the tubing. Bradycardia and heart block are reversible by decreasing rate or stopping administration if diagnosed early. Phenytoin will also cause phlebitis, and skin loss at the site of infiltration has been seen.

Phenobarbital is a very safe drug with few side effects. Its major drawback is the excessive sedation seen in some patients.

Carbamazepine (Tegretol) is becoming increasingly popular as a general anticonvulsant. However, it has caused aplastic anemia in a few isolated cases, and frequent monitoring of CBC and platelet count is necessary.

Primidone is a phenobarbital analog and is metabolized to phenobarbital in the body. It is believed to have additional anticonvulsant effects and is often used with phenobarbital, especially in partial seizures.

Antifibrinolytics. *Aminocaproic acid (EACA, epsilon aminocaproic acid, Amicar).* Rebleeding from ruptured intracranial aneurysms usually occurs at day 5 to 10 after initial bleeding. This period corresponds to the amount of time normal physiologic fibrinolysis occurs in which the old clot is lysed. Aminocaproic acid has been shown to be effective in delaying rebleeding for up to 3 weeks in a large number of patients. Aminocaproic acid works by inhibiting fibrinolysis. It is rapidly excreted and unchanged in the urine, and doses must be given frequently. It is available in oral tablet and syrup forms.

The adequacy of therapy can be monitored by measuring serum aminocaproic acid levels, or through bioassay, such as streptokinase clot lysis time. The dose required to achieve a therapeutic level of aminocaproic acid (300 mg/ml) is given in 12 divided doses or by continuous intravenous infusion.

Side effects include dehydration due to the administration of 48 g of solute a day. Oral administration frequently causes diarrhea. Reports of increased incidence of hypercoagulability and pulmonary emboli have not been substantiated. Clinical trials with tranxinamic acid are currently under way, and it also shows promise as an effective antifibrinolytic.

Antivasospasm agents. Delayed mortality from subarachnoid hemorrhage can be caused by cerebral vasospasm. Multiple agents have been tried in an attempt to reverse the spasm. The most successful therapy is volume expansion and induced hypertension in an attempt to increase blood flow through the spastic segment. This, of course, carries an increased risk in an untreated ruptured aneurysm. Histologic and pharmocologic studies have demonstrated adrenergic fibers on cerebral vessels, which constrict to alpha-stimulation and dilate with beta-adrenegic stimulation. Use of alpha-adrenergic blockade with phenoxybenzamine (Dibenzyl-ine) or phentolamine has not been successful except when applied locally. Beta-stimulants, such as Isuprel, or phosphodiesterase inhibitors, such as theophylline or papaverine, also work well locally. Isoproterenol (Isuprel) and theophylline infusions are used postoperatively at several medical centers to decrease vasospasm.

Direct vasodilation with nitroprusside or nitroglycerin is difficult because the associated hypotension tends to defeat the dilation's effect.

Serotonin, which has been used experimentally, will cause significant vasospasm. Use of antibiotics to kill serotonin-producing organisms in the gastrointestinal tract and reserpine to deplete serotonin from the cells has been shown in primate models to prevent vasospasm when used prophylactically. There is no currently available therapy that safely and consistently reverses ischemia from vasospasm. Treatment of vasospasm remains one of the most active areas of neurosurgical research.

Antibiotics. The effectiveness of antibiotics in CNS infection is related not only to the susceptibility of the organism to the drug but also to the drug's ability to cross the blood-brain barrier (BBB). The BBB, as mentioned earlier, acts to prevent access to cerebral tissue of a large number of substances in the blood. The barrier is lipid in content, and lipid-soluble substances tend to cross rapidly. The astrocytes also selectively transport certain chemicals. Often large intravenous doses of antibiotics are necessary to achieve adequate concentration in the cerebrospinal fluid (CSF). If adequate concentration of antibiotics cannot be achieved with IV administration, then intrathecal administration through lumbar puncture is indicated.

Antibiotics that have demonstrated adequate CSF penetration include penicillin G and semisynthetic analogs—nafcillin, methicillin, and ampicillin—although the presence of an impaired BBB (from meningitis) is necessary for adequate penetration of semisynthetic penicillins.

Carbenicillin penetrates only moderately.

However, adequate CSF levels have been reported with ticarcillin. Chloramphenicol concentrates in the CSF and brain. Sulfanilamides cross well.

Tetracyclines, erythromycin, streptomycin, amphotericin B, and vancomycin cross the BBB to a lesser extent, and intrathecal administration is necessary. Aminoglycosides, cephalosporins, and clindamycin all are unable to cross the barrier and require intrathecal administration if their use is indicated.

Antibiotic therapy for suspected CNS infection should begin immediately. The choice of antibiotics is based on the most frequent organisms and their local susceptibility. Antibiotics should always be given parenterally.

If a history of trauma or previous surgery or known CSF fistula exists, then a penicillinase-resistant semisynthetic penicillin—nafcillin or oxacillin—should be added to listed antibiotics for those organisms most frequently isolated and their local susceptibility.

Fungal infections are treated with amphotericin B both intravenously and intrathecally. Amphotericin is highly toxic, and may have many serious side effects, including renal failure and liver toxicity. It crosses the BBB only moderately. Severe thrombophlebitis and generalized chills frequently seen can be lessened by administration of hydrocortisone and slow intravenous infusion.

Response of cryptococcus to flucytosine, through oral administration either alone or in combination with amphotericin B, has been reported.

Herpes simplex encephalitis therapy with adenine arabinoside holds promise for decreasing mortality. The drug must be given early, before onset of coma, if it is to be effective. Long-term toxicity of the drug is unknown, and most authorities recommend confirmation of infection through brain biopsy. The drug is only minimally soluble and requires administration of large volumes of fluid. This can complicate the management of the coexisting cerebral edema.

Hormones. Patients with diseases around the

hypothalamus or pituitary often have deficits in levels of natural hormones. The most common include cortisone; the thyroid hormones T_3, or triodothyronine, and T_4, or thyroxine; and vasopressin. Lesions or surgery around the hypothalamus or pituitary will cause deficits in corticotropin-releasing factor (CRF) (hypothalamus) or adrenocorticotropic hormone (ACTH). This will be reflected in a decrease in circulating adrenocorticoids.

Glucocorticoid replacement is usually with cortisone acetate, given orally. Patients are instructed to increase this dose twofold to fourfold for minor infections or stress. Preoperative management of patients with deficits of adrenocorticoids requires intramuscular administration of cortisone acetate or intravenous administration of hydrocortisone. As stress lessens, the doses can be decreased toward maintenance levels. Mineralocorticoid replacement is seldom necessary in patients with primarily CNS-caused hypoadrenalism. However, if indicated, fludrocortisone is given orally. The dose is titrated to the individual. Alternatively, desoxycorticosterone can be used.

Thyroid hormone replacement may also be necessary as a result of impairment of manufacture or release of thyroid-stimulating hormones (TSH) or thyrotropin-releasing factor (TRF) from the hypothalamus. Hypothalamic and pituitary hormones are not available in oral form, and either desiccated thyroid or synthetic L-thyroxine (levothyroxine, Synthroid) is used. The maintenance dosage of desiccated thyroid is 1 to 3 grains daily. The onset of action of thyroid replacement hormones is 3 to 7 days and therefore must be started before a stressful situation (for example, surgery) occurs. Adequacy of therapy can easily be measured by radioimmunoassays of circulating levels of thyroid hormones.

Vasopressin (ADH) (antidiuretic hormone) is normally manufactured in the hypothalamus, transported through the hypophyseal portal circulation, and secreted from the posterior pituitary. Vasopressin acts to maintain serum osmolality around 285 to 290. A patient with hypo-

thalamic or pituitary dysfunction that affects secretion of ADH develops diabetes insipidus (DI). Such a patient will often excrete large amounts of urine—as high as 10 to 12 L/day. Thirst is controlled by another region of the hypothalamus but is usually not affected in hypothalamic dysfunction unless the condition is severe. Patients with mild DI will be able to control their own water balance quite well, using their thirst mechanism to tell them when they need to increase their intake of water. More severe DI requires replacement of the hormone. Extracts of ADH (vasopressin, Pitressin) are available as aqueous Pitressin or as Pitressin tannate in oil. Both must be given parenterally. The aqueous solution has a half-life of approximately 6 hours, and administration must be repeated every 3 to 6 hours. This allows dose control of circulating ADH levels and is useful in the initial period in the postoperative patient whose DI is often transient and whose level of natural vasopressin fluctuates. Pitressin tannate in oil was previously used for treatment of chronic DI because of its half-life of 3 to 7 days. An analog, arginine vasopressin (Pirped), is available. It can be administered as a nasal spray. It lasts only several hours, and administration every 4 hours is routine. Another analog, DDAVP (1-deamino, 8-D-arginine vasopressin), has increased activity and longer half-life. It is usually administered as a nasal drop and is now the drug of choice for severe DI. Patients with mild partial DI can usually be treated with oral agents. The oldest such agent is chlorpropamide, an oral hypoglycemic agent, that appears to enhance the renal response to endogenous ADH. It may also stimulate the neurohypophysial system to release an increased amount of ADH. Its major drawback is hypoglycemia, which usually can be controlled with diet.

Clofibrate (Atromid-S) is also effective. It appears to increase release of endogenous ADH. In combination with chlorpropamide, it is effective in many patients. Hydrodiuril, a thiazide diuretic, also acts to enhance water reabsorption at the tubule.

Oral control has several advantages, including ease of administration and enhancing natural fluctuation of ADH in response to changes in osmolality. Overdosage of drugs used to control DI can lead to hyponatremia and excessive water retention, which can be symptomatic; the symptoms must be closely monitored, with frequent electrolyte measurements and accurate input and output measurements, during initiation of therapy.

REFERENCES

1. Adams, R.D., and Victor, M.: Principles of neurology, ed. 3, New York, 1985, McGraw-Hill Book Co.

2. Afifi, A.K., and Bergman, R.A.: Basic neuroscience, Baltimore, 1980, Urban & Schwarzenberg.

3. Anthony, C.P., and Thibodeau, G.A.: Textbook of anatomy and physiology, ed. 11, St. Louis, 1983, The C.V. Mosby Co.

4. Arey, L.B.: Developmental anatomy: a textbook and laboratory manual of embryology, ed. 7, Philadelphia, 1974, W.B. Saunders Co.

5. Ausman, J.I., et al.: Intracranial neuroplasms. In Baker, A.B., and Baker, L.H.: Clinical neurology, vol. 1, New York, 1974, Harper & Row, Publisher.

6. Barnes, C.D., and Kercher, C.: Readings in neurophysiology, New York, 1968, John Wiley & Sons.

7. Barr, M.L., Kiernan, J.A.: The human nervous system, an anatomical viewpoint, ed. 4, New York, 1983, Harper & Row, Publishers, Inc.

8. Barrows, H.S.: Guide to neurological assessment, Philadelphia, 1980, J.B. Lippincott Co.

9. Becker, D.P., et al.: The outcome from severe head injury with early diagnosis and intensive management. J. Neurosurg. 47:491, 1977.

10. Bender, M.B.: Neuro-ophthalmology. In Baker, A.B., and Baker, L.H., editors: Clinical neurology, vol. 1, New York, 1974. Harper & Row, Publisher, Inc.

11. Benson, D.F., and Greshwind, N.: The aphasius and related disturbances. In Baker, A.B., and Baker, L.H., editors: Clinical neurology, vol. 1, New York, 1974, Harper & Row, Publisher, Inc.

12. Boshes, B.: Trauma to the spinal cord. In Baker, A.B., and Baker, L.H., editors: Clinical neurology, vol. 3, New York, 1974, Harper & Row, Publisher, Inc.

13. Brain, R.: The physiological basis of consciousness, Brain 81:426, 1958.

14. Butler, A.B., and Netsky, M.G.: Classification and biology of brain tumors. In Youmans, J.R., editor: Neurological surgery, vol. 3, Philadelphia, 1973, W.B. Saunders Co.

15. Carpenter, M.B., and Sutin, J.: Human neuroanatomy, ed. 8, Baltimore, 1983, Williams & Wilkins.

16. Chusid, J.C.: Correlative neuroanatomy & functional neurology, ed. 18, Los Altos, Calif., 1982, Lange Medical Publications.

17. Clark, K., and Watts, C.: The multiple injury patient with head or spine injuries. In Youmans, J.R., editor: Neurological surgery, vol. 2, Philadelphia, 1973, W.B. Saunders Co.

18. Conway-Rutkowski, B.L.: Carini and Owens' neurological and neurosurgical nursing, ed. 8, St. Louis, 1982, The C.V. Mosby Co.

19. Craig, C.R., and Stitzel, R.E.: Modern pharmacology, Boston, 1981, Little Brown & Co.

20. Cushing, H.: Concerning a definite regulatory mechanism of the vasomotor centre which controls blood pressure during cerebral compression, Bull. Hopkins Hosp. 12:290, 1901.

21. Dalessio, D.J.: Wolff's headache and other head pain, ed. 4, New York, 1980, Oxford University Press.

22. Daly, D.D.: Cerebral localization. In Baker, A.B., and Baker, L.H., editors: Clinical neurology, vol. 1, New York, 1974, Harper & Row, Publisher, Inc.

23. Davis, J., and Mason, C.B.: Neurologic critical care, New York, 1979, Van Nostrand Reinhold Co., Inc.

24. DeJong, R.W.: Case taking and the neurological exam. In Baker, A.B., and Baker, L.H., editors: Clinical neurology, vol. 1, New York, 1974, Harper & Row, Publisher, Inc.

25. DeJong, R.W.: The neurologic examination: incorporating the fundamentals of neuroanatomy and neurophysiology, ed. 3, New York, 1979, Harper & Row, Publisher, Inc.

26. DeMyer, W.: Anatomy and clinical neurology of the spinal cord. In Baker, A.B., and Baker, L.H., editors: Clinical neurology, vol. 3, New York, 1974, Harper & Row, Publisher, Inc.

27. Dodge, P.R., and Swartz, M.N.: Bacterial meningitis: a review of selected aspects. 2. Special neurologic problems, postmeningitis complications and clinicopathological correlations, N. Engl. J. Med., 272:954, 1965.

28. Drake, C.: On the surgical treatment of ruptured intracranial aneurysms, Clin. Neurosurg. 13:122, 1966.

29. Drake, C.: The surgical treatment of vertebral-basilar aneurysms, Clin. Neurosurg. 16:114, 1969.

30. Eliasson, S., et al.: Neurological pathophysiology, ed. 2, New York, 1978, Oxford University Press.

31. Farber S.D.: Neurorehabilitation. A. Multisensory approach, Philadelphia, 1982, W.B. Saunders Co.

32. Forster, F.M.: The epilepsies and convulsive disorders. In Baker, A.B., and Baker, L.H., editors: Clinical neurology, vol. 2, New York, 1974, Harper & Row, Publisher, Inc.

33. Freeman, A.: Properties of neuronal elements. In Selkurt, E.E., editor: Basic physiology for the health sciences, ed. 2, Boston, 1978, Little, Brown & Co.

34. French, L.A., and Seljeskog, E.L.: Arteriovenous mal-

formations of the brain. In Youmans, J.R., editor: Neurological surgery, vol. 2, Philadelphia, 1973, W.B. Saunders Co.

35. Galbraith, J.G.: Extracranial arterial occlusive disease. In Youmans, J.R., editor: Neurological Surgery, vol. 2, Philadelphia, 1973, W.B. Saunders Co.

36. Ganong, W.F.: Review of medical physiology, ed. 10, Los Altos, Calif., 1981, Lange Medical Publications.

37. Gowan, J.C.: Altered states of consciousness: a taxonomy, J. Alt. States Consciousness 4(2):141, 1978-1979.

38. Gregory, D.H., et al.: Metastatic brain abscess: a retrospective appraisal of 29 patients, Arch. Intern. Med. 119:25, 1967.

39. Guyton, A.C.: Organ physiology structure and function of the nervous system, ed. 2, Philadelphia, 1976, W.B. Saunders Co.

40. Guyton, A.C.: Textbook of medical physiology, ed. 6, Philadelphia, 1981, W.B. Saunders Co.

41. Hall, P.: Personal communication, Dec., 1985. Associate Professor of Medicine, Indiana University.

42. Haymaker, W., and Kuhlenbeck, H.: Disorders of the brainstem and its cranial nerves. In Baker, A.B., and Baker, L.H., editors: Clinical neurology, vol. 3, New York, 1974, Harper and Row, Publisher, Inc.

43. Heilman, K.H., et al.: Handbook for differential diagnosis of neurologic signs and symptoms, New York, 1977, Appleton-Century-Crofts.

44. Hild, W.: Neurosecretion in the central nervous system. In Fields, S.W., et al.: Hypothalamic-hypophysial interrelationships, Springfield, Ill., 1956, Charles C Thomas, Publisher.

45. Kernohan, J.W., and Sayre, G.P.: Tumors of the central nervous system, Washington, D.C., 1952, Armed Forces Institute of Pathology, Section 10.

46. Kertesz, A.: Aphasia and associated disorders: taxonomy, localization and recovery, New York, 1979, Grune & Stratton, Inc.

47. Lance, J.W.: Mechanism and management of headache, ed. 4, Boston, 1982, Butterworth Publishers.

48. Lance, J.W., and McLeod, J.G.: A physiological approach to clinical neurology, ed. 3, Boston, 1981, Butterworth Publishers.

49. Langfitt, T.W.: Increased intracranial pressure. In Youmans, J.R., editor: Neurological surgery, vol. 1, Philadelphia, 1973, W.B. Saunders Co.

50. Langfitt, T.W.: Possible mechanisms of action of hypertonic area in reducing intracranial pressure, Neurology 11:196, 1961.

51. Langfitt, T.W., and Kassell, N.F.: Acute brain swelling in neurosurgical patients, J. Neurosurg. 24:975, 1966.

52. Langfitt, T.W., et al.: Cerebral blood flow with intracranial hypertension, Neurology 15:761, 1965.

53. Langfitt, T.W., et al.: Cerebral vasomotor paralysis produced by intracranial hypertension, Neurology 15:622, 1965.

54. Lenman, J.: Clinical neurophysiology, Oxford, England, 1975, Blackwell Scientific Publications.

55. Lougheed, W.M., and Barnett, H.J.M.: Lesions producing spontaneous hemorrhage. In Youmans, J.R., editor: Neurological surgery, vol. 2, Philadelphia, 1973, W.B. Saunders Co.

56. Lundberg, N.: Continuous recording and control of ventricular fluid pressure in neurosurgical practice, Acta Psychiatr. Scand. (suppl. 149)36:1, 1960.

57. Lundberg, N., et al.: Reduction of increased intracranial pressure by hyperventilation, Acta Psychiatr. Scand. 34:4, 1959.

58. MacBryde, R.S.: MacBryde's signs and symptoms: applied pathologic physiology and clinical interpretation, ed. 6, Philadelphia, 1983, J.B. Lippincott Co.

59. McNealy, D.E., and Plum, F.: Brainstem dysfunction with supratentorial mass lesions, Arch. Neurol. 7:10, 1962.

60. Marshall, L., and Shapiro, H.: Barbiturate control of intracranial hypertension in head injury and other conditions: Iatrogenic coma. In Ingvar, D.H. and Lassen, N.A., editors: Cerebral function, metabolism and circulation, Copenhagen, 1977, Munksgaard.

61. Marshall, W.J.S., Jackson, J.L.F., and Langfitt, T.W.: Brain swelling caused by trauma and arterial hypertension, Arch Neurol. 21:545-533, 1969.

62. Meldrum, B.S., Horton, R.W., Physiology of status epilepticus in primates, Arch. Neurol. (Chicago) 28:1, 1973.

63. Meldrum, B.S., Horton, R.W., Bloom, S.R., Butler, J., Keenan, J., Endocrine factors and glucose metabolism during prolonged seizures in baboons, Epilepsia 20:527, 1979.

64. Mettler, F.A., Neuroanatomy, ed. 2, St. Louis, 1948, The C.V. Mosby Co.

65. Miller, J.D., et al.: Significance of intracranial hypertension in severe head injury, J. Neurosurg. 47:503, 1977.

66. Morley, T.P.: Intrinsic tumors of the cerebral hemispheres. In Youmans, J.R.: Neurological surgery, vol. 3, Philadelphia, 1973, W.B. Saunders Co.

67. Morley, T.P.: Tumors of the cranial meninges. In Youmans, J.R. Neurological surgery, vol. 3, Philadelphia, 1973, W.B. Saunders Co.

68. Mullan, S. and Dawley, J.: Antifibrinolytic therapy for intracranial aneurysms, J. Neurosurg. 28:21, 1968.

69. Newman, P.P. Neurophysiology, Jamaica, 1980, Spectrum Publications.

70. Ojemann, R.G.: Intracerebral and intracerebellar hemorrhage. In Youmans, J.R. Neurological surgery, vol. 2, Philadelphia, 1973, W.B. Saunders Co.

71. Ottoson, D.: Physiology of the nervous system, New York, 1983, Oxford University Press.

72. Patten, B.M.: Human embryology, ed. 2, New York, 1968, McGraw-Hill Book Co.

73. Petersdorf, R.G.: Harrison's principles of internal medicine, ed. 10, New York, 1983, McGraw-Hill Publishing Co.

74. Plum, F., and Brennan, R.W.: Differential diagnosis of altered states of consciousness. In Youmans, J.R., editor: Neurological surgery, vol. 1, Philadelphia, 1973, W.B. Saunders Co.

75. Plum, F., and Posner, J.B.: Diagnosis of stupor and coma, ed. 2, Contemporary neurology series, vol. 10, Philadelphia, 1972, F.A. Davis, Publishers.

76. Popp, A.J., et al.: Neural trauma. In Seminars in neurological surgery (series), New York, 1979, Raven Press.

77. Purpura, D.P.: Operations and processes in thalamic and synaptically related neural subsystems. In Schmitt, F.O., editor: The neurosciences, second study program, New York, 1970, Rockefeller University Press.

78. Raimondi, A.J., and Wright, R.L.: Cranial and intracranial infections. In Youmans, J.R., editor: Neurological surgery, vol. 3, Philadelphia, 1973, W.B. Saunders Co.

79. Ransoholl, J., and Goodgold, A.L.: Nonoperative management of aneurysms. In Youmans, J.R.: Neurological surgery, vol. 2, Philadelphia, 1973, W.B. Saunders Co.

80. Resch, J.A., and Sung, J.H.: Brain abscess and diffuse suppurative encephalitis. In Baker, A.B., and Baker, L.H., editors: Clinical neurology, vol. 2, New York, 1974, Harper & Row, Inc.

81. Ropper, A.H., et al.: Pyramidal infarction in the medulla: a cause of pure motor hemiplegia sparing the face, Neurology 29:91, 1979.

82. Rosati, G., and DeBastiani, P.: Pure agraphia: a discrete form of aphasia, J. Neurol. Neurosurg. Psychiatry 42:266, 1979.

83. Russell, D.S., and Rubinstein, L.J.: The pathology of tumours of the nervous system, Edward Arnold.

84. Sahs, A.L., and Joynt, R.J.: Meningitis. In Baker, A.B.: and Baker, L.H., editors: Clinical Neurology, vol. 2, New York, 1974, Harper & Row, Publisher, Inc.

85. Sahs, A.L., et al.: Intracranial aneurysms and subarachnoid hemorrhage: a cooperative study, Philadelphia, 1969, J.B. Lippincott Co.

86. Samuels, M.A.: Manual of neurologic therapeutics with essentials of diagnosis, Boston, 1982, ed. 2, Little, Brown & Co.

87. Sayers, M.P., and Hunt, W.E.: Posterior fossa tumors. In Youmans, J.R., editor: Neurological surgery, vol. 3, Philadelphia, 1973, W.B. Saunders Co.

88. Schechter, M.M.: Cerebral angiography. In Youmans, J.R., editor: Neurological surgery, vol. 1, Philadelphia, 1973, W.B. Saunders Co.

89. Schechter, M.M., and Kier, E.L.: Radiology of the spine, In Youmans, J.R., editor: Neurological surgery, vol. 1, Philadelphia, 1973, W.B. Saunders Co.

90. Schottelius, B.A., and Schottelius, D.D.: Textbook of physiology, ed. 18, St. Louis, 1978, The C.V. Mosby Co.

91. Shillito, J. Jr., and Ojemann, R.G.: Hydrocephalus. In Youmans, J.R., editor: Neurological surgery, vol. 1, Philadelphia, 1973, W.B. Saunders Co.

92. Strand, F.L.: Physiology: a regulatory systems approach, ed. 2, New York, 1983, Macmillan Publishing Co.

93. Stratton, D.B.: Neurophysiology, New York, 1981, McGraw-Hill Book Co.

94. Talbert, O.R.: General methods of clinical examination, In Youmans, J.R., editor: Neurological surgery, vol. 1, Philadelphia, 1973, W.B. Saunders Co.

95. Thomas, L.M., and Gurdjion, E.S.: Intracranial hematomas of traumatic origin. In Youmans, J.R., editor: Neurological surgery, vol. 2, Philadelphia, 1973, W.B. Saunders Co.

96. Toole, J.F., and Cole, M.: Ischemic cerebrovascular disease. In Baker, A.B., and Baker, L.H., editors: Clinical neurology, vol. 1, New York, 1974, Harper & Row, Publisher, Inc.

97. Uherback, R.A.: Hemorrhagic cerebrovascular disease. In Baker, A.B., and Baker, L.H., editors: Clinical neurology, vol. 1, New York, 1974, Harper & Row, Publisher, Inc.

98. Voris, H.C.: Craniocerebral trauma. In Baker, A.B., and Baker, L.H., editors: Clinical neurology, vol. 2, New York, 1974, Harper & Row, Publisher, Inc.

99. White, R.J., and Yashon, D.: General care of cervical spine injuries. In Youmans, J.R., editor: Neurological surgery, vol. 2, Philadelphia, 1973, W.B. Saunders Co.

100. Youmans, J.R., and Albrand, O.W.: Cerebral blood flow in clinical problems. In Youmans, J.R., editor: Neurological surgery, vol. 2, Philadelphia, 1973, W.B. Saunders Co.

101. Young, G.F.: Clinical examination in infancy and childhood. In Youmans, J.R., Neurological surgery, vol. 1, Philadelphia, 1973, W.B. Saunders Co.

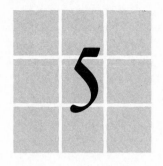

5 Fluid and Electrolytes

CHERYLL WODNIAK
JAMES SZWED

The integrity of normal physiologic functioning in the body depends on (1) the acquisition of proper nutrients and fluids and their transportation to tissue cells and (2) the removal of waste products of metabolism from these cells. When a severe illness occurs, either one or both of the above-mentioned functions is altered. These alterations are identified as fluid and electrolyte disorders or acid-base disorders. Decreased delivery of nutrients to cells leads to accumulation of lactic acid and other metabolites, resulting from an alternate route of cell functioning. This lactic acidosis begins in one tissue and will produce changes in perfusion of other organs because of decreased cardiac output and malfunction of the microcirculation. Therefore the identification of lactic acidosis is critical, and adjustments in central and peripheral cardiovascular systems, crucial to saving the organism from total collapse, must be made. Interpretation of blood gases and correct classification of the type of acidosis being dealt with are critical to successful management of the patient.

Similarly, electrolyte composition of the plasma is measured daily in a routine manner in many ill patients. The knowledge of the differential diagnosis of anion vs non-anion gap acidosis, which is perceived by careful examination of the electrolytes, results in proper treatment. In fact, acid-base and fluid-electrolyte principles are paramount to correct management in any ill patient, regardless of which major organ system is involved.

EMBRYOLOGY

Although the urinary system evolves in close approximation both structurally and temporally with the reproductive system, the emphasis of this discussion will be on the urinary system alone. However, because developmental abnormalities of the systems are often interrelated, the reproductive embryology will be discussed when appropriate.

Both urinary and reproductive systems arise from mesoderm. Mesoderm is one of the three primary germ layers that result in the early differentiation of the embryo into various types of tissues and organs. The ectoderm is the outer layer, literally the skin; the endoderm is the innermost layer; and the mesoderm is the middle layer. Both ectoderm and endoderm persist chiefly as sheets exposed on one surface (that is, the epithelial surface). The mesoderm forms most of a diffuse spongework of cells, that is, a primitive filling-tissue known as *mesenchyme*. The mesenchyme is an extraordinarily versatile tissue with many potentialities, which become actualized under the varied conditions offered during the course of development. For example, mesenchymal tissue is the basis for granulocytes, endothelial cells (in embryo), mast cells, fat cells, osteocytes, chondrocytes (which lead to the de-

337

velopment of osteocytes), osteoblasts, fibroblasts, macrophages, and the entire hematopoietic system.

Vertebrates have made three distinct experiments in the production of kidneys. Each was an improvement over the preceding type. In higher vertebrates, embryos repeat the same 3-part kidney development progressively during gestation. The earliest and simplest of the three kidneys is called the *pronephros;* it is functional today only in such animals as those of the genus Amphioxus and the myxinoid fishes. The embryos of rep-

tiles, birds, and mammals including man first develop a functionless pronephros. Then they develop a *mesonephros* (functional during part of fetal life). The final kidney is a new organ, the *metanephros.* These three kidneys develop in overlapping stages, each one caudal to the others, in the order indicated by their names (Fig. 5-1).

All three kidney types are organs composed of units known as uriniferous tubules, which have a common source of origin and exhibit somewhat the same structural plan. These tubules

Fig. 5-1. Locations and relations of the three kidney types in mammals (semidiagrammatic). **A,** Ventral dissection, the left side showing a later stage than the right. **B,** Lateral view, with the nephric system and gut showing through.

From Arey, L.B.: Developmental anatomy, a textbook and laboratory manual of embryology, ed. 7, Philadelphia, 1965, W.B. Saunders Co.

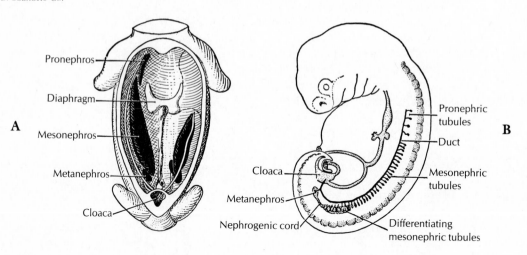

Fig. 5-2. Development of the pronephric tubule, illustrated by transverse sections of early embryos (semidiagrammatic); × 140 (approx.).

From Arey, L.B.: Developmental anatomy, a textbook and laboratory manual of embryology, ed. 7, Philadelphia, 1965, W.B. Saunders Co.

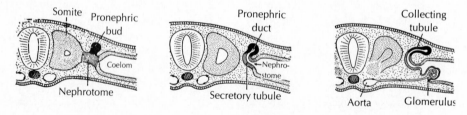

arise from mesoderm in a plate of tissue called the *nephrotome*. This plate lies just lateral to the somites (precursors of muscle and vertebrae) and connects the vertebrae with the mesoderm, which encloses the coelum (a cavity that is later subdivided into cavities for the heart, lungs, and abdominal viscera). In close relation physically to all three types of secretory nephrons is a vascular tuft, the glomerulus, which is specialized to separate urinary wastes from the blood. The collected waste products are then conducted by collecting tubules to a common excretory duct, which discharges them from the body. All three kinds of kidneys, as well as both kinds of gonads, differ from other exocrine glands in that their secretory tissue differentiates from a structureless, cellular blastema. Union with the system of excretory ducts is secondary, whereas other glands owe their origin to a direct budding and branching from the excretory duct.

Pronephros

The functional pronephros of lower vertebrates consists of paired pronephric tubules, arranged segmentally. One end of each tortuous tubule opens into the coelom; the other opens into a longitudinal pronephric duct, which is excretory in nature and drains into the cloaca. (The cloaca is the most caudal end of the endodermal tube and receives the urinary and genital ducts.) The cloaca proceeds to form the bladder and rectum. The ciliated, funnel-shaped communication with the body cavity is the nephrostome.

Nearby, but entirely separate from each tubule, arterial tufts project into the coelom. These are external glomeruli, covered only by thin epithelium; they filter wastes from the blood into the coelom. The mixture of urine and coelomic fluid is then taken up by the tubules and carried by means of ciliary current into the main excretory duct. As implied by its name, the pronephros is

Fig. 5-3. Development of the pronephric system of lower vertebrates, illustrated by models. **A,** Younger stage, with tubules still forming and linking together. **B,** Older stage, with tubules and duct completed.

From Arey, L.B.: Developmental anatomy, a textbook and laboratory manual of embryology, ed. 7, Philadelphia, 1965, W.B. Saunders Co.

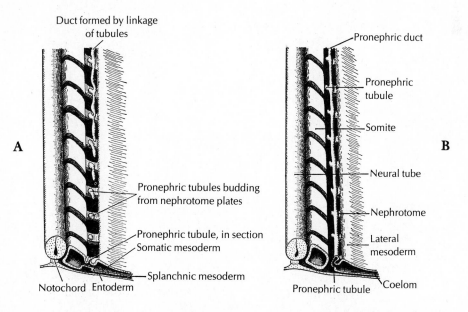

located well cephalad in the body; for this reason it has often been called the "head kidney" (Figs. 5-2 and 5-3).

Although the human pronephros is vestigial, it is as well developed as that of any reptile and better represented in humans than it is in birds and other mammals. It consists of about seven pairs of rudimentary pronephric tubules, arising as dorsolateral sprouts from those segmentally arranged nephrotomes that border on the region of junction of the future neck and thorax. The distal, or free, ends of these solid nodules bend backward, canalize, and unite into a longitudinal

Fig. 5-4. Location and composition of the human mesonephros. **A,** At 8 mm (after Shikinami; × 4.5). **B,** At 10 mm, showing the mesonephric region reconstructed in greater detail (after Felix; × 35).

From Arey, L.B.: Developmental anatomy, a textbook and laboratory manual of embryology, ed. 7, Philadelphia, 1965, W.B. Saunders Co.

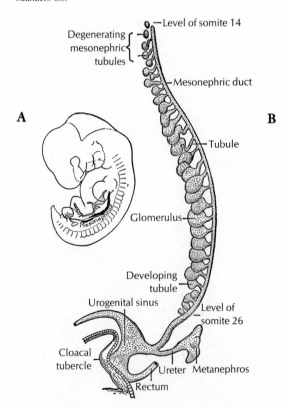

duct. Caudal to the lowest tubule, the free end of the collecting duct, by a process of terminal growth, pushes between the ectoderm and the nephrotomes until it reaches the lateral wall of the cloaca and perforates it. Thus the paired primary excretory ducts are formed, which at this period bear the name of *pronephric ducts.*

Mesonephros

The mesonephros, or wolffian body (Fig. 5-4), of vertebrates is larger than the pronephros; not only does it contain more tubules, but these tubules are also longer and more complicated. The mesonephros is located farther caudal and is appropriately named the "middle kidney." Unlike the pronephros, the primordium of the mesonephros differentiates into tubules only. These tubules drain into the pronephric duct, which is retained as the main excretory canal and is henceforth known as the mesonephric (or wolffian) duct. Whereas the pronephros is entirely functionless in higher vertebrates, the mesonephros serves the embryo as a temporary excretory organ whose activity overlaps the initial activity of the permanent kidney. In most but not all mammals, function is attained; even in man, whose mesonephros is not large, this is apparently true.

Metanephros

The permanent kidney of amniotes, the metanephros (Fig. 5-5), arises far caudal in the body. As with the mesonephros, the final kidney consists of an aggregate of tubules that drain into a common duct. Also like the mesonephros, the metanephros is of double origin. However, in the metanephros, the boundary between the two components lies midway between the uriniferous tubules. Thus the inert system of drainage ducts (ureter, pelvis, calyces, papillary ducts, and straight collecting tubules) comes from a bud growing off the mesonephric duct. On the other hand, each secretory unit or nephron (for example, Bowman's capsule, both convoluted tubules, and Henle's loop) differentiates from the substance of the caudal end of the nephrogenic cord; it thus has an origin similar to that of the entire mesonephric tubule. A collecting and secretory tubule then unites secondarily to complete a continuous uriniferous tubule. In structure and function, however, these two components remain as different from each other as their origin was.

The mesonephric duct bends sharply just before joining the cloaca. It is at this angle that the "ureteric bud" arises. The primordium appears in embryos of four weeks, which have a length of 5 mm, taking the form of a hollow bud that

first grows dorsal and then cephalad. The proximal, rapidly elongating stalk of this diverticulum is the future ureter, whereas the distal, blind end dilates at once into the primitive renal pelvis. Shortly after its appearance, the ureteric bud pushes into a mass of condensed tissue that is the most caudal portion of the nephrogenic cord. The metanephrogenic mass promptly separates from the more cranial mesonephrogenic tissue and then surrounds the pelvic dilation like a cap. Such are the early primordia that jointly give rise to the permanent kidney.

Fig. 5-5. Origin of the human metanephros and the development of its duct system, as shown by reconstructions. **A** and **B,** Origin and early relations. **A,** At 5 mm, × 35; **B,** At 11 mm, × 25. **C** through **F,** Further stages in the development of the ureteric bud into the duct system. **C,** At 15 mm, × 45; **D,** At 20 mm, × 40; **E,** At 9 weeks, × 40; **F,** At birth, × 1.5.

From Arey, L.B.: Developmental anatomy, a textbook and laboratory manual of embryology, ed. 7, Philadelphia, 1965, W.B. Saunders Co.

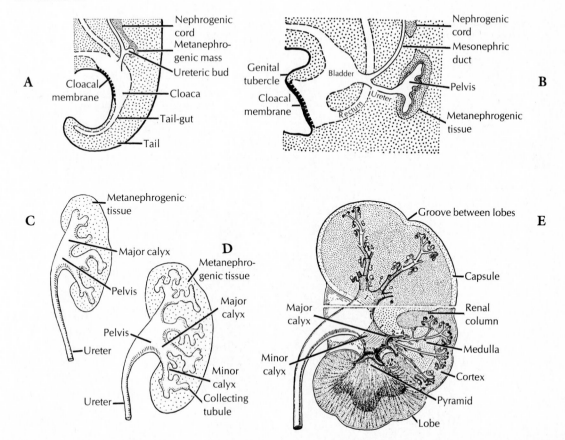

The ureteric stem elongates, and toward the end of the sixth week of gestation, the primitive renal pelvis both flattens from side to side and subdivides into the two future major calyces. From these calyces, secondary branches bud; these secondary branches in turn give rise to tertiary branches. The branching process continues until, at 5 months of gestation, twelve generations of collecting tubules have developed. The branching results in the formation of minor calyces, which open into the papillary ducts. The remaining tubules develop into the familiar structure of the tubules of the nephron.

The renal cortex consists of two kinds of territories: the pars radiata and the pars convoluta. The pars radiata, or rays, result from the massive extension of radial bundles of collecting tubules.

The pars convoluta, or labyrinth, consists of the aggregate of secretory tubules differentiated from the metanephrogenic tissue. Each tiny ball of this formative substance is the forerunner of a secretory tubule, or nephron, whose developmental course can be followed in Fig. 5-6. A ball hollows into a vesicle, which elongates and becomes tortuous. At one end, a Bowman's capsule and glomerulus differentiate, while the other end establishes communication with the nearby collecting tubule. Because the newer generations of tubules develop progressively in a capsular direction from the self-perpetuating mesonephrogenic tissue, it follows that the oldest tubules are those nearest the medulla. The differentiation of new tubules terminates about 1 month before birth in the zone just beneath the

Fig. 5-6. Composite diagram, illustrating the stages in the differentiation of nephrons and their linkages with branching collecting tubules. Progressive stages are numbered serially from 1 to 9.

From Arey, L.B.: Developmental anatomy, a textbook and laboratory manual of embryology, ed. 7, Philadelphia, 1965, W.B. Saunders Co.

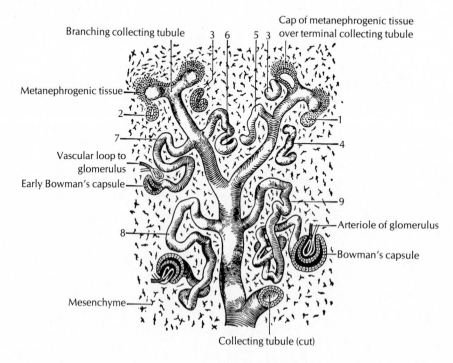

Table 5-1. Development of the urogenital tract during gestation

Age of fetus in weeks	Size (CR*) in mm	Urogenital system	Age of fetus in weeks	Size (CR*) in mm	Urogenital system
2.5	1.5	Allantois present	10	40.0	Kidney able to secrete
3.5	2.5	All pronephric tubules formed			Bladder expands as sac
		Pronephric duct growing caudad as a blind tube			Genital duct of opposite sex degenerating
		Cloaca and cloacal membrane present			Bulbo-urethral and vestibular glands appearing
4	5.0	Pronephros degenerated			Vaginal sacs forming
		Pronephric (mesonephric) duct reaches cloaca	12	56.0	Uterine horns absorbed
		Mesonephric tubules differentiating rapidly			External genitalia attain distinctive features
		Metanephric bud pushes into secretory primordium			Meson. and rete tubules complete male duct
5	8.0	Mesonephros reaches its caudal limit			Prostate and seminal vesicle appearing
		Ureteric and pelvic primordia distinct			Hollow viscera gaining muscular walls
		Genital ridge bulges	16	112.0	Kidney attains typical shape and plan
6	12.0	Cloaca subdividing			Testis in position for later descent into scrotum
		Pelvic anlage sprouts pole tubules			Uterus and vagina recognizable as such
		Sexless gonad and genital tubercle prominent			Mesonephros involuted
		Müllerian duct appearing	20-40 (5-10 mo)	160.0-350.0	Female urogenital sinus becoming a shallow vestibule (5 mo)
7	17.0	Mesonephros at height of its differentiation			Vagina regains lumen (5 mo)
		Metanephric collecting tubules begin branching			Uterine glands appear (7 mo)
		Earliest metanephric secretory tubules differentiating			Scrotum solid until sacs and testes descend (7-9 mo)
		Bladder-urethra separates from rectum			Kidney tubules cease forming at birth
		Urethral membrane rupturing			
8	23.0	Testis and ovary distinguishable as such			
		Müllerian ducts, nearing urogenital sinus, are ready to unite as uterovaginal primordium			
		Genital ligaments indicated			

From Arey, L.B.: Developmental anatomy: a textbook and laboratory manual of embryology, ed. 7, Philadelphia, 1974, W.B. Saunders Co.
*CR = Crown-rump.

Table 5-2. Total body water as a percentage of body weight in normal humans

Age	Males	Both sexes	Females
0-1 mo		76	
1-12 mo		65	
1-10 yr		62	
10-16 yr	59		57
17-39 yr	61		50
40-59 yr	55		52
60 yr and over	52		46

From Edelman, I.S., and Leibman, J.: Am. J. Med. **27**:256, 1959.

Table 5-3. Distribution of water and percentage of body weight in various tissues of a 70-kg man

Tissue	Percent of water	Percent of body weight	Liters of water/70 kg
Skin	72.0	18.0	9.07
Muscle	75.6	41.7	22.10
Skeleton	22.0	15.9	2.45
Brain	74.8	2.0	1.05
Liver	68.3	2.3	1.03
Heart	79.2	0.5	0.28
Lungs	79.0	0.7	0.39
Kidneys	82.7	0.4	0.25
Spleen	75.8	0.2	0.10
Blood	83.0	8.0	4.65
Intestine	74.5	1.8	0.94
Adipose tissue	10.0	±10.0	0.70

From Skelton, H.: Arch. Int. Med. **40**:140, 1927.

capsule. At this time, about one million tubules have been produced in each kidney. All later increases in renal size result from the enlargement of tubules already present.

The development of the urogenital tract is summarized in Table 5-1.

PHYSIOLOGY
Volume and composition of the body fluids
Body water

Water is, by far, the most abundant component of the human body, constituting 50% to 60% of body weight. Body weight and therefore water content remain constant from day to day in the normal adult with caloric balance, despite marked fluctuations in water intake. The ingestion of an extra liter or more of water induces a brisk diuresis, and the excess fluid is eliminated within the brief span of 2 to 3 hours. Variability of body water in relation to body weight among a group of individuals is largely a function of the amount of adipose tissue. Leanness is associated with a high body water fraction, and obesity, with a low. In a study of young adults, averages of 60% water in males and 50% in females are findings in accord with the greater development of subcutaneous adipose tissue in women. Table 5-2 lists total body water as a percentage of body weight. For clinical purposes, it is accurate to assume that body water is 60% of weight (in kilograms) in both men and women. Table 5-3 summarizes the percentage of water in various

tissues, the proportion of the total weight of the body that each tissue represents, and the total volume of water contained in each tissue in a relatively lean (70-kg) man (Table 5-3). As the table indicates, most of the water in the body is present in skin and muscle; the skeleton and adipose tissue contain the least water in relation to weight. Because progressive expansion of the fat stores of the body results in a small increase in water content, the percentage of water decreases as the individual becomes more obese.

Body fluid compartments

The water of the body can be considered as distributed among three compartments: an extracellular, an intracellular, and a transcellular compartment, depicted diagrammatically in Fig. 5-7.

Extracellular fluid. Extracellular fluid includes the blood plasma, which is 4.5% of body weight, and the lymph, which is about 2% of body weight. Plasma circulates rapidly in the vascular compartment, whereas interstitial fluid seeps more slowly through tissue interstices. Plasma proteins that leak through capillary walls and excess interstitial fluid are returned to the vascular compartment by lymphatic vessels.

Flow is sluggish, and volumes arrived at for the lymphatic compartment describe only a rough estimate.

More than a century ago, Claude Bernard pointed out that interstitial fluid constitutes the true environment of the body because it bathes all tissue cells, supplies their nutriments, and removes their wastes. Water and solutes, with the exception of proteins and lipids, exchange rapidly across the single-layered endothelium that makes up the capillary wall and separates the vascular from the interstitial compartments. Because diffusion distances are small, minor concentration gradients between blood plasma and interstitial fluid are adequate to supply the nutrients utilized and to remove the wastes produced by cells.

Intracellular fluid. Intracellular fluid represents neither a continuous nor a homogenous phase; rather, it is the sum of the fluid contents of all the cells of the body. Such diverse cells as erythrocytes, muscle cells, and renal tubular cells vary in water content and chemical constitution almost as much as they do in structure; therefore it is evident that representation of a single cellular compartment, such as that depicted in Fig. 5-7, is not only a gross oversimplification but also is frankly misleading. The important clinical consideration is that somewhat more than half of the total body water is contained in cells; in addition, intracellular water constitutes 30% to 40% of body weight.

Transcellular fluid. Transcellular fluid is a specialized fraction of extracellular fluid and includes cerebrospinal, intraocular, pleural, peritoneal, and synovial fluids and the digestive secretions. Digestive secretions could, in fact, be considered as extracorporeal fluid, insofar as they are contained in the open-ended digestive tract. The common factor that sets the transcellular fluids apart from extracellular fluid is that each of the several discontinuous fractions of transcellular fluids is separated from blood plasma not only by the capillary endothelial cells but also by a continuous layer of epithelial cells. These epithelial cell layers modify the composition of the transcellular fluid, with respect to extracellular fluid, in varying degrees. With the exception of the digestive secretions, their volumes are insignificant fractions of body weight. In humans, digestive secretions in the fasting state represent only 1% to 3% of body weight. For most clinical problems, transcellular fluids, with the exception of the digestive juices, are not actively dealt with.

Ionic composition of the body fluids

The ionic composition of the body fluids can be discussed cogently only in terms of chemical equivalents. When concentrations of all ionic constituents are so expressed, the sum of the concentrations of the positive ions (cations), such as sodium, potassium, calcium, and magnesium, exactly equals the sum of the concentrations of the negative ions (anions), such as chloride, bicarbonate, phosphate, sulfate, protein, and organic anion. Balance is obligatory because solutions must be electrically neutral; the number of positive charges must equal the number of negative charges.

Chemical equivalents

One equivalent of hydrogen ions consists of 6.023×10^{23} separate particles weighing 1.008 g. This quantity of hydrogen ions exactly balances, or neutralizes, one equivalent of hydroxyl ions, which consists of 6.023×10^{23} separate particles weighing 17.008 g. Neutralization results in the

Fig. 5-7. Total body water (50% to 70% of body weight).

From Szwed, J.: Fluids, electrolytes and acid-base, Indianapolis, IN, 1981, Indiana University School of Medicine.

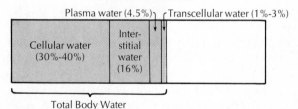

TOTAL BODY WEIGHT

Table 5-4. Average electrolyte composition of normal human blood plasma and the approximate composition of skeletal muscle intracellular fluid*

	Blood plasma			Intracellular phase	
	mEq/kg H$_2$O	mosm/kg H$_2$O		mEq/kg H$_2$O	mosm/kg H$_2$O
Cations			Cations		
Na$^+$	150	150	Na$^+$	14	14
K$^+$	5.4	5.4	K$^+$	150	150
Ca^{++}	5.4	2.7	Ca^{++}	2	1
Mg^{++}	2.2	1.1	Mg^{++}	40	20
Total cations	163.0	159.2	Total cations	206	185
Anions			Anions		
Cl$^-$	113.0	113.0	Protein$^-$	50	(5)
HCO$_3^-$	27.0	27.0	HCO$_3^-$	10	10
Protein$^-$	17.0	0.8†	A$^-$ (Phosphates and other nonprotein ions)	146	(103)
Total anions	163.0	143.0	Total anions	206	(118)
TOTAL	326.0	303.0	TOTAL	412	(303)

*Values given per 1000 g of water: plasma water, 93%; intracellular water, 74%.
†The normal plasma albumin and globulin concentrations are 4.0 g and 3.0 g, respectively, per 100 ml.

formation of 18.016 g, or one mole of water. One equivalent of hydrogen ions also combines with one equivalent of chloride ions (35.5 g) to form one mole of hydrochloric acid. Each hydrogen ion carries a unit positive charge; each chloride and hydroxyl ion carries a unit negative charge. Ions carrying a unit charge are termed *univalent* and balance each other in a 1:1 ratio. Because the concentrations of ions in the body fluids amount to fractions of an equivalent per liter, it is more convenient to express them in terms of milliequivalents (mEq) to handle whole numbers rather than decimal values. One milliequivalent of a univalent ion is equal to 1/1,000 of an equivalent and consists of 6.023 × 10^{20} particles. One milliequivalent of hydrogen ions weighs 1.008 mg, and 1.0 mEq of hydroxyl ions weighs 17.008 mg.

Certain cations such as calcium and magnesium are divalent, that is, each carries two unit positive charges. Sulfate is a divalent anion and carries two unit negative charges. Each calcium or magnesium ion can therefore combine with two chloride ions. Similarly, one sulfate ion can combine with two hydrogen ions. Accordingly,

1.0 mEq of divalent calcium ions consists of just one half the number of particles (3.012 × 10^{20}) of a milliequivalent of hydrogen ions and weighs 20 mg. One milliequivalent of sulfate ions consists of 3.012 × 10^{20} particles and weighs 48 mg. The rule is that 1.0 mEq of positive cations exactly balances or neutralizes 1.0 mEq of negative anions. If the ion is univalent, 1.0 mEq consists of 6.023 × 10^{20} particles and weighs 1/1,000 of a gram in atomic weight; if it is divalent, it consists of 3.012 × 10^{20} particles and weighs 1/2,000 of a gram in atomic weight. In working with clinical problems, the number of milliequivalents contained in a gram must be known. For example, 1 g of Na$^+$ contains 44 mEq of Na$^+$ [1000 mg/23 (atomic weight of Na$^+$)].

The fact that, for the most part, equivalent weights are not whole numbers (for example, hydrogen has an equivalent weight of 1.008 g) is explained as follows: oxygen was originally chosen as the standard of reference, with 8.000 g of oxygen being arbitrarily designated as one equivalent. This quantity of oxygen combines with 1.008 g of hydrogen. Deviations from whole numbers result from the fact that oxygen (the standard of reference), as well as many other elements, are mixtures of stable isotopes of differing atomic weights.

Extracellular fluid

Plasma. The major cations of blood plasma are sodium and potassium; the major anions are chloride, bicarbonate, and protein. The average normal concentrations of the several ionic species in plasma are given in Table 5-4. The sum of the concentrations of cations exactly equals the sum of the concentrations of anions. Exact balance is obligatory; however, the concentrations shown in Table 5-4 are in no sense absolute. Normal sodium concentrations range from 138 to 146 mEq/L, potassium ranges from 3.8 to 4.8 mEq/L, chloride ranges from 98 to 100 mEq/L, and bicarbonate ranges from 24 to 28 mEq/L of plasma. Other ions normally exhibit similar variations in concentration.

Protein occupies volume all out of proportion to the few milliequivalents of anion that it represents. One liter of plasma contains only 940 ml of water; the remaining volume is occupied by 60 g of protein. For the most part, ions are dissolved in the aqueous phase of plasma; concentrations in plasma water therefore exceed those in whole plasma by a factor of 1,000/940.

Interstitial fluid. Interstitial fluid is an ultrafiltrate of plasma. A simple filtrate of plasma is devoid of particulate matter such as erythrocytes, leukocytes, and platelets, whereas an ultrafiltrate is, in addition, devoid of protein. Although interstitial fluid is not entirely free of protein, concentration is low in comparison with that of plasma. It is not possible to sample normal interstitial fluid in amounts sufficient for analysis. However, edema fluid can be collected from Southey's tubes inserted into the subcutaneous tissue of patients with congestive heart failure, and lymph can be collected from both peripheral and central channels. Edema fluid and lymph from peripheral channels contain less than 1.0% protein, whereas lymph collected from the liver may contain from 2% to 3% protein. Accordingly, capillaries in different regions of the body vary in their permeability regarding protein.

Table 5-5. Electrolyte composition of muscle

Ion	mEq/L H_2O
Na	±10
K	160
Mg	35
Cl	±2
HCO	±8
Protein	55
$PO_4^=$ (organic)	140

Modified from Pitts, R.F.: The physiological basis of diuretic therapy, Springfield, IL, 1959, Charles C Thomas, Publisher.

Intracellular fluid. As pointed out earlier, there is no one composition of intracellular fluid applicable to all cells. Erythrocytes, muscle cells, and liver cells obviously contain quite different functional proteins. Their ionic compositions also differ. However, certain features of all cell fluids are qualitatively similar and distinct from those of extracellular fluid. Thus, in terms of concentration, the major cations of intracellular fluid are potassium and magnesium; the major anions are proteins and organic phosphates. The major ionic components of striated muscle are given in Table 5-5.

For many reasons, the values of intracellular ion concentrations are uncertain. It is impossible to analyze cell contents directly; tissue must be analyzed and cell composition calculated from the differences between the total quantities of ions measured and the quantities contained in interstitial fluid. Because the volume of interstitial fluid within a tissue cannot be determined with any degree of precision, the exact quantities of extracellular ions to be subtracted are unknown. The errors are greatest for those ions, such as chloride and sodium, that are present in highest concentrations in interstitial fluid and in lowest concentration in intracellular fluid. Chloride, the major anion of extracellular fluid, is present in very low concentration in muscle cells. Some investigators claim that it is absent. However, certain other cells, including erythrocytes, gastric mucosa, gonads, and skin, contain significant quantities of chloride. Chloride cannot be said to be exclusively an extracellular ion. The major intracellular anions are protein and organic phosphates, including adenosine mono-, di-, and triphosphates, glycerophosphate, and creatinine phosphate. The total osmolar concentration of intracellular fluid, to be discussed in the following subsection, is generally considered to be essentially the same concentration as that of extracellular fluid.

Polarization of cell membranes

Cells are electrically polarized: negative inside, positive outside. Polarization is largely a function of the difference in potassium concentration on the two sides of the membrane, and the potential difference (PD) is described in a roughly quantitative manner by the simple Nernst equation:

$$PD \text{ (in mV)} = 61 \times \log\frac{Ki^+}{Ke^+}$$

In this equation, Ki^+ is the intracellular concentration of potassium and Ke^+ is the extracellular concentration.

The potential difference is predominantly a

potassium diffusion potential modified by the restricted movements of less permeable ions. In Fig. 5-8, curve 2 illustrates the effect of progressive substitution of potassium for sodium in the medium bathing a muscle fiber on the potential difference across the sarcolemma membrane.

When the extracellular concentration of potassium is in the normal range of 3.8 to 4.8 mEq/L and the ratio Ki^+/Ke^+ = 40-60, the potential difference is about 80 to 90 mV. As Ke^+ is increased, the ratio is reduced. The potential difference decreases, reaching zero when Ki^+/Ke^+ = 1.0, that is, when the external potassium concentration equals the internal.

The origin of the potential difference is explained as follows: the cell membrane is absolutely impermeable to the large polyvalent protein and organic phosphate anions contained within the cell. The cell membrane is effectively, although not actually, impermeable to sodium as a result of the operation of the ion pumps, which continuously eject sodium. As a first approximation, one can consider the cell as permeable only to potassium and chloride ions. Positively charged potassium ions tend to diffuse out of the cell down a concentration gradient. They are restrained by the increasing negative charge left within the cell. A state is reached in which the outward diffusion of potassium, driven by concentration difference, is just balanced by increasing cell negativity, restraining further diffusion. This state is described by the Nernst equation and in Fig. 5-8 by the broken line, l. If the intracellular concentration of potassium were 10 times the extracellular concentration, the potential difference would be 61 mV (log 10 = 1.0). If the intracellular and extracellular concentrations were equal, the potential difference would be 0.0 mV (log 1.0 = 0). Values of the potential difference for most mammalian cells vary from 60 to 90 mV when exposed to normal concentrations of potassium in extracellular fluid. From such potential difference values, intracellular potassium concentrations 10 to 30 times higher than extracellular concentrations would be predicted. In a number of in-

Fig. 5-8. The relationship between the potential across the sarcolemma and the logarithm of the ratio of the concentration of potassium inside/outside skeletal muscle fibers. *Curve 1,* calculated from the Nernst equation; *Curve 2,* observed.

From Szwed, J.: Fluid, electrolytes and acid-base, Indianapolis, IN, 1981, Indiana University School of Medicine.

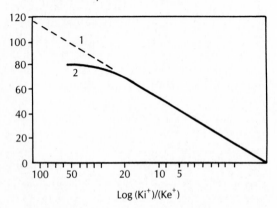

stances, the intracellular concentrations were observed to be higher, a fact that suggests that potassium is actively accumulated within cells—that is, potassium is pumped into cells. Furthermore, it is evident from Fig. 5-8 that the potential difference predicted by the Nerst equation *(curve 1)* exceeds the measured potential difference *(curve 2)*. Other ions, for example, sodium and chloride, no doubt diffuse into cells with sufficient ease to alter the relationship from that of a strict potassium diffusion potential. More complicated formulas have been devised that account for the shunting effects of other ions, but their consideration is not necessary here.

Osmotic pressure and water distribution between cells and extracellular fluid

Osmotic forces are of prime importance in determining the distribution of water among the several fluid compartments of the body. It is important, therefore, to have a clear appreciation of their operation. When a solution and pure solvent are separated by a membrane that is permeable to solvent but not to solute, the solvent passes into the solution by osmosis. The osmotic pressure is the particular hydrostatic pressure that must be applied to the solution to prevent the entry of solvent.

Cell membranes are permeable to water but effectively impermeable to many crystalloid solutes such as sodium, chloride, and bicarbonate. Cells therefore behave as tiny osmometers.

Isosmotic versus isotonic solutions

When red cells are placed in distilled water, they swell and hemolyze, that is, discharge their hemoglobin. If they are placed in 0.93% (0.16M) saline solution, they undergo no change in volume. The osmolar concentration of the saline solution (0.30 osmols/L) is exactly equal to that of the cell contents; the two solutions have the same osmotic pressure—in other words, they are isosmotic. Because no swelling or shrinking occurs, they are also isotonic. Basically, an isotonic solution is one that is physiologically isosmotic with cell fluid; that is, when a solution

is separated from cell contents by a semipermeable cell membrane, no transfer of water occurs.

A solution containing 1.8% urea has the same osmotic pressure as a solution containing 0.9% sodium chloride; the two solutions are therefore isosmotic. However, the urea solution is not isotonic because if red cells are added, they swell and hemolyze exactly as they do in distilled water. The reason for this is that the membrane of erythrocytes, like that of most cells, is nearly as permeable to urea as it is to water. Therefore, urea exerts no osmotic effect when separated from cell contents by membranes permeable to it. A solution of urea is physiologically equivalent to distilled water.

The capillary endothelium is permeable to water and to all solutes of blood plasma other than proteins and lipids. Therefore only transient osmotic forces develop across capillary walls when solutions of crystalloids that are higher or lower in osmolar concentration than interstitial fluid are introduced into the circulation.

Nature of osmotic forces

To state that a concentrated solution has a higher osmotic pressure than a dilute solution is a bit ambiguous. In isolation a solution, no matter how concentrated, has no osmotic pressure. An osmotic pressure develops only when a solution is separated from pure solvent or a more dilute solution by a semipermeable membrane. Furthermore, the force developed depends on the diffusion of solvent and not necessarily on the presence of solute except as it influences the concentration or, more accurately, the activity of the solvent in a solution.

Magnitude of osmotic forces

The osmotic forces that develop when blood plasma, interstitial fluid, and cell fluid are separated from pure water by semipermeable membranes are surprisingly large. They are of the order of magnitude of 6.7 atmospheres (atm), or 5100 mmHg. The essential equality of the osmolar concentrations of extracellular and intracellular fluids is a direct result of the rapid distribution of water through capillary walls and cell membranes, driven by forces of potentially great magnitude. Water distributes so that its escaping tendency, or activity, is the same in all body fluid compartments.

The osmotic concentrations of plasma, interstitial fluid, transcellular fluids, and intracellular fluid are all roughly equal and vary around 300 mosm/kg of water. Because 1.0 mosm/kg of water exerts an osmotic effect equivalent to 17 mmHg, the osmotic pressure of the body fluids averages $300 \times 17 = 5100$ mmHg. The osmotically active solutes of the body fluids are in large part electrolytes. The univalent ions sodium, chloride, and bicarbonate account for 90% to 95% of the osmotic activity of blood plasma and interstitial fluid. Other ions and organic compounds, such as glucose, amino acids, and urea, account for the remainder. The osmolality contributed by the blood urea nitrogen is found by dividing the concentration of blood urea nitrogen (BUN) by the atomic weight of the two nitrogens found in each urea molecule.

$$NH_3-\overset{\overset{\textstyle O}{\textstyle \|}}{C}-NH_3$$

A BUN of 150 mg/L (15 mg%) divided by 28 (each nitrogen having an atomic weight of 14) = osmolality of urea in a solution. For the sake of convenience, 30 is substituted for 28. Therefore the BUN in *mg/L* is divided by 30; the BUN in *mg%* is divided by 3 to obtain the osmolality, that is:

$$\frac{150 \text{ mg/L}}{30} = 5 \text{ mosm/kg,}$$

or

$$\frac{15 \text{ mg\%}}{3} = 5 \text{ mosm/kg}$$

The same principle applies for glucose and its osmolality. To determine the osmolality of a solution—for example, serum—the following equation may be employed:

1. Osmolality = [(Concentration of sodium) $\times$ 2] + $\dfrac{\text{Blood urea nitrogen}}{3}$ + $\dfrac{\text{Blood glucose concentration}}{18}$

For example, a patient has a serum sodium concentration of 140 mEq/L, a BUN of 15 mg%, and a blood glucose of 90 mg%.
Substituting in Equation *1* we get:

2. $(140 \times 2) + \dfrac{15}{3} + \dfrac{90}{18}$

3. $280 + 5 + 5 = 290$ mosm/kg of water

Because normal serum osmolality is 285 to 295, this patient has a normal osmolality. These equations provide a clinically useful tool and can be applied to any body fluid.

Total body stores of ions

It is evident that the total body water is a function of the total body store of ions. Furthermore, the distribution of water between cells and intracellular fluid is related to the distribution of ions. Finally, because sodium is largely an extracellular ion, whereas potassium is largely an intracellular one, the distribution of water ultimately depends on the quantities of these ions contained within the body.

Sodium. The total body sodium of a normal adult man averages 60 mEq/kg of body weight; for example, there are 4200 mEq in the body of a 70-kg man. Bone contains between 40% and 45% of the total store of sodium, or 1800 mEq. Of the remaining 2400 mEq, some 2000 to 2200 mEq are dissolved in extracellular fluid. Accordingly, about 50% of total body sodium is extracellular, 40% is associated with bone, and 10% is intracellular. Such figures are derived from postmortem chemical analyses of the body.

Potassium. The total potassium content of a normal adult man averages 42 mEq/kg of body weight. There are 2980 mEq in the body of a

70-kg man, nearly all of which is intracellular. *Only about 2%, or 60 mEq, is distributed in extracellular fluid.* The normal plasma concentration of potassium averages 4.3 mEq/L. *The shift of only a very small fraction of the intracellular store of potassium into extracellular fluid causes plasma concentration to rise to a dangerous and perhaps lethal level of 8-10 mEq/L.* Acidosis is associated with loss of cell potassium; in this condition, hydrogen ions enter cells in exchange for potassium ions. Potassium depletion is also of paramount clinical importance because the signs and symptoms may mimic serious organic diseases. Potassium depletion manifests itself in the neuromuscular signs of diminished deep tendon reflexes and muscular weakness, progressing to flaccid paralysis and mental confusion. In the gastrointestinal tract, anorexia may be the principal symptoms along with obstipation, abdominal distension, and paralytic ileus. In the renal tract, there are signs of isosthenuria, or loss of concentrating power of the kidneys; in the cardiac system, there are signs of rapid and irregular rhythm.

In the acidosis of chronic renal failure, the ability of the kidneys to excrete potassium is reduced and plasma potassium may rise. More precipitous rises occur in acute renal failure, in which urine formation may be completely suppressed. The major manifestations of hyperkalemia are cardiovascular, although muscular weakness, areflexia, and flaccid paralysis may develop *in much the same way as they do in potassium depletion.* When plasma concentration rises to 7 to 8 mEq/L, characteristic electrocardiographic changes occur. The T waves become high and peaked, the QRS complexes become broad and slurred, the P waves disappear, and arrhythmias develop. Eventually, the electrocardiogram shows complete disorganization, the heart becomes hypodynamic, and death occurs because of circulatory collapse precipitated by ventricular fibrillation.

Chloride. The total body chloride of a normal adult man averages 33 mEq/kg of body weight. In all, there are about 2300 mEq in the body of a 70-kg man. The major fraction, about 70%, is contained in the plasma and interstitial fluid. Although primarily an extracellular ion, chloride is not exclusively distributed in extracellular fluid. The remaining 30% of body chloride is in part intracellular and in part localized in connective tissue, perhaps bound to collagen. Of all cells, the erythrocytes contain the most chloride. Other tissues, such as gonads, gastric mucosa, and skin, contain lesser amounts; muscle probably contains the least.

Bicarbonate. Bicarbonate is unique in that it has no permanence. Its existence is fleeting, lasting merely as a step in the transfer of carbon dioxide between cells and lungs. The total body bicarbonate averages 10 to 12 mEq/kg of body weight. About one half is distributed in the extracellular compartment; the other half is distributed in cells. The carbon dioxide in bone is largely in the form of carbonate, bound in the crystal lattice. Cell concentrations are not known with any certainty because the distribution of carbon dioxide between ionic and carbamino combinations is unknown.

Magnesium. Knowledge of the body stores of magnesium has lagged behind that of other ions. However, in recent years, magnesium deficiency syndromes have become clinically important. These magnesium deficiency syndromes may result in coma and often are seen in malnourished patients, particularly in chronic alcoholics in our society. Total body stores average between 12 and 17 mEq/kg of body weight. There are, in all from 850 to 1200 mEq in the body of a 70-kg man, the major fraction of which is in the cells.

Normal nephron physiology

The functional unit of the kidney is the nephron. Each nephron is composed of a glomerulus, which filters fluid out of the blood, and a long tubular system that converts the glomerular filtrate into urine as it passes to the pelvis of the kidney (Fig. 5-9).

The glomerulus and filtration

The glomerulus is a capillary network, approximately 0.2 mm in diameter, with a volume of 4×10^{-6} ml (Fig. 5-10). It is positioned within Bowman's space and is surrounded by a capsule that is the invaginated beginning of the tubular system. To form the glomerular capillary bed, the afferent arteriole divides into from four to six capillary branches, each branch giving off sub-branches to form a lobule. In each lobule, the capillaries wind around a common axis that begins at the site of branching of the afferent arterioles and extends to the periphery of the glomerulus. This axis is known as the mesangium, or glomerular stalk. The mesangium provides support for the glomerular capillaries and contains cells whose functions are poorly understood.

The filtering surface of the glomerulus consists of three elements: an endothelium, a basement membrane, and an epithelial layer. The basement consists of a three-layered sandwich and has qualities similar to those of a highly hydrated gel. Although no pores have been demonstrated by presently available techniques, clearance studies with polymers of dextran suggest that the basement membrane is heteroporous, with one population of pores having a radius of 20 to 28 Å and an additional system having a radius of up to 80 Å. Such sizes allow the passage of molecules as large as those that are the size of hemoglobin but preclude the passage of the plasma proteins. Figure 5-11 illustrates the ultrastructure of the glomerular basement membrane and its relationship to endothelial and epithelial cells. Note the endothelial

Fig. 5-9. The functional unit of the kidney: the nephron.

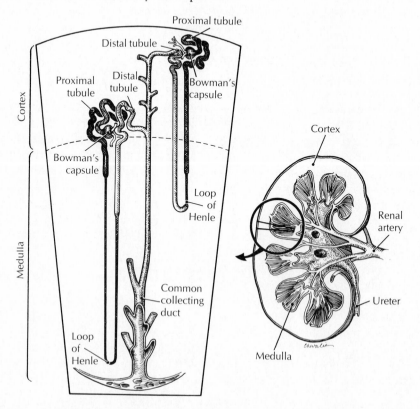

Fig. 5-10. Cross section of Bowman's capsule.

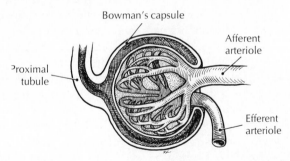

Fig. 5-11. Schematic representation of the glomerular basement membrane ultrastructure. Epithelial cell foot process, lamina rara externa, lamina densa, lamina rara interna, and endothelial cell cytoplasm.

Redrawn from Pitts, R.F.: Physiology of the kidney and body fluids, ed. 3, Chicago, 1974, Year Book Medical Publishers, Inc.

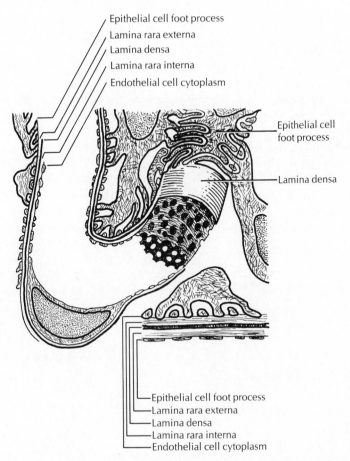

fenestrae, 500 to 750 Å in diameter; the glomerular basement membrane itself, a three-layered structure; and the visceral epithelial cells, with their foot processes.

Glomerular filtration rate. The force required for ultrafiltration is derived from the heart. The glomerular hydrostatic pressure of 60 mmHg is opposed by colloid osmotic pressure of 30 mmHg and capsular pressure of 10 mmHg, resulting in a net filtration pressure of 20 mmHg. The glomerular filtration surface is much more permeable than was previously believed. Of the 600 ml of plasma (*renal plasma flow*) that flows through the kidneys per minute, approximately 120 ml is filtered (*glomerular filtration rate*) at the glomerulus. The percent of renal plasma flow that is filtered is termed the *filtration fraction*.

$$\text{Filtration fraction} = \frac{\text{GFR}}{\text{RPF}}$$

Formation of the glomerular filtrate is the work of the glomerulus. The measurement of the glomerular filtration rate, or GFR, is accomplished with marker substances that are not acted on by the tubules in any way whatsoever. Such substances must be freely filtered, non—protein bound, biologically inert, nontoxic, and easily quantified. Inulin has long served as such a substance but first must be infused into the body. An endogenous material that closely satisfies the above criteria is creatinine, which is an anhydride of creatine and is a product of healthy muscle. Because creatinine is not acted on by the tubules, the amount appearing in the urine must equal the amount filtered. The amount filtered (filtered load) equals the plasma concentration of creatinine *multiplied by* the GFR. The amount that appears in the urine must equal the urinary concentration of creatinine the volume of urine.

$$P_{Cr} \times \text{GFR} = \text{Filtered load} \qquad U_{Cr} \times V = \text{Urinary excretion}$$

$$P_{Cr} = \text{GFR} \times U_{Cr} \times V \qquad \text{GFR} = \frac{U_{Cr}V}{P_{Cr}}$$

These principles are outlined in Fig. 5-12.

As a matter of fact, creatinine is not a perfect marker of GFR because it is very slightly secreted; however, it provides an adequate clinical measurement of GFR. An understanding by the reader of the relationship between plasma creatinine and GFR is crucial. Fig. 5-13 displays this hyperbolic relationship.

Evaluation of creatinine clearance. The normal values of GFR are 103 ± 15.8 ml/min per 1.73 m² for men and 97 ± 9.7 ml/min per 1.73 m² for women by the creatinine clearance method. An increase of the plasma creatinine from 1 to 2 mg% reflects a 50% decrease in the GFR; this decrease would result from, for example, the loss of one whole kidney. Subsequent doubling of plasma creatinine results in a further 50% decrease of GFR at each level. It must be remembered that the plasma creatinine concentration is a function of normal muscle mass. We might expect the plasma creatinine of the football player Hershel Walker to be 1.9 mg%, whereas that of singer Tiny Tim might be 0.6 mg%; however, if these amounts are correct, both individuals have a GFR in the normal range.

It can be recalled that in the previous discussion of GFR, 125 ml of plasma was filtered per minute, containing 1.25 mg of creatinine. This creatinine was completely excreted, whereas the filtrate was reabsorbed and therefore returned to the body. This filtrate had no creatinine returned with it and was therefore completely "cleared" of creatinine. The kidney functions to remove

Fig. 5-12. Principles of the measurement of glomerular filtration rate by the creatinine clearance method.

From Pitts, R.F.: Physiology of the kidney and body fluids, ed. 3, Chicago, 1974, Year Book Medical Publishers Inc.

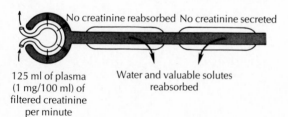

No creatinine reabsorbed No creatinine secreted

125 ml of plasma (1 mg/100 ml) of filtered creatinine per minute

Water and valuable solutes reabsorbed

many substances from the body. A measure of this function is the volume of plasma completely cleared of creatinine in 1 minute. Obviously, this is a virtual volume, not a real volume. This virtual volume (which is the volume of x cleared per minute) is defined as the quantity of x that is excreted in 1 minute divided by the plasma concentration of x.

$$C_x = \frac{U_x V}{P_x}$$

Note that if x is filtered and secreted, its clearance will exceed the GFR. If x is reabsorbed, however, its clearance will be less than the GFR.

Evaluation of blood urea nitrogen (BUN). Previously, the clearance of urea was a popular method of estimating the glomerular filtration rate. However, these measurements were unsatisfactory because urea is reabsorbed, and its reabsorption is a function of the rate of urine flow. The blood urea (expressed as BUN) is still used as a reflector of glomerular filtration rate, although those who use it keep its deficiencies in mind.

Urea production is a function of protein catabolism and requires a healthy liver. Its reabsorption is increased in situations of decreased urine flow. Therefore an elevated BUN may represent a decrease in the GFR but may also reflect dehydration, urinary obstruction, the increased protein catabolism of infection or corticosteroid therapy, or merely the consumption of several steak dinners in succession.

A low BUN, on the other hand, may represent excellent GFR, as seen in normal pregnancy, but may also indicate starvation or hepatic failure. The plasma creatinine is not subject to such effects. By comparing the BUN and plasma creatinine concentration, clues to other ongoing disorders may become apparent. Normally, BUN and plasma creatinine are present at a ratio of about 10:1.

Tubular modification of the glomerular filtrate. As the glomerular filtrate begins its descent through the nephron, it rapidly loses its original identity. The original volume is in excess of 170

L/24 hr in a normal adult; however, ordinarily less than 1.5 L of urine remain at the end of the collecting ducts. Of 1100 g of sodium chloride that are filtered, less than 10 g generally will remain in the final urine, and of the 400 mg of sodium bicarbonate filtered, only trace amounts will be excreted. Similarly, all the filtered glucose and virtually all the amino acids will be reabsorbed; 85% to 95% of the filtered solutes will be removed from the tubular fluid. On the other hand, certain substances such as ammonia, hydrogen ions, potassium, and urate will be added to the tubular fluids by secretion. Fig. 5-14 illustrates selective filtration through the tubule.

Various mechanisms of transport are available. *Passive transport* may involve a chemical concentration gradient in which a greater concentration of the solute resides on one side of the membrane than on the other, or it may involve an electric potential gradient in which one surface of the membrane is electrically positive to the other. The electric field produced will influence the movement of all charged particles. Anions tend to move toward the side where the positive charges predominate, and cations preferentially move in the opposite direction.

Fig. 5-13. The relationship between the plasma creatinine concentration and the glomerular filtration rate (GFR).

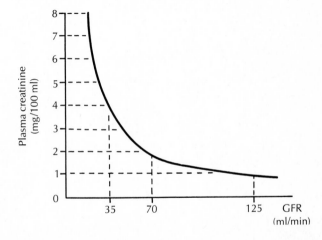

Active transport takes place "uphill" against a concentration gradient in a thermodynamic context. The energy is derived from the metabolic activity of the epithelial cells themselves. Carrier molecules form complexes with the solute; these complexes move across the finite distance of the membrane and then dissociate, releasing the transported species. The reabsorption of sodium is the principal energy-consuming process in the renal tubular epithelial cells. This transport in itself may be responsible to a major degree for establishing the conditions for the passive movement of water, chloride, urea, and possibly other solutes, including part of the secretion of hydrogen and potassium ions.

Renal regulation of sodium excretion

Claude Bernard promulgated the concept of an "internal environment" that is maintained by the body for the benefit of all the cells therein. This "internal environment" is closely regulated by the kidneys. The sodium ion is the principal cation of the extracellular fluid (ECF) that makes up the internal environment, and with its two major anions, chloride and bicarbonate, it comprises 90% of the total solute found in the ECF. The sodium content of the intracellular fluid is very low because of the cellular sodium pump. Water molecules, however, move across the cell membrane with ease in the direction of any osmotic gradient.

Therefore if there is retention of sodium ions in the ECF, there will be an attendant increase in the osmotic pressure of this compartment, resulting in a shift of water from inside to outside cells. Moreover, the rise in osmolarity of the ECF imposed by the sodium retention will result in an increase in the secretion of the antidiuretic hormone (ADH), and positive water balance will ensue. In addition, the thirst mechanism may be activated, resulting in increased water intake. Thus the overall effect of a primary increase in sodium mass will be an increase in ECF. Conversely, a decrease in sodium mass will initiate a corresponding decrease in the ECF.

Under most physiologic circumstances in man, sodium balance is well maintained; that is, the intake and output of the cation are the same. Because the amount of sodium filtered greatly exceeds the amount excreted, the nephrons must possess a highly developed system for conserving sodium.

The amount of sodium filtered, called the *filtered load,* equals the serum sodium concentration multiplied by the GFR, or approximately 23,800 mEq/24 hr. In a healthy person, more than 99% of this sodium is reabsorbed and returned to the body. The amount actually excreted approaches the amount in the diet minus slight amounts lost in the stool and through the skin.

Sodium conservation. Sodium conservation mechanisms are very finely controlled. If need be—such as in instances of severe dehydration or very low sodium intake—the amount of urine sodium falls to very low levels, for example, 1 mEq/L. In instances of greatly increased or inappropriate sodium intake, the kidneys react accordingly and can excrete large quantities of so-

Fig. 5-14. Tubular modification of the glomerular filtrate.

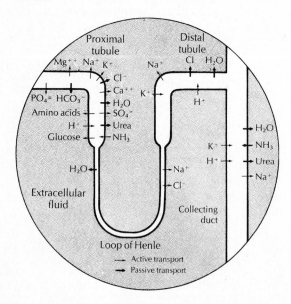

dium. Thus ECF volume and tonicity are maintained.

Hypothetically, even normal people may violate their sodium limits. If their sodium intake does not meet even the small quantities the kidneys must excrete, negative sodium balance will ensue. The ECF will contract and dehydration will result. On the other hand, if the generous excretory capacity of the kidneys for sodium is exceeded, positive sodium balance, ECF expansion, edema, and eventual pulmonary edema will result.

Approximately 65% of sodium is reabsorbed in the proximal tubule, about 25% in the loop of Henle, 6% in the distal tubule, and the final 3% to 5% in the collecting duct. There is no evidence that sodium is secreted. In humans, it appears that the major renal adjustments in maintaining sodium balance are made by changes in the tubular reabsorption.

The GFR is obviously important in sodium excretion because it is the first step in the renal elimination of sodium. The GFR is therefore sometimes referred to as *Factor 1*. Although poorly understood, it is well known that an increase in GFR, and therefore an increase in filtered sodium, is accompanied by a proportionate increase in tubular reabsorption of sodium. This phenomenon is referred to as *glomerular tubular balance*.

Aldosterone augments the rate of sodium reabsorption in the distal nephron in a loose exchange for potassium and hydrogen ions. The secretion of this hormone is under the control of the renin-angiotensin axis and, to a lesser extent, ACTH and the serum potassium concentration. Aldosterone is important in determining the quantity of sodium reabsorbed; however, all changes in sodium reabsorption cannot be explained in terms of aldosterone activity alone. Aldosterone is sometimes referred to as *Factor 2*.

Other mechanisms, loosely termed *Factor 3*, or the *Third Factor*, also influence sodium reabsorption. Some of these mechanisms, such as changes in peritubular protein, "oncotic" pressure, and alterations in cortical and medullary

blood flow, are well established. Others, such as a possible humoral factor called the "natriuretic hormone," remain elusive and are as yet unproven by scientific investigators.

It is sufficient to say that the renal regulation of sodium is intimately related to the ECF. Because most adjustments in sodium elimination are accomplished via alterations in tubular reabsorption, it is not surprising that the tubular reabsorption mechanisms are sensitive to changes in ECF. An expanded ECF results in less reabsorption and more excretion of sodium; a contracted ECF has the opposite effect. These effects may be accomplished by indirect mechanisms, including a volume receptor mechanism and an efferent system, or by a more direct action on the tubular cell. It is known that changing levels of aldosterone are not required for changes in ECF to affect the tubular cell.

Elaboration of a concentrated or dilute urine

Concentrated urine may be defined as urine in which the total solute concentration (osmolality) exceeds that of plasma. Only mammals and some birds are able to produce a concentrated urine. Humans may concentrate the urine to an osmolality of 1200 mOsm/kg of water (four times the serum osmolality). This task is accomplished by the reabsorption of filtered water, which requires the presence and maintenance of (1) an osmotic gradient and (2) the elaboration and effects on the kidney of the antidiuretic hormone (ADH).

Each juxtamedullary nephron has a segment of tubule that dips down into the medullary portion of the kidney and then doubles back on itself to form a hairpin-shaped section known as the loop of Henle. The concentration gradient pattern is a product of this loop. Isotonic fluid from the proximal tubule enters the descending limb of the loop of Henle. From the corresponding level of the ascending limb, chloride is actively extruded into the interstitium; sodium follows passively.

The concentrations of chloride and sodium

are reduced in the ascending limb and increase in the interstitium. The concentration gradient formed in the medullary interstitium occurs only because the ascending limb is impermeable to water. Sodium and chloride then freely enter the descending limb and water freely leaves, following the concentration gradient provided.

The osmolality of the fluid in the descending limb therefore progressively increases as the hairpin turn of the loop of Henle is approached. The osmolality in the ascending limb progressively decreases as fluid flows toward the cortex, and the tubular urine actually becomes hypotonic before entering the distal tubule. The flow in the loop of Henle is continuous, and chloride along with sodium are added steadily to the fluid as it descends toward the tip. This operation is referred to as the *countercurrent multiplier*.

Ultimately, equilibrium is reached, with increasing tonicity in all medullary structures as the papilla is approached. The *vasa recta* facilitate these operations, removing excess water by passive diffusion through the capillary walls. This passive process involving the vasa recta in the maintenance of medullary hypertonicity is referred to as the *countercurrent exchanger*.

The collecting ducts serve as osmotic exchangers, which permit the equilibration of the final urine with the hypertonic interstitium of the medulla and papilla. In hydropenia, during which a high titer of circulating ADH is present, the permeability of collecting ducts to water is high. Isotonic fluid, entering the collecting ducts from the distal tubule, gives up water to the hypertonic interstitium. The final urine attains an osmolar concentration equal to that of the interstitium. Fig. 5-14 provides additional explanation of countercurrent multiplication.

In establishing a dilute urine, the major requirement is the absence of ADH. Under these circumstances, even a concentrated interstitium would not prevent the excretion of a hypotonic urine; this is because in the absence of ADH, the distal nephron would not be permeable to water, and the hypotonic urine arriving there would be excreted as such.

As mentioned previously, powerful "salt pumps" reside in the ascending limb of Henle's loop, which is impermeable to water. The osmolality of tubular fluid in this segment progressively decreases as the cortex is reached until the urine is actually hypotonic to plasma. This process continues in the proximal portion of the distal tubule. In the absence of ADH, urine that is as diluted as 50 mOsm/kg of water may be achieved in man.

In the past decade, research has necessitated some modifications in the "countercurrent" model. Details do not concern us here; however, the clinician should appreciate that urea plays an important role in the generation of a concentrated urine by contributing to the gradient. Urea is resorbed in the collecting duct and reenters the loop of Henle. This medullary recycling of urea causes it to accumulate in large quantities in the medullary interstitium, where it automatically extracts water from the descending limb and thereby concentrates sodium chloride in the descending limb. Thus protein intake may influence urinary concentrating ability. "Protein-starved" individuals, who generate relatively little urea, are not able to concentrate their urine as well as individuals who ingest a liberal protein intake and produce larger quantities of urea.

Electrolyte regulation

Potassium excretion. Of the approximately 3300 mEq of potassium in the body, 98% is contained *within* cells. The amount acquired in the diet varies from 50 to 100 mEq/day. Small amounts are lost in the stool and sweat, the predominant route of excretion being the kidney. Potassium is freely filtered and almost completely reabsorbed in the proximal tubule. The potassium in the final urine is derived almost exclusively by distal tubular secretion. The determinants of potassium secretion are poorly understood. One of the determinants is the amount of potassium in the diet, but how the kidney is "made aware" of the amount ingested is not completely clear. Two factors appear to be involved. First, when a high-potassium diet is ingested, potassium in most body cells (including the distal convoluted tubule cells) increases. The increased intracellular potassium concentration favors secretion in the kidney. Second, elevated plasma potassium (or more likely, increased potassium in the adrenal cortical cells) increases the production of aldosterone. This hormone favors potassium secretion by the distal nephron. The amount of potassium secreted bears some relationship to the amount of sodium delivered to the distal tubule; however, this is not a precise stoichiometric relationship. This loose sodium-potassium exchange is modulated by aldosterone.

Hydrogen ion is also a participant in potassium excretion. There is generally an inverse relationship between the potassium ion and the hydrogen ion secreted by the distal tubular cell. In the presence of acidemia, relatively less potassium is secreted, whereas in states of alkalemia, the initial response is an increase in potassium excretion. During potassium depletion, potassium secretion is diminished even with alkalemia, whereas hydrogen ion is secreted. Thus, despite extracellular alkalemia, after a time the urine is acid (paradoxical aciduria).

Calcium and phosphorus. The ultrafilterable calcium is almost completely reabsorbed by the nephron. The mechanism of reabsorption is similar to that of sodium and occurs actively in those areas where sodium is actively reabsorbed as well. Although the reabsorption of both cations is decreased with volume expansion and increased with contraction, some important differences exist. Calcium reabsorption is augmented by parathyroid hormone without influencing sodium reabsorption. Aldosterone influences sodium reabsorption but has no effect on calcium.

Phosphate is filtered and reabsorbed. In situations of phosphate depletion, this anion may disappear from the urine. Its clearance is a function of the parathyroid hormone concentration, that is, increased hormone activity results in decreased reabsorption, or phosphaturia.

Endocrine and metabolic functions

The kidney serves in the regulation of certain biologic systems by nonexcretory functions. Several hormone activators are produced within the renal parenchyma. One of these activators is thought to act on a plasma substrate to produce an erythropoietic hormone. This material, called *erythropoietin*, is found within the kidney; however, details concerning its formation are unknown. There is evidence that it is a low-molecular-weight glycoprotein, possibly with an associated active polypeptide side chain. Erythropoietin acts to increase both the rate of red cell production in, and the rate of release of red cells from, the bone marrow and spleen. Adequate synthesis of erythropoietin requires intact kidneys and is subject to various stimuli. Three erythropoietin-mediated stimuli have been shown to increase the rate of production of erythrocytes: anemia, reduction in inspired oxygen pressure (PO_2), and the administration of salts of cobalt.

The kidney's role as an endocrine organ in calcium-phosphorus metabolism has only recently been recognized. The precursor of active vitamin D, cholecalciferol, is hydroxylated first by the liver at the 25 position and then by the kidney at the 1 position, resulting in 1,25 di (OH) cholecalciferol, the active form of this hormone. Intact kidneys are required for this function, explaining the appearance of apparent vitamin D resistance in renal failure.

Renin is a proteolytic enzyme produced by cells of the juxtaglomerular apparatus, which reacts with a plasma substrate, angiotensinogen, to produce a weakly active pressor decapeptide, angiotensin I. The decapeptide is converted into a highly active pressor octapeptide, angiotensin II, by a chloride-activated enzyme in plasma (converting enzyme). Angiotensin II has important blood pressure regulatory effects not only in a direct way but also via its effect on aldosterone release. Furthermore, angiotensin II stimulates both thirst and ADH secretion by a direct effect on the brain (Fig. 5-15). Angiotensin II is subsequently destroyed by angiotensinase, which is present in circulating blood plasma and in many organs including the kidneys, the intestine, and the liver. Renin production is mediated either by sensors in afferent arterioles, intraluminal chloride sensors at the macula densa, or both. Therefore a decrease in afferent arteriolar pressure, an increase in chloride transport, or both result in renin release. Stimulation of renal sympathetic nerves also causes renin release.

In addition, there are lipid-filled cells in the renal medulla that appear to represent a site of synthesis of prostaglandins. The effects of prostaglandins are widespread and varied. The nor-

mal physiologic functions of these biologically active compounds and the control system regulating their synthesis and release are currently under close scrutiny. Those found within the kidney appear to have an effect in lowering blood pressure. It is conceivable that the occurrence of high blood pressure seen in chronic renal disease or (rarely) after bilateral nephrectomy, when it is called *renoprival hypertension,* may be a result of an alteration in prostaglandin function.

Finally, the kidneys also participate in kinin production. Urinary kallikrein serves to generate

Fig. 5-15. Renin-angiotensin system.

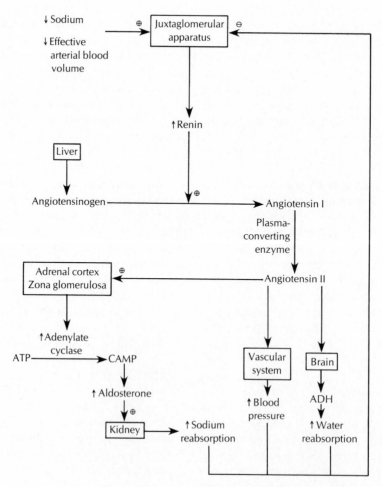

bradykinin, a peptide that has vasodilatory and natriuretic properties. The renin-angiotensin system, renal prostaglandins, and kallikrein-kinin system are all closely interrelated in the maintenance of systemic blood pressure.

Acid-base balance

The physiology of acid-base balance is concerned primarily with the mechanisms maintaining the concentration of hydrogen ions within normal limits.

Concentration of hydrogen ions and pH

The concentration of hydrogen ions is represented by the symbol (H^+) when expressed in moles per liter. The higher such a concentration is, the more acid a solution is, and vice versa. Therefore the obvious way to express the acidity of a solution should be by the concentration of hydrogen ions in moles, millimoles, or similar units per liter. Unfortunately, it is customary to express acidity in terms of pH rather than as hydrogen ion concentration, and because the concept of pH is so deeply entrenched in our chemical and biologic terminology, it is almost impossible to avoid its use, despite its obvious disadvantages.

The pH notation expresses the concentration of hydrogen ions of a solution in exponential fashion and uses the exponent alone as indicator of acidity. Because biologic solutions have a very low concentration of hydrogen ions, the exponent is always negative; therefore the sign of the exponent is inverted to make it positive. For instance, if we have a solution whose hydrogen ion concentration is 0.0001 mol/L (or 0.0001 M), it can be written in exponential form:

$$(H^+) = 0.0001 = 10^{-4} \text{ M}$$

According to the pH notation, such concentration would be presented by pH 4. Thus pH, by definition, is the negative logarithm (on the base 10) of the concentration of hydrogen ions. Actually, the true concentration of H^+ is unknown, and only the H^+ activity can be measured.

Normal pH

The normal concentration of hydrogen ions in the extracellular fluid is approximately 0.00000004 M, which can be expressed as 4 × 10^{-8}. The negative logarithm of this figure, that is, the pH, is 7.4.

If we wish to express the concentration of hydrogen ions as (H^+) rather than as pH, it is preferable to use smaller units such as nanomoles instead of moles. The normal extracellular H^+ concentration is about 40 nmol/L (40 nM). It is higher inside the cell, particularly in organelles such as the mitochondria, where oxidation and the generation of hydrogen ions take place.

pH range

The concentration of hydrogen ions in the extracellular fluid can vary in extreme cases from as low as 10 to as high as 160 nmol/L, which is roughly equivalent to a pH range of from 8.0 to 6.8. These are the limits compatible with sustaining human life. In the healthy person, however, the range is much narrower, usually from 7.38 to 7.42; this corresponds to an H^+ concentration of from 42 to 38 nmol/L.

Normal acid load

The ingestion and metabolism of food are constantly adding a load of hydrogen ions to the body's supply. The largest acid load is found in CO_2 and results from oxidation of various foodstuffs. The CO_2 acid load approaches 20,000 mmol/24 hr for the normal adult who eats an average diet and engages in routine activity. This huge amount of acid, however, is easily eliminated through the lungs, provided no impairment of ventilation is present. If ventilation is inadequate, a respiratory type of acidosis will follow.

On the other hand, a much smaller but very important amount comprised of acids other than CO_2 is added every day to the metabolic pool. CO_2 is the only volatile acid formed by metabolism; for this reason, all acids other than CO_2 are sometimes called "fixed," or nonvolatile, acids. The "fixed acids" are chiefly derived from metabolism of proteins and, to a lesser extent, fat and carbohydrates. The amount of fixed acids formed in 24 hours is approximately 50 to 30 mmol. About $\frac{2}{3}$ of this amount is derived from sulphur- and phosphate-containing metabolic substrates. Sulphuric acid results from the oxidation of methionine and cystine; phosphoric acid results from phosphate-protein complexes and phosphate-containing lipids. Another $\frac{1}{3}$ of the fixed acid load is comprised of organic acids (such as uric, lactic, and pyruvic) derived from intermediate metabolism.

Although fixed acids are produced in a much smaller quantity than CO_2 (60 mmol/24 hr), they present a special problem because they cannot be eliminated by the lungs. The body has special and sophisticated mechanisms that deal with the load of fixed acids, initially by neutralization and finally by elimination through the kidney. Although 60 mmol of fixed acid may seem like a small amount, it actually is quite large and can cause a very serious disturbance in neutrality if its elimination is impaired. If it is recalled that the normal hydrogen ion concentration in extracellular fluid is only 40 nmol/L, 50 to 80 mmol formed in 24 hours is a huge amount of acid indeed.

If a state of balance is to be maintained, the amount of acid formed or ingested every day must be the same as that which is excreted by the kidney.

Mechanisms that regulate extracellular concentration of H^+

Any situation of acid-base imbalance should be understood as a deviation above or below the normal H^+ concentration of 40 nmol/L (pH 7.4). Because under normal circumstances acid is continuously produced, the physiologic defense mechanisms are primarily geared to cope with an acid excess, or acidosis. Occasionally, however, a hydrogen ion deficit, or alkalosis, may arise, and there are also mechanisms of defense against these possibilities.

Three major mechanisms handle the normal

acid production. The same mechanisms can adapt themselves to handle an abnormal situation of acid-base imbalance. They are:

1. Neutralization of body buffers
2. Pulmonary regulation
3. Renal regulation

Neutralization by buffers. A buffer may be defined as a substrate capable of neutralizing an excess or deficit of hydrogen ions. Buffers are either weak acids or the salts of weak acids. The salt buffers neutralize acids, whereas the weak acids neutralize bases. The important and significant effect of a buffer is that the addition of a strong acid or strong alkali to a well-buffered solution will produce a change in pH much smaller than the change that would have occurred had the solution not been buffered.

Most buffering takes place intracellularly. If an H^+ ion is added to a biologic system, that ion is bound to intracellular proteins in exchange for Na^+ and K^+ ions that leave the cell. Although probably more Na^+ than K^+ leaves the cells, the relative change in K^+ concentration is more important because the normal low extracellular concentration of this cation can be increased rapidly, and dangerous hyperkalemia may result. Although buffering by proteins is most important qualitatively, the bicarbonate buffer system has a unique and important role because bicarbonate can be regenerated, and CO_2 can be excreted. Buffering by phosphates is of minor importance in the extracellular fluid, although phosphate is a very important urinary buffer.

An important concept to grasp is that the concentration of H^+ in a solution is determined by the relative proportion of the acidic and basic components of the buffer systems present in the solution. For instance, in a mixture of Na HPO and NaH PO in 4:1 ration, the resultant pH is 7.4. For the bicarbonate system, pH 7.4 is obtained when $NaHCO_3$ and H_2CO_3 are in the systems in a solution in equilibrium among themselves; that is, each buffer system will be dissociated in a ratio appropriate to produce the same concentration of hydrogen ions. Where "f" means "function of,"

$$[H^+] = f\frac{Pr^+}{Pr} = f\frac{H_2CO_3}{HCO_3^-} = f\frac{H_2Po_4^-}{HPO_4^-}$$

If the above equation is expressed logarithmically, pH instead of $[H^+]$ and pK's instead of f's will be obtained. An important consequence is that only the measurement of the components of a single buffer system (for instance, bicarbonate) is needed to know the acid-base status of the body, even though there are other buffers present. In fact, measurements of bicarbonate and CO_2 provide sufficient information in most clinical situations.

The buffers constitute the first line of defense against acid-base imbalance resulting from a large acid load. As buffers neutralize acid, they are consumed by it. Such consumption is reflected in the falling concentration of bicarbonate, as well as other basic buffers that are not measured and with which bicarbonate is in equilibrium. When bicarbonate concentration falls to very low levels, the buffering reserve is almost exhausted, and any further gain of acid will result in a sharp fall in pH. This situation also means that the basic buffers need to be replaced either by the body itself or by a doctor. If the doctor chooses to administer bicarbonate, not only will the bicarbonate reserve increase, but because of the equilibrium principle, the other basic buffers will increase as well.

In summary, the buffers permit a vital, if only temporary, neutralization of acid until a more definite acid excretion by the kidney can take place.

Pulmonary compensation. When the $[H^+]$ is higher than normal (as in acidosis), the alveolar ventilation is stimulated, with increases in both rate and depth of the respiratory movements. The resulting hyperventilation accomplishes two things: (1) CO_2 formed during neutralization of acid by bicarbonate is eliminated and (2) an additional amount of CO_2 is eliminated, which helps to change the pH to more acceptable levels by decreasing pCO_2 below normal levels.

If, on the other hand, the $[H^+]$ is lower than normal (as in alkalosis), there may be a slight degree of hypoventilation, which will tend to increase the pCO_2. This compensation is usually much less effective than the respiratory compensation to acidosis because ventilation continues to be driven by hypoxia.

Renal compensation. The kidney is the only organ that is truly able to excrete hydrogen ions. Neutralization by buffers or pulmonary compensation are mechanisms that, although very important and sometimes lifesaving, are only temporary and cannot continue indefinitely. Therefore the body has another mechanism to effectively rid the body of hydrogen ions. This mechanism, which achieves permanent correction, is the renal excretion of $H.^+$

The kidney of a normal person on an average diet adjusts the excretion of hydrogen ions to match exactly the amount of acid derived from metabolism. The metabolic acid load varies between 50 and 80 mmol in 24 hours, and an equal amount is lost by renal excretion. Approximately 40% of hydrogen ion is excreted, buffered by certain salts, particularly phosphate; 60% combines with NH_3 to form ammonium.

In cases of acidosis, the renal excretion of hydrogen ions can be enhanced many times, although it may take several days for the kidney to reach its maximal excretory capacity, which can be more than 500 mmol of H^+ in 24 hours.

Renal mechanisms for hydrogen ion excretion. A brief examination of the mechanisms of renal hydrogen ion excretion follows. Neutralization of strong acids by buffers result in depletion of extracellular bicarbonate, as well as other basic components of the buffer system. Because of these depletions, neutralization of strong acids cannot continue indefinitely unless the depleted bicarbonate stores are replenished. Fortunately, there are physiologic mechanisms in the kidney that permit bicarbonate replenishment simultaneously with hydrogen ion excretion. In addition, the kidney must conserve filtered bicarbonate by reabsorption.

BICARBONATE REABSORPTION. The normal bicarbonate concentration is about 25 mmol/L, and this is mostly matched against sodium. Assuming GFR of 120 ml/min, the amount of bicarbonate filtered in 24 hours would be:

120 ml/min $\times$ 0.025 mmol/ml $\times$ 1440 minutes = 4320 mmol/24 hr

The tubular reabsorption of bicarbonate is so perfect that no more than 1 or 2 mmol are lost in the urine during a 24-hour period.

The mechanism of bicarbonate reabsorption is believed to be indirect, involving simultaneous secretion of H^+:

1. The filtered bicarbonate is mostly matched against Na^+. As it proceeds along the tubule, bicarbonate binds the H^+ excreted by tubular cells, with formation of CO_2 and water:

$$HCO_3^- + H^+ \rightarrow CO_2 + H_2O$$

2. CO_2 diffuses into cells of the tubules. The conditions of the cell then favor a shift in the direction of the reaction that forms HCO and H^+, and at least in the proximal tubule, this reaction is catalyzed by the enzyme carbonic anhydrase (E):

$$CO_2 + H_2O \overset{(E)}{\rightarrow} H^+ + HCO_3^-$$

The HCO_3^- ion has now been saved from excretion and diffuses into the peritubular blood, whereas the H^+ ion is available to capture another bicarbonate (Fig. 5-16).

The magnitude of bicarbonate reabsorption can be influenced by factors affecting sodium reabsorption, as well as by K^+ and H^+ secretion. Among these factors are:

1. Concentration of extracellular chloride
2. Total body potassium stores
3. Extracellular volume status
4. CO_2 tension (pCO_2)

A decrease in either the first, second, or third of these factors leads to increased proximal tubular reabsorption of bicarbonate ion and therefore an elevation of the serum $[HCO_3]$. In addition, an increase in the pCO_2 of the blood leads to an increase in proximal tubular bicarbonate reabsorption and therefore an elevation of the serum $[HCO_3]$. This phenomenon of increased serum bicarbonate is clinically most commonly seen in patients taking diuretic agents, patients on nasogastric suction, and some patients with chronic lung disease who have elevated pCO_2s. It is unclear what mechanism is responsible for increased proximal tubular bicarbonate reabsorption under the conditions listed above.

In venous blood, chloride concentrations in the intracellular compartment of the red cells are higher than those on the arterial side. The significance of the chloride shift with increased hydrogen ion concentration on the venous side is uncertain when related to alterations in HCO_3^- threshold (Fig. 5-17).

Fig. 5-16. Renal bicarbonate buffer system.

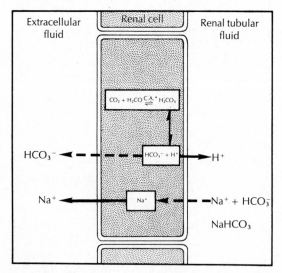

*Carbonic anhydrase

→ Active transport

- - → Osmosis

Excretion of titratable acid. This is the renal process by which hydrogen ions are excreted in the urine by combining with urinary buffers at the same time that bicarbonate is generated. This operation can be described as acidification of the urine, excretion of titratable acid, or regeneration of bicarbonate. Actually, these three descriptions emphasize different aspects of the same operation.

Hydrogen ions excreted by tubular cells into the lumen are neutralized by buffer salts, particularly Na_2HPO_4, which are in turn converted to acid salts. This process allows a large quantity of H^+ to be excreted in the urine with a relatively minor fall in urinary pH:

$$H^+ + Na_2HPO_4 \rightleftarrows NaH_2PO_4 + Na^+$$

Many years ago, it was demonstrated that venous blood coming from the kidney contained more ammonia than the arterial blood perfusing this organ. This obviously means that the kidney synthesizes ammonia, or NH_3.

Ammonia is synthesized in the tubular cells from glutamine and other amino acids. Being a gas, it diffuses easily in all directions; it goes to the luminal urine, as well as to the peritubular blood. The relative magnitude of the diffusion toward either side is highly variable and mainly depends on the urinary pH. If the urine is acid, ammonia is combined with hydrogen ions and converted into ammonium, or NH_4. Ammonium, in contrast to ammonia, does not diffuse easily back into the cells and therefore does not return to blood. As long as there are free hydrogen ions in the tubular urine, ammonia will be trapped and its concentration as free gas will be low, which in turn will allow a continuation of NH diffusion to the urine rather than toward the blood. If, on the other hand, the urine is alkaline, the lack of hydrogen ions to bind ammonia will cause most NH_3 to diffuse back to the blood.

The importance of ammonia synthesis and secretion by the tubular cells rests in the fact that it permits continuous secretion of hydrogen ions

far beyond the limits imposed by the formation of titratable acid. The tubular cells cannot secrete hydrogen ions against a gradient higher than approximately 800 between blood and urine. In other words, if the $[H^+]$ in the blood is 40 nmol/L (pH 7.4), excretion of hydrogen ions can continue until its concentration in the urine is about 800 times higher (pH 4.6). At that point, hydrogen ion secretion ceases. Secretion of ammonia binds hydrogen ions and lowers the tubular concentration of H^+ ions, therefore permitting secretion of H^+ by the tubular cells to continue.

Fig. 5-17. The chloride shift. Chloride ions diffuse into the cell to preserve electrical neutrality.

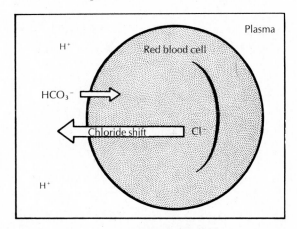

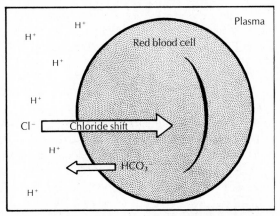

Evaluation of renal performance in acid-base balance. The ability of the kidney to excrete acid can be measured by determining the total amount of hydrogen ions excreted in 24 hours and the maximal gradient that can be established between blood and urine.

The gradient, as discussed above, is reflected in the lowest pH that urine can achieve after a proper challenge with an acid load. It is standard to use ammonium chloride (0.1 g/kg of body weight) as the acid load. The total amount of hydrogen ions excreted in the urine is determined by measuring the titratable acid and the ammonium salts. Normally, titratable acidity is 30 to 40 mEq/24 hr, and the ammonium excretion is 40 to 50 mEq/24 hr. If bicarbonate is present in the urine, the amount present should be subtracted.

The pH of the urine reflects the concentration of free H^+. Free H^+, however, constitutes an insignificant part of the total H^+ normally excreted by the kidney. Most H^+ by far is bound to buffers and ammonia. Even if the pH of the urine were as low as 4.4. (which it never is), the urine would contain 40 μmol of H^+/L (1000 more than the blood contains at pH 7.4). In 1.5 L of urine, 60 μmol of H^+ would be excreted; this is only 1/1000th of the 60 mmol that must be excreted every day.

Integration of regulatory mechanisms. The compensatory responses (buffers, lung, and kidney) are integrated in such a way that the pH, as well as the buffer content of the body, are maintained as close to normal as possible. In case of metabolic acidosis, bicarbonate and other basic buffers neutralize acid, preventing an excessive drop in the pH. This is reflected in a low bicarbonate. At the same time, the pulmonary response causes hyperventilation, and as a result, CO_2 is eliminated at a higher rate. This is reflected in a fall of partial pressure of CO_2, or pCO_2. The renal response, which takes a longer time to develop, consists of enhanced excretion of H^+ mainly in the form of NH_4 but also as titratable acidity. At the same time, bicarbonate is regenerated in the kidney and serves to replenish the exhausted stores of buffer.

Therefore in a well compensated case of metabolic acidosis the characteristic chemical changes are low pH, low bicarbonate, low pCO_2 in the arterial blood, and decreased NH_4 and total H^+ in the urine.

On the other hand, in case of chronic lung disease with hypercapnia (respiratory acidosis), CO_2 accumulates in the body and pCO_2 will be elevated. Compensation by body buffers is relatively minor, and most of it will be renal. This compensation consists of an increased ceiling for reabsorption of bicarbonate. Therefore a typical case of well compensated chronic respiratory acidosis presents with low pH, high bicarbonate, and high pCO_2 in the arterial blood, as well as high NH_2 and H^+ excretion in the urine. The opposite changes take place in respiratory alkalosis (high pH, low bicarbonate, low pCO_2 in the arterial blood, and low NH_4 and H^+ excretion in the urine).

Disturbances of acid-base balance: primary disturbances and their compensation

It is evident from the preceding discussion that changes in bicarbonate concentration, as well as in pCO_2, can be either primary or secondary (compensatory). Therefore in chronic respiratory acidosis the primary change is an elevation of pCO_2, usually followed by a secondary rise of blood bicarbonate. On the other hand, in metabolic alkalosis the bicarbonate concentration rises and, at the same time, there may or may not be a secondary rise of pCO_2. Therefore if high values of bicarbonate concentration and pCO_2 are made available to physicians without any other information, it is impossible for them to know to what extent a combination of respiratory acidosis and metabolic alkalosis is present. A similar problem exists in differentiating metabolic acidosis and respiratory alkalosis.

To delineate the participation of metabolic and respiratory components in any given disturbance, it is necessary to have the clinical information provided by the patient's history and physical examination, in addition to measurement of bicarbonate, pCO_2, and pH. Measurement of pH is important because it indicates if compensation has occurred and to what extent. It also suggests the nature of the dominant component in a mixed disturbance. Because compensation is never perfect, the pH is likely to deviate—to a variable degree—toward the side of the primary disturbance.

Some practitioners have the mistaken notion that measurement of the "standard bicarbonate" and "base excess" or "base deficit," as described by Astrup, provides information enabling them to distinguish the chemical changes of metabolic origin from those of respiratory origin without further clinical information. This is not the case, as Astrup himself has repeatedly declared. There is no magic laboratory test sufficient in itself to tell which part of the alterations in bicarbonate and pCO_2 is primary or secondary. *Only by thorough knowledge of the patient and by experience with many patients of this type can the physician arrive at a correct interpretation of the laboratory data.*

The realization of this fact has caused a great deal of interest, during the last few years, in defining precisely the range of compensatory responses that can be expected for the four primary disturbances. We will review very briefly the features of the major disturbances and some of the work done in the area of expected compensatory responses to the primary disturbances in a later section of this unit.

ASSESSMENT
History

The diagnosis and subsequent treatment of fluid and electrolyte disturbances may be facilitated by taking a comprehensive history of the patient. It is difficult, if not impossible, to separate and isolate the symptoms with which these patients present. There is considerable overlap, and no system is immune. Table 5-6 summarizes the most common complaints.

Most critically ill people are also subject to acid-base disorders. Although a thorough history is invaluable in establishing the cause of the disturbance, isolation of the presenting symptoms is, once again, a difficult task. Table 5-7 outlines the symptoms most characteristic of acid-base imbalance.

The kidney is most responsive to alterations in fluid and electrolyte balance. This organ also performs a vital function in restoration of acid-base equilibrium. Therefore renal function must be closely monitored in acutely ill people to facilitate preservation of homeostasis. The history serves as an invaluable tool in identifying potential problems. A detailed history is mandatory because a large number of diseases can cause renal dysfunction; the list seems endless.

Because the urinary tract consists of organs and structures that serve various functions, the practitioner must be alert to recognize the association of two or more related signs and symptoms. Symptoms normally referrable to the renal system include blood in the urine, reduced or absent urination, excessive urination, incomplete urination, urinary retention, urinary hesitancy, a need to arise from sleep to urinate, fluid retention, abdominal pain, flank pain, or tender bladder. Other, more nebulous behavioral, mental, and neurologic symptoms may also be linked to renal disease.

Blood in the urine (hematuria)

Blood in the urine may be *gross,* that is, visible to the naked eye, or it may be *microscopic,* that is, detectable only by a chemical test or direct visualization.

Macroscopic or significant microscopic hematuria requires a complete evaluation to determine the cause. Initially, it is a good idea to rule out the use of any drugs, food pigments, or metabolites that may color the urine red; such substances include azo dyes, phenolphthalein, indole alkaloids, beets, and prophyrins. Once this has been done, other questions are appropriate to determine whether the hematuria is caused by systemic causes, trauma, nonrenal parenchymal pathology, or renal parenchymal causes.

A thorough medication history, accompanied by a complete review of systems, may uncover some systemic cause of bleeding. Some of the more common causes of bleeding include

Text continued on p. 371.

Table 5-6. Symptoms of fluid and electrolyte disturbances obtained during the history

System	Volume deficit	Volume overload	Sodium excess	Sodium deficiency
Cardiovascular	Unexplained weight loss Palpitations Postural hypotension	Unexplained weight gain Swelling High blood pressure Pounding pulse	Rapid heart rate	
Respiratory	—	Shortness of breath Lung congestion		
Neurologic	Weariness	—	Lethargy Irritability Seizures Loss of consciousness	Lethargy Headaches Apprehension Confusion Seizures Loss of consciousness
Musculoskeletal	—	—	Muscular rigidity Tremors	Fatigue Muscle weakness Tremors
Renal	Decreased urine output	—	Decreased urine output	Decreased urine output Loss of appetite
Gastrointestinal	Thirst	—	Thirst	Nausea Vomiting Diarrhea Cramps
Integument	Dry skin Dry mouth Dry lips Furrowed tongue Fever	—	Dry, sticky mucous membranes Rough, dry tongue Dry skin Decreased tearing Fever	

System	Potassium excess	Potassium deficiency	Chloride excess	Chloride deficiency	Calcium excess
Cardiovascular	Slow heartbeat	Palpitations (skipped heartbeats)	Rapid deep breathing		
Respiratory	—	Weakness Shallow breathing		Slow, shallow breathing	
Neurologic	Confusion Abnormal sensations (numbness, prickling, tingling)	Drowsiness Confusion Apathy Loss of consciousness Abnormal sensations (numbness, prickling, tingling)	Altered level of consciousness	Nervousness Apprehension Irritability	Drowsiness Lethargy Depression Loss of memory Confusion-disorientation Loss of consciousness Bone pain
Musculoskeletal	Muscle weakness Hyperexcitability Flaccid paralysis	Irritability Muscle weakness Muscle cramps Muscle tenderness Muscle pain Intermittent muscle spasms Paralysis	Muscle weakness	Muscle weakness Intermittent muscle spasms	
Renal		Increased urine output Nocturia			Increased urine output Kidney stones
Gastrointestinal	Diarrhea Intestinal cramps Abdominal distention	Nausea Vomiting Loss of appetite Cramps Abdominal distention Thirst			Loss of appetite Nausea Vomiting Thirst Constipation

Continued.

Table 5-6. Symptoms of fluid and electrolyte disturbances obtained during the history—cont'd

System	Calcium deficiency	Phosphate excess	Phosphate deficiency	Magnesium excess	Magnesium deficiency
Cardiovascular				Low heart rate Low blood pressure Shallow breathing Apnea	High blood pressure
Respiratory	Stridor	Stridor			
Neurologic	Seizures Depression Loss of contact with reality	Abnormal sensations, numbness and tingling Depression Loss of contact with reality Seizures	Lethargy	Depression Drowsiness Loss of consciousness	Apathy Depression Confusion Irritability Loss of contact with reality Seizures
Musculoskeletal	Bone fractures	Muscle cramps Intermittent muscle spasms Carpopedal spasms	Muscle weakness	Muscle weakness Paralysis	Muscle weakness Tremors Muscle spasticity Intermittent muscle spasms
Renal	Nausea Vomiting Cramps Diarrhea				
Gastrointestinal		Nausea Vomiting Diarrhea Cramps		Nausea Vomiting	Loss of appetite Nausea
Integument		Dry skin Brittle nails Hair loss Numbness around mouth Corneal ulcers			

Table 5-7. Symptoms of acid-base disturbances reported or documented during history

System	Acid-base disturbances			
	Respiratory acidosis	Respiratory alkalosis	Nonrespiratory acidosis	Nonrespiratory alkalosis
Cardiovascular	Rapid heart rate	Low blood pressure Irregular heartbeat	Low blood pressure Irregular heartbeat	Irregular heartbeat
Respiratory	Slow, shallow breathing Shortness of breath	Rapid deep breathing Shortness of breath	Shallow, blowing breathing (Kussmaul respirations)	Slow, shallow breathing
Neurologic	Headache Apprehension Restlessness Confusion Disorientation Drowsiness Loss of consciousness	Confusion Dizziness Anxiety Nervousness Syncope Seizures Abnormal sensations, such as tingling	Headache Confusion Drowsiness Loss of consciousness Seizures	Belligerence Irritability Seizures
Musculoskeletal	Fatigue Uncoordination Muscle weakness Muscle tremors	Muscle cramps Intermittent muscle spasms	Fatigue	Intermittent muscle spasms
Renal	—	—	—	—
Gastrointestinal	—	—	Nausea Vomiting Loss of appetite	Nausea Vomiting Diarrhea
Integument	Cyanotic discoloration	Numbness around mouth	—	—

anticoagulant therapy with either heparin or vitamin K antagonists, blood dyscrasias, coagulation factor disturbances, generalized vascular bleeding associated with hyperglobulinemic syndromes, and sickle cell disease.

A history of a recent trauma must not be overlooked as a possible source of hematuria, nor should recent instrumentation be ignored.

Questions regarding the coexistence of urinary frequency, painful urination, flank pain, or bladder tenderness, as well as the relationship between the time of onset of hematuria and the act of micturation, may help distinguish nonrenal parenchymal pathology from renal parenchymal pathology. Noting whether blood with urination is seen initially (initial), throughout (total), or at the end of urination (terminal) may

be valuable in the localization. Initial hematuria occurs with urethral lesions. Terminal bleeding suggests the bladder neck or prostatic urethra as the source, whereas total hematuria indicates the presence of red blood cells throughout the urinary system and may involve the kidney, ureter, or bladder.

Reduced urination (oliguria) or absent urination (anuria)

A daily urine output of less than 500 ml/24 hr is called *oliguria;* the total absence of urine production (clinically less than 100 ml/24 hr) is called *anuria.* Both may occur in a number of conditions (Table 5-8).

An accurate history and review of systems will often help establish the cause as prerenal,

Table 5-8. Possible causes of oliguria or anuria

Prerenal	Renal	Postrenal
Shock	Acute glomerulonephritis	Bilateral ureteral obstruction
Hypovolemia	Vasculitis	Urethral obstruction
Congestive heart failure	Cortical necrosis	Rupture of bladder
Hepatic cirrhosis	Papillary necrosis	Bladder catheter obstruction
Hepatorenal syndrome	Acute tubular necrosis	
Bilateral renal artery obstruction	Acute interstitial nephritis	
Bilateral renal vein obstruction	Accelerated nephrosclerosis	
Peripheral vasodilation	Atheroembolic renal disease	
	Acute hyperuricemic nephropathy	
	Myeloma kidney	

Adapted from Mabbry, S.G., and Glassock, R.J.: Textbook of nephrotology, Baltimore, 1983, Williams and Wilkins.

renal, or postrenal. The past history may reveal the existence of chronic disease that may predispose the patient to renal disorders, or it may disclose a significant illness requiring adjunct pharmacologic therapy. A recent surgical procedure or blood transfusion may also be important factors.

The pattern of urine flow could also be helpful in determining a diagnosis. A history of difficult voiding or a pattern of oliguria or anuria, alternating with polyuria, may suggest obstruction.

In a significant number of patients, however, the history must be combined with a physical exam and a complete laboratory workup to establish a cause.

Excessive urination (polyuria)

Excessive urination amounting to 3 to 5 L/24 hr (in the absence of excessive fluid intake) is referred to as *polyuria*. There are many causes of polyuria (see box on p. 373). The history may provide some information that will be valuable in determining the cause. It may also be helpful in differentiating excessive urination caused by water diuresis from that caused by an osmotic diuresis or in detecting a combination of both.

The patient's past history will identify the existence of any underlying disease that might predispose the person to polyuria. In addition,

the family history may assist in determining if there is a genetic predisposition, whereas the review of systems and social history may identify hypochondriac traits.

A description of the onset and pattern of urination is also necessary. Polyuria because of psychogenic polydipsia has a gradual onset that is vaguely described, whereas excessive urine output caused by central diabetes insipidus occurs suddenly. Diabetes insipidus that is nephrogenic is present in infancy. Psychogenic polydipsia causes polyuria primarily during daytime hours, whereas diabetes insipidus of both central and nephrogenic origins produces continuous polyuria.

A drug history is important because certain pharmacologic agents can induce polyuria. In addition to certain diuretics, substances such as lithium carbonate, amphotericin B, methoxyflurane, and glyburide can cause excessive urinary output.

Urinary retention—incomplete urination

An inability to pass any urine spontaneously leads to urinary retention. When the patient has such a complaint, questioning should be directed toward any neurologic injuries and diseases of the spine that may result in retention of urine, particularly in cases of severe trauma such as automobile accidents and blunt trauma from

CAUSES OF POLYURIA

Water diuresis (urine-to-plasma osmolal ratio, < 0.7, C_{osm}* < 3 ml/min)

Excessive ingestion of hypotonic fluid
    Psychogenic (compulsive) polydipsia
    Potassium depletion
    Hypercalcemia
    Hyperreninemia†
    Hypothalamic polydipsia†
Impaired tubular reabsorption of water
    Central diabetes insipidus
    Hereditary nephrogenic diabetes insipidus‡
    Acquired nephrogenic diabetes insipidus‡
        Potassium depletion
        Hypercalcemia
        Obstructive uropathy
        Amyloidosis
        Sjögren's syndrome
        Sickle cell disease
        Chronic renal failure‖
        Drugs (lithium, methoxyflurane, demethylchlortetracycline, amphotericin B)

Osmotic diuresis

Endogenous solute
    Diabetes mellitus (glucose)
    Chronic renal failure (urea)
    Postrelief of obstruction of uropathy (urea, NaCl)
    Hypercatabolism (urea)
    Diuretics (NaCl)
    Diuretic phase of acute renal failure (urea, NaCl)
    Postrenal transplantation (urea)
Exogenous solute
    Saline infusion
    Mannitol infusion
    Hypertonic glucose infusion

Combination of water and osmotic diuresis (urine-to-plasma osmolal ratio > 0.7, C_{osm} > 3 ml/min)

Postrelief of obstructive uropathy
Chronic renal failure

From Flamenbaum, W., and Hamburger, R.J.: Nephrology: an approach to the patient with renal disease, Philadelphia, 1982, J.B. Lippincott.
*C_{osm}, osmolar clearance.
†Rare.
‡Resistance to the action of ADH on the renal tubule.
‖Mainly tubulo-interstitial diseases such as pyelonephritis, polycystic kidney disease, medullary cystic disease, analgesic nephropathy, and gouty nephropathy.

beatings or in cases of degenerative diseases of the central nervous system such as diabetes mellitus and multiple sclerosis.

Occasionally the problem involves an inability to completely empty the bladder. Individuals with the problem complain of a feeling of fullness after urination. Patients with neurologic defects who have this problem may have a self-catheterization program and describe an increased need to catheterize. Of significance is the time interval between the last voiding and self-catheterization, as well as the frequency of self-catheterization.

Hesitancy (slow stream)

Male patients in particular may complain of a decrease in the size and velocity of the urinary stream. They will not offer this information readily, and only subtle questioning will elicit useful information in this area. Because the force (velocity) of the stream may have decreased over many years in a subtle way, careful attention to this symptom will prevent the patient from developing urinary retention, which is very painful and can damage renal function.

Necessity to arise from sleep to urinate (nocturia)

When a sleeping person is aroused because of an urge to empty the bladder, the condition is referred to as *nocturia*. Although some people empty the bladder at night on occasion, normally urine is voided during the day. Relevant information derived from the patient history includes data regarding the normal fluid intake, the use of long-acting diuretics, or the administration of short-acting diuretics at bedtime. Also of possible significance is the presence of certain disorders such as congestive heart failure, hepatic cirrhosis, and renal failure.

Water retention (edema)

Successful therapy for the edematous patient requires an understanding of the mechanism that leads to an expansion of the interstitial space. Some valuable information can be gleaned from the history. A review of accompanying symptoms (such as shortness of breath, coughing, or production of pink frothy sputum) may pinpoint pulmonary edema secondary to heart failure. Questions about the location of the swelling may help differentiate cardiac edema from renal edema. Renal edema produces periorbital swelling, whereas cardiac edema does not. A report of any unexplained weight gain, as well as the period of time over which the weight was gained, is important. A description of the onset of edema could facilitate identification of the nephrotic syndrome, characterized by a slow onset of fluid retention over a 5- or 6-day period with no other signs or symptoms. Questions asked regarding the patient's recent medical history and the color and appearance of the urine may suggest inflammatory disease. Edema may occur in glomerular nephritis and is associated with dark urine and a previous history of a recent viral or bacterial infection.

The intake and output record provides another source of data. Too much fluid over a short period of time, especially in the presence of underlying circulatory or renal disease, can overload the vascular space. Infants and young children are particularly susceptible to volume overload because they normally have little extravascular fluid reserve. Elderly people are also at risk because of the reduced distensibility of their blood vessels. The nonjudicious use of blood, plasma, plasma expanders, and albumin can also cause fluid overload.

Abdominal pain, flank pain, and tender bladder

Because a variety of conditions can cause abdominal and flank pain, and the site of some pain is far removed from the actual site of the disorder, a thorough history can help lead to the correct diagnosis.

Determining the cause of such pain is difficult due to extensive and variable distribution of nerve fibers to the urinary tract and the close proximity of the urinary organs to other intraperitoneal structures. In an effort to differentiate abdominal or flank pain of renal origin from that which emanates from the gastrointestinal tract or cardiovascular system, the pain should be described according to (1) location, (2) quality, (3) onset, (4) temporal characteristics, (5) intensity, (6) circumstances that cause it or modify it, and (7) associated symptoms.

Pain of renal origin is usually experienced in the posterior subcostal or costovertebral areas. It is normally described as aching, although it may also be described as severe or boring (that is, like it is being made by a drill). Radiation of this pain from the flank to the ipsilateral lower abdomen and groin is common. Rarely is pain referred to the contralateral side. Generalized abdominal pain along with spasm of the abdominal muscles is characteristic, along with severe discomfort. Hyperesthesia, nausea, and vomiting are often present.

Acute ureteral pain is severe and is felt as crescendo waves of colic. It is experienced over the lower quadrant on the afflicted side. Bladder pain is usually suprapubic or low-abdominal and is associated with complaints of urgency, painful urination, and a sensation of a need to urinate without results.

The physical examination

The physical examination of the patient with fluid and electrolyte imbalance, acid-base disturbances, and renal disorders must proceed systematically.

General data

Initially, it is important to evaluate the patient's overall appearance and assess for signs of distress. Factors such as apparent age, stature, weight, nutrition, posture, motor activity, and mental status, although not restricted to a specific body system, provide general information regarding the state of health.

A great discrepancy may exist between the apparent age of the patient and actual chronologic age. Hereditary influences, the effects of chronic disease, different life-styles, and a number of physical changes associated with the aging

process (such as hypertension and reduced pulmonary reserve) may be the culprits if patients look older than they actually are.

Stature and growth and development can also be affected by serious illness and adjunct therapy. Early epiphyseal closure and growth lag, for example, have been noted with prolonged steroid therapy.

A comparison of the patient's actual and ideal weights, as well as a comparison between the patient's past and present actual weight, may reveal an unexpected weight gain or loss. Weight gain may reflect fluid retention, whereas an unexplained weight loss may indicate infection, hypovolemia, metabolic imbalance, neoplastic disease, or depression.

The state of a patient's nutrition is normally fairly obvious. Because it is influenced by numerous factors, including electrolytes and vitamins, evaluation of nutritional status provides an excellent mechanism for looking at total body health.

General nutrition is evaluated in terms of the patient being overweight or underweight. Obesity is either *exogenous,* related to an excessive calorie intake, or *endogenous,* secondary to endocrine abnormalities. Both forms of overweight must be differentiated from edema, an accumulation of fluid in the interstitial spaces. In edema an indentation is formed when the tissues are pressed with a finger; this does not occur with obesity. Edema is a common finding in the presence of nephritis, heart failure, malnutrition, and a variety of other conditions.

Underweight ranges from mild to severe underweight, or cachexia, and may accompany a number of wasting disorders and volume deficiencies.

The condition of the hair, nails, and dentition also provides an indication of the adequacy of nutrition. Patchy alopecia, brittle nails, tooth decay, and mouth odor could reflect a fluid and electrolyte disequilibrium or acid-base disturbance.

The patient's posture may provide significant information. Although good posture requires minimal muscular effort, postural abnormalities are not uncommon and may represent pathologic conditions. Fatigue, weakness, and lethargy, which are all relatively common manifestations of electrolyte imbalance and acid base disturbance, may lead to slumped posture.

Observation of motor activity and, if possible, gait may reveal involuntary movements such as tremors, fasciculations, ataxia, or even paralysis, all of which may indicate electrolyte abnormalities.

The evaluation of the patient's mental status is important and can be integrated into the history. By skillful questioning and observation it is possible to determine, among other things, the patient's orientation to time, place, and person. In the confused or disoriented individual, additional examination is necessary to identify the level of consciousness. Confusion and other disorders of mentation such as memory loss, loss of consciousness, feelings of unreality, delusions, illusions, and hallucinations may represent electrolyte derangement, acid-base abnormalities, or chronic renal failure.

Vital signs

Determination of the temperature, pulse, respiratory rate, and blood pressure provide valuable data in the identification and evaluation of many disease conditions. Fever may accompany hypernatremia. Hypovolemia and dehydration are associated with a decrease in body temperature. Tachycardia occurs with hypovolemia, respiratory acidosis, and hypernatremia, whereas a bradydysrhythmia is characteristic in hyperkalemia and hypermagnesemia. The heart rate may also be "slow" in patients being treated with beta blockers. Hypervolemia is associated with a bounding pulse. The pulse is weak in hypokalemia.

Blood pressure changes are also characteristic. Elevations are reported in hypervolemia, hypomagnesemia, and hypertensive kidney disease, whereas the blood pressure is normally low in metabolic acidosis, respiratory alkalosis, hypermagnesemia, and hypovolemia. Postural hypotension is also described with hypovolemia.

A change in the pattern of breathing might also be significant. Hyperventilation is seen in respiratory alkalosis. Metabolic acidosis leads to Kussmaul respirations. Respirations are slow and shallow in metabolic alkalosis, respiratory acidosis, hypokalemia, and hypermagnesemia. Periods of apnea may occur in hypermagnesemia.

Face

Inspection of the skin is significant in the facial exam. Initially, it is important to look at the shape of the face. Facial edema may first be evident in the eyes because the loose subcutaneous tissue of the eyelid permits fluid accumulation. Periorbital edema is manifest as puffiness around the eyes and eyelids. Edema of the face may occur in kidney disease.

Changes in color should also be noted. Facial pallor occurs in prolonged illness or may be caused by malnutrition, hemorrhage, or shock.

The lips, oral cavity, and tongue should be inspected for color and moisture content. The oral mucosal surfaces are usually light pink and moistened by saliva. Lips that are dry and cracked, a dry tongue with longitudinal furrows, and dry mucose membranes are common findings in dehydration.

Attention should also be paid to the presence of mouth odors during examination of the oral cavity. Detection of certain odors is a quick diagnostic tool. Acetone can be detected on the breath as a fruity smell even before its presence in the urine is identified by the usual chemical tests. Acetone breath signifies ketonemia in diabetic or starvation acidosis. Ammonia on the breath can be detected in some uremic patients.

Thorax

The chest exam begins with the observation of respiratory movements. Rate, rhythm, and the character of respiration are described during the exam. Inspiration may be accompanied by a high-pitched sound called *laryngeal stridor*. This sound can occur with hypocalcemia and hyperphosphatemia. The lungs are examined to judge their volume and extensibility and to identify the presence of any abnormal secretions in the airways. The latter finding is most significant in fluid and electrolyte disturbances. Vibratory palpation and auscultation are used to identify lung congestion. Moist rales can often be found in hypervolemia.

Abdomen

Abdominal examination is usually unremarkable in renal failure unless the cause of the failure is some abdominal catastrophe such as a ruptured appendix, perforation of a diverticulum, or a blunt trauma—for example, a gunshot wound in the abdomen. Exceptions are the palpably large kidneys of polycystic disease and the large kidneys associated with invasion of the kidneys by lymphoma or leukemia. Abdominal distention and even paralytic ileus may occur in some electrolyte disorders such as potassium imbalance.

In the hypertensive patient, auscultation in the costovertebral angle and upper quadrant during deep inspiration may reveal cystolic bruit suggestive of renal artery stenosis or aneurysm.

Rectum

The rectal exam is crucial in patients who have difficulty initiating the urinary stream or difficulty in holding urine at night or when coughing. Examination is conducted to detect prostatic enlargement, which is a fairly common cause of hesitancy and urinary retention in men.

Genitalia

The penis can develop obstructions to outflow. Careful inspection is necessary to detect these alterations, which can if untreated lead to obstructive changes in the genitourinary tract and cause renal failure.

Skin

The turgor of the skin is evaluated by pinching the skin over the sternum or another body prominence. Normally, turgid skin rapidly resumes its customary shape after being released. Dehydration results in a loss of skin turgor.

Extremities

Inspection of the lower extremities may reveal massive swelling, suggesting nephrotic syndrome. Edema in this instance is most significant when patients are in a dependent position.

Muscle weakness, cramping, rigidity, spasticity, and abnormal muscle movements are characteristic in a number of acid-base and fluid and electrolyte alterations. Some abnormalities frequently encountered include:

Tremors—Involuntary muscle contractions producing oscillating movements that may be rhythmic or irregular at one or more joints. All tremors disappear during sleep.

Fasciculations—Twitching in a resting muscle that occurs with spontaneous firing of motor units or bundles of fibers.

Tetany—Intermittent involuntary tonic spasms, either painless or painful, that are induced by changes in the pH and extracellular calcium; they lead to increased nervous and muscular excitability.

Carpopedal spasms—Contractions of the hands and feet; a common occurrence in latent tetany.

Trousseau's sign—A carpal spasm induced by occlusion of the brachial artery; it is characteristic of tetany.

Chvostek's sign—A contraction of facial muscle produced by tapping the facial nerve against the bone in front of the ear; occurs in latent tetany.

Episodic paralysis—Periodic loss or diminution in motor power of muscle; can occur in hypokalemia.

Evaluation of the muscle stretch reflexes elicits a graded response that may be helpful in evaluating electrolyte balance. Reflexes are often hyperactive in hypocalcemia, hyponatremia, and hyperphosphatemia. Hyporeflexia is characteristic in respiratory acidosis and hypokalemia, whereas in hypermagnesemia the deep reflexes are either diminished or lost.

Laboratory analysis

A variety of derangements can alter the normal homeostatic mechanisms that regulate fluid and electrolyte balance. Laboratory data is essential in establishing the cause of a particular disturbance because multisystem involvement is not uncommon.

In reviewing the overall state of fluid and electrolyte equilibrium, a number of determinations can supplement serum electrolyte measurements. Calculations of urine volume, specific gravity, and osmolality indicate the state of hydration, whereas measurement of urine electrolytes may aid in clarification of the cause of the alteration. Analysis of arterial blood gases provides a mechanism to evaluate oxygenation and to determine the acid-base status, concentrating on either the respiratory component, the metabolic (nonrespiratory) component, or both. Although arterial blood is traditionally sampled because it contains a mixture of blood from various parts of the body and gives additional information about how well the lungs are oxygenating the blood, mixed venous blood may also be of interest. Such blood samples tell if the tissues are receiving enough oxygen.

Numerous tests are performed to evaluate the renal system. Classification according to functional nephrology provides a clear-cut way to organize these procedures. Because the nephron's function is to clear the blood of unneeded substances via glomerular filtration, tubular reabsorption, and tubular secretion, it is helpful to describe tests that evaluate glomerular filtration and tubular transport.

Fluid and electrolyte balance

Plasma electrolytes. Currently the electrolyte panel provides measurements for sodium (Na^+), potassium (K^+), chloride (Cl^-), and carbon dioxide (CO_2) content. Because the role of magnesium (Mg^{2+}), phosphorus (PO_4), and calcium (Ca^{2+}) in electrolyte disorders is also recognized, it is probable that these panels will be expanded to include all seven values.

An electrochemical balance is maintained in the resting cell between the intracellular and extracellular ions. Regulation is accomplished via several mechanisms that involve the kidneys,

lungs, and endocrine system, with the hypothalamus and neurohypophysis intricately involved. Selective tubular reabsorption and secretion, the countercurrent mechanism, the renin angiotensin mechanism, and several feedback systems operate to maintain electrolyte balance. Therefore determinations should include the whole series to obtain an accurate picture.

Electrolyte analysis determines the ionic concentration of selected extracellular electrolytes. Because these values vary from moment to moment, they are only capable of providing a general indication of the total body content of these ions. Intracellular values cannot be measured directly. The ECG, however, does reflect the ratio of intracellular to extracellular electrolytes (Unit 2).

Sodium. Sodium is the principal cation in the extracellular fluid. The serum sodium concentration is held fairly constant, being regulated primarily by the intake and excretion of water. Renal regulation of urinary sodium excretion is determined by the difference between the rate of sodium reabsorption by the glomerulus and the rate of tubular reabsorption. Approximately 70% of sodium is reabsorbed in the proximal tubule, with the remainder reabsorbed in the distal tubule under the influence of aldosterone.

Numerous metabolic activities depend on sodium. The $Na^+ - K^+$ ATPase system that transports potassium into the cell and sodium out of the cell is an integral component of many energy-dependent transport mechanisms.

Potassium. The major intracellular cation is potassium. Its role as a major determinant of the transmembrane potential makes it vital to nerve and muscle cellular function.

Potassium balance is maintained by several mechanisms. The kidney is the major organ responsible for maintaining potassium levels via selective tubular reabsorption. The gastrointestinal tract also plays a regulatory role. Although only a small proportion of the amount of potassium is excreted in the stool on a daily basis, in some disease states this value may be increased up to threefold. Because of its influence on the distal tubule, aldosterone also regulates potassium, increasing its urinary excretion.

Chloride. Chloride balances plasma cations, serving as the principal extracellular anion. Because it is the most reabsorbable of biologically available anions, chloride plays the most important role in the preservation of electroneutrality.

Carbon dioxide. The carbon dioxide determined during electrolyte analysis is composed mainly of bicarbonate and, to a lesser extent, dissolved CO_2 gas. The CO_2 content is normally dissolved in solution. Bicarbonate is regulated chiefly by the kidneys and CO_2 by the lungs. The role of bicarbonate and CO_2 in acid-base balance is reviewed in detail in this unit and in Unit 3.

Calcium and phosphorus. Most of the calcium and phosphorus in the body is found in the skeleton. The concentration of calcium and phosphorus ions in the extracellular fluid is only a fraction of the total body level. Approximately one half of the serum calcium is ionized; the remainder is bound to protein. Calcium ions affect neuromuscular excitability and membrane permeability. They are also necessary for blood coagulation. Phosphorus is essential in the storage and release of energy and in carbohydrate and lipid intermediate metabolism. Because free phosphorus does not exist, serum inorganic phosphorus levels are measured in terms of the phosphate ion.

Both calcium and phosphorus are absorbed from the small intestine. Small amounts of vitamin D are necessary to increase the efficiency of intestinal transport.

Calcium and phosphorus levels are regulated reciprocally by the parathyroid glands. Parathormone can mobilize calcium from the bone via direct action on osteoclasts or can raise serum calcium by increasing intestinal absorption or by promoting urinary excretion of phosphate. Another hormone from the thyroid gland, calcitonin, increases renal calcium clearance.

Magnesium. Magnesium is a cation that is required in several membrane functions and enzymatic reactions. Although magnesium is found primarily in the intracellular fluid, reliance on extracellular levels is mandatory to determine deficiency states. Magnesium is found in equally divided amounts in the skeleton and soft tissues. Some in the blood is bound to proteins, whereas the rest is readily diffusible. The majority of diffusible magnesium consists of free ionized magnesium. The kidneys play an important role in maintaining the plasma concentration of magnesium within a narrow range.

Specific gravity. The concentration of urine is determined by measuring the specific gravity, that is, the relative amounts of solute and water. One of the oldest methods of calculating the specific gravity uses a float or urinometer that is precalibrated against distilled water. Simpler procedures employ urine refractometers that are calibrated to translate the refractive index directly to the specific gravity. The refractometer measures total solids, giving values comparable to those obtained by more traditional means. Automated urinalysis instruments may also be used to calculate the specific gravity. The urine may be abnormally concentrated after instrumentation, requiring the injection of contrast media.

Osmolality. The osmolality of urine provides an indication of the amount of osmotic work done by the kidney. It is determined largely by ADH, which is secreted by the neurohypophysis and acts to enhance reabsorption in the collecting ducts. Osmolality depends on the number of moles of various solutes present in urine, such as urea, sodium, and chloride. Measured with an osmometer, the osmolality is determined by comparing the freezing point of urine with the freezing point of water. When substances are dissolved in a solvent, they change some of the properties of that solvent. Freezing-point depression is one such change that can be measured. Osmolality measurements usually parallel specific gravity unless there is a good deal of protein present. In that situation, a correction must be made in the specific gravity. Osmolality as specific gravity will be increased with glycosuria.

Plasma osmolality is equivalent to the sum of the individual osmolalities of plasma solutes. It is normally maintained within a narrow limit, despite variations in salt and water intake, because the kidneys can excrete urine with a wide range of concentrations. Clinically, the importance of osmolality lies with the plasma sodium concentration. Hypoosmolality occurs with hyponatremia and can be produced by sodium or potassium loss or by water retention. Hyperosmolality is found with hypernatremia caused by sodium gain or water loss. The toxicity of hyperkalemia prevents retention of enough potassium ions to cause an elevation in the plasma sodium.

Urine electrolytes. Determination of the concentration of urinary electrolytes (sodium, potassium, and chloride) is helpful in the evaluation of electrolyte and acid-base disorders, as well as organic renal disease.

Sodium. Because the kidney varies the rate of sodium excretion to maintain the effective circulating volume, urinary sodium concentration provides an estimate of the patient's volume status. Generally, a low urine sodium concentration may reflect hypovolemia. This fact is useful in differentiating hyponatremia from acute renal failure.

The two principal causes of hyponatremia are *effective volume depletion* and the *syndrome of inappropriate antidiuretic hormone secretion (SIADH)*. The urine sodium remains low with volume depletion but is greater than 20 mEg/L in SIADH, a condition characterized by water retention and volume expansion.

Acute renal failure (ARF) can be explained similarly. The cause of ARF is frequently *volume depletion* or *acute tubular necrosis (ATN)*. Urine sodium exceeds 20 mEg/L in ATN because the tubules cannot maximally reabsorb sodium.

There are some situations in which it is misleading to rely on urinary sodium levels as a reflection of volume status. In normovolemic patients who have renal or glomerular ischemia caused by bilateral renal arterial stenosis or acute glomerulonephritis, urine sodium may be low. On the other hand, in the presence of defective tubular function (for example, with aldosterone

deficiency or advanced renal failure), it may be inappropriately high.

The urine sodium is also affected by the rate of water reabsorption. In the absence of ADH (such as in diabetes insipidus) the volume of urine output can exceed 10 L/day while the urine sodium remains low, incorrectly suggesting volume depletion. On the other hand, hypovolemia may be masked by a high rate of water reabsorption, which raises the concentration of urinary sodium. The renal handling of sodium can be evaluated by determination of the fractional excretion of sodium.

Urine sodium determinations may also be of value in monitoring dietary compliance in hypertensive patients who are placed on sodium restrictions. Normally, the urine sodium excretion is approximately equivalent to the dietary intake. With restricted intake, excretion of sodium should be less than 100 mEg/day. Concurrent diuretic therapy does not interfere because, although some diuretics initially increase sodium and water excretion by reducing reabsorption in the distal tubule, the ensuing volume depletion enhances sodium's reabsorption in the distal nephron (via aldosterone) and in the proximal tubule.

Potassium. The urine potassium concentration is helpful in the differential diagnosis of hypokalemia. Potassium excretion also varies with intake. This response is mediated by aldosterone and the direct effect of changes in plasma potassium. Low urine potassium levels in the presence of potassium depletion suggest either extrarenal losses (such as those from the gastrointestinal tract) or diuretic therapy.

Determination of potassium excretion may also be helpful in hyperkalemia, although less so. Normally, an individual is able to increase the urinary excretion of potassium as K^+ intake increases slowly to prevent significant serum elevations. Consequently, hyperkalemia is almost always caused by a failure of the kidneys to adequately excrete potassium.

Chloride. Because chloride ions are reabsorbed with sodium throughout the nephron, measurement of urine chloride adds minimal information to that obtained by determining urinary sodium concentration. However, some studies have shown that chloride conservation can occur independent of sodium, mediated partially by the active transport of the chloride ion in the inner medullary collecting tubule.

It may be helpful to determine the level of urine chloride in those with depleted volume but with an elevated urine sodium concentration because these individuals have also been shown to exhibit a difference between the urine sodium and chloride levels. This occurs most often in nonrespiratory alkalosis, when urinary excretion of excess bicarbonate can increase urinary sodium excretion and mask an underlying hypovolemia.

Acid-base balance

pH determination. pH is determined by electrometric methods that measure the potential generated across a membrane separating two solutions of unequal hydrogen ion concentrations. The pH represents the negative log of the hydrogen ion concentrations. Simply, it is a way of representing the free hydrogen ions in solution on a scale from 0 to 14. Mathematically, it is inversely proportional to the concentration of hydrogen ions in solution. Calculation of the pH is necessary to identify acidemia and alkalemia and to determine the presence of any compensatory mechanisms. Both arterial and mixed venous blood samples may be used, although values vary according to the origin of the sample.

Pa_{CO_2}. The tension exerted by carbon dioxide in its gaseous state in arterial blood is the Pa_{CO_2}. Any deviation from the normal partial pressure of CO_2 reflects an acid-base disturbance, either primary or compensatory. Because the Pa_{CO_2} is inversely related to ventilation, it serves as a good index of pulmonary function. (See Unit 3 for a more detailed discussion.)

Standard bicarbonate. The standard bicarbonate is the plasma bicarbonate concentration measured at $37°$ C ($98.6°$ F) on blood that has been equilibrated to a P_{CO_2} of 40 mmHg. This corrects any respiratory abnormalities that might have existed in the patient when the blood was drawn. Any deviation that remains represents nonrespiratory acid-base changes. The standard bicarbonate does not quantify the degree of abnormality of the buffer base, nor does it reflect the actual buffering capacity of the blood. Bicarbonate concentrations can also be calculated in the laboratory indirectly by measuring the pH and Pa_{CO_2}. From these values the bicarbonate level can be calculated, using the Henderson-Hasselbalch equation.

$$pH = pK^+ \log \frac{[HCO_3^-]}{[H_2CO_3]}$$

Base excess/deficit. This determination provides a mechanism to quantify the patient's total base excess or deficit. Expressed in mEq/L, it is the amount of strong base (or acid) that is added to a liter of blood. Calculation is made from pH, Pa_{CO_2}, and hematocrit measurements. The red blood cells contain the major blood buffers. *Normal* is arbitrarily fixed at 0. Base excess or a deficit of acid is characterized by a positive value, whereas a negative value represents a deficit of base or an excess of acid. Because the addition of nonvolatile acids affects the buffer base, whereas changes in carbonic acid concentration do not, this parameter is a reflection of nonrespiratory acid-base balance.

Carbon dioxide. The total CO_2 content represents the amount of CO_2 gas that can be extracted from the plasma in the presence of a strong acid.

Plasma electrolytes. Changes in the serum electrolytes sodium, potassium, chloride, and calcium reflect physiologic alterations that can also affect acid-base balance. Usually, sodium or potassium serve as the primary urinary cations. When a sodium ion is reabsorbed from the tubule, a potassium ion is excreted in its place; the reverse also occurs. Hydrogen ions compete with potassium. Consequently in hypokalemia or conditions of hydrogen ion excess, hydrogen ions are excreted to replace sodium.

Renal function

Routine urinalysis. The often overlooked routine urinalysis describes the color, concentration, and pH of the urine; microscopically examines the formed elements normally present; and searches for pathologically significant elements that are not usually present, such as glucose, protein, blood, ketones, and bile pigments.

Macroscopic urine examination

URINE pH. Test strips measure urine pH roughly within one half of a pH unit, ranging from 4.5 to 9.

Urine pH is regulated metabolically by the kidneys, which selectively reabsorb H^+ ions, reconstitute the bicarbonate ion, and excrete ammonium ions and free hydrogen ions. If a person has good renal function, the urine pH reflects the plasma pH, compensating where necessary. However, with altered tubular function, abnormalities may remain uncorrected. The urine may be inappropriately acidic during metabolic alkalosis because of excess hydrogen ion excretion associated with hypokalemia. The urine is usually strongly acidic with nearly all forms of acidosis. Acid urine may also be produced by diets containing high quantities of meat and by acidifying drugs.

Alkaline urine is unusual. If a freshly voided specimen is alkaline, it should be tested for evidence of a urinary tract infection because ammonia-splitting bacteria convert urine from acid to alkaline.

COLOR. Normal urine is usually clear, ranging in color from pale yellow to deep amber depending on the concentration of solutes. Urine may become cloudy on standing if urates precipitate in acid urine or phosphates precipitate at an alkaline pH. Color changes occur in the presence of blood, hemoglobin degradation products, or bilirubin and its metabolites.

Fresh blood imparts a smoky reddish-brown color to urine. The color may be brownish gray if urinary acidity converts hemoglobin to acid hematin or methemoglobin. Myoglobinuria may also give a reddish-brown discoloration to urine. Myoglobin is released with severe muscle destruction.

Bilirubin and related pigments color the urine orange to greenish brown. Other discolorations, although uncommon, are diagnostically significant. Clear urine that becomes red on standing may indicate porphobilinogen excretion, found in intermittent porphyria. Clear urine that turns brown or black on standing suggests either homogentisic acid, which is a substance excreted in alkaptonuria (a disorder in amino acid metabolism) or melanogen, which is excreted in disseminated malignant melanoma.

Drugs and dietary substances may also change normal urine color. Pyridium, which is used in the treatment of bladder discomfort, and riboflavin in large doses turn the urine bright orange. Alkaline urine turns red in the presence of phenolsulfonphthalein and bromsulfophthalein, two compounds used in renal function testing and liver function testing, respectively. The analgesic phenacetin may impart a brownish-gray or black discoloration to urine, whereas dilantin, an anticonvulsant occasionally used in the treatment of ventricular dysrhythmias, colors the urine pink to reddish brown.

GLUCOSE. Glucosuria is abnormal. Less than 100 of glucose is normally excreted in 24 hours, even though approximately 250 g pass through the kidneys daily. Glucose spills into the urine when high blood glucose levels produce a glucose load in the filtrate that surpasses the kidney's reabsorptive capacity or when tubular reabsorption is altered.

KETONES. Normal urine does not contain ketone bodies. Ketonuria occurs when available glucose supplies are inadequate to meet tissue demands, necessitating fat combustion for energy. Fat metabolism produces three ketone bodies found in the urine: betahydroxybutyric acid, acetoacetic acid, and acetone. Ketonuria can be found in any condition accompanied by acute metabolic demand with reduced intake. In children, it may be precipitated by stress. In adults, it most frequently accompanies episodes of uncontrolled diabetes in which glucose is present but not functionally available for metabolism.

PROTEIN. Small amounts of proteinuria are not unusual and often follow exercise. Protein excretion of 150 mg/day or greater is usually significant. Most of the protein is albumin and represents abnormal glomerular permeability resulting from intrinsic glomerular disease, alterations in blood pressure, preeclampsia, or abnormalities of the renal veins. Massive proteinuria (greater than 4 g/day) suggests the nephrotic syndrome.

Albumin is not the only protein excreted in the urine. Bence Jones protein of multiple myeloma may also be detected, as well as the proteins or protein components in heavy chain disease, macroglobulinemia, and various tubular defects.

Microscopic urine examination. Microscopic examination of the urine should be carried out within 1 to 2 hours after voiding for best results. Sediment of normal urine may contain occasional white blood cells and squamous epithelial cells but should be free of red cells. Improper cleansing and collection procedures often introduce contaminants such as leukocytes, epithelial cells, bacteria, and even red blood cells from menstruating women.

Significant or repeated leukocytosis indicates acute infection and may necessitate further evaluation. The white cells tend to be associated with cellular or granular casts, bacteria, and renal epithelial cells if the infection is in the kidney. Red cells are uncommon. Bladder infections, on the other hand, frequently produce red cells in addition to leukocytes and large epithelial cells but do not produce casts because the process occurs below the level of the renal tubule, where casts are normally formed. Significant leukocyturia and hematuria are characteristic of acute glomerulonephritis, although hematuria predominates. Moderate white cells may also be found in a variety of noninfectious inflammatory diseases of the kidneys, ureters, and bladder.

Red cells in the urine generally indicate bleeding into the urinary tract. This may be caused by trauma, infection, tumors, systemic diseases, aspirin ingestion, or anticoagulant therapy.

Casts are composed primarily of cells, and most originate in the distal convoluted tubule. Casts also have been seen to form in the collecting tubules, although normally the flow of urine in these ducts is too fast for them to form. Therefore development of broader casts from the collecting tubules suggests severe slowing of the urinary stream and significant renal malfunction. Desquamated epithelial cells may aggregate as casts during a patient's recovery from acute tubular damage.

Minimal significance is given to most crystals or amorphous materials. Crystalluria becomes important in some disorders of amino acid metabolism and in patients being treated with poorly soluble sulfa drugs or other medications.

Urine electrolytes. For more on urine electrolytes, see Unit 2.

Specific gravity. The specific gravity provides an index of concentration that may help detect impaired concentrating ability, which is an early sign of renal damage, before measurable changes occur in the glomerular filtration rate or renal perfusion rate or before gross signs of damage are visible. Because the complex functions of concentrating and diluting urine require interaction among the tubular system, medullary interstitium, posterior pituitary, and other whole-body volume regulators, this procedure provides only general information.

Osmolality. Because urinary concentration varies with the state of hydration, a random measurement of osmolality has little diagnostic significance. Although this procedure is helpful in the differential diagnosis of hyponatremia and hypernatremia and may be of use in renal failure, it should be reviewed in relation to the GFR for most patients with intrinsic renal disease. Concentrating ability normally varies with the GFR. Most patients having intrinsic renal disease have a concentrating ability that is reduced proportionally to the GFR. This may be attributed in part to the increase in solute excretion per functioning nephron and possibly to resistance to ADH. Consequently, urine and plasma osmolality become similar. On the other hand, volume depletion may lead to decreased renal perfusion and a subsequent reduction in the GFR. ADH release will be stimulated by the hypovolemia, resulting in a more concentrated urine. Thus urine osmolality may be one of the valuable tests used in differentiating between intrinsic renal disease and hypovolemia as a cause of decreased GFR.

Measurement of glomerular filtration rate (GFR). The GFR measures the sum of the filtration rates from each of the functioning nephrons. Clinically, it is the best index of renal function. Measurement of the GFR is also helpful in deciding the proper dosage of drugs, which will be excreted by the kidney. Determination of the GFR necessitates calculation of the rate of urinary excretion of certain compounds, such as creatinine and urea.

Creatinine. Creatinine is derived from the metabolism of creatine phosphate, a high-energy compound in skeletal muscle that functions in reversible energy reactions involving ATP and creatine phosphokinse. Creatine is released at a relatively constant rate into the plasma. Consequently, the serum creatinine remains stable, varying only minimally during a 24-hr period. People with large muscle mass have higher serum creatinine than those who have less muscle. Creatinine is freely filtered across the glomerulus. It is neither reabsorbed nor metabolized by the kidney, although some creatinine is secreted into the urine in the proximal tubule. Because of this, the amount of creatinine excreted slightly exceeds the amount filtered.

The most widely used method of evaluating the GFR is the creatinine clearance. It indicates the efficiency with which the kidneys remove creatinine from the blood. The creatinine clearance can be calculated by comparing the serum creatinine concentration with the total quantity excreted within a given time. As renal function declines, the serum creatinine rises, but the rise is less acute than the changes in BUN. The serum creatinine may be normal in some cases of acute uremia or mild chronic renal disease. When elevated, however, it represents long-standing kidney disease.

Urea. Urea is the end product of the hepatic metabolism of amino acids not used in protein synthesis. As these amino acids are deaminated, ammonia is produced. To prevent toxic levels from accumulating, the ammonia is converted into urea. Urea travels through the blood to the kidneys, where it is excreted.

Because urea is excreted primarily by glomerular filtration, the concentration urea in the blood (BUN) provides an index for assessing renal function.

Usually the BUN varies inversely with the GFR. There are, however, some notable exceptions. Urea production may not be constant. When protein metabolism is accelerated (because of such factors as high-protein diets, enhanced tissue breakdown resulting from trauma, steroid therapy, or decreased protein synthesis), urea production and therefore the BUN may increase. On the other hand, a low protein intake and/or severe liver disease can significantly decrease urea production and the BUN.

In addition, urea excretion is not determined only by glomerular filtration. Some filtered urea is passively reabsorbed aftr sodium is reabsorbed from the tubules. Therefore, in volume-depleted states, sodium and ultimately urea reabsorption is enhanced, leading to an elevation of the BUN without a prior fall in the GFR.

Although the urea clearance can be used to appraise the GFR, it is not as accurate as the plasma creatinine or BUN. This can be attributed to the variability in urea production and reabsorption.

Radiologic studies. A number of radiologic studies can be useful in the diagnostic evaluation of patients with kidney disease. Frequently they are used in conjunction with other laboratory tests to confirm or refute a diagnosis.

Abdominal film (KUB). Kidney size and shape and the presence of any gross structural changes or stones are normally visible on a routine radiograph of the abdomen. Such a film is particularly helpful in following patients with recurrent disorders.

Intravenous pyelogram (IVP). An intravenous pyelogram (IVP) is a roentgenogram that permits visualization of the renal pelvis and ureters after the intravenous injection of a radiopaque contrast medium. This procedure can be used to demonstrate the size and location of the kidneys, to confirm the presence or absence of any masses or obstruction within the kidneys, to visualize filling of the renal pelvis, and to outline the ureters and bladder. Therefore the IVP evaluates excretory function and patency of the urinary tract.

Radioisotope renogram. A radioisotope renogram is used to monitor blood supply and blood flow to the kidneys following the intravenous injection of a preparation containing a tracer dose of a radioactive isotope. The radioactively labeled compound enters the tubule by proximal tubular secretion and, to a lesser extent, by glomerular filtration. Continuous monitoring of intrarenal activity and the rates of renal uptake and excretion permit measurement of the rates of blood flow and urine flow. Scintillation scanning techniques can be used to visualize the outline of the kidneys.

This procedure can be of value in the detection of obstructions in the upper urinary tract and in the identification of acute renal failure shortly after the onset of oliguria. It is also used to monitor kidney function after transplantation and to evaluate the effectiveness of treatment in patients with renal disease.

Renal arteriogram. Renal angiography employs a contrast material. The material is injected into the renal arteries via a femoral artery catheter, which has been inserted into the aorta to outline the renal vasculature. This procedure is used diagnostically to detect renal artery stenosis, renal infarction, or polyarteritis nodosa; this last condition is manifested as aneurysms and narrowed areas in the medium-sized renal arteries. Renal arteriograms are also helpful in the identification of renal neoplasms. Although the procedure can be used to differentiate a benign avascular cyst from carcinoma that is highly vascular, the use of less invasive procedures may be more appropriate.

Ultrasonography and CT scanning. Ultrasonography and CT scanning are useful in the evaluation of masses and in the detection of hydronephrosis. The CT scan provides a better resolution, but ultrasound studies are more widely available and may be preferred because they do not involve radiation. CT scanning may be necessary in the obese patient because adequate visualization of the kidneys by ultrasonography may be impossible.

ALTERATIONS
Fluid and electrolytes

Fluid and electrolyte disorders are characterized by a myriad of multisystem symptoms. Many of these symptoms are among the most common complaints motivating people to seek help. Sometimes it is difficult to distinguish between those symptoms that are normal physiologic responses to stress and those caused by a pathologic process. In addition, determination of a cause is difficult because of the multiplicity of etiologies.

It is simpler to understand the pathophysiology of the effects of fluid and electrolyte imbalance by looking at each alteration separately and by briefly reviewing normal electrolyte physiology.

Volume abnormalities

Dehydration—water loss. Dehydration occurs when the fluid intake fails to keep up with the rate of water loss. When water is lost from the body, the volume is reduced in all body fluid compartments, and the osmolality increases. Osmoreceptors, excited specifically by changes in the extracellular fluid concentration, respond to an increased osmolality in the ECF by pulling water out of the osmoreceptors, causing them to shrink and increase their rate of discharge. This promotes ADH secretion and subsequent renal tubular water reabsorption. If water intake remains inadequate, this mechanism may be unable to restore normal fluid balance.

One of the first signs of lack of water in the body is thirst. This symptom can be traced to either extracellular or intracellular fluid dehydration, hemorrhage, or low cardiac output. All of the stimuli seem to directly affect neurons of the thirst center (drinking center), which is located on each side of the hypothalamus. The exact mechanism by which thirst is promoted is open to speculation. One theory is that ECF loss may cause dehydration of the neurons in the thirst center. The manner in which ICF dehydration stimulates thirst remains questionable. In the case of circulatory failure, it is possible that an inadequate nutrient supply could alter active transport mechanisms involved in the maintenance of normal intracellular electrolyte compositions. This could lead to a loss of intracellular electrolytes, resulting in intracellular dehydration.

Other symptoms associated with dehydration include dryness of the mouth and other mucous membranes, diminished sweating, and reduced skin turgor. All of these signs are related to the volume reduction in all body fluid compartments. A lowered volume of highly concentrated urine is characteristic and can be attributed to the effects of ADH. With severe hypovolemia, although there is increased sympathetic and angiotensin II–mediated vasoconstriction, blood pressure can only be maintained in a recumbent position. Therefore postural hypotension tends to occur in an upright position. Intense sympathetic vasoconstriction shunts blood to preserve cerebral and coronary blood flow. If more fluid is lost, marked hypotension and shock can develop.[20]

Fluid overload—water excess. Normally, an excessive water intake results in polyuria without an increase in total body water. The kidneys can excrete up to 30 L or more a day without any severe degree of fluid retention. Consequently, an increase in total body water indicates the presence of an abnormality in the kidney's ability to excrete water. The impairment may involve elevation in the circulating levels of ADH, intrinsic renal disease, or both. The impairment may be traced to hyperaldosteronism, excessive administration of adrenal cortical hormones, or the simple overloading of the body by oral or parenteral infusion of excessive quantities of an isotonic solution of sodium chloride. It may also be attributed to underlying hepatic or cardiac dysfunction or hypoproteinemia.

The primary alteration will dictate the sequence of events that lead to an increase in the extracellular fluid volume. With increased circulating ADH, water is reabsorbed from the distal tubules and collecting ducts. If ADH release is not inhibited, sodium is retained in an attempt to maintain normal solute concentrations in the ECF. The cycle continues with water reabsorption and sodium retention until proper tonicity is reached. Because there is free movement of sodium and water into the interstitium, both plasma and interstitial volumes increase.

A reduction in renal perfusion promotes renin release from the juxtaglomerular apparatus, resulting in the increased formation of angiotensin II, enhanced aldosterone secretion, and renal sodium retention. This leads to water reabsorption and extracellular fluid volume expansion.

An excessive use of adrenal cortical hormones and hyperaldosteronism result in tubular sodium reabsorption. Body tonicity sensors, in response to increased solute concentration, provide the driving force for water reabsorption.

The influx of excessive quantities of an isotonic solution of sodium chloride may present no problems to the healthy person with normal kidney function. In the oliguric phase of acute renal failure, the body is unable to excrete excess fluid.

Hepatic venous outflow obstruction and elevated hepatic intrasinusoidal pressure lead to altered renal handling of salt and water.[71] With obstruction to hepatic venous outflow, there is an increase in hepatic lymph formation. When the rate of lymph formation exceeds the rate of thoracic duct drainage, ascites develops. The subsequent loss of intravascular volume signals volume receptors, which trigger the retention of sodium and extracellular fluid volume expansion.

In the presence of cardiac dysfunction, a reduced cardiac output or diversion of blood flow through arteriovenous shunts diminishes blood flow to critical areas of the arterial circuit. Sensors perceive the diminished blood flow, which signals for renal sodium retention and ultimate extracellular fluid volume expansion. This leads to elevated atrial pressures, which promote systemic and pulmonary congestion, decreased lymphatic drainage, edema formation, and the loss of intravascular volume into the interstitial space. Elevated pressures in the atria also give rise to chronic dilation of the cardiac chambers. As a result, the natriuretic response is attenuated and sodium is retained.[71]

Water and electrolytes move from the plasma to the interstitium when the plasma albumin is depressed. Following hemorrhage, water and electrolytes move from the interstitial space to the plasma in an attempt to replace water and electrolytes that were lost. This type of shift also occurs when the plasma oncotic pressure has been increased by the administration of excessive amounts of blood, plasma, or other volume expanders.

The clinical symptoms that appear are acute weight gain (usually in excess of 5% of the total body weight), systemic and peripheral edema that may be pitting in nature, periorbital edema, shortness of breath, and moist rales in the lungs. These symptoms are caused by the increased interstitial volume. A bounding pulse and hypertension are related to the increase in plasma volume.

Laboratory findings, including the hematocrit, hemoglobin, and red cell count, are below normal because of the abnormally large increase in extracellular fluid volume.

Electrolyte disturbances

Sodium. Sodium is the most important extracellular cation. It is an integral component of numerous metabolic reactions. The sodium-potassium pump plays an important role in the maintenance of the ionic composition and volume of the interstitial fluid and in the entry of nutrients into the cell. This pump is essential for the movement of some solutes across the cell membrane against a concentration and/or elec-

---

CAUSES OF HYPERNATREMIA

Water loss

1. Insensible water loss
   Febrile illness, diaphoresis
   Burns
   Respiratory infections
2. Renal loss
   Central diabetes insipidus
   Nephrogenic diabetes insipidus
   Osmotic diuresis
3. Gastrointestinal loss
   Diarrhea
   Lactulose
4. Hypothalamic disorders
   Hypodipsia
   Essential hypernatremia
   Primary mineralocorticoid excess—osmostat reset
5. Water loss into the cells
   Seizures
   Severe exercise

Sodium retention

1. Administration of hypertonic NaCl or $NaHCO_3$
2. Excessive ingestion of NaCl
3. Inhalation of sea water

Modified from Rose, B.D.: Clinical physiology of acid-base and electrolyte disorders, ed. 2, New York, 1984, McGraw-Hill Book Co.

---

trical gradient and participates in the generation of the membrane potential. Sodium is also essential for neuromuscular transmission.

Hypernatremia. Hypernatremia can result from sodium retention or water loss. To cause hypernatremia, the loss of water must exceed the loss of solute.[20] Then, because sodium is an effective osmole, an increase in the plasma osmolality caused by hypernatremia creates an osmotic gradient that effectively pulls water out of the cells into the extracellular fluid until equilibrium is established. Causes of hypernatremia are found in the box above.

Hypothalamic osmoreceptors stimulate both ADH release and thirst in an attempt to defend

CAUSES OF HYPONATREMIA

Impaired renal water excretion

1. Depletion of effective circulating volume
   Gastrointestinal losses: vomiting, diarrhea, gastrointestinal suction, bleeding, intestinal obstruction
   Renal losses: potent diuretics, hypoaldosteronism, sodium wasting renal disease
   Skin losses, burns, cystic fibrosis
   Edematous states, heart failure, hepatic cirrhosis, nephrotic syndrome
   Potassium depletion
2. Renal failure
3. Diuretics
   Thiazides
   Furosemide
   Ethacrynic acid
4. Presence of ADH
   Syndrome of inappropriate ADH secretion
   Effective circulating volume depletion
   Cortisol deficiency
   Hypothyroidism

Normal renal water excretion

1. Primary polydipsia
2. Reset osmostat

Modified from Rose, B.D.: Clinical physiology of acid-base and electrolyte disorders, ed. 2, New York, 1984, McGraw-Hill Book Co.

the body against the development of hypernatremia. Even though ADH release occurs first, it is thirst that ultimately protects against the development of sodium excess.

Clinical findings related to the water loss include dry, sticky mucous membranes; flushed skin; rough, dry tongue; depressed lacrimation; oliguria or anuria; and fever. Cellular dehydration in the brain leads to lethargy, weakness, and irritability that can progress to twitching, seizures, coma, and death. Patients with sodium overload may show signs of volume expansion or volume depletion.

Hyponatremia. Either solute loss or water retention can cause hyponatremia, although water retention leading to an excess of fluid in relation to the solute is most common.[20] Hyponatremia essentially occurs only when there is a deficit in renal water excretion. An exception to this occurs in patients with primary polydipsia. Causes of this disorder are described in the box at left.

Because the sodium amount is deficient, there is a decrease in the osmotic pressure of body fluids. Therefore hyponatremia reflects hypoosmolality.[4,20] As a result of the changes in tonicity, water shifts from the extracellular fluid to the inside of the cell. With the loss of ECF, plasma protein concentration increases. Interstitial fluid is subsequently drawn into the plasma through the osmotic pull created by the elevated protein concentration. This movement partially restores the plasma volume.

The symptoms associated with hyponatremia are primarily a result of water movement into the brain and other cells.[19,20] Complaints of nausea and malaise accompanied by headache, lethargy, and obtundation may be seen. Seizures and coma usually are not noted until the plasma sodium concentration is reduced substantially.

Potassium. Potassium is basically an intracellular cation, with 98% of all body potassium located in the cells. It has two major physiologic functions. First, potassium plays an important role in cell metabolism, participating in the regulation of protein and glycogen synthesis. Second, the ionic concentrations of potassium in the cell and the extracellular fluid are the principle determinants of the resting membrane potential across the cell membrane. Therefore potassium is vital in the body, being needed for the transformation of carbohydrate into energy, the reassembly of amino acids into proteins, the maintenance of normal fluid and electrolyte content of the intracellular fluid, and the establishment of a resting membrane potential.

Hyperkalemia. Hyperkalemia occurs when there is an excess of potassium in the extracellular fluid. Because the kidneys remove potassium from the body so efficiently, an accumulation is less common than a deficit. Chronic hyperkalemia is always associated with an impairment in urinary potassium excretion.[65]

The sequence of imbalance that occurs varies with the cause of the disorder. An excess can occur with increased intake, movement of the ions from the intracellular space to the extracellular fluid, or decreased urinary excretion.[19] The box at right summarizes the causes of hyperkalemia.

The changes induced by hyperkalemia are primarily muscular weakness and abnormal cardiac conduction.[65] Muscle weakness associated with hyperkalemia can be attributed to the concentration changes that occur in the resting membrane potential. The resting potential is decreased because of the reduced ratio of intracellular to extracellular potassium. An action potential cannot be sustained when the resting potential falls to or below threshold; this leads to muscle weakness or paralysis.

Changes in atrial and ventricular depolarization and repolarization occur with hyperkalemia and can lead to disturbances in the conduction sequence. Ventricular fibrillation or standstill pose the greatest threat. The earliest ECG signs of hyperkalemia are peaked, narrow T waves and shortened QT intervals, reflective of more rapid repolarization. The most prominent additional changes as potassium concentration exceeds 8 mEq/L are caused by delayed depolarization and include widening of the QRS complex. The final changes are a sine wave pattern that is characteristic when the QRS complex merges with the T wave, followed by fibrillation or asystole.

Other symptoms that occur in the presence of hyperkalemia are related to an underlying disease, such as polyuria and polydipsia in uncontrolled diabetes and weight loss, or to failure to thrive in infants with hypoaldosteronism.[18,65]

Hypokalemia. The body has no efficient mechanism for conserving potassium. Therefore hypokalemia or potassium deficit can occur when the dietary intake is inadequate or as a result of excessive losses of potassium-rich secretions or excretions. The causes of hypokalemia are listed in the box on p. 390.

CAUSES OF HYPERKALEMIA

Increased intake*

Oral
Intravenous

Movement from cells into extracellular fluid

Pseudohyperkalemia*†
Metabolic acidosis
Insulin deficiency and hyperglycemia*
Tissue catabolism, such as severe trauma*
Beta-adrenergic blockade
Severe exercise
Digitalis intoxication
Periodic paralysis
Cardiac surgery
Succinylcholine
Arginine

Decreased urinary excretion

Renal failure*
Depletion of effective circulating volume*
Hypoaldosteronism*
Distal renal tubular acidosis
Selective potassium secretory defect

Modified from Rose, B.D.: Clinical physiology of acid-base and electrolyte disorders, ed. 2, New York, 1984, McGraw-Hill Book Co.
*Most common causes.
†Disorder in which hyperkalemia occurs as a result of movement of K^+ out of the cell after the blood specimen is drawn.

Hypokalemia can cause muscle weakness and paralysis.[18,20] The mechanisms by which this occurs can be described as follows: hypokalemia initially causes hyperpolarization of the cell membrane by increasing the rate of the intracellular potassium concentration to that in the ECF. This reduces membrane excitability because the resting potential is farther away from the threshold that must be reached to generate an action potential. As a result, there is decreased responsiveness of the membrane to exciting stimuli.[65]

Severe hypokalemia leading to muscle weakness and paralysis is apparently associated with depolarization rather than hyperpolarization. As the resting membrane potential falls, the muscle

CAUSES OF HYPOKALEMIA

Decreased intake

1. Low potassium diet
2. Intravenous infusion of potassium-free fluids
3. Clay ingestion

Increased entry into cells

1. Alkalemia
2. Increased insulin availability
3. Elevated beta-adrenergic activity
4. Periodic paralysis-hypokalemic form
5. Treatment of anemia (with folic acid or vitamin B_{12})
6. Pseudohypokalemia
7. Delirium tremens
8. Hypothermia

Increased gastrointestinal losses*

1. Diarrhea
2. Bowel fistula
3. Vomiting
4. Nasogastric tube

Increased urinary loss

1. Primary mineral-corticoid excess
2. Enhanced distal flow (diuretic therapy + salt-wasting nephropathies)
   Hypercalcemia
   Acute leukemia
3. Sodium reabsorption with a nonreabsorbable anion
   Vomiting +
   Nasogastric suction +
   Metabolic acidosis +
   Carbenicillin or other penicillin derivative
4. Miscellaneous
   Hypomagnesemia +
   Polyuric states
   L-dopa therapy

Increased sweat loss dialysis

Modified from Rose, B.D.: Clinical physiology of acid-base and electrolyte disorders, ed. 2, New York, 1984, McGraw-Hill Book Co.
*Most common causes.

cell is unable to sustain an action potential. Although the cause for this is uncertain, one study suggests that depolarization could be caused by an increase in membrane permeability to sodium or a decrease in permeability to potassium. This would permit sodium entry and limit potassium exit and could result in the generation of an action potential.[42]

Potassium depletion can also induce cardiac dysrhythmias. Abnormalities, including premature atrial and ventricular beats, sinus bradycardia, paroxysmal atrial or junctional tachycardia, atrioventricular block, and ventricular tachycardia or fibrillation, have been documented and are related to the effects of potassium in impulse conduction and muscle contractility.[34,73] Hypokalemia also potentiates the action of digitalis and may therefore result in the development of arrhythmias.

The ECG manifestations of hypokalemia are characteristic, primarily because of delayed ventricular repolarization. Hypokalemia results in ST segment depression, decreased amplitude or inversion of the T wave, increased U wave height to greater than 1 mm, and prolongation of the QU interval. With severe depletion, the amplitude of the P wave increases, the PR interval becomes prolonged, and the QRS widens.[73]

Hypokalemia can also interfere with renal functions, causing renal insufficiency, impaired urinary concentration (leading to polyuria and polydipsia), increased ammonia production, impaired urinary acidification, increased bicarbonate reabsorption, and abnormal sodium chloride reabsorption.

Mild hyperglycemia can also occur with hypokalemia; it is probably caused by impaired insulin secretion.[32]

Chloride. Chloride is one of the major extracellular anions. It plays an important role in the maintenance of electrolyte balance (electrical neutrality), hydration, and osmotic pressure. It plays a passive role in the generation and propagation of an action potential. Chloride is also essential for the formation of gastric hydrochloric acid.

Hyperchloremia. High concentrations of chloride ions are usually found in dehydration, in certain types of renal tubular acidosis, and in patients who lose carbon dioxide by hyperventilating following stimulation of the respiratory center.

Hypochloremia. Decreases in the concentration of chloride ions in the extracellular fluid occur in metabolic acidosis of various types. In uncontrolled diabetes mellitus, there is an overproduction of keto acids whose anions replace chloride ions. Phosphate ion retention accompanies impaired glomerular filtration in renal disease and is associated with a concomitant decrease in the extracellular chloride level. Prolonged vomiting leads to a deficit of body chloride whether the etiology is pyloric stenosis, intestinal obstruction, or some other cause. Gastric suction without adequate fluid and electrolyte replacement can result in chloride deficiency because these secretions contain a high concentration of hydrogen and chloride ions. Low values also occur in salt-losing nephritis and in metabolic alkalosis when bicarbonate is increased and chloride drops reciprocally. Both sodium and chloride levels are low during a crisis in patients with Addison's disease.

Calcium. Calcium is an important extracellular cation that is indispensable in several physiologic processes. It influences the cardiac action potential and helps to control myocardial function and contractility through the protein calmodulin. Calcium affects neuromuscular transmission by altering the excitability of nerve and muscle tissue. It participates in the regulation of many enzyme systems, serving as a second messenger for many secretory processes. This ion is a necessary factor in blood coagulation and in activation of the complement system, a circulatory group of protein moieties in the blood. Calcium is also responsible for providing a portion of the matrix structure of bone and is vital to the integrity of membranes.

Hypercalcemia. The primary alteration in hypercalcemia is an excess of the ionized portion of the total plasma calcium. This excess is precipitated by parathyroid overactivity, causing an excessive removal of calcium from the bones, or by prolonged calcium mobilization. Hypercalcemia depends on factors that either increase calcium absorption or prevent adequate renal excretion.[46]

Elevated serum calcium levels produce symptoms related to decreased neuromuscular transmission and muscle contraction.[20] Clinical symptoms include fatigue, muscle weakness, muscle hypotonicity, drowsiness, lethargy, disorientation, memory loss, depression, and loss of consciousness. Rarely does the calcium level become high enough to significantly affect the heart because, as calcium excess develops, it is precipitated in the bones and other tissue. However, rapid administration of calcium intravenously can decrease the conduction velocity and shorten the refractory interval, predisposing to the onset of cardiac dysrhythmias. These changes are seen on the ECG as shortened PR and ST intervals with a somewhat prolonged QRS interval. When urinary calcium is excessive, stones may form. Bone pain also occurs, resulting from cavitation.

Hypocalcemia. Hypocalcemia is a deficit of the ionized portion of the extracellular calcium. Calcium deficiency leads to enhanced neuromuscular transmission, producing the following symptoms: numbness and tingling in the extremities, circumoral paresthesia, muscle cramps affecting both abdominal and skeletal muscle, tetany, positive Chvostek's and Trousseau's signs, and seizures. Carpopedal spasms, hyperreflexia, and mental depression also occur. Pathologic fractures can occur with sustained deficiency because calcium is withdrawn from the osteoid tissue to replenish extracellular fluid, leaving bone porous and brittle.

Phosphate. The phosphate ion participates in numerous biochemical reactions. It is the major inracellular anion of most cells. Phosphate is a constituent of several high-energy metabolic intermediates and takes an active part in the metabolism of carbohydrates, lipids, and nucleic acids. It participates in oxidative phosphorylation and is one of the determinants of red blood cell production at ATP and 2,3-diphosphoglycerate, which is involved in oxygen delivery. Phosphate compounds aid in the intestinal absorption of glucose and glycerol. Phosphate also functions as an effective extracellular buffer. It is integral in maintaining calcium homeostasis and the structural integrity of the cell wall and in providing bone with structural strength.

Hyperphosphatemia. *Hyperphosphatemia* is an excess of phosphate in the extracellular fluid. It is most often related to renal dysfunction but can occur in hypoparathyroidism, pseudohypoparathyroidism, excessive oral ingestion or parenteral infusion of phosphate salts, overingestion of vitamin D metabolites, neoplastic disorders, or catabolic states.[39]

Because there is a reciprocal relationship between phosphate and calcium, an excess of phosphate produces clinical symptoms of hypocalcemia.[20]

Hypophosphatemia. A deficiency of phosphate is called *hypophosphatemia.* Renal loss of phosphate is most often responsible for clinical phosphate deficiency and can be traced to tubular reabsorption defects. Other causes include hyperparathyroidism, chronic metabolic acidosis, hypokalemia, administration of phosphate binders, prolonged use of phosphate-free parenteral solutions in fasting patients, vitamin D deficiency, alcohol withdrawal, and body processes during the recovery phase of malnutrition.

The clinical signs of deficiency are principally neurologic and musculoskeletal and inclulde muscle cramping, carpopedal spasms, and bone pain.

Magnesium. Magnesium has many physiologic functions. Extracellular magnesium is important in neuromuscular transmission, acting as a mediator of neural transmission in the central nervous system and at the myoneural junction. Intracellular magnesium is a component of bone matrix and is an essential cofactor in many enzyme reactions including glycolysis, oxidative phosphorylation, protein, and nucleic acid synthesis. In addition, this cation is necessary for helical stability in ribosomal RNA and DNA.

Hypermagnesemia. An excess of magnesium leads to *hypermagnesemia.* This condition occurs when renal excretion is decreased, as in renal failure and eclampsia. Because the kidneys can normally excrete large quantities of the cation, other causes are rare. Some factors that can lead to magnesium excess include adrenal insufficiency, shock, hypothermia, and increased intake. Increased intake can occur with prolonged parenteral therapy using magnesium-containing solutions, with repeated use of oral laxatives containing magnesium, or with the administration of enemas that contain magnesium.[47]

Elevated plasma levels of magnesium produce variable symptoms, depending on the severity of the imbalance. Few symptoms occur with mild hypermagnesemia. Serum levels greater than 4 mEq/L can block neuromuscular transmission, leading to decreased tendon reflexes and muscle weakness. Hypoventilation, respiratory paralysis, heart block, and coma can occur at levels above 10 mEq/L. With extreme elevations (above 15 mEq/L), cardiac arrest has been noted.[20]

Hypomagnesemia. A deficiency in magnesium results in *hypomagnesemia.* Deficits can be attributed to decreased intake, impaired intestinal absorption, excessive loss of body fluids, increased renal excretion, and a number of miscellaneous factors.[47]

Decreased intake may occur during protein-calorie malnutrition, starvation, or with prolonged parenteral therapy using magnesium-free solutions.

Altered intestinal absorption is found in several malabsorption syndromes, after bowel resection, and in some hereditary defects.

Prolonged gastric suctioning, chronic use of enemas and nonmagnesium laxatives, severe diarrhea, and the presence of intestinal or biliary fistulas result in magnesium loss via body fluids.

Chronic alcoholism, diuretic therapy, hyperaldosteronism, and hypercalcemia, especially in conjunction with primary hyperparathyroidism, increase magnesium loss via the kidneys. Increased renal excretion also occurs in certain neoplastic diseases, with vitamin D toxicity, in hyperthyroidism, in renal tubular acidosis, and in ketoacidosis; in addition, it could be related to gentamycin toxicity.

Miscellaneous factors that lead to hypomagnesemia include hypoparathyroidism, acute pancreatitis, the syndrome of inappropriate antidiuretic hormone (ADH SI), and multiple transfusions using citrated blood.

The clinical symptoms associated with hypomagnesemia vary. When magnesium deficiency is severe and the plasma level is very low, parathormone secretion is impaired.[20] These factors together act to decrease calcium mobilization from the bone. Therefore severe hypomagnesemia is associated with hypocalcemia. The clinical signs associated with this type of deficiency are similar to those appearing with calcium deficiency and include muscular twitching and tremor, a positive Chvostek's sign, and numbness and tingling. Less commonly seen are muscle weakness, convulsions, apathy, depression, delirium, and ventricular cardiac dysrhythmias. Rare findings include vertigo, ataxia, tetany, and a positive Trousseau's sign.[13,20]

Manifestations of acid-base disorders depend in part on the primary disease. In addition, there may be symptoms specifically referable to the acidotic or alkalotic state that can affect other body systems. Consequently, it is difficult if not impossible to identify a symptom or symptoms that are representative of acid-base disturbance and review the pathophysiology. Therefore each specific pathologic alteration in acid-base balance will be discussed separately.

Metabolic acidosis

A combination of low arterial pH and low serum bicarbonate suggests metabolic acidosis as a diagnosis. Bicarbonate is low because it either has been consumed in the neutralization of acid or because of direct loss, depending on the cause. An additional feature usually present is a low P_{CO_2}. Serum chloride is usually elevated in those cases without *anion gap,* which is described below. Potassium may be high, particularly if the renal function is poor.

The most frequent causes of metabolic acidosis are:

Excessive acid load
  Diabetic ketoacidosis
  Lactic acidosis
  Ingestion of such substances as methanol, salicylate, ethylene glycol, ammonium chloride, and paraldehyde
Inability to excrete normal acid load
  Uremia
Bicarbonate loss
  Renal tubular acidosis
  Severe diarrhea, particularly in infants
  Pancreatic drainage, ileostomy, colostomy
  Ureterosigmoidostomy
  Carbonic anhydrase inhibitors

To establish the cause of the acidosis, it is advisable to determine if a significant "anion gap," or amount of nonmeasured anions, is present. This is done by matching the milliequivalents of Na^+ against the sum of the milliequivalents of CL^- and HCO_3. Normally, there is a small difference because of anions that are not routinely measured, which may include organic, as well as mineral, anions.

Serum electrolytes are used for these measurements. For example,

Serum $[Na^+]$ = 142 mEq/L; Serum $[Cl]$ = 105 mEq/L

$$\text{Serum } [HCO_3] = \frac{+26 \text{ mEq/L}}{131 \text{ mEq/L}}$$

"Anion gap" = 142 − 131 = 11 mEq/L

The normal gap is less than 13 mEq/L. A larger gap suggests the presence of unidentified anions, which probably correspond to the acid causing the problem (such as lactic acid and ketone bodies).

With "anion gap"	Without "anion gap" (with hyperchloremia)
Uremia	Ammonium chloride administration
Diabetic ketoacidosis	Renal tubular acidosis
Lactic acidosis	Bicarbonate losses
Salicylate poisoning	Carbonic anhydrase inhibitors
Methyl alcohol	
Ethylene glycol	
Paraldehyde	

Causes of acidosis without "anion gap" are usually present with hyperchloremia.

Compensation of metabolic acidosis

Compensation of metabolic acidosis may occur by means of the three mechanisms already mentioned: buffers, pulmonary compensation, and renal compensation.

As discussed previously, a great deal of buffering takes place in the cells, as well as in the extracellular fluid. However, the easiest change to detect in the laboratory is the consumption of bicarbonate, which to some extent reflects the overall buffering action. Bicarbonate consumption always occurs in metabolic acidosis, and low bicarbonate concentration is characteristic of metabolic acidosis.

Respiratory compensation is particularly efficient in mild or moderate degrees of acidosis. It seems that pulmonary hyperventilation is somewhat more efficient in acute than in chronic metabolic acidosis, although this concept is not accepted by all authors.

Renal compensation consists of enhanced excretion of hydrogen ions. Such enhancement results from increased synthesis and excretion of ammonia in the urine. Maximal synthesis of ammonia is reached after 5 or 6 days. Low urinary pH permits more ammonia to diffuse into the urine, where it will bind with H^+. Excretion

of titratable acid does not increase as much as ammonia formation in response to acidosis because the former operation depends mainly on the availability of basic phosphate.

Symptoms of metabolic acidosis

Metabolic acidosis can cause changes in pulmonary, cardiovascular, neurologic, and skeletal functions. Hyperventilation attendant to respiratory compensation produces a four- to eight-fold increase in minute volume; therefore complaints of dyspnea on exertion and shortness of breath at rest with severe acidemia are not unusual. Hyperpnea may be the only finding on physical examination.

Ventricular dysrhythmias, some of which may be fatal, can occur with a low pH[28] and can reduce both myocardial contractility and the inotropic response to catecholamines.[77]

A fall in the pH of the cerebrospinal fluid may be responsible for the neurologic symptoms that develop, which range from lethargy to coma.[60] Other factors, such as the toxic effects of ingestions and hyperosmolality caused by hyperglycemia in diabetic ketoacidosis, may also produce neurologic alterations.[26,61]

The negative calcium and phosphate balance associated with chronic acidemia, such as occurs in renal failure or renal tubular acidosis, may lead to bone problems. Impaired growth and rickets have been noted in children.[62] Other abnormalities have also been reported; these include osteitis fibrosis (from secondary hyperparathyroidism) and osteomalacia and osteopenia in adults.[9,16]

Nonspecific symptoms including anorexia, nausea, weight loss, muscle weakness, and listlessness have been documented in infants and young children with acidemia.[49]

Metabolic alkalosis

Metabolic alkalosis is a condition in which there is either excessive loss of fixed acids or ingestion of alkaline substances such as bicarbonate. The arterial blood pH is high, the HCO_3 is high, and the arterial blood Pco_2 is normal or somewhat elevated. The most frequent causes are

Vomiting

Gastric drainage (such as through a naso-gastric tube)

Diuretic therapy

Treatment with adrenal corticoids

Excessive ingestion of Na^+ bicarbonate

Physiologic changes following correction of ventilatory insufficiency

It should be emphasized that in most of these clinical situations, one or more of the following factors are present: (1) potassium depletion, (2) hypochloremia, (3) hypovolemia, and (4) excessive mineralocorticoid activity.

Alkalosis caused by gastric loss

The alkalosis of persistent vomiting or stomach drainage is one of the most severe forms of metabolic alkalosis. Although this is a multifactorial situation in which hypovolemia and hypokalemia play a role, the most important factor is the loss of HCl per se. Gastric fluid contains approximately 90 mmol of HCl, 50 mmol of Na^+, and 10 mmol of K^+ per liter. For each mole of HCl that is secreted in the stomach, 1 mole of bicarbonate is generated and released to the bloodstream. If HCl is lost, this bicarbonate remains unchecked.

The alkalosis of gastric loss is maintained by several factors but principally by volume depletion resulting from loss of water and sodium. Volume contraction in itself enhances proximal reabsorption of bicarbonate, as discussed earlier. In addition, the loss of chloride forces Na^+ to be reabsorbed with a relatively higher fraction of bicarbonate. Another effect of volume contraction is enhanced mineralocorticoid secretion, which is also known to cause metabolic alkalosis.

The hypokalemia that is usually present in gastric loss does not result from loss of K^+ in the gastric fluid; a better reason is the renal loss of K^+ that takes place in alkalosis. Despite severe K^+ depletion, the kidney continues excreting large amounts of potassium. It is known that the distal secretion of K^+ is en-

hanced in alkalosis, but the mechanism is under debate. The traditional concept, that K^+ and H^+ compete among themselves for exchange with sodium, has been challenged. The most important characteristics of gastric alkalosis are the extremely small amount of chloride and the relatively large amount of potassium in the urine.

Diuretic therapy functions to produce hypovolemia, hypokalemia, hypochloremia, and metabolic alkalosis in severe circumstances. The factors enhancing bicarbonate reabsorption and producing metabolic alkalosis, such as potassium depletion, hypochloremia, hypovolemia, and excessive mineralocorticoid activity, are explained in detail in preceding sections.

Compensation of metabolic alkalosis

The kidney is responsible for the maintenance of metabolic alkalosis except on those rare occasions when excessive amounts of alkali have been administered to the patient. Consequently, any compensatory mechanisms must originate in the respiratory system. Normally the lungs compensate by hypoventilation; this not only leads to an increase in carbon dioxide but also promotes a decline in the Po_2. The latter would serve to stimulate ventilation.

Compensatory hypoventilation may also be inhibited by the intracellular acidosis in the brain brought about by hypokalemia. Therefore it is obvious that whatever mechanism is involved is not very effective.

Symptoms of metabolic alkalosis

The symptoms associated with metabolic alkalosis are variable. Some patients may be asymptomatic. Others may describe symptoms related to volume depletion, such as weakness, muscle cramps, and postural dizziness, or problems caused by hypokalemia, including polyuria, polydipsia, and muscle weakness. Neurologic symptoms of paresthesia, carpopedal spasm, and lightheadedness, although characteristic in respiratory alkalosis, occur infrequently in metabolic alkalosis. This may be explained by the fact that the bicarbonate ion crosses the blood-brain

Table 5-9. $PaCO_2$—pH in acute and chronic hypercapnia

$PaCO_2$ (mmHg)	pH*	
	Acute	Chronic
40	7.40	7.40
50	7.30	7.38
60	7.25	7.36
70	7.20	7.34
80	7.15	7.32
90	7.10	7.30†
100	7.05	—

*Values are ± 0.05 for pH > 7.2, 0.03 for pH < 7.2. pH of chronic COLD with ARF will fall between acute and chronic levels. pH values will be altered by simultaneous metabolic acidosis (↓) or metabolic alkalosis (↑).

†Rare to see a patient with COLD, breathing room air, who has a $PaCO_2$ higher than 80 mmHg.

barrier more slowly than carbon dioxide, creating a lesser increase in the pH of the cerebrospinal fluid.

Respiratory acidosis

Respiratory acidosis occurs in any situation in which the ability of the lungs to eliminate CO_2 is reduced. In most cases, it is caused by hypoventilation, which is secondary to central nervous system problems, neuromuscular problems, chest wall or pleural disease, airway obstructions, or severe impairment of lung parenchyma or pulmonary vasculature. Chronic hypercapnia can occur in patients with emphysema, chronic bronchitis, kyphoscoliosis, and the alveolar hypoventilation syndrome associated with obesity. Chronic hypercapnia is particularly common in patients with chronic obstructive lung disease. With progression of pathologic changes in emphysema and bronchitis, the patient's effort in respiration and work of breathing will be increased. This mechanical impairment interferes with the patient's ability to increase ventilatory effort in response to an increased central respiratory drive. As carbon dioxide is retained, the central responsiveness to an increase in carbon dioxide becomes impaired. If the airway obstruction is caused by broncho-

constriction and can be relieved, then carbon dioxide responsiveness improves. Severe ventilation-perfusion imbalance, as can be seen in patients with chronic obstructive lung disease (COLD), can contribute to hypercapnia.

Compensation of respiratory acidosis

In response to hypercapnia, kidneys retain bicarbonate. Several days (4 to 5) are required to achieve maximal renal compensation and respiratory acidosis. A patient with acute hypercapnia will not have an elevated serum bicarbonate level and will have a lower pH at any $PaCO_2$ than will a patient with chronic hypercapnia (Table 5-9).

The relationship between $PaCO_2$ and pH in Table 5-9 can help us differentiate between acute hypercapnia and chronic hypercapnia. Patients with chronic hypercapnia who become acutely decompensated will have pH values that are intermediate for any given $PaCO_2$. Simultaneous metabolic acidosis will lead to a lower serum bicarbonate and therefore lower pH, whereas metabolic alkalosis with be associated with a higher bicarbonate and higher pH.

Because of compensatory bicarbonate retention in those with chronic hypercapnia, lowering their $PaCO_2$ to normal with a mechanical ventilator can lead to profound metabolic alkalosis. This in turn can result in seizures and further suppression of patients' respiratory drive.

A pH below 7.2 is associated with mental obtundation and impaired cardiovascular function. Intravenous bicarbonate can be given to raise arterial pH above 7.2, but this must be done with extreme caution. If excess bicarbonate is given, patients are in danger of developing metabolic alkalosis as their $PaCO_2$ is improved with medical management. Another danger of excess bicarbonate administration is suppression of ventilatory drive. With increasing serum bicarbonate levels, ventilatory responsiveness to carbon dioxide decreases. The bicarbonate level in a cerebrospinal fluid seems to be particularly important in determining the carbon dioxide responsiveness in the brainstem.

A potential complication of chronic respiratory acidosis is potassium depletion. During acidosis, potassium and bicarbonate are shifted out of cells into plasma while hydrogen ions and chloride move into cells. In a patient with COLD and chronic hypercapnia, there may be a 15% to 40% total body potassium depletion in spite of a normal serum potassium level. If there is superimposed acute acidosis, the serum potassium may actually be elevated and may fall significantly as the acute acidosis is corrected. Potassium depletion aggravates respiratory failure by contributing to respiratory muscle weakness and increased cardiac irritability. A chloride deficit elevates the renal bicarbonate threshold, reducing excretion. Potassium deficit leads to increased hydrogen ion loss in the renal tubules. The combination causes a hypokalemic, hypochloremic metabolic alkalosis. Potassium chloride replacement helps to correct excess bicarbonate retention.

Symptoms of respiratory acidosis

Most of the clinical manifestations in respiratory acidosis are nonspecific and are the result of the combined effects of hypoxia,* hypercarbia, and acidemia. Neurologic symptoms are most abundant in respiratory acidosis.[37] Initial complaints consist of headache, blurred vision, restlessness, and anxiety; these may progress to asterixis, delirium, and drowsiness. Papilledema may be noted in a funduscopic exam. The increased cerebrospinal fluid pressure may be traced to an elevation in cerebral blood flow triggered by acidemia.[23] Both the neurologic symptoms and the increase in cerebral blood flow have been shown to result from changes in the pH of the CSF (or cerebral interstitial) rather than from the reduced arterial pH or elevated P_{CO_2}.[23,60]

Dysrhythmias and peripheral vasodilation may develop and combine to produce severe hypotension if the systemic pH falls below 7.1. This

occurs most commonly when respiratory acidosis is complicated by a metabolic acidosis. Blood pressure control may be difficult without raising the pH because acidemia diminishes the inotropic response to catecholamines.[77]

Chronic respiratory acidosis is frequently associated with both cor pulmonale and edema. Although the cardiac output and GFR remain normal or near normal in these conditions, patients usually have severe lung disease and are hypercapnic. This suggests a relationship between CO_2 and sodium retention. Both the compensatory reabsorption of sodium bicarbonate and a reduction in renal blood flow may contribute to chronic respiratory acidosis.[65,67]

Respiratory alkalosis

Respiratory alkalosis is caused by hyperventilation and an excessive loss of CO_2. Patients have a low arterial P_{CO_2} and high arterial pH.

The fall in arterial P_{CO_2} produces a reduction in cerebral blood flow. Bronchoconstriction can occur, which increases the work of breathing and may lead to hypoxemia in spite of hyperventilation. The alkalosis is associated with a decrease in ionized calcium in the serum and leads to changes in cell membrane potential in muscles and heart. The arterial P_{CO_2} is reduced to 30 or even 20 mmHg, with an increase in pH of 7.5 to 7.6. Hyperventilation can result from (1) functional or psychogenic changes, (2) normal physiologic responses to exercise, high altitude exposure, or overventilation on a mechanical ventilator, or (3) pathologic changes. Pathology can be pulmonary, including pulmonary emboli, restrictive lung disease, pneumothorax, and atelectasis. It can also be cardiac in origin, such as left ventricular failure. Organic lesions in the brain such as meningitis and encephalitis, cerebral hemorrhage, or tumor can be associated with hyperventilation. Excessive ingestion of drugs such as salicylates can lead to the syndrome, as can hypermetabolic states such as hyperthyroidism, fever, or Gram-negative sepsis. Hypocapnia is also seen in patients with acute pain or hypotension of any etiology.

---

*Since hypercarbia usually results from hypoventilation, hypoxia is normally an associated finding unless oxygen therapy is being administered.

Compensation of respiratory alkalosis

There are two types of compensatory responses that attempt to minimize the effects of an elevated pH: tissue buffering and renal mechanisms.

Within a short period of time after the onset of respiratory alkalosis, hydrogen ions move from the cells into the ECF where they combine with bicarbonate ions to form carbonic acid, which dissociates into water and carbon dioxide. The H^+ comes from protein, phosphate, and hemoglobin buffers in the cells. Some acids are derived from increased lactic acid production, which is induced by the alkalotic state.[29] Cell buffering is not very efficient, lowering the plasma bicarbonate concentration only slightly.

If hyperventilation is chronic, that is, if it lasts more than 2 or 3 days, there will be a renal response in the form of increased bicarbonate excretion. This results in a decreased net acid excretion.

Symptoms of respiratory alkalosis

There are generally no symptoms in chronic respiratory alkalosis because the arterial pH is either normal or close to normal. The clinical manifestations of acute respiratory alkalosis are numerous and are induced by a reduction in cerebral blood flow caused by a low Pco_2 and concomitant hyperventilation. Symptoms of hyperventilation are dizziness; dyspnea; blurred vision; palpitations; tachycardia; discomfort in the throat, precordium, or epigastric area; numbness in the hands, feet, and perioral region; and associated apprehension. Patients usually are unaware of their excessive ventilation even if it is obvious to others around them. If the episodes are prolonged, patients can lose consciousness and experience muscular irritability manifested by carpopedal spasm.

Renal disorders

The pathogenesis of symptoms precipitated by renal dysfunction is fairly specific. Each symptom depends on the pathology of the disease process and the manner in which it alters the anatomic or physiologic function of underlying systemic structures. Those symptoms occurring most frequently in acutely ill people are reviewed in the pages that follow.

Blood in the urine (hematuria)

The presence of abnormal quantities of red blood cells in the urine is referred to as hematuria. There are multiple causes of hematuria that can be categorized into 3 groups: (1) renal parenchymal causes, (2) urinary tract causes, and (3) systemic coagulation disturbances.

It is difficult to locate the origin of erythrocytes in the urine in renal parenchymal disorders. Localized tears in the glomerular capillary walls, rupture of the basement membrane, and invasion of blood vessels and tubules by tumors may be aggravated by locally impaired thrombus generation and/or excessive thrombolysis.[30]

Historical symptomatology may be helpful in finding the site and origin of hematuria when the urinary tract is the cause, whereas the character of systemic symptoms or the presence of recognizable underlying disease may provide the needed data when the cause is a coagulation disturbance.

The pathogensis of hematuria can be linked to specific functional derangements induced by injury, neoplasia, or defects in coagulation.

Although the injurious agent—for example, trauma or infection—may vary, the mechanism and place of attack are often well defined. In each situation, the integrity of the capillary network is interrupted, and erythrocyte exudation occurs. For example, in acute poststreptococcal glomerulonephritis, the glomeruli are damaged secondary to a hypersensitivity reaction. The glomerular capillary, which is the site of the immunologic reaction, is injured and permits the escape of red blood cells. In the calyces and pelvis, injurious agents erode the capillary wall, leading to leakage of red cells into the urinary tract.

The manner in which neoplasia is produced in hematuria is somewhat different. Neoplasms develop their own blood supply. They have an extensive capillary network that proliferates and ruptures, permitting the extravasation of red blood cells into the surrounding areas.

Defects in coagulation also produce hematuria. The mechanism that causes hematuria in this instance is related to the specific interruption in the clotting cascade.

Reduced or absent urination (oliguria or anuria)

Oliguria may be caused by a reduction in the glomerular filtration rate, an obstruction to the flow of urine, or leakage of urine along the excretory tract.[44] When the problem becomes severe enough, anuria may ensue. The mechanisms producing oliguria and anuria are commonly organized into prerenal, renal, and postrenal causes.

Prerenal diminished urine output occurs secondary to hypoperfusion. When the intravascular volume is significantly depleted, a number of protective mechanisms are instituted to maintain adequate perfusion of critical organs. Renal vasoconstriction, mediated by increased production of angiotensin and catecholamines and possibly by a decrease in the secretion of hormonal vasodilators, results in a reduction in the renal blood flow. This decrease produces a concurrent fall in the glomerular filtration rate.

A marked increase in tubular salt and water reabsorption also occurs and is apparently related to an alteration in peritubular physical factors. Mechanisms that operate in the distal segments are most important. Increased levels of aldosterone, precipitated by volume depletion, enhance distal tubular fluid reabsorption, as does the nonosmolar release of ADH.

Oliguria produced by prerenal causes also occurs in disorders in which there is a reduction in the effective intravascular volume even though the total intravascular volume remains normal or elevated (such as in hepatic cirrhosis, ascites, or heart failure). People with these disorders respond as if they have true volume depletion and consequently exhibit many of the

same physiologic alterations as previously described.

Renal perfusion is also compromised if the patient is in shock from any cause. The mechanism is the same as that which occurs in volume depletion.

Obstruction may also be the cause of inadequate renal blood flow. Obstruction of the renal artery must be bilateral to cause oliguria. Bilateral obstruction of the renal vein can also diminish urine output.

The renal causes of reduced urine output include acute tubular necrosis, acute glomerulonephritis, and various systemic and nonsystemic glomerulopathies.

The mechanisms producing oliguria in acute tubular necrosis remain highly controversial. Four possibilities are proposed: (1) defective tubular epithelium, leading to back leak of filtered tubular fluid; (2) tubular obstruction, resulting from the deposition of tubular debris; (3) a change in renovascular dynamics, that is, a decrease in renal blood flow with concurrent GFR reduction; and (4) an alteration in the permeability barrier of glomerular filtration.[3,15] These mechanisms continue to be the subject of an intense study.

In end-stage renal failure, oliguria or anuria occur very late in the disease process and signify total nephron loss.[3]

Oliguria during acute glomerulonephritis is caused by direct glomerular damage that results in a decrease in the GFR. Enhanced tubular reabsorption may also occur.[3]

Postrenal causes of oliguria or anuria are related to urinary tract obstruction. Some of the possible causes include urethral obstruction resulting from, for example, stricture; ureteral obstruction above or within the bladder; bladder catheter blockage; or in rare cases, rupture of the bladder.[3,11]

Excessive urination (polyuria)

Polyuria occurs in the presence of a renal concentrating mechanism that does not work properly. Large volumes of dilute urine with a low specific gravity are produced. This urine may arise as a consequence of increased water excretion (water diuresis), increased solute excretion (osmotic diuresis), or both. An increased water intake, or polydipsia, may also be involved.[66]

Water diuresis results from the excessive ingestion of hypotonic fluids, the complete or partial lack of ADH (as in central diabetes insipidus), or the resistance to the renal action of ADH (as in hereditary or acquired nephrogenic diabetes insipidus).[66] In the last situation, the failure of the hormone to trigger cellular events necessary for enhanced tubular permeability to water or the loss of medullary hypertonicity may be responsible.[66]

Osmotic diuresis can be found in clinical disorders in which there is enhanced urinary excretion of endogenous solutes or following the parenteral administration of exogenous solutes. The excretion of additional solute requires water to keep the solute concentration stable. The urine is hypotonic and the osmolality low in pure water diuresis, whereas the urine is isotonic or slightly hypotonic in pure osmotic diuresis.

People who consume large volumes of water or other hypotonic fluids may also exhibit excessive urination. This large consumption is usually caused by a psychogenic disorder.[11]

Urinary retention—incomplete urination

Retention begins when outlet obstruction reaches a critical pressure and the bladder muscle cannot overcome it; therefore no urine can be excreted. When the urethral channel is partially obstructed, resulting from such conditions as prostatism or bladder neck contracture, the urinary stream will be slow and frequently will result in dribbling after the cessation of micturation.

Hesitancy

Prostatic obstruction usually presents with hesitancy. Hesitancy is the inability to initiate the urinary stream within 30 to 60 seconds after an attempt. In females, congenital valves may cause hesitancy.

Necessity to arise from sleep to urinate (nocturia)

Because most of the urine volume is excreted during the day, nocturia constitutes an alteration in the normal diurnal pattern. The pathogenesis of this disorder is uncertain, although it seems to occur in conjunction with congestive heart failure, hepatic cirrhosis, and renal failure. In some cases, it may be caused by the administration of diuretics before bedtime.

Fluid retention (edema)

Edema occurs when there is an abnormal accumulation of interstitial fluid in the body that results in detectable swelling in the tissues. The increase in interstitial volume is produced ultimately by the translocation of fluid from the intravascular to the interstitial compartments. The volume may increase as much as 5 L in an adult before clinical signs of generalized edema become visible.

The kidneys play a dominant role in edema formation. When significant amounts of intravascular fluids are lost, they must be replaced by renal conservation of sodium and water to avoid the deleterious effects of reduced plasma volume. The effectiveness of the circulating blood volume is monitored by receptors located throughout the body. If stimulated, these sensors trigger a series of activities. The mechanisms mediating renal reabsorption of salt and water involve alterations of intrarenal hemodynamics and augmented tubular reabsorption of filtrate as a result of increased sympathetic activity that includes catecholamine release and activation of the renin angiotensin aldosterone system.[33] Other humoral factors, natriuretic hormones, prostaglandins, and kinins are also involved, although their exact roles remain the subject of investigation. If these compensatory mechanisms are successful in the restoration of an effective circulating volume, the stimulus for further sodium and water conservation is removed.

Generalized edema can also develop in primary renal disease as a direct consequence of sodium and water retention. The diseased kidney's impaired ability to excrete salt and water in accordance with intake leads to an increase in the extracellular volume, circulatory congestion, hypertension, and edema. Frequently, edema formation is associated with an increase in the effective circulating volume, which acts to suppress the compensatory activities of the sympathetic nervous system and the renin angiotensin aldosterone mechanisms.

Pain (abdominal and flank)

Pain emanating from the upper urinary tract is often confused with abdominal or back pain. The kidney is innervated by afferent nerve fibers that emerge from cord levels T11 to T12. Pain can be elicited by stretching the viscera distention of a hollow structure; traction on the peritoneum, mesentery, or mesenteric blood vessels; inflammation; or ischemia.[1] Pain of renal origin may be caused by inflammation or distention of the renal capsule, ischemia, stretching of the intrarenal blood vessels, or distention of the collecting system itself.[11]

Inflammatory pain, usually secondary to infection, causes edema that leads to capsular stretching.

Ischemic pain can be traced to occlusion of the renal blood vessels, usually the arteries. Arterial occlusion may be caused by embolization or arteriosclerosis, resulting in thrombi and capsular distention secondary to parenchymal edema. Venous obstruction also causes capsular distention.

An obstruction of the collecting system can also lead to distention and pain. The occlusion may be located at the intrarenal infundibulum, the ureteropelvic junction, the ureter, or the ureterovesical junction. Lesions in the calyx do not obstruct the infundibulum and therefore do not usually produce pain.

Renal pain can also be referred and therefore perceived as being of somatic origin. Referred pain can be explained by the fact that afferent fibers from the upper urinary tract stimulate the central nervous system, causing pain to be felt at the corresponding dermatome level. Irritation of adjoining structures may also occur and lead to pain that is referable to another area.

INTERVENTIONS

Medications and fluid therapy may play major roles in fluid and electrolyte balance, either contributing to or correcting an imbalance. The cause of imbalance may be internal or external; regardless of etiology, however, vital systems may become impaired with time and degree of imbalance. The kidney will not be able to sustain compensatory mechanisms if the demand is too great or if the kidneys themselves are malfunctioning. When a vital system function becomes impaired, external therapeutic regimens will be necessary.

Interventions for dealing with fluid and/or electrolyte abnormalities will depend on etiology and the nature of onset of the problem, as well as on the age and overall general well-being of the patient with fluid and electrolyte problems.

Fluid replacement

The goal in fluid replacement is to correct electrolyte or water deficits while attempting to prevent creation of new disturbances as a result of replacement therapy. The type and amount of fluid necessary to correct deficits will depend on

1. Amount and type of fluid lost from the body.
2. Cause of deficit and impact on other body systems.
3. Other pre-existing physiologic problems.

Several methods exist for determining the amount of fluid lost and the amount necessary to correct the situation. Three different methods for calculating fluid needs are presented here.

One method that may be employed is related to the presence of water loss symptoms. In the presence of thirst and other minimal symptoms such as irritability, dry skin, and dry mucous

Table 5-10. Ranges of daily water requirements of infants and children at different ages under normal conditions

Age	Average body weight (kg)	Total water requirements/ 24 hours (ml)	Water require-ments/kg/24 hours (ml)
3 days	3.0	250-300	80-100
10 days	3.2	400-500	125-150
3 months	5.4	750-850	140-160
6 months	7.3	950-1100	130-135
9 months	8.6	1100-1250	125-145
1 year	9.5	1150-1300	120-135
2 years	11.8	1350-1500	115-125
4 years	16.2	1600-1800	100-110
6 years	20.0	1800-2000	90-100
10 years	28.7	2000-2500	70-85
14 years	45.0	2200-2700	50-60
18 years	54.0	2200-2700	40-50

From Vaughn, V.C., and McKay, R.J.: Nelson's textbook of pediatrics, ed. 10, Philadelphia, 1975, W.B. Saunders Co.

membranes, estimating 2% of the body weight can yield an approximation of fluid loss; that is, in a 70 kg person the approximate fluid loss would be 1.4 L. In the presence of marked thirst, dry mouth, and oliguria resulting from 3 to 4 days without water, estimating 6% of the body weight would yield approximate fluid loss.

When significant physical weakness and severe mental changes are added to the previous symptoms, fluid loss may be estimated by calculating 7% to 14% of the body weight. When 12% of the body weight has been lost, a patient loses swallowing capabilities, and when 15% to 25% of body weight has been lost, the usual consequence is death.

Another method for determining amount of fluid loss uses daily weights during the acute period of dehydration. Each kilogram of weight loss represents approximately 1 L of fluid loss.

The previous two methods provide only estimates of losses. When replacing fluids, the average daily maintenance requirements should be added to estimated losses along with any other intervening variables. The daily fluid requirement for an average adult is between 1500

and 2000 ml. Pediatric requirements will vary according to size (Table 5-10). In the presence of a high fever, 500 to 1500 ml should be added to the total amount to be infused. With moderate sweating, 500 ml should be added; with profuse diaphoresis, 1000 ml should be added.

The third method employs body surface area. By estimating body surface area from height and weight indexes through the use of a simple nomogram, it is possible to use a formula to determine fluid requirements. An approximation of body surface area may be determined from weight alone, as indicated in Table 5-11.

Once body surface area has been determined, the data are incorporated into appropriate formulas according to the clinical status of the patient. These formulas are as follows:

Fluid needs	Formula
Maintenance	1500 ml/m² body surface/day
Presence of moderate deficit	2400 ml/m² body surface/day (incorporates daily maintenance requirements)
Presence of severe deficit	3000 ml/ml² body surface/day (incorporates daily maintenance requirements)

The presence of other physiologic problems occurring along with fluid loss may have a significant impact on when and how fast fluid is replaced and what type of replacement is used.

Concomitant renal or cardiac problems may have a harmful impact because these systems are intricately involved in the use of fluid replacement. When initiating fluid replacement, the practitioner may present a challenge of fluids to the patient and observe responses that are made. Renal suppression often accompanies dehydration. A urine specific gravity above 1.030, less than three urinary voidings in 24 hours, or absence of urine in the bladder are all factors that may indicate suppression, which may or may not be related to dehydration. A challenge solution administered at 8 ml/m² body surface area/min for 45 minutes should restore urine flow suppressed from dehydration. If urine flow is restored, the challenge administration is discontinued and the replacement regimen begun. If urine flow is not restored, the challenge administration is decreased to 2 ml/m² body surface area/min for 1 hour. If urine flow is not restored at this time, renal impairment is indicated. Fluid administration should then be decreased, and concurrent renal management activities should be initiated.

Cardiovascular hemodynamics should also be monitored during fluid challenge. Although the basic parameters of blood pressure and pulse yield valuable information, more discriminate information may be gained through vascular pressure monitoring. Many clinicians rely on central venous pressure monitoring as a major index of patient response to fluid replacement endeavors, reducing the fluid infusion as the pressure rises above 15 cm. Measurement of pulmonary arterial pressure in conjunction with determinations of cardiac output can be extremely useful in discriminating early impact of fluid replacement on the hemodynamic system.

The infusion should proceed at a recommended rate of 3 ml/m² body surface area/min after challenge has been made. The fluid replacement usually may be corrected within 2 days, administering one half of the calculated needs in the first 24 hours.

The patient who has suffered a severe burn poses a great challenge. Several formulas are available to determine fluid need and replacement quantification. A split appears evident between those formulas advocating initial use of colloids and those negating such use in preference to crystalloid solutions. Although colloid solutions may maintain intravascular osmolarity, they may also enter the interstitial fluid compartment because of increased capillary permeability. An additional factor for debate is that initial use of crystalloids may lead to later pulmonary complications resulting from the preferential collection of crystalloids in the interstitial space of the lung. There are indications that colloids exert no more measurable effect in expanding plasma volume than lactated Ringer's solution does in

Table 5-11. Chart for converting weight to surface area*

Pounds	Surface area (square meters)
4	0.15
6	0.20
10	0.27
15	0.36
20	0.45
30	0.60
40	0.72
50	0.87
60	0.97
70	1.10
80	1.21
90	1.33
100	1.40
125	1.60
150	1.75
175	2.00
200	2.20
250	2.70

From Methany, N.M., and Snively, W.D.: Nurses' handbook of fluid balance, ed. 3, Philadelphia, 1979, J.B. Lippincott Co.
*Figures are approximate and apply only to people of average build.

the first 24 hours. Some advocates of initial colloid use incorporate concomitant crystalloids in their formulas. Formulas recommending crystalloid use in the first 24 hours do advocate colloid use on all other days subsequent to the burn to return plasma volume to normal. Regardless of debate, a formula is in order that will quantify fluid replacement and will take into account burn surface, weight of the individual patient, and concomitant evaporated losses.

The proponents of initial colloid use recommend, for the first 24 hours after the burn:

Colloid—between 0.5 and 1 ml/kg of body weight/ each % burn
±
Concomitant crystalloid—between 1 and 1.5 mL/kg of body weight/ % body area burned
+
Electrolyte-free solution (D5W)—2000 ml

Table 5-12. Intravenous solutions

	Na (mEq/L)	Cl (mEq/L)
Sodium chloride (0.9% NaCl)	154	154
Sodium chloride (3% NaCl)	513	513
Sodium chloride (5% NaCl)	855	855
Dextrose and water (5% D₅W)	—	—
Dextrose and water (10% D₅W)	—	—
Dextrose and water (20% D₅W)	—	—
Dextrose and water and sodium chloride (D₅W/0.45 NaCl)	77	77
Lactated Ringer's solution	130	109
Osmitrol - 5%	50 mg/ml of mannitol	
Osmitrol - 10%	100 mg/ml of mannitol	

*3.4 kcal/g; depends on purity of solution.

Colloid proponents also advocate initial use of a nonelectrolyte solution such as D₅W to replace insensible losses (Table 5-12).

Proponents of crystalloid solution use recommend, for the first 24 hours after the burn:

Four mL lactated Ringer's solution/kg of body weight/each % burn

No colloid; may be added after 24 hours

No dextrose solution; may be added after 24 hours

Dextrose solutions are avoided initially because of attendant stress-induced pseudodiabetes, which may result from burn trauma.

Additional factors when considering the type of solutions to administer and when to administer them include:

1. The capillary defect. This defect, in which plasma escapes into the surrounding interstitial fluid, resolves in approximately 24 hours after the burn. Plasma contains sodium, which may assist in correction of sodium deficits, but it also carries the disadvantages that accompany blood products. The use of dextran solutions does not change acid-base balance, nor does it add any caloric value. The attendant presence of clotting factors in fresh plasma may not be necessary or desired because of slow blood flow from hemoconcentration occurring in the burn patient; therefore aged plasma may be preferred. With the occurrence of hemoconcentration, the use of blood in initial fluid resuscitation is rarely advocated.

2. Anemia accompanies burn trauma, but because of early hemoconcentration, it may not be evident. In fact, the hematocrit may be elevated from the hemoconcentration. The hematocrit may be more reflective of blood loss after initial fluid resuscitation has occurred.

3. A sodium deficit initially results from entrapment of sodium in edema and exudate. After initial fluid resuscitation, a sodium deficit may occur from diuresis. Both lactated Ringer's solution and plasma contain sodium. Sodium has been noted to be a critical determinant in burn

K (mEq/L)	Glucose (mEq/ml)	Lactate (mEq/L)	Kcal/L
—	—	—	0
—	—	—	0
—	—	—	0
—	50	—	170 = 200*
—	100	—	340 = 400*
—	200	—	680 = 800*
—	50	—	340 = 400*
4	3	28	9

resuscitation by proponents of the use of hypertonic saline solution in the initial fluid resuscitation phase. Isotonic saline may be used to supply sodium, but it also has the disadvantage of supplying excess chloride in an amount that could contribute to acidosis.

4. Potassium losses may be high because of intracellular escape from damaged cells and from cells having impaired membrane potentials. Evidence of hyperkalemia may be deceiving because potassium is lost to the cells and excreted in urine. The deception is also exaggerated by the aldosterone mechanism, conserving sodium through reabsorption with resulting potassium excretion. The treatment of potassium losses may be carried out more adequately after initial fluid resuscitation has occurred. As potassium reenters the intracellular compartment, frequently on the fourth or fifth day after the burn, hypokalemia necessitating correction may be noted.

5. Early calcium deficits may also be noted in patients with burns because of saponification of fat at the burn site in subcutaneous adipose tissue. Later, calcium deficits may be noted, resulting from immobilization of calcium at the burn site.

After the amount of replacement solution that is needed has been calculated, a judicious rate of delivery must be considered to prevent further insult and overloading. The rate of delivery must be at a sufficient speed to prevent further physiologic deterioration from hypovolemia. Frequently, one half of the total calculated amount is delivered in the first 8 hours; the remaining one half is then spread out over the following 16 hours.

It is important to note that the formulas cited in this unit are not absolute but may vary depending on the institution and medical staff using them, their underlying philosophy, and their experiential and theoretical knowledge bases.

In summary, the type of solution used will

depend upon the specific disorder being treated and the electrolyte and nonelectrolyte deficits or excesses that exist. Table 5-12 lists some current preparations being used.

During the total replacement effort, close observation of the patient and of her unique response to the treatment regimen is paramount and includes frequent total-system physical assessments along with accurate intake and output, vital signs, weights, and monitoring of laboratory values.

Diuretics

The category of drugs used most frequently for fluid overload is that of the *diuretics*. There are other drug classifications besides the diuretics that have diuresing effects. When drugs with diuresing side effects are used for an indication other than the promotion of diuresis, it should be kept in mind that they will contribute to the overall balance of fluids.

Fluid overload as evidenced by edema is an increase of extracellular fluid volume in the interstitial compartment and/or a maldistribution of extracellular fluid between the intravascular and interstitial spaces. The kidney's avidity for sodium reabsorption can perpetuate and further increase an already high extracellular fluid volume.

Overall, many of the diuretics work by a process of decreasing sodium reabsorption by the kidney and increasing sodium excretion via the urine (natriuresis). It can be said that where sodium goes, there also goes water. The relationship between sodium and extracellular fluid and the principles of sodium conservation have been discussed earlier in the unit.

Diuretics can be categorized in many ways. Some classifications are made according to mechanism of action, whereas others are reviewed according to chemical composition. These two types of classification do not always closely correlate. In addition, the cellular mechanism of action for many of the diuretics is not always completely known or understood.

Diuretics will be discussed according to their

effects in the nephron. Not all diuretics work by natriuresis, as evidenced by the discussions of osmotic diuretics that follow.

In the proximal tubule

In the proximal tubule, approximately 60% to 70% of filtered sodium and water is reabsorbed. Both sodium chloride and sodium bicarbonate are reabsorbed, with practically all sodium bicarbonate reabsorbed at this point. The sodium reabsorption is an active process, pulling equivalent amounts of chloride with it, and is based on a hydrogen- or potassium-ion exchange process. The sodium bicarbonate reabsorption depends on hydrogen ion secretion, which requires carbonic anhydrase enzyme activity. Along with inhibition of carbonic anhydrase activity comes a subsequent decrease in sodium bicarbonate reabsorption; with the distal tubule having a limited capacity for sodium bicarbonate reabsorption, the sodium bicarbonate is excreted. The loss of sodium bicarbonate can result in hyperchloremic metabolic acidosis. Potassium excretion may occur along with sodium reabsorption inhibition because, when sodium reabsorption is blocked proximally to the more distal potassium secretory sites, the increased sodium flow through the tubule stimulates potassium secretion into the tubule and urine. The loss of potassium in the urine may ultimately lead to hypokalemia. Other substances reabsorbed by the proximal tubule and affected by a decrease in sodium reabsorption are calcium, phosphate, glucose, uric acid, and amino acids. Although inhibitions of sodium reabsorption in the proximal tubule do not result in aminoaciduria, glucosuria, or uricosuria, phosphaturia is common, which reflects a distal nephron's limited ability to reabsorb phosphate.

The principle group of diuretics acting on the proximal tubule is that of the carbonic anhydrase inhibitors, such as acetazolamide and dichlorphenamide. These diuretics are potent carbonic anhydrase inhibitors but generally weak diuretics because they inhibit sodium bicarbonate reabsorption, which only accounts for a small portion of the filtered sodium load. The carbonic anhydrase inhibitors have proven useful in glaucoma because the aqueous excess humor is high in bicarbonate. With carbonic anhydrase inhibition, the rate of aqueous formation is decreased, thereby reducing intraocular pressure.

Other agents that exert a proximal diuretic effect are albumin and xanthine derivatives, particularly theophylline. Albumin is frequently given to patients to expand extracellular fluid volume, which in turn has a rebound effect of inhibiting sodium reabsorption in the proximal tubule. The effect of theophylline appears to be an impairment of sodium transport in the proximal tubule through renal vasodilation. Along with affecting an increased blood flow, xanthines also appear to directly act on the tubule, with a resulting increase in sodium and chloride excretion rates.

In the ascending limb—loop of Henle

In the ascending limb, chloride is reabsored through active transport, and sodium follows passively. The diuretics affecting reabsorption in the ascending limb are furosemide, ethacrynic acid, and the mercurials; they do this by inhibiting active chloride transport.

Both furosemide and ethacrynic acid are potent, rapid-acting natriuretics, capable of eliminating ion transport in the ascending loop and of creating natriuresis even in the presence of renal insufficiency.

Because of the action exhibited by these drugs and the inability of the more distal nephron to reabsorb excess delivered sodium, the sodium is accompanied by chloride ion excretion. The presentation of excess sodium to the more distal potassium secretory sites also results in increased potassium excretion. Both furosemide and ethacrynic acid also effect increases in calcium excretion and may be used in the treatment of hypercalcemia. Furosemide has been noted to have some proximal tubule effect through carbonic anhydrase inhibitory activity, thereby producing a slight bicarbonate diuresis.

Mercurial diuretic action is somewhat different in that metabolic alkalosis diminishes the diuretic effect, and mercurials appear to have a separate inhibitory action at the potassium secretory site so that potassium depletion is nonexistent. Whereas furosemide and ethacrynic acid may be administered either orally or parenterally, mercurials are only administered parenterally. Side effects related to toxicity of the mercuric ion, which results in acute renal failure or nephrotic syndrome, appear to be related to injudicious use of the mercurial diuretics.

A new drug that has recently become available is bumetanide; it is a potent loop diuretic. Bumetanide may also have additional effects in the proximal tubule, but the action does not appear related to inhibition of carbonic anhydrase. As with the other loop diuretics, potassium excretion may be enhanced, with resulting hypokalemia.

In the distal convoluted tubule

Toward the end of the thick portion of the ascending limb of Henle's loop and toward the beginning of the distal tubule lies the cortical diluting segment. The diuretics that have an effect on this portion of the nephron are two of the benzothiadizide derivatives, chlorthalidone and metolazone. Chlorthalidone's actions approximate those of the thiazides. Metolazone's actions are also similar to the thiazides', but in addition metolazone appears to have an effect on the proximal tubule, thereby increasing its natriuretic effect. The action is again through inhibition of sodium and chloride transport. The thiazide diuretics have a corresponding modest carbonic anhydrase inhibitory effect with attendant excretion of bicarbonate, but the effects are variable according to each specific drug. The thiazides effect excretion of sodium and have some effect on arteriolar dilation. The natriuretic effect is self-limited with chronic administration; that is, after a few days of administration, provided that the sodium intake is relatively constant, the sodium balance is reestablished and no longer negative. The process is thought to result from stimulation by volume contraction on the proximal tubule to reabsorb sodium. The net result is a stabilized but lower extracellular fluid volume and body weight. With an increased amount of sodium presented to the distal potassium secretory sites, large amounts of potassium may be lost in the urine; this process is known as *kaliuresis*. The amount of kaliuresis occurring with these drugs is variable and appears to be related to dosage and duration of treatment. High doses appear to augment excretion of potassium, whereas in chronic use significant total body potassium has appeared uncommon. Attendant to thiazide use are (1) decreased glomerular filtration rate from a direct action on renal vasculature; (2) decreased uric acid excretion with resultant hyperuricemia; (3) decreased calcium excretion with resultant hypercalcemia; (4) hypomagnesemia through enhancement of magnesium excretion; (5) increased iodine and bromide excretion, which is indistinguishable from chloride excretion; and (6) hyponatremia, which is unrelated to volume contraction and mimics SIADH.

In the distal tubule and collecting duct

The secretory sites for potassium and hydrogen ion, as well as aldosterone activity, are located in the distal tubule. The diuretics that have the primary action within this section of the nephron are the "potassium-sparing" diuretics, such as spironolactone and triamterene. Both drugs block potassium secretion and to a lesser extent hydrogen ion secretion, with a resulting modest natriuresis. The method by which they block potassium secretion is different. Triamterene exhibits a direct action on tubular transport in the distal nephron independent of aldosterone. Sodium reabsorption is blocked with a resultant decrease in the transtubular electrical-potential difference, which is necessary for potassium secretion. With inhibited potassium secretion, potassium excretion is decreased. Spironolactone affects aldosterone and other mineralocorticoids through competitive inhibition. Aldosterone augments sodium and chlo-

ride reabsorption and increases potassium secretion through enhancement of the sodium-potassium exchange process. By inhibiting aldosterone, the net result is sodium excretion and conservation of potassium. Because the action of spironolactone is through competitive inhibition, the inhibition can be overridden by the presence of high levels of mineralocorticoids. In addition, because spironolactone's action is based on the presence of aldosterone, its diuretic effect is nonexistent in an adrenalectomized person.

Most sodium is absorbed in the proximal nephron, therefore suggesting that drugs affecting the distal portion of the nephron are not potent natriuretics. The efficacy of these drugs is predominantly in combination with other potent diuretics, partly for their added natriuresis but more importantly for their potassium-conserving capabilities, which prevent hypokalemia.

Osmotic diuretics

Osmotic diuretics operate in a manner quite dissimilar from the diuretics discussed so far. The function of osmotic diuretics is to promote water diuresis rather than sodium. Their action depends on concentrations of osmotically active particles in solution, which when elevated in urine produce an increased urine volume. When the glomerular filtration rate decreases, there is a corresponding, more complete reabsorption of particles, resulting in a large decrease in urine flow rate and solute excretion. Normally, the administration of a normal solute could restore renal output but is contingent on good renal hemodynamics. The natriuretics are ineffective in the presence of impaired renal hemodynamics, a decreased glomerular filtration rate, decreased urine flow, and solute excretion because the degree to which they inhibit reabsorption is insufficient to override the effects of a reduced filtered load. With these conditions the osmotic diuretics such as mannitol and urea can be useful.

Through osmosis, the osmotic diuretics attract water in the nephron to remain within the nephron. Because of the dilutional effect within the nephron, there is a possibility of a resulting increase in sodium, chloride, and potassium excretion, but this effect appears to be associated with the administration of large doses of osmotic diuretics.

Pediatric considerations

Some differences exist between adult and infant renal function, especially between adult and infant renal function during periods of stress, that need to be considered, particularly with diuretic therapy.

Differences in the urine-concentrating mechanism exist between adults and newborn infants. Newborn infants are unable to fully concentrate urine; the solute concentration is different partially because the infants are in an anabolic state, and they tend to excrete small amounts of urea. Urea is an important factor in the normal concentrating mechanism. As a newborn is given protein, more urea is formed, and the capacity to concentrate urine approaches that of an adult. The length of the loop of Henle, a factor in the ability to concentrate urine, increases with age.

Infants are capable of eliminating urine that is relatively sodium-free, and they can compensate for wide variations in salt intake under stress. But under salt-loading conditions, infants tend to retain excess sodium, with an increase in extracellular fluid volume and resulting mild edema formation. Contributing factors to this tendency are as follows:

1. The glomerular filtration rate is lower in infancy.
2. There appears to be preferential renal blood flow to the juxtamedullary nephrons, which may be sodium retaining, rather than to the outer cortex nephrons.
3. Compared to an adult, the newborn has increased concentrations of renin, angiotensin, and aldosterone, and the increased aldosterone concentrations relate to sodium reabsorption.

It is most important to evaluate children and their responses to diuretics at various ages because of the developmental changes in glomerular filtration rate, renal blood flow, and tubular processing of sodium chloride. Water and organic anions may affect the diuretic response at different ages.

Guidelines to diuretic use

In the diuretic selection process, certain guidelines should be considered and are as follows:

1. Initiation of diuretic therapy should begin with a medium-potency natriuretic drug, except in emergency situations.
2. With all but the potassium-sparing diuretics, kaliuresis and possible hypokalemia should be anticipated.
3. With a decreased glomerular filtration rate or renal blood flow, there is decreasing intratubular concentration of administered medication and diminished drug response. As renal function further diminishes, there is increased tubular sodium reabsorption inclusive of the proximal site, so that a decreasing amount of sodium is presented to the distal nephron and natriuresis diminishes. To interrupt the spiraling and diminishing effect, the dose of a single diuretic may be increased, or the diuretic may be changed or augmented with a drug having a more proximal site of action in the nephron.
4. Measurement of urine volume and weight are extremely important in monitoring drug response.
5. Nothing is gained by administering two drugs of the same type.
6. When the intravascular volume cannot be maintained because the rate of sodium loss from diuretics is so high, tachycardia, hypotension, and azotemia may result. Certain conditions, such as the nephrotic syndrome or hepatic cirrhosis, will by virtue of their pathology diminish intravascular oncotic pressure, causing fluid to leave the intravascular space and enter the

extravascular space. With a decreased intravascular volume, use of diuretics may result in hypotension and shock. A general rule for rate of diuresis is not to exceed 1 to 2 kg of weight loss/day. In cirrhotic patients with ascites and little or no edema, weight loss should not exceed 0.5 kg/day.

7. Diuretics are nephron site specific. Nephron sites unaffected by a diuretic tend to compensate at a level to counteract the diuretic effect, which may lead to metabolic complications. Many diuretic therapy complications arise from compensatory mechanisms in tubular segments unaffected by a diuretic.

8. Strategies for treating the refractory patient include the following:
   a) A response to previously ineffective diuretics may be realized by adding an inotropic agent, which increases cardiac output and renal blood flow.
   b) Long-acting nitrates or arterial vasodilators change cardiac preload and afterload, improving cardiac output. With administration of these drugs, the cardiac output may be increased sufficiently to realize a response from previously ineffective diuretics.
   c) The addition of low oral doses of metolazone in patients receiving high doses of loop diuretics may restore diuresis, suggesting a metolazone proximal site of action. Bumethanide, although predominantly a loop diuretic, appears to have a proximal tubule effect. Administration has been indicated in patients allergic or refractory to furosemide, and there are suggestions that effective responses may be realized.

Recognizing that drug dosage ceilings are available for specific diuretics, practitioners should tailor dosage of drugs according to specific individual response.

Dialytic therapy

Dialysis management is employed when kidneys fail to function at an adequate level or when toxic elements have been introduced into the body, posing a life-threatening situation. Reduction in kidney function may be chronic or of sudden onset. Regardless of the nature of the problem, there is a need to maintain fluid and electrolyte balance or to clear toxins from the body. Dialytic therapy uses principles of filtration, osmosis, and diffusion to remove these toxins. Fig. 5-18 provides a schematic illustration of dialysis.

Two basic forms of dialysis exist: hemodialysis and peritoneal dialysis. Remarkable advances in both forms continue to be made.

Hemodialysis

The basic purpose of hemodialysis is to correct and/or maintain fluid and electrolyte bal-

Fig. 5-18. Physiologic view of dialysis. Small particles are seen diffusing through "pores" from the blood to the extravascular milieu. Water molecules, as well as urea and creatinine, are easily removed from the blood because of their small molecular weights and steric configurations. Large particles such as cells and proteins are unable to leave the circulation.

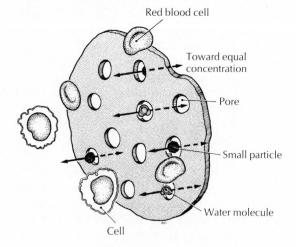

Red blood cell

Toward equal concentration

Pore

Small particle

Water molecule

Cell

ance and remove toxic materials. Hemodialysis has five basic functions:

1. To remove waste products of protein metabolism; desired when the creatinine is greater than 10 mg/dL and the BUN level rises over 100 ng/dL.
2. To remove excess fluid.
3. To correct electrolyte imbalance, primarily imbalances of potassium, sodium, chloride, magnesium, calcium, and phosphorus.
4. To correct acid-base balance.
5. To correct a situation in which ingestion of exogenous toxic substances has occurred.

Because the hemodialysis machine acts as a kidney, anything excreted by a kidney can normally be dialyzed in the procedure. Hemodialysis operates on the principles of diffusion and mass transfer, osmosis, and filtration. There are many variations of the hemodialysis mechanism with a wide range of complicated-appearing attachments designed for specific functions, such as pressure alarms and special solution infusers. Basically, however, the system is comprised of three major components: a blood compartment, a solution or dialysate compartment, and the semipermeable membrane that separates the two, allowing for water and solute transference. In hemodialysis, diffusion occurs between blood and dialysate, resulting in a solute level difference establishing a concentration gradient. Higher concentration gradients allow greater diffusion to occur. The passage and amount of solute moving across a semipermeable membrane at any one time is referred to as *mass transfer*. The rate at which mass transfer occurs may be varied or controlled. The solute concentration gradient is normally greatest at the beginning of dialysis; this is also when it is possible for the mass transfer rate to be greatest. Rate control can also be affected by the amount of dialysis membrane surface and the rate and flow pattern of blood and dialysate during dialysis. The flow pattern approximates normal kidney function, establishing an osmotic gradient and countercurrent mechanism.

Osmosis occurs through the establishment of an osmotic gradient occurring between blood and the dialysate. The movement of water from blood will flow toward the higher-concentrated dialysate solution.

The transmembrane pressure created between negative pressure on the dialysate side and positive pressure on the blood side is the hydrostatic pressure difference, which is responsible for the filtration mechanism and is the predominant mechanism for removal of fluid from blood during hemodialysis.

For hemodialysis to occur, an access to the patient's vascular system must first be established. If a patient requires hemodialysis before establishment of a hopefully permanent access site, a temporary access site may be instituted via percutaneous cannulation. For many years, quick access was established through insertion of Shaldon catheters into the large femoral or subclavian vessels. Preferably, two sites were used, one of them allowing blood flow to the machine and the other blood flow away from the machine. Single access sites may be used, alternating in-and-out blood flow cycles, but this technique has not been as efficient as the two-site technique. More recently, refinement and progress have been made in the use of a double lumen cannula and single access site, in conjunction with development of a special machine designed for acute use.

Permanent access sites may be established for chronic hemodialysis use. There are two basic types of permanent access sites: the arteriovenous (AV) fistula (Fig. 5-19) and the arteriovenous (AV) shunt (Fig. 5-20). In creating an AV fistula a vein and artery are anastomosed, either side to side or end to end, so that increased blood flow dilates the vessels, creating access to large-bore needles. In preparing the patient for dialysis, a local anesthetic is used and large needles are inserted. The needle entrance sites require rotation within the area each time to prevent complications. Besides the complications that may develop from not rotating sites, venipuncture with large-bore needles for each dialysis is psychologically unpleasant. Recently, work has been done on a vascular access device that resembles a button on the patient's skin. This device is implanted into a graft between artery and vein; without needles, the hemodialysis line, so to speak, "plugs into" the device. With the more recently introduced dual-lumen device, the process is as efficient as and similar to the two-needle dialysis process.

The life expectancy of an AV fistula is variable, and the fistula is subject to many different sources of insult. Patients may acquire a systemic infection and, through the infectious process, clot off their access site. It is not uncommon to go through a variety of locations in successvie attempts to create and maintain an access site. Further attempts to create an AV fistula may include vein grafting. Vein grafting may include attempts to use the patient's own saphenous vein, to use bovine vessels, or even more recently to graft with the human umbilical cord.

Another mechanism for providing an access site is through an AV shunt. With this method, an appliance is inserted between vein and artery and lies outside the skin. The outside portion of the appliance is separated for dialysis and "plugged" into the dialysis machine. With an apparatus lying outside the skin, there are attendant complications such as infection and accidental separation. Although shunt devices are designed to minimize clotting, the very presence of a foreign body can increase its incidence; therefore AV fistulas are the preferred method of access site. The AV shunt does allow for quick, easy access and may utilize sites that are unsuitable for fistulas.

One of the major obstacles to pediatric hemodialysis is access site. Because of vessel immaturity, it is very difficult to locate vessels of sufficient size for children to undergo hemodialysis. It has also been hypothesized that the hemodynamic impact of hemodialysis is far greater on children than is the impact of the more preferred and gentler pediatric alternative, peritoneal dialysis.

Dialyzers. Dialyzers fall into three basic but different types of categories: coil, parallel plate, and hollow-fiber. Each category has attendant advantages and disadvantages. The criteria for type selection are predicated on:

1. Efficiency in solute clearance.
2. Degree and predictability of ultrafiltration that is possible.
3. Amount of extracorporeal blood volume caught up in machine, and lines and retrieval capability.
4. Degree to which membrane rupture is possible.
5. Degree of incidence in blood path leakage.
6. Potential for reuse.
7. Amount of contingent equipment necessary.
8. Amount of heparinization necessary.

How each type lies within a specific machine and the number and degree of modifications and attachments used will vary the advantages and disadvantages associated with any one of the basic designs. The choice of dialyzer may also be influenced by individual preference and/or setting.

The coil dialyzer is a plastic core surrounded

Fig. 5-19. Arteriovenous (AV) fistula.

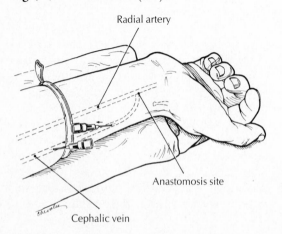

Radial artery

Anastomosis site

Cephalic vein

by a spiral cuprophane or cellophane membrane sheet supported by mesh screening. A sterile coil sits in a tank, which holds the coil in the dialysate. Blood lines from the coil allow blood to flow from the patient and through the coil, with the dialysate being pumped between coil layers on both sides of the blood flow; then the blood is returned to the patient. High rates of ultrafiltration may be made possible through blood compartment pressure adjustment.

The parallel plate dialyzer is comprised of alternating layers of cuprophane membranous sheets supported by rigid or semirigid plates. Additional layers increase the dialyzing surface area. Blood flows between the membranes while the dialysate flows, in either the same or the opposite direction as the blood, between the outer side of the membrane and the supporting plate. Ultrafiltration is controlled by adjusting dialysate compartment pressure or venous flow resistance, both of which are negative pressure adjustments.

The hollow-fiber dialyzer is comprised of thousands of tiny semipermeable membranous tubes bundled together in a plastic cylinder. A pump forces blood through the tiny tubes as dialysate is pumped countercurrently on the opposite side of the membranes through the closed system. Ultrafiltration is controlled through negative pressure adjustment.

The dialysate or bath solution is comprised of 34 parts of water to 1 part of dialysis concentrate. The dialysis concentrate contains chemically pure solutes. Along with water, the composition of the bath includes sodium, potassium, chloride, calcium, magnesium, glucose, and either sodium acetate or bicarbonate. Both sodium acetate and bicarbonate have been used as the dialysate base buffer to attain normal blood pH. Although acetate baths are easier to use, requiring no mixing, they have been associated with hypotension and decreased stroke volume. The trend appears to be a return to bicarbonate baths, which are more compatible with newer machines that are currently able to mix the appropriate proportions. The water used in the

bath must meet established standards, necessitating a purification system because water constituents vary according to location. The purification system must be able to remove high inorganic salt concentrations, suspended solids, organic impurities, microorganisms, dissolved gases, and industrial-product or agricultural-waste trace elements. A continuous pressure of water delivered at 40 pounds/sq in will also be necessary. Once the right proportion of water to dialysis concentrate is achieved, the solution approximates that of normal plasma. Tailoring the electrolyte concentrations, most frequently potassium and calcium, within an individual bath solution will affect the diffusion of those specific particles from the blood. In addition, the dialysate will need to be warmed to prevent blood cooling.

Batch, proportioning, and regenerative systems refer to the actual process of bath mixing, whether automatic or manual and whether recyclable or not. Each system has attendant advantages and disadvantages having to do with ease, speed, expense, complicated equipment, portability, space requirements, and human error. Hemodialysis is a relatively quick technique associated with rapid hemodynamic changes and technical complications and therefore is not suited for all people. An alternative to hemodialysis, now receiving greater prominence and promising better effects than in the past, is peritoneal dialysis.

Fig. 5-20. Arteriovenous (AV) shunt.

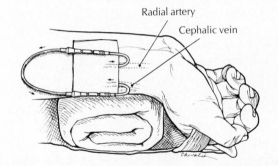

Radial artery

Cephalic vein

Peritoneal dialysis

Peritoneal dialysis operates on the principles of diffusion and osmosis, using the peritoneum as a membrane for filtering out toxic wastes and fluid from the body. The process is passive, requiring no cell energy expenditure. The principles have been discussed earlier in this unit. Solvent moving across the membrane tends to pull solute with it, and this becomes more pronounced as solvent movement increases. The result is equalization of solutes and solvents on both sides of the peritoneal membrane. As equalization occurs, solutes and solvents may be reabsorbed into the bloodstream; it is then necessary to introduce fresh dialysis solutions to achieve the greatest effect.

To prepare for peritoneal dialysis, an entry into the peritoneum must be established. The advent of the Tenckhoff catheter has eliminated the need for repeated needle punctures into the abdominal cavity. The Tenckhoff catheter may be left in the abdomen for long-term chronic use. The physician, using aseptic technique, inserts the catheter through the layers of the peritoneal cavity and tunnels the end to embed along one side of the lower pelvic region. The underlying principles for any peritoneal dialysis program are essentially the same. A dialysate solution is infused and allowed to dwell; as a result, equilibration of solutes and solvents occurs, after which the dialysate solution is allowed to run off or out of the patient. Commercial dialysate solutions are available for peritoneal dialysis and are composed of various electrolytes and dextrose. Dextrose is used to promote osmotic pressure in the removal of fluid. The 1.5% dextrose concentrated solution promotes very little fluid removal, but solutions with greater than 1.5% dextrose increase osmotic pressure and therefore result in fluid removal. Patients who have normal or low potassium levels may need to have extra potassium added to the dialysate to prevent hypokalemia. Heparin may be added to prevent fibrin formation around the catheter. Routine prophylactic addition of antibiotics is not recommended because doing so could mask the devel-

opment of an infectious process. In addition, in chronic ambulatory peritoneal dialysis, most patients first present with Gram-positive infections; repeated infections are Gram-negative, however.

Variations in time frames and equipment in peritoneal dialysis occur according to the type of program a patient is undergoing and his particular fluid and electrolyte balance needs.

Peritoneal dialysis programs are generally divided into two different types: *intermittent* and *continuous*.

Intermittent peritoneal dialysis may be either manual or automated. The manual method provides gentle and quick dialysis for a patient in acute need of dialysis, particularly when only simple equipment may be available. Manual intermittent peritoneal dialysis may be initiated quickly, although the process may proceed over several hours. A standard commercial dialysate solution is infused into the peritoneal cavity by means of gravity over a period of a few minutes. Before infusion, other elements may be added, and the solution is warmed to body temperature. The solution is then allowed to dwell in the cavity over a period of approximately 30 minutes. After the dwell time, the solution is allowed to drain out of the cavity, again by means of gravity. One cycle normally takes 1 hour, being followed with another cycle of exchange. The cycles of exchange are continuous up to the number of cycles or hours prescribed and may go on for 48 hours before being discontinued. The dialysis process resumes once waste products start accumulating again.

Two basic automated methods of intermittent peritoneal dialysis exist. One type of automated equipment uses standard commercial dialysate solution fed through a cycling device, which operates by gravity. The cycling device includes a timer to determine installation, dwell, and drain times. A heating device is also incorporated to bring the dialysate to body temperature before infusion. The other type of automated equipment uses proportioning pumps to mix the appropriate ratio of dialysate concentration to sterile deionized water, which the machine processes itself. The process again occurs by means of gravity, but a timing device regulates the time frame for installation, dwelling, and draining.

Intermittent manual peritoneal dialysis may be implemented for chronic use, but the automated forms are considered more efficient and certainly more convenient.

The use of continuous ambulatory peritoneal dialysis has risen in recent years and shows promise in efficiency and convenience for the patient. Dialysis occurs via infusion of 500 to 2000 ml of dialysate, by means of gravity, over approximately 10 minutes. The solution is then allowed to dwell for 4 to 8 hours. During the first 160 minutes of dwell time, the greatest exchange of solutes and solvent occurs and will continue for up to 8 hours, followed by a leveling-off effect. At the end of the dwell time, the dialysate is drained into the bag used for infusion of dialysate. Drainage occurs by means of gravity for over 25 to 30 minutes. At the end of drainage, the dialysate drainage bag is removed and a new one attached. Although the bag exchange system is considered relatively simple and safe, it has inherent risk for development of peritonitis. Patients normally are placed on an exchange program using 3 to 5 bags/day, with an overnight dwell. Patients on a continuous peritoneal dialysis program are unhampered by machines and are relatively unencumbered when carrying out their activities of daily living.

Dietary management

Dietary management is twofold. It consists of attempting to control accumulation of nitrogen metabolism end products by minimizing protein, electrolyte, and fluid intake, while at the same time attempting to maintain nutrition through replacement of protein, carbohydrates, and fats as they are metabolized. There is no single, overall diet plan for patients with renal failure or insufficiency; rather, a diet must be tailored according to the amount of renal impairment of patients, their fluid and electrolyte needs, each patient's unique physiologic processing of metabolites, and any concomitant dialysis plan. Dietary planning is further complicated for children with renal impairment because attempts must be made, in designing a diet, to account for their growth and developmental needs. It is not so much the renal impairment but the balance of fluids and electrolytes that is the critical determinant for approximating normal growth in the pediatric patient.

Nutritional therapy for renally impaired patients is predicated on the following goals:

1. Retaining remaining renal function.
2. Maintaining a positive nitrogen balance.
3. Maintaining safe physiologic parameters, such as blood pressure, that are necessarily related to the consequences of nutritional deficiencies and overloads. The impact of nutritional deficiencies and overloads on physiologic parameters is explained earlier in this unit.
4. Promoting a sense of general well-being in the patient, which also relates to nutritional deficiencies and overloads. The diet will deviate considerably from the patient's original eating habits and style, which will have a profound effect on his psychosocial status and attendant compliance. The more the diet can be adjusted to the patient and his eating preferences, the better the patient will feel overall.

Dietary management basically consists of a reduction in protein, potassium, sodium, and fluid intake, which are the major components that the kidney, when not functioning optimally, is inefficient in eliminating. A low-protein diet allows the caloric intake to be high enough to maintain a nitrogen balance, thereby preventing a breakdown of endogenous protein with resultant muscle wasting. As the glomerular filtration rate, in decreasing amounts, approaches 3 ml/min, the protein, potassium, sodium, and fluid restrictions in the diet may be rather severe. When dialysis management is initiated, the dietary restrictions are modified, and some increases in the patient's well-being may be realized. Diet control is still an important aspect of management even when a patient is receiving dialysis at the same time as the dietary changes; this is because the patient still accumulates metabolic end products between dialysis episodes.

Protein

With an accompanying hemodialysis program, dietary protein intake is often restricted to 60 to 80 g/day. With renal insufficiency, it is not uncommon for a patient's sodium intake to be restricted to 20 to 40 g/day. Too much protein is evidenced by nausea, diarrhea, capillary bleeding, and other signs of accumulated urea. With insufficient protein intake, endogenous protein from muscle tissue may be broken down to supply the essential amino acids necessary for enzyme synthesis. The patient then experiences protein depletion, with symptoms of increased urea, nausea, and weight loss.

The dietary management of a patient on intermittent peritoneal dialysis which can be seen in the critical care setting, is similar to dietary management of the patient on a hemodialysis program.

With continuous ambulatory peritoneal dialysis, patients lose a significantly large amount of protein, from 6 to 12 g/day. Patients will need a protein intake of approximately 1.5 g/kg of body weight/day.

High-quality protein foods, such as whole eggs and red meat, more adequately achieve the goal of meeting a positive nitrogen balance. When low-quality protein is used, more is needed to achieve the positive balance.

In chronic renal failure the plasma concentration of essential amino acids decreases, and the nonessentials are normal or increased. The low essentials of tyrosine, serine, citrulline, and methylhistidine appear to be related to the chronic renal failure process and uremia rather than to nutritional status.

With renal insufficiency, it is not uncommon for a patient to be on sodium restrictions before and during a concomitant dialysis program. The restrictions may be mild or severe and will depend on the patient and etiology of renal impairment. Some renal pathologies are associated with salt wasting, which may necessitate sodium supplementation, but more often than not patients will need to be restricted in sodium intake, which reduces urinary sodium excretion and preserves sodium balance. Frequently children and infants are restricted to 50 mg of sodium, or 2 mEq/kg of body weight/day, whereas adults and adolescents are restricted to around 2 g, or 90 mEq/day.

Potassium is often restricted to approximately 1500 mg/day; again, restrictions depend on individual renal response. Serum potassium levels that are too high or too low have several severe implications, but a high serum potassium level is not necessarily an indicator of dietary indiscretion. If the patient does not have sufficient caloric intake, a breakdown in body tissue may ensue, resulting in potassium movement from the intracellular to the extracellular areas.

Fluid restriction is also geared to the individual. Physiologically, an individual will lose 600 ml in fluid/day from nonrenal routes, that is, respirations, perspiration, and feces. Often an anephric patient will be allowed at least 600 mL in fluid/day to account for these insensible losses. Accommodations to the 600 mL limit may need to be made for patients experiencing increases in insensible losses, such as increased perspiration in the summertime with no air conditioning.

Patients with some remaining renal function may be allowed, in addition to the 600 mL, the equivalent of whatever amount of fluid is passed as urine per day.

Sufficient attention needs to be directed toward maintaining sufficient energy intake. An inadequate intake may lead to protein catabolism, with a resultant nitrogen imbalance and an accumulation of nitrogen waste products. Energy intake in the form of carbohydrate supplements without due consideration of other energy production forms may increase the incidence of hypertriglyceridemia for these patients. Hypertriglyceridemia, with or without hypercholesterolemia, has been frequently noted in renal failure patients, along with an increased incidence of arteriosclerotic heart disease. Both lipoprotein lipase activity and triglyceride clearance are decreased. The elevated triglyceride levels are related to plasma insulin levels and the supplemental carbohydrate. Unsaturated fats may be used for energy needs; they can be effective in lowering plasma triglyceride levels. An accompanying exercise program may also effect a reduction in plasma insulin levels, improve glucose clearance, and decrease plasma triglyceride levels, as well as improve blood pressure control and the patient's sense of well-being. Adequate caloric intake improves the possibility of achievement of a positive nitrogen balance.

Caution should be exercised in increasing or supplementing caloric intake in patients whose energy intake is presently sufficient. The additional calories may increase the incidence of hypertriglyceridemia and obesity. Obesity can be especially problematic for patients on peritoneal dialysis, who may in addition absorb glucose from the dialysate.

Decreased renal function also leads to calcium and phosphorus imbalances. A low calcium level in chronic renal failure results from anorexia and dairy-product diet restrictions. Dairy products are restricted because of their phosphorus and protein content and also because many of them contribute to fluid intake, which is also restricted. In addition, calcium absorption in the gastrointestinal tract is impeded by a decreased renal cortex production of 1, 25-dihydroxycholecalciferol, which is necessary for gastrointestinal calcium transport (box at right).

As the body attempts to return calcium and phosphorus levels to normal, the compensatory mechanisms lead to bone demineralization and secondary hyperparathyroidism. Therefore administration of phosphate-binding gels is of paramount importance in controlling parathyroid hormone (PTH) secretion.

Phosphate-binding gels may limit gastric phosphate absorption, but their use may result in development of taste fatigue and subsequent noncompliance.

DECREASED RENAL FUNCTION

↓ Renal function →↓ Renal phosphate excretion
With ↑ plasma
phosphorus
↓
↓ Plasma calcium
↓
Stimulates parathyroid
↑ Parathyroid hormone
secreted
↓
↑ Renal calcium reabsorption ↑ Calcium and
phosphorus
↓ Renal phosphate reabsorption Reabsorption
from bone

Patients who are on nonprotein, restricted diets and acquire attendant hyperphosphatemia may develop metastatic calcification through increased calcium-phosphate solubility. As calcification metastasizes through the remaining nephrons of an already compromised kidney, there is further renal function deterioration. Plasma calcium levels are low, and renal failure patients may require calcium supplements. However, before calcium supplements are initiated, the phosphorus levels need to be returned to normal to prevent calcification. Prevention efforts should begin when kidney function, that is, GFR, has dropped no lower than 50% of normal.

The intake of water-soluble vitamins is problematic because (1) foods higher in water-soluble vitamins are also high in potassium, and if the potassium is restricted, the vitamin intake will be inadequate; and (2) water-soluble vitamins will be dialyzed off in patients undergoing hemodialysis.

Plasma levels of fat-soluble vitamins have not been noted to be reduced except for vitamin D, which is somewhat associated with calcium. A good multivitamin along with a folic acid supplement will be necessary to maintain normal levels in the renally compromised patient.

When enteral intake of nutrients is curtailed because of other pathologic states existing within a patient, nutrients may be provided parenterally. Total parenteral nutrition will need to incorporate guidelines similar to those for enteral nutrition. Consideration will need to be given to sodium, potassium, amino acid, and fluid intake. Dramatic changes in recent years have occurred, and continue to occur, in the degree of sophistication of standardized TPN solutions available. TPN solutions are available for the renally impaired patient that incorporate less nonessential amino acids and less fluid volume than other solutions. However, the designation of essential nonessential amino acids has been changing, and there has been some evidence of success in nutritional achievement in renal failure patients using standardized nonrenal TPN solutions. Attention to lipid emulsion and trace metal supplements is just as important in the renal failure patient as in those patients without renal compromise.

Renal failure, especially if congenital, retards the growth process by virtue of the physiologic disease process. Special attention needs to be directed toward the first 2 years of life, when 30% of growth occurs. When the glomerular filtration rate drops below 50% of normal, growth velocity decreases. Growth failure occurs when glomerular filtration rate drops below 25% of normal. The decrease in growth and weight gain is related to the renal failure metabolic abnormality, as well as dietary intake. The dietary restrictions and supplements necessary for the pediatric renal-failure patient parallel those of an adult. But in relationship to meeting the extra growth considerations of a child, close monitoring will be important. Pediatric growth and nutrition parameters to be monitored, and their frequency, include:

Height: 2 times a year

Weight: each visit

Skinfold thickness and midarm circumference: each visit

Radiographs of left hand, wrist, and knee: 2 times a year

Dietary intake analysis: once a month

Plasma levels of glucose, triglycerides, cholesterol, albumin, and transferrin: on a regular basis

With some modification, these parameters should be paralleled for the adult when evaluating adult nutritional status.

REFERENCES

1. Aach, R.D.: Abdominal pain. In Blacklow, R.S.: MacBryde's signs and symptoms applied pathologic physiology and clinical interpretation, ed. 6, Philadelphia, 1983, J.B. Lippincott Co.

2. Adler, S., Fraley, D.S.: Acid-base regulation: cellular and whole body. In Arieff, A.I., and DeFronzo, R.A.: Fluid, electrolyte, and acid-base disorders, New York, 1985, Churchill Livingstone.

3. Alexander, E.A.: Oliguria and anuria. In Massry, S.G., and Glassock, R.J.: Textbook of nephrology, Baltimore, 1983, Williams and Wilkins.

4. Alvis, R., Geheb, M., et al.: Hypo- and hyperosmolar states: diagnostic approaches. In Arieff, A.I., and DeFronzo, R.A.: Fluid, electrolyte, and acid-base disorders, New York, 1985, Churchill Livingstone.

5. Arey, L.B.: Developmental anatomy: a textbook and laboratory manual of embryology, ed. 7, Philadelphia, 1974, W.B. Saunders Co.

6. Bailie, M.D., Linshaw, M.A., et al.: Diuretic pharmacology in infants and children, Pediatric Clinics of North America 28(1):217, 1981.

7. Beck, L.H.: Edema states and the use of diuretics, Medical Clinics of North America 65(2):291, 1982.

8. Berger, B.E., and Warnock, D.G.: Sites of action and clinical uses of diuretics. In Arieff, A.I., and DeFronzo, R.A.: Fluid, electrolyte, and acid-base disorders, New York, 1985, Churchill Livingstone.

9. Brenner, R.J., et al.: Incidence of radiographically evident bone disease, nephrocalcinosis and nephrolithiasis in various types of renal tubular acidosis, New England Journal of Medicine 307:217, 1982.

10. Brundage, D.J.: Nursing management of renal problems, St. Louis, 1976, The C.V. Mosby Co.

11. Bruskewitz, R.: Urinary tract signs and symptoms. In Franklin, S.S.: Practical nephrology, New York, 1981, John Wiley & Sons.

12. Burrell, Z.L., and Burrell, L.O.: Critical care, St. Louis, 1977, The C.V. Mosby Co.

13. Carroll, H.J., and Oh, M.S.: Water, electrolyte, and acid-base metabolism, diagnosis and management, Philadelphia, 1978, J.B. Lippincott Co.

14. Ceccarelli, C.M.: Hemodialysis therapy for the patient with chronic renal failure, Nursing Clinics of North America 16(3):531, 1981.

15. Conger, J.D., and Anderson, R.J.: Acute renal failure including cortical necrosis. In Massry, S.G., and Glassock, R.J.: Textbook of nephrology, Baltimore, 1983, Williams and Wilkins.

16. Cunningham, J., et al: Chronic acidosis with metabolic bone disease, American Journal of Medicine **73**:199, 1982.

17. Danovitch, G.M., Bourgoignie, J.J., et al: Reversibility of the "salt-losing" tendency of chronic renal failure, New England Journal of Medicine **296**:14, 1977.

18. DeFronzo, R.A., and Thier, S.O.: Fluid and electrolyte disturbances: hypo- and hyperkalemia. In Martinez-Maldonado, M.: Handbook of renal therapeutics, New York, 1983, Plenum Book Co.

19. DeFronzo, R.A., and Thier, S.O.: Fluid and electrolyte disturbances: hypo- and hypernatremia. In Martinez-Maldonado, M.: Handbook of renal therapeutics, New York, 1983, Plenum Book Co.

20. Dubois, G., and Arieff, A.I.: Clinical manifestations of electrolyte disorders. In Arieff, A.I., and DeFronzo, R.A.: Fluid, electrolyte, and acid-base disorders, New York, 1985, Churchill Livingstone.

21. Edelman, I.S., and Leibman, J.: Anatomy of body water and electrolytes, American Journal of Medicine **27**:256, 1959.

22. Farber, M.O., et al: Abnormalities of sodium and H_2O handling in chronic obstructive lung disease, Archives of Internal Medicine **142**:1236, 1982.

23. Fencl, V., Vale, J.R., et al.: Respiration and cerebral blood flow in acidosis and alkalosis in humans, Journal of Applied Physiology **27**:67, 1969.

24. Fine, L.G., et al: Functional profile of the isolated uremic nephron: impaired water permeability and adenylate cyclase responsiveness of the cortical collecting tubule to vasopressin, Journal of Clinical Investigation **61**:1519, 1978.

25. Flamenbaum, W., and Hamburger, R.J.: Nephrology: an approach to the patient with renal disease, Philadelphia, 1982, J.B. Lippincott.

26. Fulop, M., Tannenbaum, H., et al: Ketotic hyperosmolar coma, Lancet **2**:635, 1973.

27. Galligan, E.D., and Trebbin, W.M.: Intensified ambulatory chronic peritoneal dialysis, a case report, Contemporary Dialysis **4**(3):13, 1983.

28. Gerst, P., Fleming, W., et al: A quantitative evaluation of the effects of acidosis and alkalosis upon the ventricular fibrillation threshold, Surgery **59**:1050, 1966.

29. Giebish, G.E., Berger, L., et al.: The extrarenal response to acute acid-base disturbances of respiratory origin, Journal of Clinical Investigation **34**:231, 1955.

30. Glassock, R.J.: Hematuria and pigmenturia. In Massry, S.G., and Glassock, R.J.: Textbook of nephrology, Baltimore, 1983, Williams and Wilkins.

31. Goldberger, E.: A primer of water, electrolyte and acid-base syndromes, Philadelphia, 1980, Lea & Febiger.

32. Gorden, P., Sherman, B.M., et al: Glucose intolerance with hypokalemia: an increased proportion of circulating proinsulin-like component, Journal of Clinical Endocrinology and Metabolism **34**:235, 1972.

33. Guyton, A.C.: Textbook of medical physiology, ed. 6, Philadelphia, 1984, W.B. Saunders Co.

34. Holland, O.B., Nixon, J.V., et al: Diuretic-induced ventricular ectopic activity, American Journal of Medicine **70**:762, 1982.

35. Holliday, S.: Chronic ambulatory peritoneal dialysis. Presented at the "Get the Inside Line" seminar sponsored by the Indiana Association for Practitioners in Infection Control, Aug. 4, 1982.

36. Hussey, J.L.: Conduit placement for hemodialysis experience with the human umbilical cord, Contemporary Dialysis **4**(2):24, 1983.

37. Kilburn, K.: Neurologic manifestations of respiratory failure, Archives of Internal Medicine **116**:409, 1965.

38. Kleeman, C.R., Adams, D.A., et al: An evaluation of maximal water diuresis in chronic renal disease. I. Normal solute intake, Journal of Laboratory and Clinical Medicine **58**:169, 1961.

39. Knochel, J.P.: Fluid and electrolyte disturbances: treatment of hypophosphatemia and phosphate depletion. In Martinez-Maldonado, M.: Handbook of renal therapeutics, New York, 1983, Plenum Book Co.

40. Kreye, V.A.W., and Ziegler, F.W.: Anions and vascular smooth muscle function, Advances in Microcirculation **11**:114, 1982.

41. Lassiter, W.E., and Gottschalk, C.W.: Volume and composition of the body fluids. In Mountcastle, V.B.: Medical physiology, ed. 14, St. Louis, 1980, The C.V. Mosby Co.

42. Layzer, R.B.: Periodic paralysis and the sodium-potassium pump, Annals of Neurology **11**:547, 1982.

43. Luke, R.G.: Effect of adrenalectomy on the renal response to chloride depletion in the rat, Journal of Clinical Investigation **54**:1329, 1974.

44. Mabbry, S.G., and Glassock, R.J.: Textbook of nephrotology, Baltimore, 1983, Williams and Wilkins.

45. Martinez-Maldonado, M.: Handbook of renal theapeutics, New York, 1983, Plenum Medical Book Co.

46. Martinez-Maldonado, M., and Garcia, A.: Fluid and electrolyte disturbances: Hypo- and Hypercalcemia. In Martinez-Maldonado, M.: Handbook of renal therapeutics, New York, 1983, Plenum Medical Book Co.

47. Martinez-Maldonado, M., and Garcia, A.: Fluid and electrolyte disturbances: Hypo- and hypermagnesemia. In Martinez-Maldonado, M.: Handbook of renal therapeutics, New York, 1983, Plenum Medical Book Co.

48. Marvin, J.: Acute care of the burn patient, Critical Care Quarterly **1**(3):25, 1978.

49. McSherry, E.: Renal tubular acidosis in childhood, Kidney International **20**:799, 1981.

50. Methany, N.M., and Snively, W.D.: Nurses' handbook of fluid balance, ed. 3, Philadelphia, 1979, J.B. Lippincott Co.

51. Meyers, F.H., Jawetz, E., et al: Review of medical pharmacology, Los Altos, CA, 1980, Lange Medical Publications.

52. Miller, T.R., et al: Urinary diagnostic indices in acute renal failure: a prospective study, Annals of Internal Medicine 89:47, 1978.

53. Mudge, G.H.: Drugs affecting renal function and electrolyte metabolism. In Goodman, L.S., and Gilman, A., editors: The pharmacological basis of therapeutics, New York, 1975, MacMillan Publishing Co., Inc.

54. Neff, T.A., and Petty, T.L.: Tolerance and survival in severe chronic hypercapnia, Archives of Internal Medicine 129:591, 1972.

55. Nissenson, A.R., Higgins, R., et al: No-needle hemodialysis biocarbon vascular access device, Contemporary Dialysis 2(10):39, 1981.

56. Oh, M.S., and Carroll, H.J.: Regulation of extra- and intracellular fluid composition and content. In Arieff, A.I., and DeFronzo, R.A.: Fluid, electrolyte, and acid-base disorders, New York, 1985, Churchill Livingstone.

57. Pascoe, D.J., and Grossman, ,M., editors: Quick reference to pediatric emergencies, Philadelphia, 1973, J.B. Lippincott Co.

58. Pitts, R.F.: The physiological basis of diuretic therapy, Springfield, IL, 1959, Charles C. Thomas, Publisher.

59. Pitts, R.F.: Physiology of the kidney and body fluids, ed. 3, Chicago, 1974, Year Book Medical Publishers, Inc.

60. Posner, J., and Plum, F.: Spinal-fluid pH and neurologic symptoms in systemic acidosis, New England Journal of Medicine 277:605, 1976.

61. Posner, J.A., Swanson, A.G., et al.: Acid-base balance in cerebrospinal fluid, Archives of Neurology 12:479, 1965.

62. Potter, D.E., and Greifer, I.: Statural growth of children with renal disease, Kidney International 14:334, 1978.

63. Raymond, K.H., Reineck, H.J., et al.: Sodium metabolism and maintenance of extracellular fluid volume. In Arieff, A.I., and DeFronzo, R.A.: Fluid, electrolyte, and acid-base disorders, New York, 1985, Churchill Livingstone.

64. Reed, G.M., and Sheppard, V.F.: Regulation of fluid and electrolyte balance: a programmed instruction in physiology for nurses, Philadelphia, 1971, W.B. Saunders Co.

65. Rose, B.D.: Clinical physiology of acid-base and electrolyte disorders, New York, 1984, McGraw-Hill Book Co.

66. Schrier, R.W., and deTorrente, A.: Polyuria and nocturia. In Massry, S.G., and Glassock, R.J.: Textbook of nephrology, Baltimore, 1983, Williams & Wilkins.

67. Schwartz, A.B., and Lyons, H., editors: Acid-base and electrolyte balance, normal regulation and clinical disorders, New York, 1977, Grune & Stratton.

68. Sherman, R.A., and Eisinger, R.P.: The use (and misuse) of urinary sodium and chloride measurements, Journal of the American Medical Association 247:3121, 1982.

69. Siegel, N.J., and Lattanzi, W.E.: Fluid and electrolyte therapy in children. In Arieff, A.I., and DeFronzo, R.A.: Fluid, electrolyte, and acid-base disorders, New York, 1985, Churchill Livingstone.

70. Skelton, H.: Storage of water by various tissues of the body, Archives of Internal Medicine 40:152, 1927.

71. Skorecki, K.L., and Brenner, B.M.: Edema forming states: congestive heart failure, liver disease and nephrotic syndrome. In Arieff, A.I., and DeFronzo, R.A.: Fluid, electrolyte, and acid-base disorders, New York, 1985, Churchill Livingstone.

72. Sorrels, A.J.: Peritoneal dialysis: a rediscovery, Nursing Clinics of North America 6(3):515, 1981.

73. Surawicz, B.: Relationship between electrocardiogram and electrolytes, American Heart Journal 73:814, 1967.

74. Szwed, J.: Fluids, electrolytes & acid-base, Indianapolis, IN, 1981, Indiana University School of Medicine.

75. Vaughn, V.C., and McKay, R.J.: Nelson's textbook of pediatrics, ed. 10, Philadelphia, 1975, W.B. Saunders Co.

76. Wassner, S.J.: The role of nutrition in the care of children with renal insufficiency, The Pediatric Clinics of North America, 29(4):973, 1982.

77. Wildenthal, K., Mierzwiak, D.S., et al.: Effects of acute lactic acidosis on left ventricular performance, American Journal of Physiology 214:1352, 1968.

78. Zschoche, D.A.: Mosby's comprehensive review of critical care, ed. 3, St. Louis, 1986, The C.V. Mosby Co.

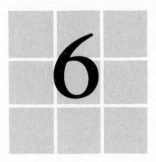

6 Alimentation

MARY ROPKA

Gastrointestinal diseases are the cause of major morbidity and mortality in all age groups and populations. Gastroenteritis, ulcer disease, gallstones, inflammatory bowel disease, and intestinal cancer are common diseases that take a significant toll.

The last several years have brought great advances in both diagnostic and therapeutic approaches to gastrointestinal disease. Fiberoptic endoscopy is replacing barium techniques in many areas. Endoscopy has a clearly superior diagnostic accuracy, although these procedures are more costly and have slightly higher complication rates. A variety of therapeutic endoscopic techniques are now widely applied. These include endoscopic sclerosis of esophageal varices, sphincterotomy and gallstone extraction, electrocautery of GI bleeding, laser coagulation of GI bleeding, laser vaporization of tumors, and colonoscopic polypectomy. These therapeutic techniques have decreased the need for surgery in many settings and decreased patient morbidity and mortality. Numerous advances have occurred in the area of liver and biliary tract disease. Oral agents for gallstone dissolution are now available; however, their efficacy is somewhat limited. Endoscopic methods for gallstone extraction were mentioned earlier in this paragraph. A wide variety of hepatitis antigens and

antibodies have now been identified. An effective vaccine is now available for hepatitis B; hyperimmune serum globulin is also available. Liver transplant is clearly more successful, especially with the availability of cyclosporin A for immunosuppression.

Peptic ulcer therapy has undergone a great change with the availability of H_2-type antihistamines. Cimetidine has become the most widely prescribed drug in the world. Second and third generation H_2 blockers are now available or in testing. Other effective ulcer therapeutic agents such as cytoprotective drugs are also available.

The ongoing developments in gastroenterologic medicine and nursing make the present an exciting time for involvement.

EMBRYOLOGY

The gut and its derivatives develop from the three basic divisions of the embryological digestive system—the foregut, midgut, and hindgut—which are formed by the yolk sac endoderm. The endoderm of the embryo gives rise to the epithelial cells and glands, while the encasing mesoderm gives rise to connective tissue, muscle, and visceral and parietal peritoneum portions of the gut. Cephalocaudal and lateral folding of the embryo results in the endoderm-lined cavity being partially incorporated into the embryo to form the primitive gut.

The foregut lies caudal to the tracheo-bronchial diverticulum and extends caudally to the liver outgrowth. The midgut begins caudal to the liver and extends to the posterior intestinal portal (the point where the right two thirds and left one third of transverse colon is formed in adults). The hindgut extends from the posterior intestinal portal to the cloacal membrane (anus).

Knowledge regarding the embryologic origins of the digestive tract is significant when considering nervous and circulatory supplies to its various segments, as well as possible anomalies.

The foregut

The cranial portion of the foregut gives rise to the mouth, pharynx, and associated structures. The esophagus, stomach, a portion of the duodenum proximal to the entrance of the bile duct, liver and gallbladder, and pancreas, are formed from the caudal portion of the foregut. Kuppfer cells and connective tissue cells are of mesodermal origin.

The midgut

The midgut begins immediately distal to the entrance of the bile duct into the duodenum and terminates at the junction of the proximal two thirds of the transverse colon with the distal one third. It forms the primary intestinal loop.

The hindgut

The hindgut gives rise to the distal third of the transverse colon, descending colon, sigmoid, rectum, and upper part of the anal canal. The endoderm of the hindgut also forms the internal lining of the bladder and urethra. The caudal hindgut is divided by the urorectal septum, resulting in the rectum and anal canal posteriorly and urinary bladder and urethra anteriorly.

Fig. 6-1 illustrates the early development of the digestive system, and Table 6-1 describes each stage.

PHYSIOLOGY

Each part of the gastrointestinal tract is adapted for specific functions: (1) carrying food from one area to another, (2) digestion of food, (3) absorption of nutrients, fluids, and other digestive end products, and (4) storage of food or fecal matter. This reveiw of the physiology of the gastrointestinal tract discusses the role of ingestion, digestion, and excretion in alimentation.

Ingestion

Ingestion of food involves hunger, appetite, mastication, and swallowing. The amount of food that a person actually consumes is controlled by two mechanisms: maintenance of normal quantities of nutrient stores in the body and immediate effects of feeding on the alimentary tract.

Hunger

Hunger—the intrinsic desire for food—is the major determinant of the amount of food that a person consumes. Objective sensations such as hunger pains or increasing tension and restlessness may be associated with hunger. Satiety, the opposite of hunger, is the feeling of fulfillment in the quest for food and usually results from ingestion of a meal.

The lateral nuclei of the hypothalamus is the *feeding center,* and the ventromedial nuclei of the hypothalamus is considered to be the *satiety center*. It is thought that the feeding center is continually activated, resulting in the emotional drive to search for food, while the satiety center primarily inhibits the feeding center. Thus the hypothalamus functions to control the quantity of food intake as well as to excite the lower centers to activity. The hypothalamic feeding center is concerned with the nutritional status of the body. Centers in the brain stem control the actual mechanics of feeding.

Cortical regions of the limbic system, such as the intraorbital regions, the hippocampal gyrus, and the cingulate gyrus, can increase or decrease feeding when stimulated. It is thought that they also operate in the neural regulation of appetite, affecting the quality or type of food that is preferentially sought.

Appetite

Appetite determines the desire for specific types of food, instead of food in general. Control of appetite occurs in centers higher than the hypothalamus, particularly amygdala and the cortical areas of the limbic system. These are closely connected to the hypothalamus. When the amygdala is destroyed on both sides of the brain, "psychic blindness" in the choice of foods is a problem.

It is thought that size of body fat deposits, environmental temperature (cold stimulates, heat depresses), distention of the gastrointestinal tract, cultural factors, environment, and past experience all potentially effect appetite. Ideally, the appetite-regulating mechanisms in

Fig. 6-1. Human embryos in the third and fourth weeks show the establishment of the digestive system. **A,** 16 days. **B,** 18 days. **C,** 22 days. **D,** Toward the end of the first month.

From Patten, B.M.: Human embryology, ed. 3, 1968, New York, McGraw-Hill Book Co.

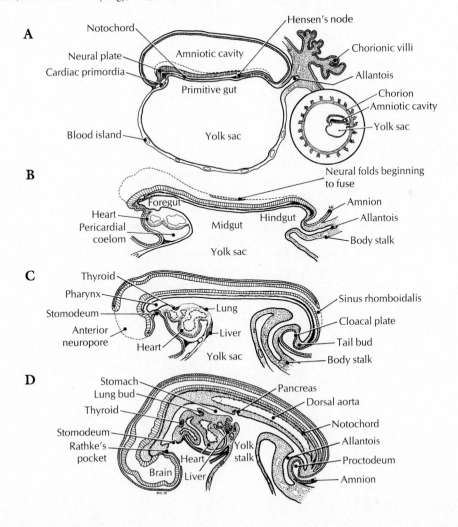

Table 6-1. Human development of the mouth, pharynx and derivatives, and digestive tubes and glands

Age (in weeks)	Size (in mm)	Mouth	Pharynx and derivatives	Digestive tube and glands
2.5	1.5	—	—	Gut not distinct from yolk sac.
3.5	2.5	Mandibular arch prominent. Stomodeum a definite pit. Oral membrane ruptures.	Pharynx broad and flat. Pharyngeal pouches forming. Thyroid indicated.	Fore- and hind-gut present. Yolk sac broadly attached at mid-gut. Liver bud present. Cloaca and cloacal membrane present.
4	5.0	Maxillary and mandibular processes prominent. Tongue primordia present. Rathke's pouch indicated.	Five pharyngeal pouches present. Pouches 1-4 have closing plates. Primary tympanic cavity indicated. Thyroid a stalked sac.	Esophagus short. Stomach spindle-shaped. Intestine a simple tube. Liver cords, ducts and gall bladder forming. Both pancreatic buds appear. Cloaca at height.
5	8.0	Jaws outlined. Rathke's pouch a stalked sac.	Phar. pouches gain dors. and vent. diverticula. Thyroid bilobed. Thyro-glossal duct atrophies.	Tail-gut atrophies. Yolk stalk detaches. Intestine elongates into a loop Cæcum indicated.
6	12.0	Lingual primordia fusing. Foramen cæcum established. Labio-dental laminæ appearing. Parotid acid submaxillary buds indicated.	Thymic sacs, ultimobranchial sacs and solid parathyroids are conspicuous and ready to detach. Thyroid becomes solid and converts into plates.	Stomach rotating. Intestinal loop undergoes torsion. Hepatic lobes identifiable. Cloaca subdividing.
7	17.0	Lingual primordia merge into single tongue. Separate labial and dental laminæ distinguishable. Jaws formed and begin to ossify. Palate folds present and separated by tongue.	Thymi elongating and losing lumina. Parathyroids become trabeculate and associate with thyroid. Ultimobranchial bodies fuse with thyroid. Thyroid becoming crescentic.	Stomach attaining final shape and position. Duodenum temporarily occluded. Intestinal loops herniate into cord. Rectum separates from bladder-urethra. Anal membrane ruptures. Dorsal and ventral pancreatic primordia fuse.

From Arey, L.B.: Developmental anatomy, ed. 7, Philadelphia, 1974, W.B. Saunders Co.

Table 6-1. Human development of the mouth, pharynx and derivatives, and digestive tubes and glands—cont'd

Age (in weeks)	Size (in mm)	Mouth	Pharynx and derivatives	Digestive tube and glands
8	23.0	Tongue muscles well differentiated. Earliest taste buds indicated. Rathke's pouch detaches from mouth. Sublingual gland appearing.	Auditory tube and tympanic cavity distinguishable. Sites of tonsil and its fossæ indicated. Thymic halves unite and become solid. Thyroid follicles forming.	Small intestine coiling within cord. Intestinal villi developing. Liver very large in relative size.
10	40.0	Fungiform and vallate papillæ differentiating. Lips separate from jaws. Enamel organs and dental papillae forming. Palate folds fusing.	Thymic epithelium transforming into reticulum and thymic corpuscles. Ultimobranchial bodies disappear as such.	Intestines withdraw from cord and assume characteristic positions. Anal canal formed. Pancreatic alveoli present.
12	56.0	Filiform and foliate papillæ elevating. Tooth primordia form prominent cups. Cheeks represented. Palate fusion complete.	Tonsillar crypts begin to invaginate. Thymus forming medulla and becoming increasingly lymphoid. Thyroid attains typical structure.	Muscle layers of gut represented. Pancreatic islands appearing. Bile secreted.
16	112.0	Hard and soft palate differentiating. Hypophysis acquiring definitive structure.	Lymphocytes accumulate in tonsils. Pharyngeal tonsil begins development.	Gastric and intestinal glands developing. Duodenum and colon affixing to body wall. Meconium collecting.
20-40 (5-10 mo.)	160.0-350.0	Enamel and dentine depositing (5). Lingual tonsil forming (5). Permanent tooth primordia indicated (6-8). Milk teeth unerupted at birth.	Tonsil structurally typical (5).	Lymph nodules and muscularis mucosæ of gut present (5). Ascending colon becomes recognizable (6). Appendix lags behind cæcum in growth (6). Deep esophageal glands indicated (7). Plicæ circulares represented (8).

normal humans should result in a balance of food intake so that caloric intake matches energy expenditure and nutritional needs are met.

Mastication (chewing)

Chewing, occurring most effectively in the person with healthy dentition, results in the breakup of large food particles as well as mixing the oral secretions of the salivary glands with the chewed food particles, which are smaller and thus have greater surface area. The smaller particles pass more easily through the remainder of the gastrointestinal tract and are also less likely to cause excoriation.

Most of the muscles involved in chewing are innervated by the motor branch of the fifth cranial nerve. Nuclei in the hindbrain control the chewing process, much of which is caused by the chewing reflex, initiated by the presence of a bolus of food in the mouth.

Deglutition (swallowing)

During swallowing, the pharynx, which serves several functions, is temporarily converted into a tract for carrying food from the mouth to the stomach. There are three stages of swallowing. The first is the voluntary stage, which initiates the process and involves the voluntary act of propelling the oral contents toward the back of the pharynx where the swallowing

Fig. 6-2. The swallowing mechanism.

From Berne, R.M., and Levy, M.N.: Physiology, St. Louis, 1983, The C.V. Mosby Co.

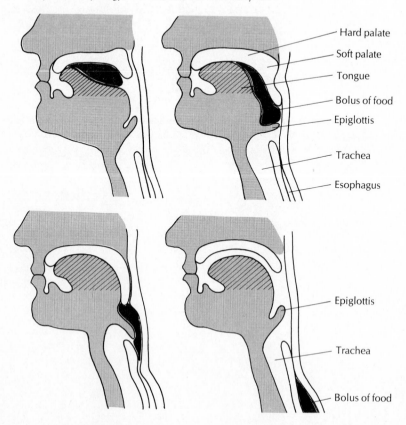

reflex is activated. The second is the pharyngeal stage, which is involuntary and involves the passage of food through the pharynx to the upper esophagus. Brief interruption of respiration and closure of the glottis are part of this reflex response. The swallowing center inhibits the respiratory center of the medulla during this time. The third stage of swallowing is the esophageal stage, which is involuntary and promotes the passage of food from the pharynx to the stomach. Fig. 6-2 illustrates the swallowing mechanism.

The movement of the esophagus assists in transporting the food from the pharynx to the stomach. Peristalsis of the esophagus is controlled almost entirely by the vagal reflexes. The two types of movement are *primary peristalsis* and *secondary peristalsis*. Primary peristalsis, beginning at the pharynx and continuing down the esophagus, is aided by gravity. Secondary peristalsis orginates in the esophagus, rather than the pharynx, as a result of distention of the esophagus by food remaining in the esophagus. It continues until all the food is moved into the stomach.

As the esophageal peristaltic waves pass toward the stomach, a wave of relaxation precedes constriction and both the stomach and the lower esophageal sphincter relax, allowing passage of the food bolus into the stomach.

Lower esophageal sphincter (LES). The lower esophageal sphincter is located at the lower end of the esophagus, 2 to 5 cm above the gastroesophageal junction. Although this area is not anatomically or morphologically different from the rest of the esophagus, it functions differently. The LES area remains tonically constricted, relaxing only following swallowing when a peristaltic wave formed behind the swallowed material passes down. Reflux of stomach contents is prevented by the lower esophageal sphincter and by the valvelike mechanism of the portion of the esophagus that lies right under the diaphragm. Increases in intra-abdominal pressure (such as walking, coughing, and breathing) caves the esophagus inward at this point.

Digestion and absorption

Digestion is the process by which food is broken down, mechanically and chemically, in the gastrointestinal tract and is converted into absorbable forms. Various gastrointestinal secretions, as well as motility of the GI tract, are involved in this process. Absorption, or the passage of these resulting substances through various surfaces within the GI system into body fluids and tissues, can then follow. Motility, secretion, and absorption will be discussed for the following anatomic parts of the gastrointestinal tract, proceeding cephalocaudally.

The mouth

The initial steps of digestion occur in the mouth and involve chewing and swallowing (see previous page).

Secretion of saliva. The three major salivary glands include the parotid glands, submaxillary glands, and sublingual glands. Approximately 1000 to 1500 ml of saliva normally is secreted each day. Ptyalin (salivary amylase), which begins the breakdown of large polysaccharides, and mucin, which lubricates food, are found in saliva. The pH of saliva ranges from 6.0 to 7.4. Saliva is loaded with large quantities of potassium and bicarbonate, so that any condition that results in large losses of saliva externally may cause serious potassium depletion. Secretion of saliva is neurally controlled, with parasympathetic stimulation resulting in profuse secretion of watery saliva. Atropine and other anticholinergics reduce salivary secretion. In humans stimulation of the sympathetic nervous system causes the release of small amounts of saliva with organic constituents from the submaxillary glands. Food in the mouth and stimulation of vagal afferent fibers of the distal esophagus cause reflex salivary secretion.

Saliva has a number of important functions: increasing the ease of swallowing, maintaining moisture in the mouth, facilitating movements of the lips and tongue when speaking, and maintaining good oral hygiene. It is thought that mucus-type salivary secretions assist in maintaining good oral hygiene by (1) washing away pathogenic bacteria and food particles, (2) containing protein antibodies that destroy oral bacteria, and (3) containing thiocyanate ions and proteolytic enzymes that destroy bacteria. In the absence of saliva, oral tissues are likely to become ulcerated and infected, and dental caries increase.

The esophagus

Motility. Peristaltic waves move a food bolus into the stomach (p. 427).

Secretions. Secretions in the entire esophagus are mucoid in nature, providing lubrication for swallowing. Large compound glands, which provide mucus to prevent mucosal excoriation from entering food proximally or refluxing gastric contents distally, are located at the initial portion and gastric end of the esophagus. The remainder of the glands lining the esophagus are simple mucous glands.

The stomach

The primary function of the stomach is to store the contents of a meal. Several other activities also occur: the hormone gastrin is synthesized and released, food is mixed with various digestive enzymes and juices, some digestion and absorption occur, and the contents of the stomach are released at a controlled, stable rate into the small intestine for further digestion and absorption.

The stomach is composed of the corpus or body (including the fundus) and the antrum (Fig. 6-3). Shape and size of the stomach may vary considerably, depending on body build, body position, and gastric filling. There are three layers of smooth muscle in the wall of the stomach. In addition to an external longitudinal layer and an inner circular layer as in the rest of the digestive system, there is an oblique layer located inside the circular one from the fundus to the pyloric antrum. From interior to exterior the layers of the stomach are mucosa, submucosa, oblique muscular layer, circular muscular layer, longitudinal muscular layer, and serosa. Different types of cells are found in different areas of the mucosa of the stomach, and different glands are found in various areas of the stomach.

Storage in the stomach. Food from the esophagus enters the body and fundus of the

---

Fig. 6-3. Anatomy of the stomach.

From Berne, R.M., and Levy, M.N.: Physiology, St. Louis, 1983, The C.V. Mosby Co.

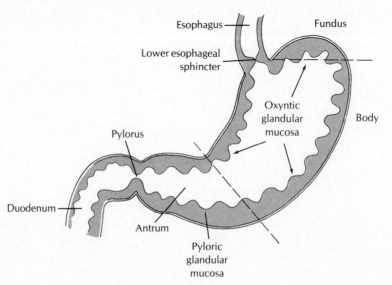

stomach through the lower esophageal sphincter and exits through the pylorus into the duodenum. The food that has entered most recently is closest to the esophageal opening, while the older food is nearest the wall of the stomach. The empty stomach has a volume of about 50 ml. The smooth muscle in the body of the stomach relaxes as food enters to allow the volume of the lumen to increase with minimal increase in pressure. Neural mechanisms mediated by the vagus nerve and coordinated by the swallowing center facilitate this change in muscular tone.

Mixing in the stomach. Rhythmic peristaltic waves (3 waves/min) begin near the entry of the esophagus and proceed over the body of the stomach. Initially, these waves produce only a weak ripple. They become more powerful upon approaching the larger muscle mass that surrounds the antrum. The antral contents are forced toward the pylorus under high pressure by intense peristaltic waves or *peristaltic constrictor rings*. Small amounts of the antral contents move through the pylorus into the duodenum, whereas the majority is "squirted" back toward the body of the stomach. The rhythmicity of peristalsis can be traced to spontaneously discharging pacemaker cells located in the longitudinal muscle layer near the esophagus. Depolarizations of these cells are propagated along the longitudinal muscle layer of the stomach. Similar waves occur in the overlying circular muscle layer. Since these waves alone are too small to cause the muscle membrane to reach threshold and fire an action potential, this action, in combination with the effects of neurotransmittors and hormones, acts upon the muscle to depolarize the membrane so that action potentials can be generated. Vagal afferent signals to the medulla oblongata reflexly inhibit tone in the storage area of the stomach, resulting in an increased rate of digestion and removal of stored food.

Gastric secretion. The stomach mucosa is lined by *mucus-secreting cells* to protect and lubricate and has two different types of tubular glands, the *oxyntic glands* (fundic or gastric glands), and the *pyloric glands* (antral glands)

(Fig. 6-4). The oxyntic glands are located in the mucosa of the body and fundus of the stomach with the exception of the lesser curvature; they secrete hydrochloric acid from the parietal cells (Fig. 6-5), mucus from the mucous neck cells, and pepsinogen* from the chief cells. The pyloric glands are located in the antrum of the stomach and secrete mucus, a different pepsinogen from that from the chief cells, and gastrin. They are structurally similar to the oxyntic glands but contain few peptic and oxyntic cells and many mucous cells. Located very near the gastroesophageal junction are a few mucus-secreting cardiac glands. Small quantities of gastric lipase and gastric amylase are secreted as well. Intrinsic factor, which is essential for absorption of vitamin B_{12} in the ileum, is secreted by the oxyntic cells. Destruction of the parietal cells results in the absence of intrinsic factor, associated with pernicious anemia, and the absence of hydrochloric acid, or achlorhydria. Between meals little or no secretion occurs, but that which does occur is mostly of the nonoxyntic type (mostly mucus, a little pepsin, and little or no acid). Emotional stress may increase gastric secretion at any time.

Regulation of gastric secretion. Regulation of gastric secretion can be described in three phases: the cephalic phase (before food reaches the stomach), the gastric phase (when food is in the stomach), and the intestinal phase (when gastric contents are released into the duodenum).

The cephalic phase of gastric secretion is mediated principally by parasympathetic vagal fibers. Chemoreceptors activated by the sight and smell of food and mechanoreceptors stimulated by chewing and swallowing transmit afferent impulses to the CNS. Vagal efferents acting primarily through the myenteric plexus and, to a lesser extent, via the submucosal plexus cause the release of acetylcholine (ACh). The release of ACh near parietal and chief cells causes the se-

---

*Pepsinogen is the inactive form of pepsin, an enzyme involved in proteolysis.

Fig. 6-4. Structure of gastric mucosa. **A,** Reconstruction of part of the gastric wall. **B,** Schematic depiction of a gastric gland showing the different cell types.

From Berne, R.M., and Levy, M.N.: Physiology, St. Louis, 1983, The C.V. Mosby Co.

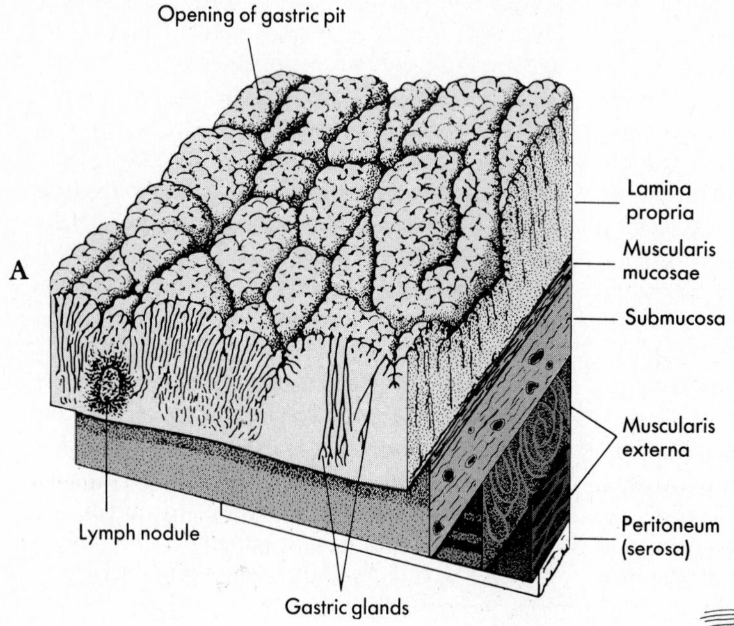

Opening of gastric pit

A

Lamina propria

Muscularis mucosae

Submucosa

Muscularis externa

Peritoneum (serosa)

Lymph nodule

Gastric glands

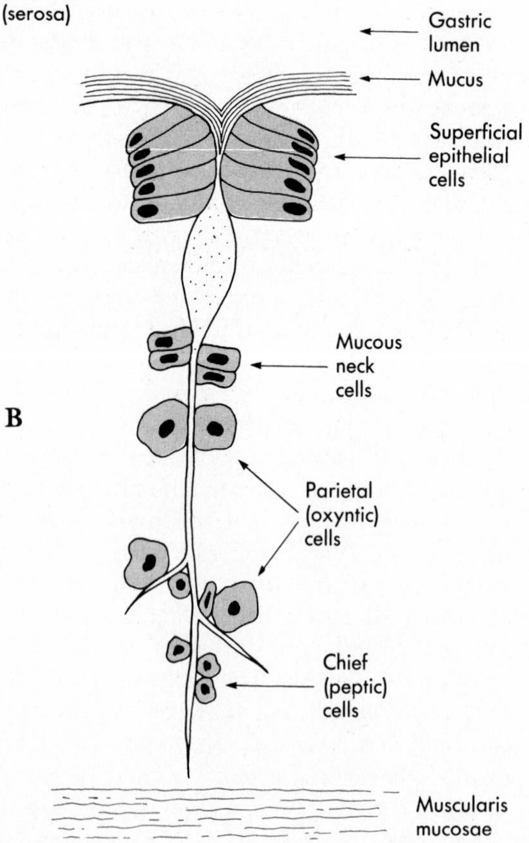

Gastric lumen

Mucus

Superficial epithelial cells

Mucous neck cells

B

Parietal (oxyntic) cells

Chief (peptic) cells

Muscularis mucosae

cretion of HCl and pepsinogen, respectively, while G cells respond by secreting gastrin. Gastrin subsequently stimulates the parietal cells to secrete more acid.

The gastric phase begins when food enters the stomach. Gastric distention in different regions of the stomach stimulates mechanoreceptors that cause the release of ACh via both local and central reflexes. ACh near G cells results in increased gastrin release. Parietal cells respond by additional release of HCl. The presence of amino acids and peptides from protein degradation also stimulates the parietal cells directly to produce HCl.

Stimulation of acid secretion continues during the intestinal phase of digestion via two mechanisms. The presence of intraduodenal stimuli (peptides and amino acids) trigger G cells located within the mucosa of the proximal duodenum to release gastrin, which is carried by the blood to the stomach where it elicits acid release by the parietal cells. Another mechanism involving the release of a local hormone in response to the presence of chyme in the duodenum acts directly upon the parietal cells to increase HCl secretion and potentiate the effect of gastrin.

Gastric secretion is inhibited by the presence of acid in the duodenum and fat digestion products or hypertonicity in the duodenum and proximal jejunum. Duodenal acidity triggers the release of secretion, which reduces gastric acid by directly inhibiting the parietal cells and by inhibition of gastrin release. Two hormones, gastric inhibitory peptide and cholecystokinin, are released in response to fatty acids and other fat digestion by-products in the duodenum and jejunum. Gastric inhibitory peptide suppresses gastrin release and inhibits the parietal cells from secreting acid. Cholecystokinin inhibits the parietal cells, but its action may be physiologically insignificant. Hyperosmotic solutions in the duodenum elicit the release of another hormone, not yet identified, that also appears to inhibit gastric secretion.

Absorption in the stomach. Very little absorption occurs in the stomach because the epithelial cells are very close together and the absorptive membrane, such as in the villus, is missing. However, quantities of lipid-soluble substances, such as alcohol and aspirin, are absorbed.

Emptying of the stomach. Gastric emptying is a function of gastric volume, motility, and secretion. The rate of evacuation decreases progressively with emptying of the stomach. Gastric wall distention stimulates mechanoreceptors in

Fig. 6-5. Mechanism of hydrochloric acid release.

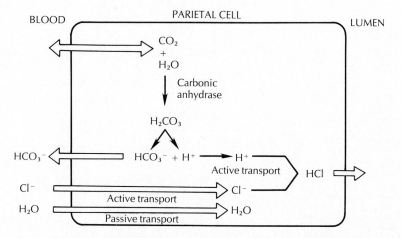

the wall of the stomach, resulting in augmentation of peristalsis in proportion to the degree of distention. This activity is mediated by long reflexes over the vagi and short reflexes through the internal nerve plexus. These fibers release ACh, and this in turn determines the rate of firing of action potentials and the ultimate strength of peristalsis. Gastric motility is also augmented by the hormone gastrin from the pyloric antrum in the presence of intraluminal stimuli found during digestion.

Some of the mechanisms that participate in the regulation of gastric emptying are initiated in the duodenum. Duodenal receptors respond to intraluminal stimuli to initiate hormonal and reflex inhibition of gastric motor activity (see previous page).

The small intestine

The small intestine, especially the duodenum and jejunum, is the site where the majority of digestion and absorption occurs. It is in this area that chyme is mixed with digestive juices and brought into contact with absorptive surfaces or propelled toward the colon.

Motility of the small intestine. Mixing contractions and propulsive contractions occur in the small intestine. These mixing contractions,

also referred to as segmentation contractions, occur when a portion of the small intestine is distended with chyme, causing the wall to stretch and initiate concentric contractions spaced at intervals along the intestine. New contractions form at different points as the old contractions fade out (Fig. 6-6). Chyme is chopped 7 to 12 times per minute by these mixing contractions, which also help propel food to a small extent as they travel caudally.

Propulsive movements are waves of peristalsis that propel chyme. They move faster in the proximal intestine and slower in the distal intestine. These propulsive movements, initiated by distention after a meal, are usually weak and die out after traveling a few centimeters. While the propulsive movements push chyme towards the ileocecal valve, they also spread chyme along the intestinal mucosa.

The villi of the small intestine also contract, agitating fluids so that new areas are exposed for absorption.

The ileocecal valve prevents the backflow of fecal contents from the colon into the small intestine. It is usually mildly constricted, slowing emptying of the ileocecal contents, which consist of about 750 ml of chyme daily. Relaxation of the ileocecal valve occurs as a result of (1) the gastroileal reflex after a meal, which intensifies peristalsis in the ileum, (2) the direct relaxant effect of gastrin, and (3) reflexes from the cecum. If the cecum is distended or irritated (such as from an inflamed appendix), contraction of the ileocecal valve is intensified.

Contractile activity is influenced by both intrinsic and extrinsic mechanisms, although the latter are not required for the initiation and maintenance of intestinal motility. Movement in the small intestine is dependent in part on short reflexes mediated by the internal nerve plexus to the intestinal wall smooth muscle. Local reflex stimulation occurs in response to mechanical and chemical receptor stimulation by intestinal contents. A direct response to stretching of the muscles also occurs. Extrinsic innervation of the intestine mediated by both parasympathetic (via

Fig. 6-6. Segmentation movements of the small intestine.

From Guyton, A.C.: Textbook of medical physiology, ed. 6, Philadelphia, 1981, W.B. Saunders Co.

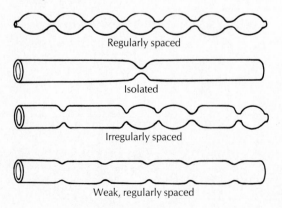

Regularly spaced

Isolated

Irregularly spaced

Weak, regularly spaced

the vagus nerve) and sympathetic (via the celiac and superior mesenteric plexuses) also modifies intestinal movements. Vagal stimulation generally increases intestinal motility, and sympathetic innervation produces inhibition of intestinal motor activity.

Secretion of the small intestine. Mucus and digestive juices are secreted by the small intestine. Secretion of mucus is from the *Brunner's glands* and *goblet cells.* Brunner's glands, compound mucous glands, are located in the first few centimeters of the duodenum, their secretions functioning to protect the duodenal wall. They are stimulated to secrete by (1) direct tactile stimulation or irritating stimuli over the mucosa, (2) intestinal hormones (especially secretin), and (3) vagal stimuli. They are inhibited by sympathetic stimuli. Goblet cells are located primarily on the surface of the intestinal mucosa and also in the intestinal pits, the crypts of Lieberkühn. They secrete mucus in response to direct tactile or chemical stimulation of the mucosa by chyme.

Daily secretion of about 2000 ml of digestive juices consisting of almost pure extracellular fluid from the small intestine comes from the crypts of Lieberkühn, located on the entire surface of the small intestine, except in the area of the duodenum where the Brunner's glands are found. Digestive enzymes including peptidases, sucrase, maltase, isomaltase, lactase, and lipase are contained in the brush border of the epithelial cells of the mucosa.

Regulation of small intestinal secretion occurs through local neural reflexes and through hormonal influences.

Absorption by the small intestine. The vast majority of absorption that occurs in the gastrointestinal tract takes place in the small intestine. The anatomy of the small intestine is especially adapted for absorption. *Valvulae conniventes* (folds of Kerckring) are folds that increase the surface area of the absorptive mucosa about three times, especially in the duodenum and jejunum (Fig. 6-7). *Villi* are found over the entire surface of the small intestine and serve to

enhance the absorptive area (Fig. 6-8). *Microvilli,* located in the intestinal epithelium brush border, further increase the surface area exposed to intestinal materials.

Removal of short segments of jejunum or ileum usually does not cause severe symptoms of malabsorption because compensatory hypertrophy and hyperplasia of the remaining mucosa results in intestinal adaptation and return of absorptive function. When more than 50% of the small intestine is resected or bypassed, absorption of nutrients and vitamins is compromised to the extent that it is difficult to prevent malnutrition and wasting. Absorption by the small intestine consists of several hundred grams of carbohydrates, 100 or more grams of fat, 50 to 100 grams of amino acids, 50 to 100 grams of ions, and 8 to 9 L of water daily.

Absorption in the small intestine occurs in numerous ways. The central lacteals absorb into the lymph. The vascular system absorbs fluid

Fig. 6-7. Valvulae conniventes (folds of Kerckring) in the duodenum and jejunum that increase the surface area for absorption in the intestine.

From Guyton, A.C.: Textbook of medical physiology, ed. 6, Philadelphia, 1981, W.B. Saunders Co.

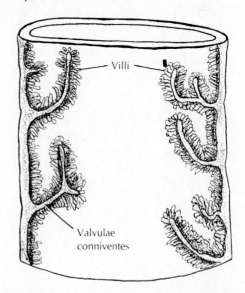

Villi

Valvulae conniventes

and dissolved substances into portal blood. Small amounts of substances are absorbed by pinocytosis. Most absorption occurs through single molecular transfer (passive diffusion) through the membrane along an electrical gradient. Some materials are absorbed by active transport through the intestinal epitheleum against an electrical gradient with energy supplied by mitochondria in the form of high energy compounds such as ATP. Active transport requires (1) a carrier, (2) energy, and (3) catalyzation by an appropriate ATPase carrier enzyme in the cell membrane.

Various substances are absorbed in different portions of the small intestine. The proximal intestine absorbs iron, calcium, fat, sugars, and amino acids. The middle of the small intestine absorbs sugars and amino acids, and the distal small intestine absorbs bile salts and vitamin B_{12}. Some surgical procedures and disease processes can affect the ability of the small intestine to absorb these nutrients.

The large intestine

The main functions of the colon are absorption of water, sodium, and other minerals in addition to storage of fecal material. Certain vitamins are absorbed, and some are synthesized by bacteria that grow in the colon. Some secretion also occurs.

Secretion by the large intestine. No digestive enzymes are secreted by the colon. Goblet cells contained in crypts of Lieberkühn lining the mucosa of the colon secrete mucus, as do goblet cells dispersed on the surface of the epithelium of the large intestine. The mucus serves to (1) protect the wall from excoriation, (2) provide an adherent substance for holding the feces together, and (3) protect the intestinal wall from bacterial activity and acids. Regulation of mucus secretion is by direct, tactile stimulation of the surface mucosal goblet cells and by local myenteric reflexes to the goblet cells in the crypts of Lieberkühn.

Water and electrolytes can be secreted by the

Fig. 6-8. Villi located over the surface area of the small intestine that enhance absorption. **A,** Longitudinal section. **B,** Cross section showing the epithelial cells and basement membrane.

From Guyton, A.C.: Textbook of medical physiology, ed. 6, Philadelphia, 1981, W.B. Saunders Co.

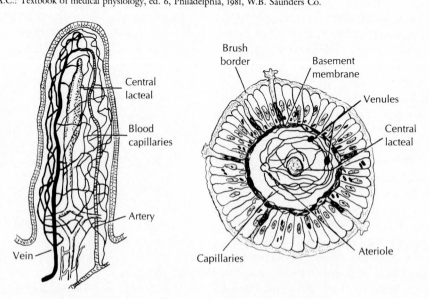

mucosa of the colon when it is irritated, such as with a bacterial infection or from use of some laxatives. In the event of infection, this can serve as a protective mechanism by diluting the irritating factors and encouraging rapid movement of the feces out of the body.

Motility of the colon. Essentially two types of movements occur in the colon to move its contents along, *mixing movements* (haustrations) and *propulsive movements* (mass movements). Haustrations are a result of large circular constrictions, similar to segmentation contractions in the small intestine, and contraction of the three longitudinal muscles, or tinea coli. All of the fecal material is thus gradually exposed to the colonic surface for absorption, and the fecal matter in the colon is mixed up. Propulsive movements from the transverse colon to the sigmoid colon occur in addition to smaller or mass action contraction peristaltic waves. They are most abundant for 15 minutes during the first hour after eating but can occur a few times each day. They are the predominant action during defecation.

Absorption in the colon. The colon, especially proximally, absorbs large quantities of water and electrolytes. Of the 500 to 1000 ml of chyme that come through the ileocecal valve daily, only about 100 ml of fluid remains to be excreted in the feces. The capacity of the colon for absorption is far greater than that. The largest amount of absorption occurs in the ascending colon, and then absorption decreases as one moves distally. Almost all ions are absorbed, with only a little sodium and chloride remaining in the feces. Sodium is absorbed by active transport, taking chloride along with it, whereas water is absorbed passively. The mucosa actually absorbs chloride ions while actively secreting bicarbonate ions. Water is absorbed as a result of the osmotic gradient across the colonic mucosa that occurs with the absorption of sodium and chloride ions.

Feces contain inorganic material, undigested plant fibers, fat, proteins, bacteria, and water. A large portion of fecal matter is of nondietary origin, thus it is little affected by diet or pro-

longed starvation. The brown color is caused by *stercobilin* and *urobilin,* both derived from bilirubin. The fecal odor is caused by the products of bacterial action, varying with the type of food eaten and the person's colonic bacterial flora. Substances formed from bacterial activity are vitamin K, vitamin B_{12}, thiamine, riboflavin, and various gases.

The pancreas

The pancreas, an endocrine and exocrine gland, is similar in structure to the salivary glands. Pancreatic juice contains electrolytes, water and enzymes. Pancreatic endocrine secretions include insulin and glucagon. The exocrine functions are limited to digestion. The acini cells secrete digestive enzymes, and the ductal epithelium produces sodium bicarbonate ions and water. Pancreatic juice adjusts the duodenal content to an alkaline pH suitable for action of the pancreatic enzymes. As acid chyme enters the duodenum during periods of food digestion, pancreatic secretion is thought to be increased by hormones such as secretin and cholecystokinin-pancreozymin (CCK-PZ). Secretin stimulates the pancreas to produce water and bicarbonate, and CCK-PZ stimulates production of pancreatic enzymes. Proteolytic endopeptidase enzymes secreted by the pancreas include trypsin (the most abundant), chymotrypsin, carboxypolypeptidase, aminopeptidases, and deoxyribonuclease. The first three enzymes are inactive when secreted. Amylase breaks down polysaccharides into disaccharides in carbohydrate digestion. Lipolytic enzymes include lipase and cholesterol esterase. Trypsin inhibitor is stored in the cytoplasm of the glandular cells of the pancreas and prevents activation of trypsin both inside the secretory cells and in the acini and ducts of the pancreas, therefore preventing autodigestion.

Pancreatic secretion is regulated by neural and hormonal signals. Chyme in the small intestine causes the release of secretin and cholecystokinin, both of which are absorbed by the blood stream. Secretin results in copious secretion of pancreatic fluid and bicarbonate, while cholecystokinin causes secretion of enzymes. In addition, the pancreas is supplied with preganglionic parasympathetic fibers, whose branches synapse with postganglionic cholinergic neurons innervating both acinar and islet cells. Postganglionic parasympathetic nerves from the celiac and superior mesenteric plexuses innervate pancreatic vessels. Parasympathetic stimulation generally increases pancreatic secretion, while sympathetic activity is inhibitory.

The liver and gall bladder

Bile secretion and storage. The liver is a highly complex organ having many functions: formation of bile, carbohydrate storage, ketone body formation, control of carbohydrate metabolism, reduction and conjugation of adrenal and gonadal steroid hormones, detoxification of drugs and toxins, manufacture of plasma proteins, inactivation of polypeptide hormones, urea formation, and fat metabolism.

Bile is secreted continuously by the parenchymal cells of the liver. The secretion enters tiny channels in the liver (bile canaliculi) and

then flows to the common bile duct into the duodenum at or near the site where the pancreatic duct empties. The sphincter of Oddi, a smooth muscle sphincter, surrounds the common bile duct where it enters the duodenum. It is usually closed during fasting to divert bile. Between meals the bile flows to and is stored in the gall bladder where it is concentrated after salt and water extraction. Following a meal, the amount of bile that enters the duodenum is increased as a result of enhanced liver secretion, the contraction of the gall bladder, and intestinal secretion of cholecystokinin (Fig. 6-9).

Human hepatic duct bile contains water (97%), bile salts, bile pigments, cholesterol, inorganic salts, fatty acids, lecithin, fat, alkaline phosphatase, and electrolytes. It contains no digestive enzymes. About 600 to 1000 ml are secreted daily. The enterohepatic circulation consists of various components of the bile, which are reabsorbed in the ileum (90% to 95% of bile salts) and then resecreted again by the liver about twenty times before finally being excreted in the feces.

Bile acids are formed in the liver, principally as cholic acid and chenodeoxycholic acid. Bacteria in the colon convert them to other acids. Lithocolic acid is insoluble and is excreted; deoxycholate is reabsorbed and transported back to the liver. Bile acids are conjugated in the liver to bile salts—glycocholic acid and taurocholic acid.

The rate of bile secretion is increased by (1) increased bile salts in the blood, (2) increased liver blood flow, (3) vagal stimulation, and (4) secretin, which stimulates the small bile ducts to secrete sodium bicarbonate solution.

Bile salts are important in various aspects of digestion. They (1) assist in emulsifying fat globules for digestion; (2) combine with lipids to form micelles, which assist in transporting the end products of fat digestion to the intestinal villi for absorption by the lymphatics; (3) activate lipases in the intestine; and (4) stimulate reesterification of fatty acids and glycerol synthesis from glucose.

Fig. 6-9. Mechanism of liver secretion and gallbladder emptying.

From Guyton, A.C.: Textbook of medical physiology, ed. 6, Philadelphia, 1981, W.B. Saunders Co.

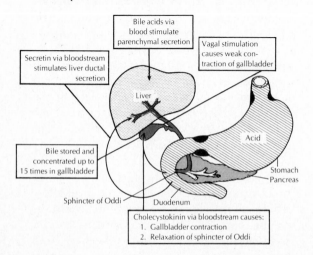

Excretion (defecation)

Defecation is a complex act consisting of voluntary and involuntary components (Fig. 6-10). The rectum is usually empty of feces. Mass movements of the colon force feces into the rectum, which increases the tension in the rectal wall and initiates the desire for defecation. Defecation involves a cord-mediated reflex, which passes from the rectum to the spinal cord and then back to the descending colon, sigmoid, rectum, and anus. This defecation reflex augments considerably the intrinsic defecation reflex that is mediated through the myenteric plexus of the sigmoid and colon wall itself. It may be lost or altered by spinal cord injuries. Contraction of the longitudinal rectal muscles cause shortening of the rectum, and relaxation of the internal anal sphincter occurs. The internal anal sphincter, which is tonically constricted, is a circular mass of smooth muscle located just inside the anus. The external anal sphincter is under voluntary control, mediated by the somatic nervous system. Reflex contraction holds the feces in until it is relaxed by voluntary processes, allowing expulsion of the feces, after which rebound closure occurs.

Two mechanisms that facilitate defecation are assuming a squatting position, which increases intra-abdominal pressure, and the Valsalva maneuver, which also increases intra-abdominal pressure by descent of the diaphragm, closure of the glottis, and contraction of the abdominal and chest muscles. These voluntary aids to defecation may be lost as a result of spinal cord injuries.

ASSESSMENT
Gastrointestinal history

Establishing the etiology of digestive disorders is often difficult since there are systemic manifestations of gastrointestinal disease and systemic diseases with gastrointestinal manifestations. Thus a good history is imperative in minimizing the confusion and complexity associated with making a definitive diagnosis. Although the patient's primary complaint may appear to be gastrointestinal, it is necessary to pursue all other complaints to make sure the etiology is not found in another system.

Many gastrointestinal disorders have similar manifestations. The cardinal GI symptoms can be categorized into four main groups: (1) symptoms resulting from depression or exaggeration of normal sensations; (2) symptoms resulting from disturbances in motility; (3) symptoms from disturbances in function; and (4) pain.

Symptoms that result from depression or exaggeration of normal sensations such as loss of appetite (anorexia), abnormal hunger, belching (eructation), regurgitation, heartburn, epigastric fullness after eating, intestinal flatulence, and spasmodic anal contractions with pain and a feeling of a need to evacuate (tenesmus) may be of pathologic significance.

Complaints stemming from a disturbance in motility include difficulty swallowing (dysphagia), painful swallowing (odynophagia), vomiting, and altered defecation. These problems, as well as those arising from a depression or exaggeration of symptoms, should be correlated with any recent changes in food patterns or habits.

Fig. 6-10. The defecation reflex, illustrating afferent and efferent parasympathetic pathways.

From Guyton, A.C.: Textbook of medical physiology, ed. 6, Philadelphia, 1981, W.B. Saunders Co.

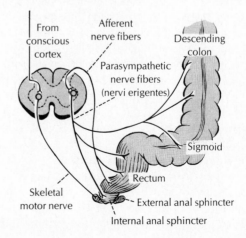

The relationship of these symptoms to eating, eliminating, position, or activity should be noted. Since this information is not always volunteered, direct inquiry may be necessary.

A thorough knowledge of normal gastrointestinal physiology will be helpful in identifying symptoms that are brought about by a disturbance in function. Included in this category are disorders of secretion, disorders of digestion, failure of absorption, and alterations in excretion. Relating these complaints to regional organ structures may provide further relevant information.

Pain occurrence should be correlated with GI function and considered chronologically. The onset, duration, frequency, and severity of pain should be noted. Notation of factors that aggravate or relieve symptoms and their timing are also important. Here, too, the relationship of symptoms to eating, defecation, position, and medication ingestion is vital. The interpretation of pain is complicated by the fact that it is not always evident directly over the suspected source of the problem but may be referred pain.

Information about the past history can provide clues to determine the likely source of current problems or help to eliminate possible sources of the problem. Also included would be information about current medications and habits. For example, the person who is taking antibiotics is likely to have diarrhea as a result of altered GI flora. The person who has recently lost 20 pounds without trying or experienced a recent aversion to particular foods is highly suspected of having a malignancy. Prior removal of an appendix eliminates appendicitis as the source of abdominal pain but might raise the suspicion of obstruction from adhesions. The person who has consumed a quart of whiskey per week for many years and has recently developed ascites would make one consider Laënnec's cirrhosis as the source of that person's problems.

Information obtained from the family history helps to identify those people with a predisposition for diseases that are thought to be passed along genetically, or along ethnic lines.

GI tumors, pernicious anemia, and Crohn's disease are examples. Identifying those individuals at risk for certain problems can raise the investigator's index of suspicion in the right direction.

The nutritional history is important because of the relationship of nutrition to health in general. In addition, it is very likely to pinpoint manifestations of GI disorders. Nutrition has received much attention recently both as a factor in causing disease and as a manifestation of disease, regardless of what the patient's major problem is. In assessing nutritional status it is important to do so with consideration of developmental factors. Different ages have different needs and problems. The person should be asked information about his actual dietary intake, as well as about his beliefs and knowledge regarding nutrition.

The nutritional history should consider assessment of psychological factors, socioeconomic status, medications, and other health problems as they relate to nutrition. Psychological factors such as depression, anxiety, and isolation should be noted. Socioeconomic information as it reflects ability to purchase and prepare food is important. Medications should be evaluated for possible effects on nutritional status and GI function. The patient's perception of his diet, in addition to how he sees himself nutritionally and weight-wise should be determined. Methods of food preparation as well as ingredients used in cooking may be inquired about.

There are a number of methods to assess actual dietary intake, but it must be remembered that it is generally difficult to do accurately. This is because recording influences intake, people may have difficulty remembering types and amounts of food eaten, and it is often impossible to evaluate the nutrient composition of the ingested food. Methods that can be used to assess dietary intake include 24-hour recall, food frequency questionnaire, dietary history, a food diary, and observation of food intake. It is most likely that when dealing with the acutely ill patient, the majority of attention is focused on assessment of current nutritional status by looking at various anthropometric measurements (discussed under physical examination) and at biochemical tests obtained from laboratory tests. It is also likely that dietary intake, if there is any, will be assessed in the hospitalized patient by direct observation. For the person who is being nourished by parenteral and/or enteral hyperalimentation, evaluation of calories and nutrients given (including vitamins and minerals) is essential. Assessment of nutritional knowledge and beliefs of the patient and family is likely to have a role of increasing importance as the patient recovers and moves toward rehabilitation.

The review of systems (ROS) looks at all complaints by body system, considering past and present status. Certain portions of the review of systems deserve especially close attention in the patient with a problem suspected to be of GI origin. In the first part of the ROS, entitled *General,* one questions the patient about usual weight, recent weight changes, weakness, fatigue, or fever. Skin changes, such as desquamation, bruising, and changes in pigmentation might be GI related. Hair texture and hair thickness change with poor nutritional status. The ROS of the mouth includes sore or bleeding gums; lesions of lips, tongue, or mucosa; use of dentures; soreness of the throat; difficulty swallowing; and taste changes. Nonspecifically, the patient is asked about appetite, bowel patterns, change in stools, diarrhea, constipation, abdominal pain, excessive flatulence, hemorrhoids, jaundice, dysphagia, changes in weight, tarry stools, anal itching, incontinence of stool, indigestion, nausea, hernia or other changes in stool pattern, previously diagnosed problems, hematemesis, and food idiosyncrasies.

In summary, a general review of the GI system should include questions about the following:

1. Pain (if positive, determine sequence and chronology, onset, location, quality, intensity, frequency, associated phenomena, aggravating factors, alleviating factors)
2. Bowel habits (frequency, character, pain, hemorrhoids)
3. Constipation (definition, frequency, treatment)
4. Diarrhea (definition, frequency, treatment)
5. Thirst
6. Change in appetite
7. Heartburn (definition, frequency, treatment)
8. Food intolerances
9. Belching
10. Flatulence
11. Prior problems, evaluations, diagnoses, treatments
12. History of jaundice

Physical examination
Examination of the mouth and pharynx

Inspection is the primary method of examining the mouth and pharynx. Abnormalities are noted and described. The lips are observed for color, moisture, lumps, ulcers, or cracking. The buccal mucosa is checked for color, pigmentation, ulcers, or nodules. The gums are inspected for inflammation, swelling, bleeding, retraction, and lesions. Abnormalities of the teeth such as cavities, displacement, and dislocation are noted, as well as their general state of repair and position. The roof of the mouth is checked for color and architecture. The tongue is observed for color and papillae and for abnormal smoothness or size. Aspects of the pharynx that are checked include the soft palate, anterior and posterior pillars, uvula, tonsils, and posterior pharynx for color, symmetry, exudate, edema, ulceration, and petechiae.

Examination of the neck

To prepare the person for examination of the neck, she is asked to raise her chin and tilt the head back. Good lighting is essential. Inspection and palpation are the primary modes of examination utilized. The neck is inspected for symmetry, masses, and scars, as well as obvious lymph nodes or lesions.

The lymph nodes are palpated in a systematic fashion, noting location, size, shape, delimitation, mobility, consistency, and tenderness. The lymph nodes of the neck include preauricular, postauricular, occipital, tonsillar, submaxillary, submental, superficial cervical, posterior cervical chain, deep cervical chain, and supraclavicular nodes (Fig. 6-11).

The trachea and thyroid are also examined. The trachea is inspected and palpated for deviation. The thyroid is inspected for enlargement and nodules. The thyroid is palpated in an anterior and posterior approach for size, tenderness, masses, and nodules. Auscultation of the thyroid is performed in an attempt to detect bruits.

Examination of the abdomen

In approaching the examination of the abdomen, for the sake of reference and description,

the abdomen can be divided into two standard systems (Fig. 6-12). One system consists of four quadrants: right upper quadrant (RUQ), right lower quadrant (RLQ), left upper quadrant (LUQ), and left lower quadrant (LLQ). The other system consists of nine areas: right hypochondriac, epigastric, left hypochondriac, right lumbar, umbilical, left lumbar, right inguinal, pubic, and left inguinal. No matter which geographic system is used when looking at the areas of the abdomen, it is most helpful to remember

Fig. 6-12. Abdominal examination using different reference systems. **A,** Four quadrants—RUQ right upper quadrant, LUQ left upper quadrant, RLQ right lower quadrant, LLQ left lower quadrant. **B,** Nine areas.

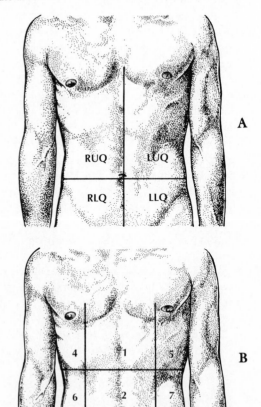

Fig. 6-11. Lymph nodes of the neck.

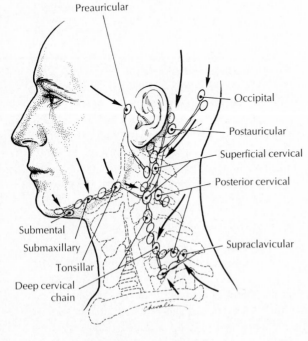

Preauricular

Occipital

Postauricular

Superficial cervical

Posterior cervical

Submental

Submaxillary

Supraclavicular

Tonsillar

Deep cervical chain

Arrows indicate direction of lymph flow

and mentally picture the organs that lie therein (Figs. 6-13 and 6-14).

In preparing for the examination of the abdomen, the following equipment needs to be acquired: stethoscope; marking pen; tape measure; and good lighting, shining across the patient's abdomen toward the examiner, such as the light from a gooseneck lamp.

Preparing the patient for the examination involves a number of considerations. First is the comfort of the patient. The room should be a comfortable temperature, considering the patient's attire, and the patient should be properly draped to preserve modesty. An opportunity to empty the patient's bladder should have been provided. The patient should be relaxed and instructed to breath quietly through her mouth.

The patient should be lying supine, with pillows under her knees and head, with arms at her sides or across the chest (not over the head or behind the head). The procedure should be explained to the patient as it is being performed. During the exam, the patient's face, not the abdomen, should be observed. If the patient is ticklish, palpation can be performed with one of the patient's hands between the examiner's hands. Tender areas should be examined last. Warm hands, a warm stethoscope, and short fingernails facilitate relaxation of the patient. The abdominal examination is performed from the patient's right side, with the examiner visualizing the organs in each region as it is examined. The abdominal examination is the only one where the order is changed—inspection, auscultation, per-

Fig. 6-13. Four quadrant abdominal reference system illustrating location of abdominal organs.

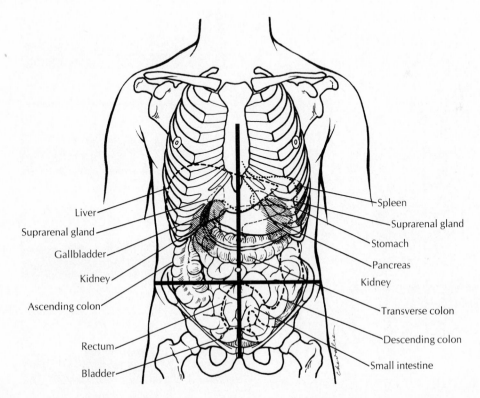

cussion, and palpation—to prevent percussion and palpation from influencing bowel activity. Each aspect of the examination will be discussed in the order the techniques should be performed.

Inspection. The skin is observed for scars, with location, length, and width described and pictured in a diagram. Size and color of striae should be described. Rashes, lesions, and moles should be noted as to location, color, and size. Presence and location of dilated veins should be noted.

The umbilicus is observed and described in terms of contour, location, inflammation, or herniation. In infants the remains of the umbilical cord are usually present for approximately 2 weeks. It should be observed for erythema, swelling, discharge, and odor.

Fig. 6-14. Nine section abdominal reference system illustrating location of abdominal organs.

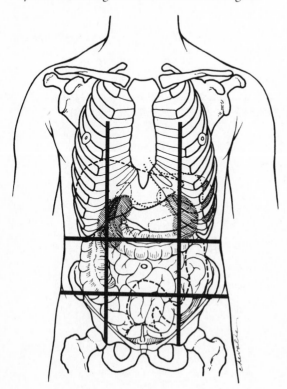

Fig. 6-15. Contour of abdomen.

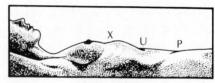

Normal profile

X = Xiphoid
U = Umbilicus
P = Pubis

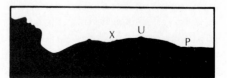

Generalized distention, with umbilicus everted

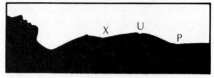

Generalized distention, with umbilicus inverted

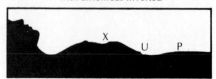

Scaphoid abdomen

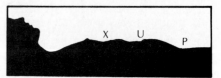

Distention of lower half

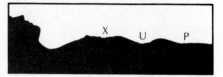

Distention of lower third

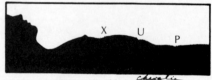

Distention of upper half

The shape or contour of the abdomen is described as flat, round, protuberant, or scaphoid (Fig. 6-15). The femoral and inguinal areas are observed for herniation.

The abdomen is also inspected for symmetry, masses, and abdominal movements (those of respiration, peristalsis, and pulsations). Look across the patient to observe peristalsis, which is most easily evident in thin people. Pulsation of the aorta in the epigastric area is most likely seen in thin adults or children. In observing movements of respiration, it should be kept in mind that men are better abdominal breathers than women. Women tend to use only their thoracic muscles, while men use both.

Auscultation. In the abdominal examination auscultation is performed before percussion or palpation in order to avoid altering the frequency of bowel sounds. Initially, it is important to listen for bowel sounds in all four quadrants and the epigastrium (Fig. 6-16). Note the frequency and character of the bowel sounds. Normally, bowel sounds occur from 5 to 34 times per minute and should be audible in all four quadrants. Three to five minutes is required before concluding the absence of bowel sounds. Bowel sounds are usually described as hypoactive, hyperactive, audible, or borborygmi (loud prolonged gurgles of hyperperistalsis). Hypoactive or absent bowel sounds are a result of decreased intestinal motility, such as with paralytic ileus, gangrenous bowel, peritonitis, intraabdominal bleeding, electrolyte disturbances, pneumonia, and appendicitis. Increased bowel sounds (hyperactive) are caused by increased motility such as occurs with gastroenteritis, diarrhea, and early mechanical obstruction. As the mechanical obstruction progresses, bowel sounds become hypoactive or absent. Note bruits (abnormal flow sounds heard over the aorta or renal or iliac arteries) (Fig. 6-17), a venous hum over the epigastric and umbilical region, or fraction rubs (grating sounds) over the liver and spleen (Fig. 6-18). A venous hum is a continuous noise indicative of increased collateral circulation between portal and systemic venous systems. Friction rubs are

Fig. 6-16. Auscultation for bowel sounds. High-pitched bowel sounds necessitate the use of the diaphragm of the stethoscope. Bowel sounds may be increased with diarrhea or early intestinal obstruction. They are decreased, then absent in paralytic ileus and peritonitis. Bowel sounds are high-pitched tinkling sounds from air under tension in a dilated bowel. Rushes of high-pitched sounds with abdominal cramping occur in intestinal obstruction.

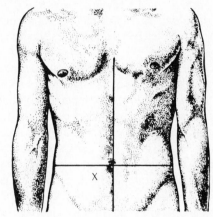

"X" indicates bowel sounds

Fig. 6-17. Sites of abdominal auscultation for systolic bruits suggestive of partial arterial obstruction or turbulent flow such as occurs in an aneurysm.

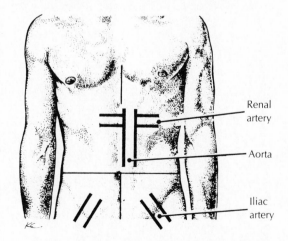

Renal artery

Aorta

Iliac artery

usually caused by liver tumor, infection, or infarction.

Percussion. Percussion is performed to (1) determine the size and location of the organs, (2) establish general orientation, and (3) detect air in the stomach and bowel. The examiner may percuss all areas of the abdomen and then palpate or may combine the two processes in each area before moving on to the next, as long as the approach is organized and systematic. Discussion here will be organized with the methods separate. Tender and painful areas should always be palpated last.

To establish general orientation, percuss all four quadrants, assessing general proportions and the distribution of tympany and dullness. The suprapubic area should be checked for the dullness of a distended bladder. Note areas full to percussion (from stool, masses, or increased fluid) as well as areas of tenderness.

Liver. Percussion of the liver only provides a gross estimate of liver size and location but probably provides the most accurate clinical method of estimating liver size. The liver is always percussed at the midclavicular line (MCL) and may also be percussed at the midsternal line (MSL).

Percussion at the midclavicular line will be discussed first. Start below the level of the umbilicus (not in an area of dullness), and percuss upward toward the liver. Find the liver border, usually located just above the right costal margin (RCM); mark with a pen. Identify the upper border of liver dullness in the midclavicular line (MCL) by percussing from lung resonance down from the right nipple toward liver dullness, usually between the fifth and seventh intercostal spaces (ICS) along the midclavicular line (MCL). Mark with a pen and measure the span. The average liver span at the midclavicular line is 6 to 12 cm. The liver can also be percussed at the midsternal line (MSL), using the same procedure. The average span is 4 to 8 cm but may be more in men and tall people (Fig. 6-19). If the liver is enlarged, it also may be desirable to measure size in the right anterior axillary line.

Spleen. The spleen is most easily percussed if it is enlarged. The primary purpose of percussing the spleen is to rule out enlargement. This is accomplished by identifying a small oval area of dullness near the left tenth rib just posterior to the midaxillary line (MAL). If the spleen is enlarged, this will change from tympany to dullness. Another method is to percuss the lowest

Fig. 6-18. Sites of abdominal auscultation. **A,** A venous hum indicative of increased collateral circulation between portal and systemic venous systems. **B,** Friction rubs that occur with inflammation of the peritoneal surface of an organ.

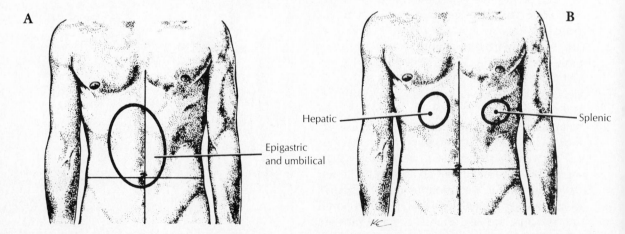

A

B

Hepatic

Splenic

Epigastric and umbilical

interspace in the left anterior axillary line. It is usually tympanitic. It should remain normal, or tympanitic, with deep inspiration unless the spleen is enlarged.

Stomach. Percussion of the gastric air bubble at the left lower anterior rib cage is tympanitic. Its size is variable. If the size of the gastric air bubble is increased and accompanied by upper abdominal distention, gastric dilatation is suggested.

Palpation. Palpation is performed in order to (1) locate the abdominal organs, (2) determine the presence of masses or distention, and (3) detect tenderness. Two types of palpation are performed—light and deep. The patient's face should always be observed, as facial expression may change with discomfort. Discomfort or pain may also provoke muscle guarding by the abdominal muscles.

Light palpation is performed in order to (1) identify muscular resistance, (2) identify superficial organs and masses, and (3) identify abdominal tenderness. The palmar surfaces of the fingertips are used. Press the hand lightly and systematically over all four quadrants. Proceed systematically, using a gentle dipping motion and moving smoothly. Using light palpation, check for tenderness, increased muscle tone, abdominal stiffening, organs or masses. Malingering can be detected by pressing the stethoscope on the abdomen, producing a pressure similar to that of light palpation. To differentiate voluntary muscle spasm in the abdomen from involuntary spasm, such as that from peritoneal inflammation, may involve two possible approaches. Try all maneuvers to make the patient and his abdomen relax. In addition, check for normal relaxation of the rectus muscle with expiration. If it remains rigid even with all suggested maneuvers, the spasm is probably involuntary.

Deep palpation is used to delineate the deep abdominal organs and masses and to elicit deep pain. All four quadrants are explored, using the palmar surfaces of the fingers. It is essential that the patient be relaxed. He should be warned that the deep palpation may cause some discomfort. Deep abdominal breathing may help to relax the patient. Deep palpation is difficult to perform on the obese or resistant person. The use of two hands may help, pressing with the top hand and feeling with the bottom hand.

All areas should be checked systematically and carefully for masses and for tender areas. Masses should be described in the following aspects: location, size, consistency, pulsations, tenderness, contour, and mobility. Tender areas should be noted, and the abdomen should be checked specifically for rebound tenderness by pressing deeply and then quickly letting go. If the pain increases when quickly released, rebound tenderness is present (+), indicating peritoneal inflammation.

Deep palpation is performed on the liver to detect enlargement or tenderness. Two techniques exist and whatever is going to be done should be explained previously to the patient. In the first method (Fig. 6-20, *top*), the left hand is placed on the posterior thorax at the eleventh or twelfth rib. Press upward to support. The right hand is placed on the right abdomen at a 45-degree angle to the right rectus muscle along

Fig. 6-19. Percussion of the liver.

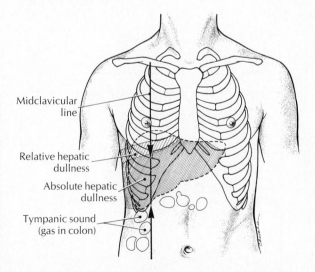

Midclavicular line

Relative hepatic dullness

Absolute hepatic dullness

Tympanic sound (gas in colon)

the rib cage, with the fingertips below the lower border of liver dullness pointing toward the right costal margin (RCM). The patient inspires deeply, causing the liver edge to descend. As the patient inhales, the examiner slides a finger under the costal margin, pressing in and up. The normal liver edge is felt during inspiration as a firm sharp regular ridge with a smooth surface. Sometimes only increased resistance is felt. The liver edge is followed medially and laterally.

With the second method, called *hooking* (Fig. 6-20, *bottom*), stand at the patient's right and face caudally. Place both hands, side by side, on the right abdomen below the border of liver dullness. Press in and up while the patient takes a deep breath.

Even when the liver is not palpable, it is important to check for tenderness. The examin-

er's left hand is placed flat on the patient's lower right rib cage, while the ulnar surface of the right fist is used to strike the left hand. The patient is asked to compare the sensations on both sides.

An attempt is made to palpate the spleen in the following manner, although it is highly unlikely that it will be palpable unless it is three times its normal size (Fig. 6-21). With the left hand reach over and around the patient for support and press the lower left rib cage anteriorly. Place the right hand below the left costal margin and press in toward the spleen. Have the patient inspire deeply. The tip or edge of the spleen may be felt as it descends during inspiration. To facilitate palpation this procedure may be repeated with the patient on her right side with the legs flexed at the hips and knees.

The kidneys are usually not palpable except in a child or very thin adult. The right kidney is more likely to be palpable than the left. The purpose of palpation of the kidneys is to feel the lower pole of the kidney between the palpating hands to determine kidney size. Enlarged kidneys may be caused by hyponephrosis, neoplasm, or polycystic disease.

Place one hand along the inferior edge of the costal margin on the right anterior abdominal area. Place the other hand on the posterior thorax at the same place. As the patient inspires deeply, push both hands together. The kidney

Fig. 6-20. Palpation of the liver illustrating two techniques. See text for explanation.

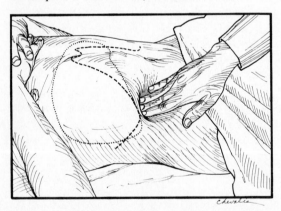

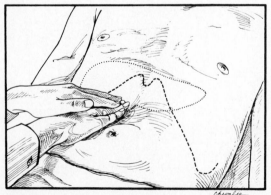

Fig. 6-21. Palpation of the spleen.

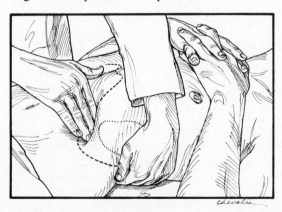

descends with inspiration and the pole, if felt, will be felt between the hands (Fig 6-22). The same process is used for the other side.

Costovertebral (CVA) tenderness may be caused by kidney inflammation. Although it is appropriate for the convenience of the patient to postpone checking it until examining the back, it will be discussed here. Place the palm of the left hand over each costovertebral angle while striking lightly with the ulnar surface of the right fist. The patient without kidney inflammation should experience a jar or thud, but not pain.

The aorta is felt as a tube structure to the left of the umbilicus in the epigastric area. To palpate the aorta, press firmly deep into the upper abdomen, slightly left of the midline to detect the pulsation of the aorta. Try to place the thumb along one side and the fingers along the other side, feeling for expansile pulsation. Prominent pulsation plus lateral expansion is indicative of an aortic aneurysm. The normal aorta or an aorta covered by a mass produces a pulsation forward without lateral movement.

Physical signs of malnutrition

Practically all areas of the body can be affected by malnutrition, so that when the patient is examined by the astute observer, different signs specific to various deficiencies can be detected and are of great use in diagnosis. Areas to be observed include the hair, face, eyes, lips, tongue, teeth, gums, glands, skin, nails, subcutaneous tissue, muscular and skeletal systems, cardiovascular system, gastrointestinal system, and nervous system. Table 6-2 is a summary of information about physical signs of malnutrition.

Diagnostic studies used with the acutely ill GI patient

Many types of studies are employed to identify the source of problems in GI patients. Some are useful in evaluating the prognosis and monitoring the patient in the course of therapy. These tests often include laboratory, radiologic, cytologic, and endoscopic procedures. Descriptions of some of them follow.

Complete blood count (CBC)

The CBC consists of a series of tests of the peripheral blood that provides invaluable data about many organ systems, including the GI system. For a review of these tests the reader is referred to Units 2 and 7.

Fasting blood sugar (FBS)

This test is performed prior to eating breakfast to measure glucose, the principle fuel for all body activities, in the blood. Disease processes as well as certain normal physiologic variables (age, sex, emotional state, dietary pattern, exercise, and time since last meal) can affect the fasting blood glucose levels.

Hyperglycemic values are associated with the following:
Mild hyperglycemia (120 to 150 mg/100 ml)
 Hypertension
 Acute shock, injury, trauma, stress, infection
 Overweight
 Thiazide diuretics
Moderate hyperglycemia (300 to 500 mg/100 ml
 Anesthesia
 Infectious diseases
 Intracranial diseases and cerebral lesions
Marked hyperglycemia (>500 mg/100 ml)
 Diabetes mellitus

Fig. 6-22. Palpation of the kidneys.

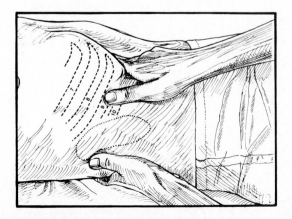

Table 6-2. Physical signs indicative or suggestive of malnutrition

	Normal appearance	Signs associated with malnutrition	Possible disorder or nutrient deficiency	Possible non-nutritional problem
Hair	Shiny; firm; not easily plucked	Lack of natural shine; dull and dry Thin and sparse Silky and straight; fine Dyspigmented Flag sign Easily plucked (no pain)	Kwashiorkor and, less commonly, marasmus	Excessive bleaching of hair Alopecia
Face	Skin color uniform; smooth, pink, healthy appearance; not swollen	Nasolabial seborrhea (scaling of skin around nostrils) Swollen face (moon face) Paleness	Riboflavin Iron Kwashiorkor	Acne vulgaris
Eyes	Bright, clear, shiny; no sores at corners of eyelids; membranes a healthy pink and moist; no prominent blood vessels or mound of tissue or sclera	Pale conjunctiva Red membranes Bitot's spots Conjunctival xerosis (dryness) Corneal xerosis (dullness) Keratomalacia (softening of cornea) Redness and fissuring of eyelid corners Corneal arcus (white ring around eye) Xanthelasma (small yellowish lumps around eyes)	Anemia (e.g., iron) Vitamin A Riboflavin, pyridoxine Hyperlipidemia	Bloodshot eyes from exposure to weather, lack of sleep, smoke, or alcohol
Lips	Smooth, not chapped or swollen	Angular stomatitis (white or pink lesions at corners of mouth) Angular scars Cheilosis (redness or swelling of lips and mouth)	Riboflavin	Excessive salivation from improperly fitting dentures

Krause, M.V., and Mahan, K.: Food, nutrition and diet therapy: a textbook of nutritional care, ed. 7, Philadelphia, 1984, W.B. Saunders Co.

Table 6-2. Physical signs indicative or suggestive of malnutrition—cont'd

	Normal appearance	Signs associated with malnutrition	Possible disorder or nutrient deficiency	Possible non-nutritional problem
Tongue	Deep red in appearance; not swollen or smooth	Scarlet and raw tongue	Nicotinic acid	Leukoplakia
		Magenta (purplish) tongue	Riboflavin	
		Swollen tongue	Niacin	
		Filiform papillae atrophy or hypertrophy	Folic acid Vitamin B_{12}	
Teeth	No cavities; no pain; bright	Mottled enamel	Fluorosis	Malocclusion
		Caries (cavities)	Excessive sugar	Periodontal disease
		Missing teeth		Health habits
Gums	Healthy; red; do not bleed; not swollen	Spongy, bleeding Receding gums	Vitamin C	Periodontal disease
Glands	Face not swollen	Thyroid enlargement (front of neck swollen)	Iodine	Allergic or inflammatory enlargement of thyroid
		Parotid enlargement (cheeks become swollen)	Starvation	
Skin	No signs of rashes, swelling, or dark or light spots	Xerosis (dryness)	Vitamin A	Environmental exposure
		Follicular hyperkeratosis (sandpaper feel to skin)		
		Petechiae (small skin hemorrhages)	Vitamin C	
		Pellagrous dermatosis (red swollen pigmentation of areas exposed to sunlight)	Nicotinic acid	
		Excessive bruising	Vitamin K	Physical abuse
		Flaky paint dermatosis	Kwashiorkor	
		Scrotal and vulval dermatosis	Riboflavin	
		Xanthomas (fat deposits under skin around joints)	Hyperlipidemia	
Nails	Firm; pink	Koilonychia (spoon-shaped)	Iron	
		Brittle; ridged		
Subcutaneous tissue	Normal amount of fat	Edema	Kwashiorkor	
		Fat below standard	Starvation; marasmus	
		Fat above standard	Obesity	

Continued.

Table 6-2. Physical signs indicative or suggestive of malnutrition—cont'd

	Normal appearance	Signs associated with malnutrition	Possible disorder or nutrient deficiency	Possible non-nutritional problem
Muscular and skeletal systems	Good muscle tone; some fat under skin; can walk or run without pain	Muscle wasting	Starvation, marasmus, kwashiorkor	
		Craniotabes (thin, soft skull bones in infant)		
		Frontal and parietal bossing (round swelling of front and side of head)		
		Epiphyseal enlargement (swelling of ends of bones)	Vitamin D	
		Persistently open anterior fontanelle (soft area on head closes late)		
		Knock knees or bow legs		
		Musculoskeletal hemorrhages	Vitamin C	
		Calf muscle tenderness	Thiamin	
		Thoracic rosary	Vitamin D; vitamin C	
		Fractures in elderly	Osteoporosis	
Cardiovascular system	Normal heart rate and rhythm; no murmurs or abnormal rhythms; normal blood pressure for age	Cardiac enlargement Tachycardia	Thiamin	
		Elevated blood pressure	Sodium?	
Gastrointestinal system	No palpable organs or masses (in children, however, liver edge may be palpable)	Hepatosplenomegaly	Kwashiorkor	
Nervous system	Psychologic stability; normal reflexes	Psychomotor changes	Kwashiorkor	
		Mental confusion	Nicotinic acid; thiamin	
		Depression	Pyridoxine;	
		Sensory loss	vitamin B_{12}	
		Motor weakness		
		Loss of position sense		
		Loss of vibration	Thiamine	
		Loss of ankle and knee jerks		
		Burning and tingling of hands and feet (paresthesia)		

Hypoglycemia (<65 mg/100 ml) may be caused by extensive liver disease, hyperinsulinism from a pancreatic lesion or insulin overdose, hypoadrenalism, hypopituitarism, hypothyroidism, vomiting, prolonged fever, or malnutrition.

The procedure for blood collection for an FBS is as follows: (1) NPO after midnight, (2) no insulin until specimen is drawn, and (3) utilize blood within 30 minutes after drawing.

Blood urea nitrogen (BUN)

Urea is the end product of protein metabolism; it is produced in the liver and carried by the blood to the kidneys for excretion. The blood urea nitrogen (BUN) test measures the concentration of urea in serum or plasma and is most commonly used as a screening test for renal disease. It is determined and reported in terms of urea nitrogen because urea alone is difficult to measure, but the nitrogen contained in the urea is relatively easy to analyze.

BUN values are slightly higher in men than in women. Multiplying BUN values by 2.14 will give urea values. Decreased BUN values may result from acute liver destruction and cirrhosis (rare until 80% to 85% of liver function is lost), hemodialysis, malnutrition or low-protein intake, or nephrosis. Elevated BUN results may be from renal disease; excess protein ingestion; cachexia; dehydration; increased protein catabolism, and decreased renal blood flow or decreased urine production (burns, massive hemorrhage); visceral damage; and pancreatitis. Elevated urinary urea nitrogen values may result from febrile conditions, GI bleeding, or malnutrition. Decreased urinary urea nitrogen values are potentially due to acidosis, cirrhosis or acute liver destruction, dehydration, or hypovolemic or surgical shock.

Serum enzymes

Serum enzymes, which will be discussed in this chapter, include amylase, lipase, LDH5, SGOT, and SGPT. Each body organ contains its own characteristic enzymes, which act as catalysts to speed the rate of many metabolic reac-tions. When tissue cells are damaged or destroyed, these enzymes enter the blood after release from the tissues and can be measured as an indicator of the size and degree of tissue damage. This is complicated by the fact that many enzymes are found in more than one type of tissue and most tissues contain more than one enzyme. Isoenzymes are enzymes with a similar function in each organ but having unique structural and physical characteristics. Each of the aforementioned enzymes will be discussed separately in the following paragraphs.

Amylase. Amylase, a digestive enzyme active in breaking down starch, is produced in the pancreas and salivary glands.

Elevated serum amylase levels may occur with acute pancreatitis, an acute exacerbation of chronic pancreatitis; carcinoma of the head of the pancreas; intestinal obstruction; perforated gastric or duodenal ulcers; renal disease with impaired excretion; some narcotic analgesics (morphine within 24 hours of blood sampling); or after upper abdominal surgery. Low serum amylase levels may be associated with extensive pancreatic destruction or severe liver damage. Falsely elevated serum and urinary amylase levels may occur within 24 hours after administration of certain drugs: bethanechol chloride (Urecholine), codeine, diatrizoate sodium (Hypaque), indomethacin, meperidine, morphine, pentazocine hydrochloride (Talwin), or thiazide diuretics.

Amylase remains stable in serum specimens at room temperature for about a week or for several months when refrigerated or frozen immediately. Blood specimens should be collected preferably before performance of any diagnostic procedures using dyes or medications. Urine specimens should be collected at accurate times and kept refrigerated or on ice until sent to the laboratory.

Lipase. Lipase is a hydrolytic enzyme secreted by the pancreas into the duodenum, where combined with bile salts and calcium ions, it splits fats and triglycerides into fatty acids and glycerol. Lipase, like amylase, is found in the blood stream after pancreatic damage has occurred. Like amylase, it is useful in diagnosing pancreatic disorders.

Elevated serum lipase levels are associated with acute pancreatitis. Lipase levels remain elevated longer than amylase—up to 10 days—and are useful in following the progress of acute pancreatitis. Other causes of elevated lipase levels include obstruction of a pancreatic duct, high intestinal obstruction, pancreatic carcinoma, renal disease involving impaired excretion, or perforated duodenal ulcers. False elevations are caused by administration of opiates or other narcotics within 24 hours of the drawing of the blood specimen. If drugs that cause false elevations have been given within 24 hours of obtaining the specimen, this should be indicated to the laboratory.

Lipase remains stable in serum for 1 week at room temperature and for around 6 weeks if refrigerated or frozen right after drawing. Preferably, the serum sample should be drawn after an overnight fast.

Lactic dehydrogenase (LDH). Lactic dehydrogenase (LDH) is found in nearly all cells of the body that undergo metabolism, with especially high concentrations in heart, liver, brain, kidney, skeletal muscle, and red blood cells (RBC). LDH levels can be elevated as a result of many pathologic processes, but are of special use in diagnosing myocardial infarction, pulmonary infarction, and liver disease.

Electrophoretic methods separate the LDH into five distinct molecular forms or isoenzymes. Isoenzyme electrophoresis gives more specific information and thus is more useful diagnostically. Each of the LDH isoenzymes occurs in different proportions and concentrations in tissues and organs of the body. They appear in the following tissues:

LDH1 —heart, brain, RBC
LDH2 —heart, brain, RBC
LDH3 —lung, spleen, pancreas, thyroid, adrenals, kidneys
LDH4 —liver, skeletal muscle, kidney, brain
LDH5 —liver, kidney, skeletal muscle

Normal isoenzyme concentrations are usually the following:

LDH1 18% to 33%
LDH2 28% to 40%
LDH3 16% to 30%
LDH4 6% to 16%
LDH5 2% to 13%

LDH5. LDH5, identified as the liver isoenzyme, can be elevated several days prior to the appearance of jaundice or with acute pancreatitis, drug-associated hepatitis, shock, and other causes of liver damage such as cirrhosis and congestive heart failure. It is not affected by purely obstructive jaundice.

Glutamic-oxaloacetic transaminase (SGOT). The liver stores many enzymes, that are released when the liver is damaged, including SGOT and SGPT. SGOT is released from liver, heart, kidney, lungs, skeletal muscle, pancreas, and kidneys when there is damage to tissue. SGOT levels serve as an indication of the extent and severity of tissue damage because SGOT leaks into the serum from dead or damaged cells. It is a sensitive indicator of tissue necrosis but does not indicate the exact site. SGOT levels are used to follow the progress of patients with myocardial and liver diseases.

Marked elevations of SGOT levels are associated with acute myocardial infarctions, infectious hepatitis, and toxic hepatitis. Slight to moderate SGOT levels are associated with acute pancreatitis; bile duct obstruction, obstructive jaundice, or cholangiolitic jaundice; cirrhosis of the liver; shock and trauma; liver abscess; and liver metastasis.

Glutamic-pyruvic transaminase (GPT). GPT is more specifically identified with the liver than is GOT. It occurs in small concentrations in kidney, heart, and skeletal muscle, in addition to occurring in high concentrations in the liver. GPT is released during liver damage in amounts paralleling the degree of hepatic necrosis. When compared to GOT levels, it can be a useful indicator for differentiating cardiac and hepatic tissue damage.

Again, normal ranges vary with the method

used and should be clarified with each laboratory used. Marked GPT elevations occur with hepatic necrosis, infectious hepatitis, toxic hepatitis, and viral hepatitis. Slight to moderate GPT elevations occur with acute pancreatitis, cirrhosis, infectious hepatitis, metastatic hepatic tumor, and obstructive jaundice.

GPT remains stable in serum for three days at room temperature; it remains stable in serum for up to a week when refrigerated. It is not stable when frozen.

Liver function tests (LFTs)

Liver function tests are performed for numerous reasons: to detect the presence of liver disease, to determine the severity of the problem, to follow the progress of the disease, and to determine the type of liver disease. Determining the complete clinical or diagnostic picture of liver disease requires the performance of a group of carefully selected tests; no one single measurement gives all of the necessary information. Frequently used liver function tests include blood ammonia, BSP excretion, fecal urobilinogen, flocculation tests, serum bilirubin, serum enzymes (alkaline phosphatase, GOT, GPT, LDH), serum protein, bilirubin, and urine urobilinogen. In the next sections we will discuss bilirubin, serum albumin, and total protein.

Bilirubin. Bilirubin is a major product of hemoglobin breakdown. Its level in serum can be estimated; when this level is elevated, it is associated with the presence of jaundice. Both bilirubin metabolism and jaundice are discussed in depth in later sections of this chapter (p. 473).

An elevated total serum bilirubin (hyperbilirubinemia) level is associated with hemolytic jaundice, hepatic jaundice, and obstructive jaundice. An elevated indirect bilirubin level is associated with acute alcoholic hepatitis, cirrhosis, hemorrhage into body cavities and soft tissues, autoimmune or transfusion-induced hemolysis, hepatitis B, or septicemia. An elevated direct bilirubin is associated with acute alcoholic hepatitis, biliary obstruction from certain medications, carcinoma of the head of the pancreas, cirrhosis, hepatitis, and obstructive disease of the biliary system. (Refer to Tables 6-7 and 6-8.)

Serum specimens for bilirubin are stable for up to 1 week when refrigerated or for 3 months when frozen. Specimens should be protected from strong light to prevent lowering of bilirubin levels.

Drugs that can cause false elevations of serum bilirubin are numerous, but include the following: androgens, chlorpromazine, erythromycin, indomethacin, isoniazid, salicylates, methanol, nitrofurantoin, oxacillin, phenothiazines, phenylbutazone, certain radiopaque contrast media, and sulfonamides.

Plasma proteins. Plasma proteins are synthesized in the liver and reticuloendothelial system, contributing antibodies, enzymes, and hormones to the blood. Their physiologic function is different from tissue proteins. Functions of plasma proteins include the following: providing a source of rapid tissue replacement during tissue depletion, maintaining osmotic pressure and water balance between blood and tissue, serving as pH buffers for acid-base balance, maintaining a reserve of protein for tissue growth and repair, transporting various blood constituents, functioning as immunologic agents, providing essential coagulation factors as well as enzymes, and providing for the body's nitrogen needs. Proteins are present in the plasma as globulins, albumin, and fibrinogen.

Total protein. Total protein is determined on serum specimens and represents a quantitative measure of combined albumin and globulins in the blood. It is useful as a screening test for diseases that alter protein balance or body hydration, especially when used with albumin values and A/G ratio calculations.

Serum protein may be elevated from dehydration, vomiting, diarrhea, hemoconcentration, or multiple myeloma. Depressed serum protein levels may occur with severe hemorrhage, malnutrition, liver damage, infectious hepatitis, cirrhosis, malabsorption, sprue, kwashiorkor, protein-losing enteropathies, renal disease, water intoxication, or severe burns.

Serum protein levels may be falsely elevated when free hemaglobin or BSP dye is in the serum specimen. Serum specimens are stable for 1 week if refrigerated at 4° C.

Serum albumin. Albumin, the smallest of the protein molecules, comprises about 52% to 68% of the total protein value. Albumin is important in maintaining colloid oncotic pressure, which regulates fluid exchange and stabilizes blood volume, as well as serving as a transport mechanism for substances not soluble in water alone (bilirubin, fatty acids, cortisol, drugs).

Hyperalbuminemia can occur from dehydration, hemoconcentration, prolonged vomiting, or diarrhea. Hypoalbuminemia may occur with chronic liver disease, malnutrition, malabsorption, protein-losing enteropathies, and acute or chronic infections.

Schilling test

The Schilling test tells if vitamin B_{12} absorption is defective or if the absorptive mechanisms are intact but intrinsic factor (IF) is deficient. Absorption of dietary vitamin B_{12} requires it to be bound to intrinsic factor. Pernicious anemia is a result of a deficiency of intrinsic factor and decreased vitamin B_{12} absorption. Vitamin B_{12} deficiency may also result from intestinal malabsorption syndromes or resective surgical procedures.

The patient is given a dose (0.5 to 1.0 μg) of radioactive ^{57}Co-tagged vitamin B_{12} by mouth after parenteral injection of 1000 mg of unlabeled vitamin B_{12}. All urine is collected for 24 hours. The amount of radiolabeled vitamin excreted is compared with the amount given. The result is expressed as a percentage of excretion.

Normally 15% to 40% of the smaller dose or 5% to 40% of the larger dose is excreted within 24 hours. Accurate test results depend on normal urinary excretion and successful collection of all urine for 24 hours.

If the initial test reveals decreased vitamin B_{12} absorption, it is necessary to determine the cause. The test is repeated with 60 mg of intrinsic factor administered by mouth along with vitamin B_{12}. Urinary radioactive ^{57}Co-tagged vitamin B_{12} excretion rises to normal when intrinsic factor is added if the problem is from an intrinsic factor deficiency. If it remains low, then the cause is intestinal disease or abnormal competition for B_{12} in the bowel lumen.

Secretin test

The secretin test is a test of pancreatic secretion, making possible the recognition of deceased pancreatic secretion for any cause. While it is standardized and sensitive as a diagnostic test, it is so sensitive that it often gives clinically insignificant information.

A double-lumen tube is positioned in the patient's duodenum under fluoroscopic guidance. Gastric secretion is aspirated through one lumen and pancreatic secretion through the other lumen. Two 10-minute collections of basal secretions are made, after which 1 unit of secretin/kilogram of body weight is administered intravenously. Following this, four 20-minute samples are collected, and the volume of bicarbonate is measured in each. Enzyme assays may also be done on pooled samples.

The total volume after administration of secretin should measure at least 2 ml/kg. After secretin is administered, the maximal bicarbonate concentration in any sample should exceed 90 mEq/L. Normal values for enzymes will vary with the laboratory.

One suggestion for interpreting results of the secretin test is as follows: (1) complete ductal obstruction leads to a marked decrease in volume bicarbonate and enzymes; (2) with partial ductal obstruction the volume will be low but bicarbonate and enzymes will be normal; (3) chronic pancreatitis will be associated with normal volume, low bicarbonate concentration, and normal or low enzyme concentration.

Lundh test meal

The Lundh test meal measures the concentration of pancreatic enzymes secreted in response to ordinary digestive stimuli and the effect of pancreatic enzymes upon the components of that meal. For example, triglycerides, fatty acids, and conjugated and unconjugated bile salts may be measured.

The proximal jejunum is intubated with a polyvinyl tube, and 300 ml of a test meal containing protein, carbohydrate, and fat is drunk after an overnight fast. The jejunal contents are aspirated in four half-hour samples and concentrations of pancreatic enzymes are measured. The results are altered when pancreatic insufficiency exists.

Gastric acid secretory studies

Measurement of gastric acid secretion is accomplished, in both resting and stimulated states, by this test. Gastric secretion mechanisms were discussed earlier in this chapter. This test is useful principally for demonstrating anacidity* (pH should be less than 6.0) and determining Zollinger-Ellison syndrome.

Gastric secretions are collected by aspiration from a tube passed through the mouth or nasopharynx into the stomach. Fluoroscopic monitoring can help to ensure good intragastric placement, with the uncurled or untwisted tube tip at the most dependent position of the stomach. This is performed in the morning after an overnight fast.

The basal collection is performed by removing the fasting contents, observing for volume, color, and gross composition. The gastric secretions are collected for a total of 1 hour at 15-minute intervals. It is best to collect the samples by continuous suction. Results are reported as milliequivalents/hour.

The stimulated collection determines maximal acid production. Histamine (histamine acid phosphate 0.04 mg/kg body weight) is given in the United States and synthetic gastrin (Pentagastrin) is given in Great Britain and Europe to stimulate maximal production. An antihistamine may be given 30 minutes prior to the histamine

injection to decrease the side effects. After the stimulant is given, 15-minute collections are withdrawn sequentially for 1 hour. The acidity of each is measured separately. Results are expressed as MAO = the total amount of acid produced in an hour after pharmacologic stimulation (milliequivalents/hour or percent increase over basal output) and PAO = the sum of the two highest consecutive 15-minute values (milliequivalents/30 minutes).

Fecal fat

Stools are analyzed to quantitate fat excretion and detect excess fecal fat, which can result in steatorrhea. It does not, however, distinguish maldigestion from malabsorption. To perform the test it is necessary to know the dietary intake of fat and have a timed stool collection.

The usual procedure involves administering a diet of 100 grams of fat daily and collecting all stools for 3 days in order to determine the total fat excretion by microscopic evaluation.

Excretion of more than 5 grams of fat per day is abnormal. Abnormal results are associated with pancreatic disease with resulting inadequate levels of lipolytic enzymes and with intestinal malabsorption of fat.

Stool for occult blood

Feces are examined to detect blood in the feces by using reagents that interact with heme compounds. Blood loss can be established but not quantitated accurately. Normally blood loss occurs in the stool at the rate of 1-3 ml per day.

Common reagents include orthotolidine and guiac. Orthotolidine is most sensitive. Benzidine gives fewer false positives, but its use is discouraged as it is a potential carcinogen. Guiac must be made up fresh monthly. It is much less sensitive but best for routine screening because it results in fewer false positives and does not require a meat-free diet. Hemocult packets are also available for use now but are probably of primary benefit for outpatients.

Common causes of positive tests for occult blood in stools include these: upper gastrointes-

---

Anacidity is extreme hyperacidity.

tinal—peptic ulcer disease, bleeding varices, gastritis, and gastric carcinoma; lower gastrointestinal—colitis, colon carcinoma, and diverticulitis. Between 2 and 5 ml of swallowed blood can give a positive occult blood report.

Patients who are eating should be on a meat-free diet for three days before stool is tested for occult blood to avoid false positive results.

Roentographic studies

X-rays. Radiologic tests used in diagnosing gastrointestinal disorders include various modalities: plain films, contrast studies, ultrasound, radioisotope studies (nuclear medicine), and angiography. X-ray examination is extremely valuable in diagnosing disorders of the gastrointestinal system. Examination by x-ray of all parts of the gastrointestinal system can be accomplished. In addition, cineradiographs of the esophagus are useful in diagnosing upper esophageal disorders. Any time multiple radiographic examinations of the gastrointestinal system are being performed, it is important to determine the appropriate sequence so that one does not interfere with the performance of another, as well as to consider any contraindications to the proposed radiologic study. Patients should be instructed regarding the purpose of the tests, any dangers or risks, special procedures, and preparation.

Barium studies. Special radiologic examinations using barium as contrast medium are invaluable in diagnosing certain gastrointestinal disorders. These include an upper GI series, with or without small bowel follow-through, and a barium enema.

An *upper GI series* or *barium swallow* visualizes (as the patient swallows the barium) the esophagus, stomach, and small intestine, all or in part, in order to detect structural or functional abnormalities. Preparation for the test simply involves not eating or drinking anything within eight hours or so of the examination, as well as eliminating smoking and medications. These restrictions should be maintained until it has been determined that the examination, which may include a small bowel follow-through, has

been completed. Various disorders may be detected using this procedure: in the esophagus—diverticula, polyps, tumors, hiatal hernia; in the stomach—ulcers or tumors; in the small intestine—obstruction, polyps, diverticuli, pressure externally, ulcerations, and motility. In terms of special manuevers, the procedure may vary depending on the area to be looked at anatomically and functionally. For instance, in order to avoid rapid transit down the esophagus, which might occur if the patient stood to drink the barium, the patient might be given a thicker barium solution to drink or might be placed supine. Trendelenberg's position might be used to detect gastric reflux. Problems with swallowing solids might be investigated by having the person swallow a barium-coated marshmallow. In evaluating the stomach, the patient will be asked to assume various positions on the x-ray table so that the barium will outline all portions of the gastric wall. Films of the small intestine may require a prolonged stay (up to 6 hours) in the x-ray department. Films are usually taken about every 30 minutes. Use of a cathartic or lubricant for 2 to 3 days and drinking lots of fluids (if possible) is helpful in assuring passage of the barium through the gastrointestinal system and out, thus preventing constipation.

A *barium enema,* or examination of the lower intestinal tract, allows visualization of the rectum, colon, and ileocecal junction. It should be performed before a barium swallow because it takes several days for the swallowed barium to pass through the gastrointestinal tract and this may alter lower colon findings. Results can also be affected if the colon and cecum are not empty of stool or mucus, or if enemas have been given within 2 or 3 hours prior to the procedure as they may irritate the colon and alter secretions and motility. Preparation for the test includes a cleansing procedure of a clear liquid diet for up to 24 hours and use of laxatives or enemas. Smoking should be avoided for a number of hours before the examination. The person should be told what to expect during the procedure and given an opportunity to ask questions.

A barium enema is useful in diagnosing many disorders of the colon. During the procedure, a thick barium solution will be instilled through a tube into the colon. It will be essential for the patient to be able to retain the barium in spite of the urge to defecate. With people who are unable to accomplish this, the barium may be administered using a French catheter and the balloon slightly inflated to prevent expulsion of the solution. The patient or table may be moved in different positions to move the barium throughout the colon. Air may be injected into the colon to detect smaller lesions or polypoid masses. This may add to the patient's discomfort. After the procedure is completed, enemas should be given until the returns are free of barium to prevent constipation and impaction from the barium solution. Any pain, fever, or bleeding should be reported.

A *cholecystogram* is commonly used to detect gallbladder disorders. The gallbladder is not well visualized on x-ray films unless orally ingested radiopaque dye is swallowed by the patient, absorbed by the small intestine, removed from the blood by the liver, excreted into the bile, and concentrated and stored by the gallbladder. Inability to visualize the gallbladder is usually indicative of biliary duct obstruction or the gallbladder's inability to concentrate the dye. The patient should be prepared both educationally and physiologically. A dye is given in the form of tablets to be swallowed the evening before with small amounts of water, and then nothing should be eaten, drunk, or smoked until the test is completed. Complications such as vomiting, diarrhea, abdominal cramps, or urinary complications, should be reported as they may alter the uptake of the dye. After the initial test, a fatty meal may be given to stimulate emptying of the gallbladder. Further, x-rays may be taken then to check patency of the ducts and emptying of the gallbladder. Because the dye contains iodine, the patient should be carefully questioned about hypersensitivity to iodine or its products. In addition, compromised liver and/or kidney status is of concern because the test dyes are primarily excreted by the liver with secondary excretion by the kidneys. Tests such as for protein-bound iodine and iodine uptake should be done prior to administering this dye.

Intravenous and *operative cholangiograms* allow visualization of the cystic, hepatic, and common bile duct and may be performed before, during, or after surgery. The procedure varies accordingly. The dye which is injected is selectively excreted by the liver into the biliary tract. Films are then made at intervals beginning after the injection, continuing until the height of concentration and the beginning of flow of the dye into the intestinal tract. Intravenous cholangiograms are useful when the patient cannot take things orally, after cholecystectomy, or when direct visualization of the ducts is desirable. Preparation for the test involves discussing the purpose and procedure with the patient, having the patient NPO, and having the intestinal tract cleared. When performed prior to surgery, the dye is given intravenously and then x-ray examinations are taken for up to 4 hours. The biliary ducts can be visualized within 10 to 30 minutes after injection and the gallbladder within 4 hours. Performed during surgery, the contrast medium is injected into the common bile duct under direct vision. This allows visualization of residual filling defects and common or hepatic duct stones. When the cholangiogram is done postoperatively, the dye is injected through a T tube or drain left in place in the common bile duct. If normal, the biliary structures fill readily and are visible immediately by fluoroscopy.

Percutaneous transhepatic cholangiogram, or "skinny needle," helps to establish the presence of obstruction in patients with jaundice, to determine the site of obstruction in jaundiced patients, and to give information about the nature of the obstruction. It is most valuable in distinguishing extrahepatic obstruction and hepatocellular disease from intrahepatic obstruction. Transhepatic cholangiography is based on the assumption that the intrahepatic ducts can be entered only when dilated from extrahepatic obstruction. The procedure itself involves administration of local anesthesia and the insertion of a long needle with fluoroscopic guidance into the liver at the right costal margin. As the needle is slowly withdrawn, constant suction is applied until a bile duct is entered. Bile can be withdrawn if a biliary radicle is dilated as a result of a mechanical obstruction. After the bile duct is punctured dye is instilled while fluoroscopy is used to monitor the filling of the hepatic and biliary trees. Information about the anatomy and physiology of the extrahepatic biliary system is thus obtained. The patient should be informed as to the potential risks and benefits of the procedure, and the procedure itself should be discussed with him. Biliary leakage or hemorrhage is a potential risk. Vital signs should be monitored regularly for 24 hours after the procedure, with careful assessment for sepsis or hemorrhage. Percutaneous transhepatic cholangiogram is contraindicated if a person has cholangitis.

Liver scans are used to obtain information about anatomic structures, changes in size, and the presence of subphrenic and subhepatic abscesses. It is also helpful in following the course of and progression of liver disease and response to treatment. The scans produce a picture giving information about the size, shape, location, and relative density of normally functioning hepatic cells. No special preparation of the patient is required, although he must be able to lay flat while the scanner moves above him. Explanation of what to expect should help the patient to be able to cooperate and not be frightened. Four different substances to carry radionuclides are currently used in liver scans: rose bengal (^{131}I), radioiodinated serum albumin (Risa-131), colloidal gold (^{198}Au), and technetium (^{99}Tc). Some are metabolized by the liver; some are taken up by the reticuloendothelial system; some are confined to the blood pool, acting as markers of the blood; and some act as markers of abnormal tissue (gallium). The radionucleide is injected, and then in 30 to 60 minutes scanning is begun. Hepatic scans cannot detect lesions smaller than 2.0 to 2.5 cm in diameter, nor do they provide histologic information. No special follow-up is required in the care of this patient after the procedure is completed.

Ultrasonography or *echography* is a relatively new diagnostic modality, used on many areas of the body with varying degrees of promise and accuracy. The quality of the results vary greatly with the experience of the person performing and interpreting the test. One of its greatest benefits is that it is noninvasive and almost without discomfort or known risks. High-frequency sound waves are emitted from a central transducer as repetitive pulses. They spread through homogeneous tissues unaltered, but when they come up against the boundary of different densities or tissues, they bounce back, causing "echoes." These are received by the receiver, which is housed in the same black box that produces the echoes. A series of dots reflects the location of an echo in the body. The brightness of each dot correlates with the strength of the echo. Abnormalities identified and preparation for the ultrasound of the abdomen and its organs varies with the exact area to be examined. No special follow-up care of the patient is necessary after completion of the examination.

Endoscopy

Endoscopy allows the direct visualization of various parts of the gastrointestinal tract through a lighted tube passed into the particular orifice to be observed. In recent years this has been greatly facilitated by the development of flexible endoscopes or flexible fiberoptic instruments. Photographs can and should be taken to document what the endoscopist sees. In addition, biopsies and cytologic specimens can be obtained, and removal of polyps can be accomplished. Upper endoscopy includes esophagoscopy, gastroscopy or examination of the first and second portions of the duodenum. Other common endoscopic procedures include colonoscopy, sigmoidoscopy, and endoscopic retrograde cholangiopancreatography (ERCP). Each will be discussed separately in terms of purpose of the procedure, preparation, the procedure itself, and follow-up care.

Esophagoscopy. Esophageal endoscopy provides direct visualization of the entire mucosa of the esophagus. It allows inspection of the lesion, biopsy, and acquiring specimens for cytology. Esophagoscopy can be used to describe a lesion suggested by x-ray, to obtain biopsies from masses or abnormal mucosa, and to obtain washings for exfoliative cytologic study. It is possible to detect inflammation, ulceration, hiatal hernia stricture, and varices. Evaluation of symptoms such as persistent dysphagia, indigestion, regurgitation, odynophagia, or substernal chest pain may be attempted.

Preparing the patient for the test includes the following: (1) allow nothing to eat or drink for about 6 hours before the test to decrease the patient's risk of aspiration; (2) remove dentures; (3) explain and discuss the purpose, risks and benefits, procedure, and follow-up care; (4) premedicate with a narcotic and/or sedative and atropine; (5) anesthetize throat and depress gag reflex by having patient suck a benzonatate (Tessalon) perle or gargle a teaspoon of intravenous diphenhydramine (Benadryl), or by spraying the back of the throat with a local anesthetic such as procaine.

During the procedure the patient will lay on his back or left side, while the esophagoscope is inserted into the mouth with the neck hyperextended and head supported. Swallowing may facilitate passage of the scope. The patient may be asked to change positions to facilitate visualizing various sections of the esophagus if the flexible esophagascope is used. Oral secretions may require suctioning.

Following the procedure, food and fluids should be withheld until the gag reflex returns. Patients should be observed for a time afterward until they are fully alert and able to swallow. A friend or relative may stay with them during this time. Observation for signs of perforation such as pain and elevated temperature should be performed.

Upper endoscopy—gastroscopy plus duodenoscopy. Upper endoscopy can include direct visualization of the esophagus, in addition to the stomach and first and second portions of the duodenum. The mucosa is observed for lesions, biopsy and brush cytology may be performed, and polyps may be removed. Like esophagoscopy, flexible instruments have greatly facilitated this procedure. Progression of disease and response to treatment can be followed. Motion pictures can be made to study gastric motility. Indications for gastroduodenoscopy include: acute and chronic gastritis, ulceration and tumors, pernicious anemia, bleeding, epigastric distress, and determination of postoperative conditions.

The preparation of the patient, procedure, and care following the procedure are essentially the same as those discussed for esophagoscopy.

Endoscopic retrograde cholangiopancreatography (ERCP). ERCP is done to visualize the pancreatic ducts and hepatobiliary tree radiologically. This procedure is not without risk, and therefore is justifiable only to seek an operable lesion or to prevent unnecessary surgery. A side-viewing fiberscope is passed into the duodenum, the papilla of Vater located, and a catheter passed through the papilla into the common bile duct and into the pancreatic duct so that dye can be injected. ERCP is most useful in the jaundiced patient in whom intravenous cholangiography cannot be carried out. ERCP is a new procedure, and much remains to be known about indications for its use and accuracy of the information obtained.

The patient is prepared for and informed about the procedure in the same manner as for an upper endoscopic procedure. Atropine and glucagon are given intravenously to induce duodenal hypotonia and relaxation of the ampullary sphincter.

Following the procedure, precautions similar to those after esophagoscopy should be taken. The patient should be observed for pancreatitis or cholangitis. Patients who have ostructed ducts or have retained dye should be covered immediately with antibiotics and drained surgically within 12 to 24 hours.

Colonoscopy. Colonoscopy is an endoscopic procedure, using a flexible fiberscope, which provides direct visualization of the entire colon including the transverse colon and often the ileocecal valve. It is possible to accomplish direct examination, biopsy of lesions or polyps, photography, excision, or fulgaration by this method. Visualization of the rectum is best accomplished through sigmoidoscopy performed before colonoscopy.

Major indications include the following: an abnormal barium enema, rectal bleeding, follow-up of patients who have previously had colonic polyps of cancer, lower bowel complaints and a normal barium enema, removal of polyps, or management of inflammatory bowel disease. Contraindications to colonoscopy include acute ulcerative colitis or diverticulitis, ischemic bowel disease, radiation colitis, pregnancy, or peritonitis.

The patient is prepared for colonoscopy in a manner similar to the following. Exact agents and process may vary from agency to agency. Thorough cleansing of the bowel is needed for adequate visualization, including clear liquid diet for 2 to 3 days before; a laxative the day before; nothing by mouth the day of the procedure; and a cleansing enema the night before and at least three hours before the procedure. The patient should be included in a discussion of the purpose of the test, the actual procedure, potential risks and benefits, and follow-up care.

During the procedure, the patient will be asked to lie in the left lateral decubitus position, although he may be asked to move into the supine position to aid insertion or passage of the colonoscope. Premedication may include meperidine, diazepam, and/or atropine. Discomfort and cramping may be experienced when air is introduced or when the colonoscope is being advanced around flexures.

Following the colonoscopy, observation for pain, temperature, rectal discomfort, bleeding, signs of sepsis or perforation, feeling of inability to pass gas, and left shoulder pain is important. The passage of flatus should be expected and encouraged.

Sigmoidoscopy (proctoscopy). Sigmoidoscopy can be performed using a flexible or rigid sigmoidoscope, of which there are many forms. With the sigmoidoscope the examiner can directly visualize the mucosa of the anal canal, rectum, and lower 15 cm of the sigmoid colon. Biopsies may be taken.

Indications for colonoscopy include intestinal, rectal, or anal symptoms and follow-up of patients who have had a neoplasm of the large bowel. Its use in routine screening for neoplasms has not been definitely established and is controversial.

Preparation for sigmoidoscopy focuses on cleansing of the colon. For adequate visualization the mucosa must be free of stool and mucus. This can be accomplished by numerous specific regimes, including increased fluid intake, cathartics the preceding day, a Fleet's enema the day of the procedure, and a light meal the evening before and morning of the procedure. This prep may be eliminated when evaluating diarrhea or ulcerative colitis.

The patient should be part of a discussion about the purpose, potential risks and benefits, preparation, and details of the procedure. The procedure itself is mildly uncomfortable and may require assuming an awkward position.

For this procedure the patient should assume a knee-chest or left lateral position unless a tilt table is used. He should be told that the instillation of air may cause some discomfort.

ALTERATIONS

Disorders in GI function can be psychologic, physiologic, or pathologic in origin. Regardless of the etiology, these disorders interrupt normal gastrointestinal tract function and consequently the nutritional status of the patient, causing both acute and chronic problems. The pathophysiology of these abnormalities is discussed in the following pages.

Dysphagia

Dysphagia is defined as difficulty swallowing; odynophagia is defined as painful swallowing. Physiologic causes of dysphagia can be divided into three categories: (1) "transfer dysphagia," which is difficulty in getting a bolus of food or fluid into the esophagus; (2) alterations in transport of the bolus of food down the esophagus; and (3) problems with the bolus entering the stomach from the esophagus (see outline in box at right).

The majority of dysphagias of the transfer type, are caused by neuromuscular incoordination due to primary neurologic or muscular disease involving the mouth, pharynx, or hypopharynx. This disorder accompanies poliomyelitis, amyotrophic lateral sclerosis, myasthenia gravis, dermatomyositis, muscular dystrophy, multiple sclerosis, and cerebrovascular disease. Other causes include pharyngoesophageal diverticulum (Zenker's diverticulum), carcinoma of the mouth, tongue, or hypopharyngeal region; cricopharyngeal dysfunction or incoordination; or retrosternal enlargement of the thyroid. Cricopharyngeal dysfunction occurs when the cricopharyngeus muscle fails to relax prior to the passage of a bolus of food. It occurs in association with thyrotoxic myopathy, poliomyelitis, and left or right recurrent laryngeal nerve paralysis. The person complains of mild dysphagia at the upper end of the esophagus, felt in the back of the throat as an inability to swallow.

The second type of dysphagia results from an alteration in passage of the bolus of food down the esophagus. Decreased, absent, disorganized or ineffective peristalsis can cause this type of dysphagia, as can obstruction of the esophagus. Scleroderma frequently is associated with loss of esophageal peristalsis. Obstruction can be extrinsic, such as from marked osteoarthritis of the cervical spine. However, extrinsic obstructions are rarely of clinical significance because of the great mobility of the esophagus. Obstruction can also be intrinsic, such as from a tumor or inflammatory stricture. Incidents of dysphagia from esophageal stricture usually occur predict-

---

TYPES OF DYSPHAGIA AND ASSOCIATED CAUSES

I. Transfer dysphagia

  A. Neuromuscular incoordination

  B. Zenker's diverticulum

  C. Carcinoma of mouth, tongue, hypopharyngeal region

  D. Cricopharyngeal dysfunction or incoordination

  E. Thyroid enlargement

II. Alterations in transport down esophagus

  A. Decreased, absent, disorganized, or ineffective peristalsis

  B. Extrinsic obstruction

  C. Intrinsic obstruction

    1. Tumor

    2. Stricture

  D. Esophageal spasm

III. Problems with bolus entering stomach

  A. LES dysfunction

    1. Achalasia

    2. Lower esophageal ring

  B. Stenosis

---

ably. Narrowing of the lumen as a result of malignancy may also interfere with the passage of food through the esophagus. Dysphagia of this type is usually noted first with solid food and may progress to liquids. At first, the difficulty is intermittent.

Esophageal spasm, primary or secondary, is another example of this second type of dysphagia. It occurs when peristaltic waves do not pass down the esophagus in a normal pattern so that several patterns occur at once. Peristalsis is normal from the pharynx to the upper esophagus; however, as the bolus of food enters the lower esophagus, whole portions contract asynchronously rather than sequentially. Peristalsis is inefficient and the passage of food is slowed as a result. Spasm is usually diffuse but can be localized. The resulting dysphagia the patient has occurs intermittently and unpredictably. When severe it may be accompanied by pain.

The third type of dysphagia, occurring as a result of problems with the bolus of food entering the stomach from the esophagus, can be caused by lower esophageal sphincter (LES) dysfunction such as with achalasia or scleroderma or by the presence of obstructing lesions, either benign or malignant, such as a lower esophageal ring.

Achalasia is a disorder of esophageal motility characterized by failure of the lower esophageal sphincter (LES) to relax and let food enter the stomach. It is primarily a disorder occurring in adults, the cause of which is unknown it is thought to be of neural origin. Usually the LES relaxes as a reflex response right after a swallow, allowing food to enter the stomach. The pressure of the LES drops to a level at least equal to the pressure of the stomach. In achalasia, the LES fails to relax and food accumulates in the esophagus until hydrostatic pressure builds up, finally forcing the esophageal contents to empty into stomach. When the LES fails to relax, it remains in a tonic state, and esophageal motility is disturbed. Achalasia may be abrupt in onset, but is usually gradual, causing slowly progressive dysphagia but not pain.

A lower esophageal ring is a concentric ring or weblike narrowing or indentation at the gastroesophageal junction, usually occurring in individuals over the age of 40. Esophageal motility is normal. The result is episodic dysphagia of short duration without heartburn. The dysphagia may be due in part to associated spasm.

Stenosis of the esophagus resulting from long-term reflux esophagitis is recognized by symptoms of hearburn changing to those of dysphagia. Such stenosis causes an obstruction that makes it difficult for the esophageal contents to move on. It usually occurs with a sliding hiatal hernia but may appear whenever the efficiency of the lower esophageal sphinctor is decreased, such as from scleroderma or prolonged gastric intubation.

In summary, the characteristics of the dysphagia may vary with the anatomic localization of the cause. An oropharyngeal location may involve symptoms of (1) regurgitation of liquid through the nose, (2) aspiration when swallowing, (3) pharyngeal pain when swallowing, or (4) inability of the tongue to move the bolus in the pharynx. When the cause of the dysphagia is located in the esophagus, symptoms may include (1) retrosternal fullness on swallowing, (2) the sensation that the bolus of food is stuck in the esophagus, or (3) the failure of the food to move and relief by regurgitation. Table 6-3 compares the symptoms and most common causes of dysphagia when the cause is located in the oropharynx and in the esophagus.

Odynophagia

Odynophagia, or painful swallowing, almost always is caused by an organic lesion of the esophagus. It may be indistinguishable from the pain of heartburn or from the chest pain of esophageal distention or esophageal contractions except when it occurs after swallowing. Pain from the esophagus usually has a burning or squeezing quality and may be localized or felt from the suprasternal notch to the xiphoid. Odynophagia may be caused by esophageal spasm or inflammation of the esophagus, such as the esophagitis of monilia or herpes.

Anorexia

Anorexia is defined in several ways: the loss of or reduced desire to eat, decreased appetite, or the inability to ingest dietary intake adequate for body needs. Anorexia, a nonspecific symptom occurring with many acute and chronic disorders, should be differentiated clinically from specific food intolerances and from sitophobia (the fear of eating because of subsequent or associated discomforts). Malnutrition, the inevitable sequela of anorexia, makes it a most worrisome occurrence. Without proper nutrition, the human body can neither maintain nor regain a healthy status.

The mechanisms that are operating in control

of feeding are not completely understood. Various theoretical explanations have been proposed. A summary of theories of appetite stimulation appear in Table 6-4. The hypothalamus interacts with the cerebal cortex, sensory stimuli, and internal chemical and physical factors, as described in the preceding physiology section and reviewed briefly here. Chemoreceptors are thought to be associated with control of the ingestive apparatus in a couple of ways. First, they serve a gating function, by selecting for ingestion those substances with high nutritive value and rejecting injurious or non-nutritive substances. Second, chemoreceptors are thought to serve a motivational or excitatory role by activating or driving the central nervous system mechanisms that control the rate of ingestion. In addition to the proposed functions of chemoreceptors, ingested substances within the GI tract are thought to counteract the excitatory effects of the stimulation of eating and result in inhibition of intake. Other factors proposed to be active in control of feeding include hypothalmic lesions, hormones, metabolites, body lipids, and amino acid concentrations in blood and extracellular fluids. Intake is thought to be increased by lesions in the ventromedial area (satiety center), which is an alpha adrenergic mechanism, and decreased by lesions in the lateral hypothalamus, involving beta-adrenergic and dopamine receptors. Intake is frequently influenced by systemic administration of some drugs. Hormones thought to be active in controlling ingestion of food include insulin, glucagon, epinephrine, enterogastrone, cholecystokinin, and polypeptides.

Hepatic disease, renal disease, and tumors are common problems of acute care patients known to be accompanied by anorexia. When evaluating the patient with anorexia, it is important to look for abnormalities of the gastrointestinal system first. When anorexia is accompanied by abdominal pain, it is likely that the disease process involves the stomach or possibly the pancreas. GI abnormalities such as decreased absorption, obstruction, hepatobiliary disease,

Table 6-3. Anatomic localization of dysphagia

Oropharyngeal	Esophageal
SYMPTOMS	
Regurgitation through nose	Sensation of bolus sticking in esophagus
Pain in pharynx when swallowing	
Aspiration with swallowing	Retrosternal fullness
Tongue unable to move food bolus in pharynx	Regurgitation does not relieve failure of bolus to move through esophagus
COMMON CAUSES	
Neuromuscular disorders (see text for more detail)	Diffuse esophageal spasm
	Strictures

Adapted from Harvey, A.M., et al.: The principles and practice of medicine, ed. 21, New York, 1984, Appleton-Century-Crofts.

motility disorders, and impaired digestion may contribute to the development of anorexia.

Various causes of anorexia in patients with tumors have been proposed and investigated. They include nonspecific disease symptoms (nausea, vomiting, fatigue, pain), altered host metabolism, psychologic factors, and treatment such as medication and surgery. The box on p. 465 gives a detailed summary.

Four possible mechanisms of the anorexia associated with liver disease have been considered: (1) a nonspecific response to sickness results in the central nervous system decreasing appetite; (2) postprandial hypoglycemia tells the central nervous system glucostats to decrease appetite; (3) the hepatic glucoreceptors become hypersensitive to incorrect messages to the central appetite control center; and (4) liver disease causes an amino acid imbalance in the plasma, and anorexia results.

Certain psychologic disorders such as depression, anorexia nervosa, and abnormal environment with its changed food preparation, different people, strange smells, and altered eating patterns affect food intake and can contribute to anorexia.

Table 6-4. Theories of appetite stimulation

Theory	Physiologic response	Effect on appetite
Glucostatic	↓ Blood sugar stimulates lateral nuclei to initiate a search for food;	Appetite increased
	↑ Blood sugar stimulates satiety center	Appetite decreased
Amino acid	↑ Blood amino acids stimulate the satiety center	Appetite decreased
Thermostat	↑ Heat from metabolism of food stimulates satiety center	Appetite decreased
Lipostatic	↑ In adipose tissue	Appetite decreased
Alimentary • Visceral receptors	Sensitivity to chemical, osmotic, and volumetric properties of food ingested	Appetite decreased
• Abdominal stretch receptors	↑ Volume in stomach—stretch receptors are stimulated and send impulses to satiety center	Appetite decreased
Hormonal • Enterogastrone • Cholecystokinin	Stimulated by fats and fatty acids secreted after food intake	Appetite decreased
• Glucagon	Stimulated by low blood sugar, causing glucogenolysis in liver and gluconeogenesis to increase blood sugar	Appetite decreased
• Insulin	Lowers plasma glucose by: ↑ Tissue utilization of glucose Promoting glucose storage as glycogen Promoting formation of fat from glucose ↓ Gluconeogenesis from amino acids	Appetite increased
• Epinephrine	Antagonizes insulin effect by causing breakdown of glycogen in the liver; inhibits insulin secretion	Appetite decreased
"Head receptors": sight, smell, taste, touch, texture	Contribute to the pleasure of eating, stimulate saliva flow, facilitate swallowing, stimulate gastric secretions	Appetite increased

Adapted from Donoghue, M., Nunnally, C., and Yaska, J.: Nutritional aspects of cancer care nursing: a self-learning module for nurses, 1980, Pennsylvania Division, American Cancer Society, p. 35.

PROPOSED CAUSES OF ANOREXIA IN PATIENTS WITH CANCER

Nonspecific manifestations of disease (fatigue)

Mechanical interference with the GI tract

Alterations of taste and/or smell perception (food aversions)

Treatment (chemotherapy, radiation therapy)

Production of lactate

Production of ketones

Hypothetical tumor toxins (small metabolites, peptides, oligonucleotides)

Direct effects on appetite center

Psychologic factors

Infection

Hypercalcemia

Uremia

Drugs (analgesics, sedatives, antiemetics, antibiotics)

Many additional systemic disturbances may contribute to anorexia, such as infection, cardiovascular disease, endocrine/metabolic disorders (for example, adrenal insufficiency, hypercalcemia, hypokalemia), lead and alcohol intoxication, constipation, nausea and vomiting, pain, and inactivity.

Nausea

Nausea and vomiting frequently go hand in hand but may occur separately. Nausea is a subjective feeling of the imminent desire to vomit. It is the conscious psychic recognition of subconscious excitation in an area of the medulla that is closely associated with or a part of the vomiting center. Nausea is frequently a prodrome to vomiting.

Nausea may be caused by irritative impulses from the GI tract, impulses from the lower brain associated with motion sickness, or impulses of the cerebral cortex to initiate vomiting. A common GI cause of nausea is distention or irritation of the duodenum or lower small intestine.

A number of physiologic responses are usually involved with nausea—hypersalivation, decreased gastric tone, diminished or absent gastric peristalsis, and increased duodenal and jejunal tone that results in reflux of duodenal contents into the stomach.

Severe nausea may involve altered autonomic activity, especially parasympathetic, resulting in pallor of the skin, increased perspiration, salivation, and occasional hypotension.

Vomiting

Vomiting, or emesis, is the forceful expulsion of the contents of the upper GI tract when any part of the GI tract becomes excessively irritated, overdistended, or overexcitable. The strongest stimulus for such vomiting is distention or irritation of the stomach or duodenum. The *vomiting center* or *emetic center,* which is thought to control the vomiting reflex, is probably located in the lateral reticular formation of the medulla at the level of the olivary nuclei, lying central to the solitary tract and its nucleus. The center is closely associated functionally and anatomically with the respiratory center, vasomotor nuclei, and a locus whose stimulation produces retching apart from vomiting. The associated activities of vomiting are thus accounted for, their activities coordinated by the vomiting center. The vomiting center is activated by afferent impulses that may arise from numerous parts of the body. Examples of these are tactile stimulation to the back of the throat; distention of stomach or duodenum to 20 mm Hg pressure; increased intracranial pressure; acceleration of the head; pain; and distention or injury of the uterus, renal pelvis, or bladder.

The vomiting act involves stimulation of the vomiting center to initiate it, resulting in (1) a deep breath, (2) raising the hyoid bone and larynx and opening of the cricoesophageal sphincter, (3) closure of the glottis, and (4) lifting the soft palate to close the posterior nares. Following this the diaphragm contracts strongly downward while the abdominal muscles contract, causing intragastric pressure to be elevated. The LES relaxes and the gastric contents are expelled up and out. Reflex elevation of the soft palate prevents reflux into the nasopharynx, while reflex closure of the glottis and inhibition of respiration prevent pulmonary aspiration.

It is thought that vomiting occurs when impulses from the various organs are carried by both vagal and sympathetic afferent fibers to the vomiting center of the medulla. Motor impulses for vomiting are then transmitted from the vomiting center through the fifth, seventh, ninth, tenth, and twelfth cranial nerves to the upper GI tract and through the spinal nerves to the diaphragm and abdominal muscles. Vomiting produced by this mechanism can result from various stimulants including copper sulfate PI; staphylococcus enterotoxin; GI, biliary, peritoneal, or mesenteric disease; pharyngeal stimulation; cardiac disease; and urogenital disease.

A second mechanism by which vomiting is thought to occur involves the chemoreceptor trigger zone (CTZ), located outside the vomit-

ing center bilaterally on the floor of the fourth ventricle in or above the area postrema. This mechanism is thought to be involved in vomiting caused by radiation sickness; electrical stimulation; administration of drugs including apomorphine, morphine, digitalis derivatives, copper sulfate given IV, and some anesthetics. Fig. 6-23 summarizes two mechanisms—those mediated through the vomiting center and those mediated through the chemoreceptor trigger zone.

A third mechanism is thought to be called into play when rapidly changing motions of the body result in vomiting. The motion stimulates receptors of the labyrinth, generating impulses transmitted by the vestibular nuclei into the cerebellum, which is then thought to stimulate the chemoreceptor trigger zone and then the vomiting center.

Cortical excitation of vomiting from psychic stimuli or psychological factors is thought to

---

Fig. 6-23. Diagram of proposed pathways in the act of vomiting.

From Greenberger, N.J., and Winship, D.H.: Gastrointestinal disorders: a pathophysiologic approach, ed. 2, Chicago, 1981, Year Book Medical Publishers, Inc.

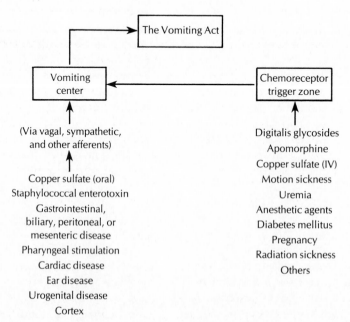

stimulate parts of the hypothalmus, also resulting in the act of vomiting.

Two major clinical concerns when severe vomiting occurs are the development of *dehydration* and *malnutrition* as a result of impaired intake and excess fluid loss, or the development of *metabolic alkalosis with hypokalemia* from the loss of gastric secretions. An acute but less common complication is traumatic rupture or tear at the gastroesophageal junction (Mallory-Weiss syndrome), often resulting in massive hematemasis. In the unconscious patient, prevention of aspiration is a priority.

When evaluating any type of vomiting in a patient, it is important to consider its occurrence in relation to time of eating and time of day, as well as the character of the vomitus—acid, feculent, bilious, or blood—and amount.

Abdominal pain

Abdominal pain is a challenge and worry to the clinician. Its assessment requires a carefully detailed history in order to establish the sequence and nature of events, and a thorough physical examination, in which a pelvic and rectal examination are essential. Abdominal pain is part of the clinical picture of a large number of illnesses, many of which share similar signs and symptoms, thus adding to the difficulty and complexity of diagnosis. This fact makes obtaining a thorough and accurate history especially important.

In considering abdominal pain, it is important to have a clear concept of the physiological mechanisms of visceral pain, parietal pain, and referred pain.

Referred pain

Pain that is felt in a part of the body distant to the tissue causing the pain is termed *referred pain*. There are essentially two types. Pain is usually referred to an area of the body surface after originating in one of the visceral organs. It is transmitted via the afferent visceral and cerebrospinal nerve fibers of the autonomic nervous system. Pain sensations are open between afferent visceral fibers and somatic dermatomes. Thus such pain is referred to areas of the body supplied by somatic nerves from the same cord segment. In addition, a viscus may be the site of origin of pain that is then referred to another deep body area not in the proximity of the viscus producing the pain.

Referred pain can be the only symptom of many visceral ailments. It is usually sharp and well-defined. In evaluating referred pain, it is important to keep in mind and apply knowledge of the anatomical course and distribution of the segmental nerves and embryological development. Those areas of the body that developed in proximity in the embryo are likely to be related by referred pain.

Visceral pain

Visceral pain, as opposed to surface pain, is rarely caused by highly localized types of damage. The pain is more likely to be dull than superficial pain, appearing as aching or burning and is diffuse. For instance, visceral tubes composed of smooth muscle fibers, such as the intestine, are not sensitive to palpation, crushing, cutting, or tearing. The stimulus required to cause pain in these organs is stretching or distention by gas or fluid of a substantial area of the tube, or excessive contraction against resistance. In general, excitation of pain nerve endings in diffuse areas of the viscera by any stimulus causes visceral pain. Examples of such stimuli include ischemia of visceral tissue, spasm of the smooth muscle in a hollow viscus, chemical damage to the surfaces of the viscera, or stretching of the ligaments. Visceral pain originating in the abdominal cavity is transmitted through sensory nerve fibers that run in the autonomic nervous system sympathetic trunks. They are small type C fibers that are capable of transmitting only burning- or aching-type pain.

Ischemia causes visceral pain by the formation of acidic metabolic end products or tissue degenerative products, such as bradykinin or proteolytic enzymes, that stimulate pain nerve endings. Spasm of a hollow viscus, such as a bile duct, the gallbladder, or the gut, can cause pain similar to that of skeletal muscle spasm. The mechanism for this is thought to be mechanical stimulation of pain endings or diminished blood flow to the muscle combined with increased metabolic need. Pain from a spastic viscus may appear as cramps, the rhythmic cycles corresponding with contraction of the smooth muscle, such as occurs with peristalsis. This type of pain may accompany gastroenteritis, constipation, menstruation, or gall bladder disease. Sometimes damaging substances, such as gastric juice, leak from the gastrointestinal tract into the peritoneal cavity. Extensive digestion of the visceral peritoneum results, stimulating very large areas of pain fibers and thus extremely severe pain. Overstretching of tissues by overfilling of a hollow viscus also results in pain.

Some visceral pain sensations are also transmitted from the viscera through nerve fibers that innervate the parietal tissue such as the peritoneum. Spinal nerve fibers that penetrate from

Table 6-5. Divisions of nervous system operative in abdominal pain categories

Category of pain	Transmission via
"True visceral pain"	Afferent visceral fibers (autonomic nervous system sympathetic trunks)
Referred pain due to viscerosensory reflex	Afferent visceral and cerebrospinal nerve fibers (autonomic-cerebrospinal nervous system)
Referred pain due to peritoneocutaneous reflex	Only via cerebrospinal nervous system

From Robins, A.H.: GI series: physical examination of the abdomen, Richmond, Va., 1978, A.H. Robins Co.

the surface of the body inward supply the parietal surfaces of the visceral cavities. The parietal wall, like the skin, is supplied with extensive innervation from the spinal nerves, as opposed to sympathetic nerves. These include "fast" delta fibers as opposed to the "slow" type C fibers active in the true visceral pain pathways of the sympathetic nerves. The resulting pain is very sharp and pricking (Fig. 6-24).

Pain transmission

Pain from the abdomen is transmitted to the central nervous system by two separate or dual pathways—the true visceral pathway and the parietal pathway—one fast and one slow. The fast one localizes the pain while the slow pathway brings information from related areas and alters response to pain. The position in the spinal cord to which visceral afferant fibers pass from each organ depends on the segment of the body from which the organ developed embryologically. As mentioned before, true visceral pain is transmitted by way of sensory fibers of the autonomic nervous system. These sensations are referred to surface areas of the body that may be distant from the painful organ. Parietal sensations are conducted directly from the parietal peritoneum, for instance. These sensations are usually located directly over the painful area (Table 6-5).

Fig. 6-24. Visceral and parietal transmission of pain from the appendix.

From Guyton, A.C.: Textbook of medical physiology, ed. 6, Philadelphia, 1981, W.B. Saunders Co.

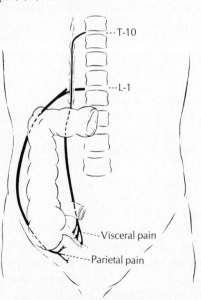

T-10

L-1

Visceral pain

Parietal pain

Table 6-6. Symptoms and possible causes of abdominal pain

Organ	Typical location of pain	Typical symptoms	Associated symptoms
Esophagus	Upper epigastrium	Dysphagia; hot searing pain that travels from stomach to throat; pain most severe 30-60 min. after meals; pain relieved by antacids	Regurgitation of food
Stomach	Upper epigastrium or left upper quadrant	Diffuse burning or gnawing pain beginning 30-60 min. after meals; pain relieved by antacids	Bloating, eructation, nausea, vomiting, hematemesis, melena
Duodenum	Upper epigastrium or right upper quadrant	More localized gnawing or burning pain before meal-time and at night, relieved by antacids; pain may radiate into the back	Nausea, hematemesis, melena
Liver	Right upper quadrant discomfort or fullness	Anorexia, nausea, vomiting, jaundice, dark urine, light stools	Fatigue, malaise
Gallbladder	Right upper quadrant	Abrupt onset of severe steady pain lasting 2-4 hours and ending abruptly	Nausea, vomiting, jaundice, fever
Small intestine	Periumbilical	Colicky pain associated with disturbance of normal bowel function (usually diarrhea)	Bloody diarrhea, fever, weight loss
Pancreas	Periumbilical or upper epigastric	Steady, sharp pain radiating into the midthoracic area	Nausea and vomiting; patients frequently either have gall-bladder disease or are alcoholics
Large intestine	Left or right lower quadrant or hypogastric region	Sharp, crampy pain associated with diarrhea or constipation; pain relieved by a bowel movement or passing gas	Tenesmus, bleeding and bloating

From Capell, P.T., and Case, D.B.: Ambulatory care manual for nurse practitioners, Philadelphia, 1976, J.B. Lippincott Co.

Abdominal pain having its origin in the abdomen may result from inflammation of the parietal peritoneum, obstruction of a hollow viscera, vascular disturbances of the abdominal wall, or it may be referred pain from the thorax, spine, or genitalia. Other causes of abdominal pain include metabolic abdominal crisis or neurogenic causes, such as that of spinal nerves or roots on psychogenic pain.

When evaluating abdominal pain it is important to obtain information about a number of aspects: sequence and chronology, location, onset, quality, frequency, intensity, associated phenomena, aggravating factors, and alleviating factors. It is also important to determine recent exposure to anyone else with similar symptoms, type and site of recent food intake, allergies, and recent life changes. Discussion of such evaluation in greater detail is found in the assessment section.

Information about manifestations of intra-abdominal disorders as well as demonstration of pain areas are found in Table 6-6 and Figs. 6-25, 6-26, and 6-27.

GI hemorrhage

GI hemorrhage is a common problem that can result from a variety of causes in the upper or lower GI tract, resulting in chronic blood loss or acute massive blood loss. In any discussion of GI bleeding it is important to clarify some commonly used terms first. An *upper GI bleed* occurs as the result of a lesion proximal to the ligament of Treitz. These lesions are more likely to cause the patient to exsanguinate than those distal to the ligament of Treitz. A *lower GI bleed* is from a lesion distal to the ligament of Treitz. *Hematemasis* is vomiting of blood, usually as a result of bleeding proximal to the jejunum. *Melena* is the passage from the rectum of black, tarry stools occurring as the result of at least 50 to 100 ml of blood rapidly entering the upper GI tract. When hematemasis occurs, there is usually also melena, lasting 1 to 3 days, while the presence of occult blood in the stool may last 3 to 8 days. *Hematochezia* is the passage of bright red blood from the rectum, usually as a result of bleeding from below the duodenum, although it may be from above when the bleeding is massive. With *occult bleeding,* the stools appear normal but blood is present in the stool when tested with guiac or orthotoluidene.

GI bleeding or hemorrhage can be looked at in terms of acute and chronic blood loss. Chronic blood loss will be discussed first. When chronic blood loss occurs slowly it causes iron deficiency anemia. The rate of development and se-

---

Fig. 6-25. Common areas where abdominal pain is referred or perceived. **A,** Anterior review. **B,** Posterior view.

From Robins, A.H.: GI series, physical examination of the abdomen, Richmond, Va., 1978, A.H. Robins Co.

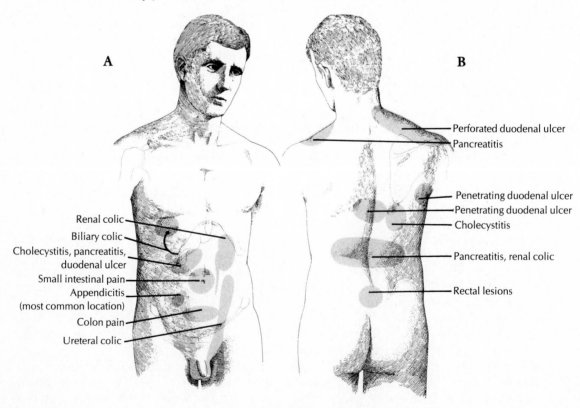

A

B

Renal colic

Biliary colic

Cholecystitis, pancreatitis, duodenal ulcer

Small intestinal pain

Appendicitis (most common location)

Colon pain

Ureteral colic

Perforated duodenal ulcer
Pancreatitis

Penetrating duodenal ulcer
Penetrating duodenal ulcer
Cholecystitis

Pancreatitis, renal colic

Rectal lesions

verity of the anemia depends on the rate of blood loss, the body iron stores, and iron intake. Severe weakness, fatigue, and symptoms of cardiovascular and cerebrovascular disease may accompany the anemia of chronic blood loss.

The physiologic changes of acute massive blood loss depend on the amount and rate of blood loss. Acute massive blood loss will usually involve loss of 25% of the circulating blood volume, or at least 1500 ml over several hours. Acute blood loss causes a decreased cardiac output, which in turn causes a decreased systolic blood pressure and then a lowered diastolic blood pressure and pulse. This is reflected originally in orthostatic changes, then occurs without any positional changes. Venous constriction assists in the maintenance of central circulation, while periph-

eral arteriole constriction results in a decreased flow to the skin, splanchnic, and renal arteries in an attempt to maintain cardiac and cerebral flow. The body adjusts physiologically to maintain the blood supply to the most vital areas. This is accomplished by increasing the heart rate and expanding the circulatory volume at the expense of the extravascular fluid, causing a volume adjustment that results in anemia (the remaining cells are diluted and the hematocrit drops over a 48- to 72-hour period). Thus it is important to keep in mind that the hemoglobin and hematocrit often do not initially reflect the severity of the blood loss. Depending on the extent of re-expansion of the plasma volume, objective signs of anemia may lag 18 to 36 hours. When attempting to correlate clinical changes

Fig. 6-26. Areas and common cause of periumbilical or midabdominal pain.

From Robins, A.H.: GI series, physical examination of the abdomen, Richmond, VA, 1978, A.H. Robins Co.

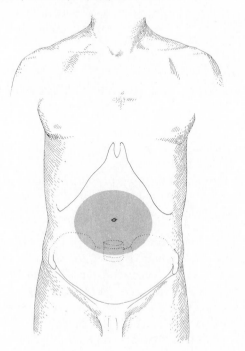

Fig. 6-27. Area and common cause of pain in the lower abdomen and suprapubic region.

From Robins, A.H.: GI series, Physical examination of the abdomen, Richmond, VA, 1978, A.H. Robins Co.

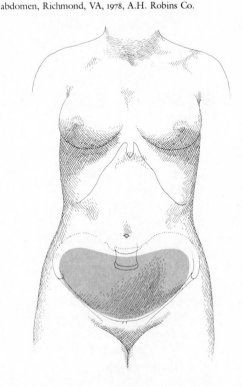

Table 6-7. Sources of gastrointestinal bleeding

Category	Upper GI tract	Lower GI tract
Inflammatory	Peptic ulcer*	Ulcerative colitis*
	Esophagitis*	Crohn's disease*
	Gastritis*	Diverticulitis
	Stress ulcer	Enterocolitis: tuberculosis, bacterial, toxic, radiation
	Pancreatitis	
Mechanical	Hiatal hernia	Diverticulosis*
	Mallory-Weiss syndrome*	Anal fissure*
	Hematobilia	
Vascular	Esophageal or gastric varices*	Hemorrhoids*
	Mesenteric vascular occlusion	Mesenteric vascular occlusion
	Aortoduodenal fistula	Aortointestinal fistula
	Malformations: hemangioma, Osler-Weber-Rendu syndrome, blue nevus bleb	Aortic aneurysm
		Malformations: hemangioma, Osler-Weber-Rendu syndrome, blue nevus bleb
		Angiodysplasia*
Neoplastic	Carcinoma	Carcinoma*
	Polyps: single, multiple, Peutz-Jeghers syndrome	Polyps: adenomatous and villous, familial polyposis, Peutz-Jeghers syndrome*
	Leiomyoma	Leiomyoma
	Carcinoid	Carcinoid
	Leukemia	Leukemia
	Sarcoma	Sarcoma
	Metastatic (e.g., melanoma)	Metastatic (for example, melanoma)
Systemic	Blood dyscrasias and clotting abnormalities	Blood dyscrasias and clotting abnormalities
	Collagen diseases	Collagen diseases
	Uremia	Uremia
Anomalies	Gastric and duodenal diverticula	Meckel's diverticulum

From Greenberger, N.J., and Winship, D.H.: Gastrointestinal disorders: a pathophysiologic approach, ed. 2, Chicago, 1981, Year Book Medical Publishers, Inc.
*Most common.

with physiologic changes, a couple of guidelines are helpful. A fall in blood pressure to less than 100 mmHg systolic and a rise in pulse greater than 100 beats/min represent approximately 20% volume depletion. Orthostatic changes in pulse of an increase of more than 20 beats/min or a blood pressure drop of more than 10 mmHg indicate a blood loss of more than 20% of the volume. Blood pressure change is thought to be a better indicator of volume depletion than pulse. In order to have systemic symptoms, a loss of at least 500 ml of blood is required. As blood loss volume approaches 40%, symptoms of shock will become evident.

Clinical manifestations bring attention to the patient but also help locate the bleeding site, depending on the extent of hemorrhage, rate of bleeding, and associated diseases. Decreased urinary output, oliguria, possibly ATN, mesenteric vascular insufficiency, bowel infarction, hepatic centrilobular necrosis, impaired coronary and cerebral blood flow, and metabolic acidosis all are potential sequelae to this circulatory response to acute blood loss. Blood lost into the lower GI tract may cause increased propulsive movements of the intestine, ultimately resulting in diarrhea. Blood loss into the upper GI tract may also cause an elevated BUN as a result of the digestion and absorption of quantities of blood protein. This person will have an elevated BUN (40 mg/100 ml), appearing 24 to 48 hours after the hemorrhage, and a normal creatinine.

The three most common causes of upper GI bleed include peptic ulceration, erosive gastritis, and variceal bleeding. Peptic ulceration most commonly occurs in the duodenum. Erosive gastritis can be precipitated by the ingestion of salicylates or other drugs, recent heavy ingestion of alcohol, or stress. Variceal bleeding results from esophageal or gastric varices of portal vein thrombosis or portal hypertension from cirrhosis. These three categories together account for 90% to 95% of all cases of upper GI hemorrhage.

The most common causes of lower GI bleed are anal lesions, rectal and colonic disease, and diverticula. Anal lesions include anal tissues or fistulas and hemorrhoids or tumors. Rectal and colonic disease include carcinoma of the rectum, rectal polyps, and ulcerative proctitis. Diverticulosis is the most common cause of massive lower GI bleeding, especially when the diverticula occur proximal to the splenic flexure. Table 6-7 lists possible sources of upper and lower gastrointestinal bleeding. The sequelae to GI bleeding are diagrammed in Fig. 6-28.

Jaundice (Icterus)

Jaundice is a yellowish tint given to the body tissues, including the skin, sclera, and deep tissues, by the presence of bilirubin. It reflects large quantities of either free or conjugated bilirubin in the extracellular fluid. The normal plasma concentration of bilirubin, mostly in conjugated form, averages 0.5 to 1.0 mg/100 ml. Jaundice is usually clinically evident when the total serum bilirubin is greater than 2.0 to 2.5 mg/100 ml.

To review briefly, hepatic metabolism of bile pigments includes hepatic uptake, conjugation, and excretion into bile. All hepatic cells synthesize small amounts of bile and then secrete it into the bile canaliculi. Bile salts are synthesized by liver cells from cholesterol, which is then converted to cholic acid and conjugated with other substances to form bile salts. Bile salts serve two important functions: (1) a detergent action that helps emulsify fat globules in the intestine and (2) the formation of micelles (fat acids and monoglycerides) to help absorption of fatty acids, monoglycerides, cholesterol, and fat-soluble vitamins like A, D, and K. Bilirubin is not synthesized by the liver, but the liver converts it from an insoluble to a soluble form.

Red blood cells are destroyed in the reticuloendothelial cells, at which time the hemoglobin is split into globulin and heme, and then bile pigments are formed from the heme. Biliverdin is the first pigment formed, and it is quickly converted to bilirubin, which is insoluble and is released into the blood where it combines with plasma albumin for transport to the liver. At the liver it is released and actively transported into the hepatic cells where it combines with another protein. There the bilirubin is conjugated with glucuronic acid or sulfates, using the microsomal enzyme UDP glucuronyltransferase, to form bilirubin glucuronides or bilirubin sulfates, both of which are soluble in bile. Some small quantities of bilirubin are returned to the plasma directly or reabsorbed from the bile duct. Both insoluble and soluble bilirubin (unconjugated and conjugated) forms are found in the plasma. Bilirubin glucuronide or bilirubin sulfate, when excreted into the bile, are carried to the intestines and converted by bacterial action to urobilinogen, a highly soluble substance. In the intestines, urobilinogen is converted to stercobilin. Part of the urobilinogen is reabsorbed into the bile and subsequently re-excreted by the liver, while a small portion is transported via the blood to the kidneys. In the kidneys, urobilinogen is oxidized to urobilin. Urobilin and stercobilin are excreted in the urine and feces (Fig. 6-29).

The pathophysiologic mechanisms that are involved in the development of jaundice include: (1) overproduction of bilirubin resulting in an elevated pigment load, such as occurs from a hemolytic disorder; (2) extrahepatic biliary tree obstruction; (3) impaired canicular excretion of

Fig. 6-28. Diagrammatic representation of the sequelae to gastrointestinal (GI) bleeding.

From Greenberger, N.J., and Winship, D.H.: Gastrointestinal disorders: a pathophysiologic approach, ed. 2, Chicago, 1981, Year Book Medical Publishers, Inc.

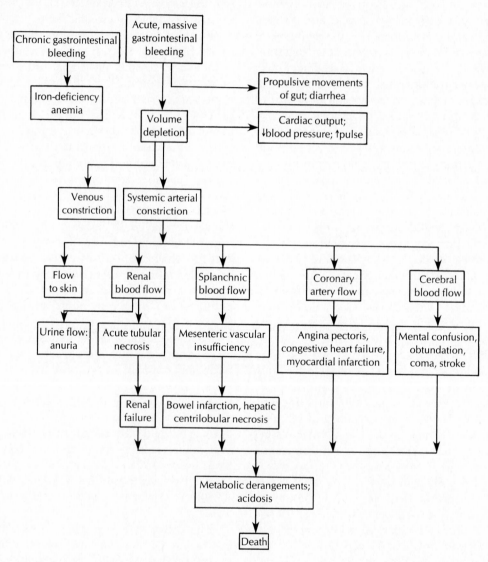

Fig. 6-29. The metabolism of bilirubin. The breakdown of aged or injured red blood cells in the reticuloendothelial system accounts for 80 to 90% of bilirubin production. A small percentage of bilirubin (10% to 20%) is derived from immature erythroid cells in the bone marrow or from nonerythroid enzymes in the liver. Bilirubin released from hemoglobin is water insoluble (free or unconjugated bilirubin) and is transported in serum as a bilirubin-albumin complex that is not filtered at the renal glomerular membrane. At the hepatic cell membrane the bilirubin-albumin complex is dissociated with selective uptake of the bilirubin, conjugation in the smooth endoplasmic reticulum and plasma membranes (see text) to a diglucuronide, and active secretion into bile (Fig. 6-9). Once in the intestine, the conjugated bilirubin is catabolized by bacteria to urobilinogens, which are reabsorbed into an enterohepatic circulation with the majority excreted by the liver into bile. A small amount (about 4 mg/day) of urobilinogen is filtered at the glomerular membrane and excreted into the urine.

From Harvey, A.M., et al.: The principles and practices of medicine, ed. 20, New York, 1980, Appleton-Century-Crofts.

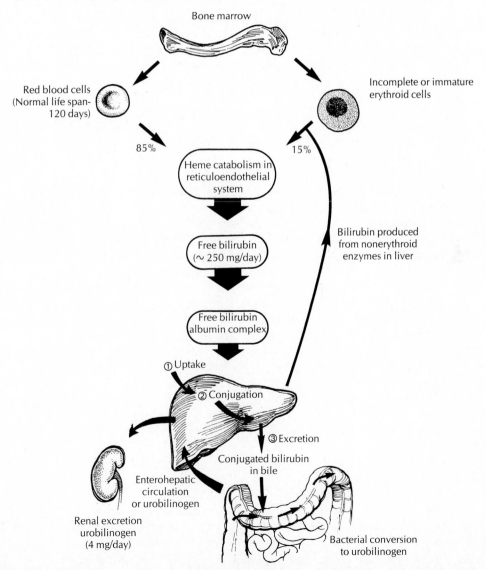

Bone marrow

Red blood cells
(Normal life span-
120 days)

Incomplete or immature
erythroid cells

85%

15%

Heme catabolism in
reticuloendothelial
system

Bilirubin produced
from nonerythroid
enzymes in liver

Free bilirubin
(~ 250 mg/day)

Free bilirubin
albumin complex

① Uptake

② Conjugation

③ Excretion

Conjugated bilirubin
in bile

Enterohepatic
circulation
or urobilinogen

Renal excretion
urobilinogen
(4 mg/day)

Bacterial conversion
to urobilinogen

Table 6-8. Jaundice: pathophysiologic mechanisms and type of hyperbilirubinemia

Pathophysiologic disorder	Resultant hyperbilirubinemia
↑ pigment load	Unconjugated
Extrahepatic biliary obstruction	Conjugated
Impaired canalicular excretion of bilirubin	Conjugated
Impaired hepatic uptake of unconjugated bilirubin	Unconjugated
Impaired hepatic conjugation of bilirubin	Primary unconjugated

bilirubin; (4) impaired hepatic uptake of unconjugated bilirubin; and (5) impaired hepatic conjugation of bilirubin. Table 6-8 lists the pathophysiologic mechanisms and types of hyperbilirubinemia that result.

Jaundice can be classified as hemolytic, obstructive, or hepatocellular. Table 6-9 summarizes bilirubin breakdown as it is effected by the various forms of jaundice. The excretory function of the liver is not impaired in hemolytic anemia. Rather, red blood cells are hemolyzed so rapidly that the hepatic cells cannot keep up to excrete bilirubin as rapidly as it is formed. As a result, the plasma concentration of free bilirubin rises quite high. In addition, the rate of formation of urobilinogen in the intestine is greatly increased. Much is absorbed in the blood and excreted in the urine. The cardinal features of hemolytic jaundice include unconjugated hyperbilirubinemia, increased fecal excretion of urobilinogen (normal is 50 to 280 mg daily), and the absence of bilirubinemia.

Obstructive jaundice can be intrahepatic or extrahepatic. It is caused by obstruction of the bile ducts or damage to the liver cells. However, the rate of bilirubin formation is normal. After formation, the bilirubin fails to get from the blood to the intestines as it usually would; instead the free bilirubin from the liver cells where it is conjugated is returned to the blood as a result of rupture of congested canaliculi and direct emptying of the bilirubin into the lymph as it leaves the liver. In this instance, bilirubin in the plasma is the conjugated type. Clinical features of obstructive jaundice include hyperbilirubinemia (predominantly conjugated bilirubin will be in the blood), bilirubinuria, and decreased fecal and urinary excretion of urobilinogen.

Hepatocellular jaundice is associated with such clinical disorders as cirrhosis of the liver, viral hepatitis, and chronic active hepatitis. It is caused by impairments in all three major hepatic processes of bilirubin metabolism—uptake, conjugation, and excretion. However, the major defect is in excretion of conjugated bilirubin. An intrahepatic block results in a normal or decreased amount of conjugated bilirubin entering the intestinal tract. Normal or decreased fecal excretion of urobilinogen occurs. At the same time, normal or decreased amounts of urobilinogen are passed through the enterohepatic circulation. Urobilinogen is taken up by the diseased liver at an abnormal rate. Clinical features of hepatocellular jaundice include normal to increased urinary excretion of urobilinogen, normal or decreased fecal excretion, hyperbilirubinemia (conjugated and unconjugated), and bilirubinuria.

When total obstructive jaundice occurs, no bilirubin reaches the intestines to be converted to urobilinogen by bacteria. No bilirubin is reabsorbed into the blood or excreted by the kidneys into the urine and no stercobilin or other bile pigments are present, resulting in clay-colored stools. When severe obstructive jaundice is the problem, conjugated bilirubin can be excreted by the kidneys. When the urine is shaken, a yellow foam can be observed.

Van den Bergh's test is used to differentiate between free and conjugated bilirubin in the plasma. Conjugated bilirubin causes an immediate reaction to the van den Bergh reagent (direct reaction), and free (unconjugated) bilirubin causes a reaction only when alcohol is added to precipitate protein from the bilirubin (indirect reaction).

Common diseases associated with the development of jaundice include the following: viral hepatitis, chronic acute hepatitis with or with-

Table 6-9. Bilirubin breakdown in various types of jaundice*

Disorder causing jaundice	Hematology		Urine		Stool		Liver function studies				
	Hct	WBC	Bilirubin	Urobi-linogen	Color	Blood	TB	DRB	SAP	SGOT	Chol
Overproduction (e.g., hemolytic anemia)	N or ↓	N	o	↑	N	o	↑	N	N	N	N
Defective uptake and storage (e.g., Gilbert syndrome)	N	N	o	N or ↓	N	o	↑	N	N	N	N
Hepatocellular disease, viral hepatitis (usual)	N	↓	↑	↑	N or ↓	o	↑	↑	N or ↑	↑↑	N
Defective excretion of bilirubin											
Intrahepatic cholestasis (for example, chlorpromazine reaction)	N	N	N or ↑	↓	N or ↓	o	↑	↑	↑	N	N or ↑
Extrahepatic biliary obstruction	N	N or ↑	↑	↓	↓	+/−	↑	↑	↑↑	N or ↑	↑
Hereditary (for example, Dubin-Johnson syndrome)	N	N	↑	N	N	o	↑	↑	N	N	N

From Harvey, A.M., et al.: The principles and practice of medicine, ed. 21, New York, 1984, Appleton-Century-Crofts.

*N	= normal		TB	= total bilirubin	
↑	= increased		DRB	= direct reacting bilirubin	
↑↑	= markedly elevated		SAP	= serum alkaline phosphatase	
↓	= decreased		SGOT	= serum glutamic oxaloacetic transaminase	
Hct	= hematocrit		Chol	= cholesterol	
WBC	= white blood cell count		o	= not useful or usually performed for this purpose	

out postnecrotic cirrhosis, drug-induced liver disease, alcoholic liver disease (fatty liver, alcoholic hepatitis, Laennec's cirrhosis), postnecrotic cirrhosis, gallstones and their complications, extrahepatic biliary obstruction from tumors, hemolytic jaundice, and disorders of bilirubin metabolism.

Ascites

Ascites, a type of "third-spacing," is the accumulation of free fluid in the peritoneal cavity caused by exudation of fluid from the surface of the liver or from the surfaces of the gut and its mesentery. Ascites can occur in isolation or along with generalized fluid retention with edema. Factors involved in the pathogenesis of ascites include (1) portal hypertension, (2) hypoalbuminemia, (3) increased sodium reabsorption in the proximal tubule, (4) impaired water excretion, and (5) increased production and flow of hepatic lymph. Two of the most important factors involved in the formation of ascites are portal venous hypertension and a decrease in serum colloid osmotic pressure. The low serum albumin levels noted in ascites, are caused by decreased hepatic synthesis or increased loss of albumin. Ascites may develop when the outflow of blood from the liver into the inferior vena cava is blocked. This causes high pressure in the liver sinusoids to develop and fluid to weep from the surfaces of the liver into the peritoneal cavity. The resulting high colloid oncotic pressure in the abdominal fluid pulls fluid from the surfaces of the gut and mesentery by osmosis. Hepatic lymph production is increased in patients with chronic liver disease and may contribute to ascites formation. Abnormalities of salt and water metabolism include increased sodium reabsorption in the proximal renal tubule and hyperaldosteronism resulting in increased distal reabsorption of sodium and decreased free water clearance. These abnormalities may contribute to the development of ascites in chronic liver disease. Metabolism of aldosterone is impaired.

The effusions of ascites are either transudative or exudative. Transudative effusions have a specific gravity of less than 1.015, a protein concentration less than 3.0 grams/100 ml, and a cell count less than 500/mm.[3] Common causes of transudative effusions include cirrhosis of the liver, congestive heart failure, constrictive pericarditis, obstruction of hepatic veins, and Budd-Chiari syndrome. Exudative effusions have a specific gravity greater than 1.015, a protein concentration greater than 3.0 gm/100 ml, an elevated cell count, and elevated peritoneal fluid LDH levels. Common causes of exudative effusions include neoplastic diseases involving the peritoneum, tuberculosis peritonitis, pancreatitis, and lymphomatous disorders. An extensive list of causes of ascites is found in the box on the next page. A few conditions that simulate ascites should be kept in mind—obesity, hydronephrosis, ovarian cyst, pancreatic pseudocyst, and pregnancy.

Physical signs of ascites include bulging of the flanks, shifting dullness of the abdomen when the person is turned from side to side, and the development of abdominal striae from stretching of the skin. Small amounts of ascites may be difficult to detect based on physical signs. Paracentesis may be done to confirm the diagnosis. The fluid should be analyzed to determine specific gravity, protein content, cell count, bacteriology, and cytology.

Constipation

Constipation, like all alterations in patterns of elimination, must be considered in relation to the person. Implicit in the term is a change in bowel habits. Constipation can be operationally defined as "too little of a too hard stool." Some would define it as "infrequent evacuation of stools," but in addition to bowel movements that are more infrequent than the person usually experiences, constipation also commonly refers to excessive straining during a bowel movement and the passage of small amounts of dry, hard stool. Small amounts of rocky, hard stools are the key to identification of the problem. In clinically evaluating for the occurrence of constipation it is important to determine how the person using the term *constipation* defines it.

Normally, defecation is a complex reflex act, initiated by distention in the rectum. The reflex can be voluntarily inhibited. When practiced habitually, this leads to diminished sensitivity of the reflex and chronic constipation. Other factors that can lead to chronic constipation include eating low residue foods or prevention of proper gastrocolic reflex. Many factors, disease-related or treatment-related, may lead to the development of constipation. Disease-related factors might include spinal cord disease or involvement; disease of the GI tract, especially with decreased GI motility; a change in performance status or decreased mobility; dehydration; hypothyroidism; dehydration; anorexia; depression; and hypercalcemia. Pregnancy is a condition frequently associated with constipation. Treatment-related factors might include use of narcotics or the CNS depressants, medication such as anticholinergics, antihypertensives, ganglionic blocking agents, and iron; use of neurotoxic

CAUSES OF ASCITES

I. **Exudative ascites**

    A. Inflammatory diseases of the peritoneum—peritonitis

        1. Ruptured viscus with or without intraabdominal abscess: peptic ulcer, diverticulitis, appendicitis, cholecystitis, intestinal infarction, etc.

        2. Tuberculous peritonitis

        3. "Spontaneous" bacterial peritonitis

        4. Pancreatitis

        5. Bile peritonitis (secondary to ruptured gallbladder, needle penetration of dilated bile duct, etc.)

    B. Tumors

        1. Metastatic to the liver and/or peritoneal lining

        2. Leukemia, lymphoma, myeloid metaplasia

        3. Primary hepatocellular carcinoma, and cholangiocarcinoma

II. **Lymphatic obstruction with chylous ascites**

    A. Trauma to the thoracic duct in the chest

    B. Mediastinal tumors

    C. Filariasis

    D. Tuberculosis (occasionally)

    E. Cirrhosis (occasionally)

III. **Transudative ascites**

    A. As part of generalized fluid retention with hypoalbuminemia

        1. Nephrotic syndrome

        2. Protein-losing gastroenteropathy

    B. Failure of return of blood to the right side of the heart

        1. Congestive heart failure

        2. Tricuspid insufficiency

        3. Constrictive pericarditis

    C. Blockage of the hepatic veins and/or vena cava

        1. Budd-Chiari syndrome, tumor, webs, etc.*

        2. Veno-occlusive disease

    D. Diffuse hepatic disease with portal hypertension

        1. Cirrhosis—all forms

    E. Infiltrative processes of the liver

        1. Tumors, lymphomas, myeloid metaplasia, etc.*

        2. Granulomatous diseases (occasionally sarcoidosis, schistosomiasis)

IV. **Conditions that may mimic ascites**

    A. Pregnancy

    B. Ovarian cyst

    C. Pancreatic cyst

    D. Mesenteric cyst

    E. Ruptured urinary tract

From Harvey, A.M., et al.: The principles and practices of medicine, ed. 21, New York, 1984, Appleton-Century-Crofts.
*Ascites may have characteristics of an exudate.

chemotherapeutic agents; surgery; treatments restricting mobility; treatments or diagnostic procedures causing a loss of appetite or decreased intake. Hospitalization alone with its change in activity, different diet and food preparation, strange surroundings, and lack of privacy can contribute to the development of constipation.

Inability to utilize the mechanisms that facilitate defecation can contribute to the development of constipation. Facilitating mechanisms include: (1) valsalva maneuver, which increases intra-abdominal pressure and increases intrathoracic pressure; (2) squatting, which increases intraabdominal pressure; and (3) the pelvic diaphragm contracting and drawing the anus up over the fecal mass.

It can be useful clinically to categorize constipation as three types: (1) imaginary, (2) spastic, and (3) rectal insensibility. Imaginery constipation involves stools that appear normal by ordinary standards but about which the person is concerned because the bowel movements do not measure up to his or her expectations. With spastic constipation, hard stools are passed with effort. The person experiences abdominal aching and a sense of incomplete evacuation (tenesmus). This is due to spasm of a small section of the sigmoid delaying the colonic contents in passage from the colon to the rectum. It also can result from painful anal disorders. If the constipation is due to rectal insensibility, the rectum is often found full of soft feces and the person does not experience the urge to defecate. The usual complaint of scybalous stools is not evident here.

GI obstruction

Obstruction occurring in the GI tract results in a failure of the progression of its contents and can occur as a consequence of an abnormality in muscular activity or from mechanical causes. GI obstruction usually refers to obstruction of some part of the intestine.

Marked distention of the intestine from accumulated gas and fluid proximal to and within the obstructed area occur as a result of small intestine obstruction. The gas that accumulates is largely swallowed, thus containing nitrogen, which is not well absorbed. The fluid consists of ingested fluid, swallowed saliva, gastric juice, biliary and pancreatic secretions, and interferes with normal sodium and water transport. After approximately 24 hours of complete obstruction, large quantities of fluids and electrolytes are secreted into the lumen. Protein lost from the blood stream into the intestinal lumen and the peritoneal cavity causes more distention, and the cycle repeats and builds. Additional loss of fluids and electrolytes occurs from vomiting, accumulation of fluid within the lumen, sequestration of fluid into the edematous intestinal wall and peritoneal cavity from impaired intestinal venous return, hemoconcentration, hypovolemia, renal insufficiency, and shock. When the obstruction is near the distal large intestine,

feces can accumulate for several weeks. If prolonged, vomiting, rupture of the intestine, or dehydration and shock may eventually develop. The pathophysiological alterations in intestinal obstruction are described in Fig. 6-30.

Types of obstruction are mechanical or nonmechanical. Nonmechanical obstructions occur as a result of neuromuscular disturbances that produce paralytic ileus. Paralytic ileus may occur after general anesthesia, after abdominal surgery or trauma, with electrolyte imbalance (especially hypokalemia), with peritoneal irritation, with metabolic imbalances, with severe pain, or with excess anticholinergic or ganglion-blocking drugs.

Common causes of mechanical obstruction are numerous. Cancer, involving a lesion intrinsic or extrinsic to the wall, may be involved. In the small intestine, 70 to 75% of obstructions are accounted for by adhesions and external hernias. In the colon, 90% of obstructions are caused by carcinoma, sigmoid diverticulitis, or volvulus.

Clinically, it is useful to consider whether the obstruction is located in the large intestine or small intestine, since the causes, symptoms, and treatment may differ. The consequences depend on where in the GI tract the obstruction is located. When at the pylorus, one can expect persistent and more severe vomiting of stomach contents leading to malnutrition and hypochloremic hypokalemic alkalosis. When the obstruction is distal to the stomach, intestinal juices reflux into the stomach and are vomited with the stomach contents resulting in a loss of water and electrolytes. While dehydration ultimately ensues, the acid/base balance may remain stable because of equal losses. When the obstruction is at the distal lower small intestine, the vomitus is more basic than acidic, resulting in acidosis. After a few days, the vomitus may become fecal from reverse peristalsis.

Symptoms vary with the type and site of obstruction. Mechanical small intestinal obstruction causes cramping, midabdominal pain (unless strangulated and then it is localized and steady); audible borborygmi; vomiting of bile and mucus, if high, and fecal contents, if low; singultus (hiccups); obstipation and failure to pass gas rectally, if complete, and diarrhea, if partial. The symptoms of mechanical chronic obstruction include daily abdominal pain that is similar to small intestinal obstruction in quality but of less intensity; vomiting in the late stages; a recent change in bowel habits; progressive constipation; and obstipation with a failure to pass gas. Adynamic ileus is associated with colicky pain; discomfort from distention; vomiting of gastric contents and bile (never feces); possible presence of obstipation; and singultus.

Common signs of obstruction include abdominal distention and auscultation of borborygmi. If strangulating, signs may include minimal tenderness and rigidity, low-grade temperature, and in the very late stages, shock.

Diarrhea

Diarrhea implies a change in bowel habits for the person involved. There is tremendous individual variation in what is normal bowel function. Simply put, diarrhea is "too much of a too liquid stool." Diarrhea usually means increased frequency, increased fluidity, or the presence of abnormal constituents (blood, pus, mucus). Usually, 100 to 200 grams of stool is excreted daily, about 75% of which is water. Diarrhea is physiologically defined as the excretion of more than 225 grams/day. Excess water is in the fecal contents. Stool weight is the most objective simple measure. In practice,

Fig. 6-30. Schematic diagram depicting the pathophysiologic alterations in intestinal obstruction.

From Greenberger, N.J., and Winship, D.H.: Gastrointestinal disorders: a pathophysiologic approach, ed. 2, Chicago, 1981, Year Book Medical Publishers, Inc.

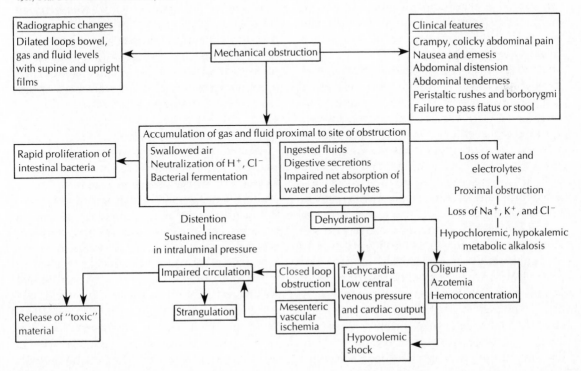

major subjective changes in frequency, fluidity, or abnormal constituents are the usual yardsticks utilized to determine diarrhea, but strictly speaking, an increased number of stools per day does not mean diarrhea.

Normally, fluids are reabsorbed from the intestine with remarkable efficiency. Ninety-nine percent of the total fluid volume is returned to the extracellular space. Fluid reabsorption begins in the jejunum in conjunction with digestion and absorption of nutrients. After the nutrients have been assimilated, the distal small bowel (ileum) continues the process of conservation of electrolytes and water. The ileum also actively reabsorbs bile acids. The colon then serves as the organ of dessication by returning the final portions of intraluminal fluid to the general circulation. Water is transported through the intestinal membrane entirely by the process of diffusion. It diffuses rapidly through the intestinal membrane, following absorbed substances (ions and nutrients) from the lumen of the gut into the blood. This tends to decrease the osmotic pressure of the chyme. About 95% of the water and most of the ions and nutrients are absorbed in this way before the chyme passes through the small intestine.

The vast majority of sodium secreted into the intestine each day is reabsorbed, playing a major role in the absorption of sugars and amino acids. Sodium is actively transported from inside the epithelial cells through the side walls into the intercellular spaces. Part of the sodium is transported along with chloride ions and part is transported in exchange for potassium ions, while part is transported with neither. The sodium that was actively transported out of the epithelial cells is replaced by diffusion of sodium from the chyme. In addition, water travels by osmosis out of the epithelial cells into the intercellular space because of the osmotic gradient caused by low sodium concentration inside the cell and high concentration in the intercellular space. In the upper small intestine chloride is transported mainly by passive diffusion, while in the distal ileum and large intestine chloride is

actively absorbed while equal amounts of bicarbonate are secreted. The absorption of chloride and sodium ions by the large intestine creates an osmotic gradient, which results in the absorption of water. The primary mechanism for fluid reabsorption proximally is solvent drag involving nutrients, fluid, electrolytes, and potassium, with water absorption being secondary to solute transport and sodium movement accompanying solute transport and bulk water movement. In the distal ileum and colon, an active sodium pump performs water movement (Fig. 6-31). Although the total volume of fluid reabsorbed by the colon is smaller than that absorbed by the jejunum or ileum, the *absorptive efficiency* of the colon is especially important in governing fecal volume. The normal water load is 10 L/day—2 to 3 L of ingested food and liquid and 7 to 8 L of endogenous secretions (salivary, gastric, biliary, pancreatic, and intestinal). The jejunum absorbs 5 L at 50% efficiency; the ileum absorbs 3 L at 60% efficiency; and the colon absorbs 1800 cc at 90% efficiency.

Knowing the mechanism involved in causing the diarrhea may help to distinguish the source early on and provide a basis for rationale therapy. The excess fluid in the stools of diarrhea is a result of decreased net absorption (osmotic), net secretion (secretory), or a combination of the two (includes hypermotility states).

Secretory diarrhea

Secretory diarrhea occurs when the normal mechanism for secretion is stimulated beyond the point for which absorption can compensate, whether electrolyte or water absorption is defective. Inhibition of absorption can also cause secretory diarrhea. More sodium than potassium is lost when secretory diarrhea occurs, resulting in a net sodium loss. Bicarbonate is also secreted, so that the stool pH remains near normal even when colonic bacteria produce acid. Secretagogues include bacterial enterotoxins, hormones, and laxatives. Secretory diarrhea also occurs with certain neoplasms, such as villous adenoma, medullary carcinoma of the thyroid,

Fig. 6-31. Mechanisms of fluid reabsorption. Major mechanism proximally is solvent drag, wherein water absorption is secondary to solute transport, and sodium movement accompanies solute transport and bulk water movement. An active Na$^+$ pump accomplishes sodium transport distally with water movement occurring in response to sodium shifts.

From Goldfinger, S., Phillips, S., and Rogers, A.: Diarrhea: a practical guide to diagnosis and management, New York, 1976, Projects in Health, Inc.

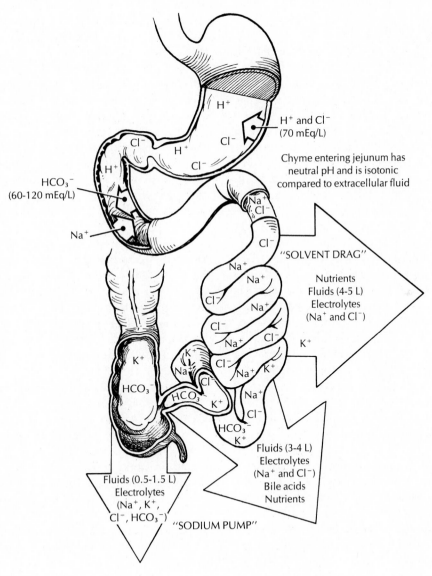

and pancreatic islet cell tumors. Additional agents include deconjugated and dehydroxylated bile salts and hydroxy fatty acids. Hormones thought to cause secretory diarrhea include VIP, prostaglandins, glucagon, calcitonin, gastric inhibitory polypeptide (GIP), secretin, and cholinergic agonists. Some laxatives work this way, including diocytil sodium sulfosuccinate, bisacodyl, oxyphenisatin, and magnesium.

Osmotic diarrhea

When unabsorbable or poorly absorbable solute is in the alimentary tract, osmotic diarrhea occurs. Impaired digestion and absorption even in the light of normal dietary consumption can result in osmotic diarrhea, as can ingestion of unabsorbable solutes. At the point when the amount of solute and water in the lumen of the bowel exceeds the absorptive capacity of the colon, diarrhea is the result. The net effect of this type of diarrhea is water and potassium depletion instead of electrolyte depletion. Because much of the solute is not electrolytes, fewer cations are lost. In addition, the colon preserves sodium but not potassium. The feces are acidic because the unabsorbed nutrients are fermented to acids by colonic bacteria. Osmotic diarrhea occurs as a result of surgical intervention (gastric dumping syndrome); diseases with histopathologic lesions (sprues, lymphomas, ulcerative colitis, giardia); biochemical mucosal diseases (lactase deficiency); immune deficiency states (IgA, IgM, IgG deficiencies); and drug ingestion (lactulose, antacids containing magnesium, colchicine, neomycin, tetracycline).

Mixed diarrhea

Mixed causes of diarrhea may occur, as when hypermotility of the alimentary tract exists. One mechanism—secretory or osmotic—may predominate. For example, solute from ingested foods may exert an osmotic effect only because of rapid intestinal transit so that normal digestion and absorption do not occur. This will appear as an osmotic-type diarrhea. Or normal amounts of secretion may not be able to be ab-

sorbed when rapid transit is an underlying problem, appearing as a secretory diarrhea. It will not always be possible to determine the predominating mechanism. Potential causes of such mixed diarrheal disorders include: cholinergic drugs, hypocalcemia, and carcinoid syndrome. Table 6-10 summarizes information about causes of the various classifications of diarrhea and pathophysiology.

People with diarrhea from different causes and locations will experience different symptoms, such as frequency of bowel movements, abdominal pain, blood or mucus in the stools, and the amount and character of the stools.

Frequency of bowel movements may vary depending on the site. Few bowel movements without urgency are most likely a result of a disorder in the small intestine or right colon, such as Crohn's disease or malabsorption. Frequent stools with urgency and tenusmus are most likely a result of a problem in the left colon or rectum, such as ulcerative colitis or amebiasis.

Diarrhea occurring at night is a result of organic disease such as ulcerative colitis. This is in contrast to diarrhea occurring during the day, especially after a normal stool or after meals, which is most likely from functional disease such as irritable colon.

Presence of blood in the stools is always a concern that needs further attention. Bright red blood is usually (depending on transit time) a result of a problem in the distal colon such as ulcerative colitis, carcinoma, or diverticulitis, as opposed to melena, which is usually from a disorder in the right colon or proximal to the right colon such as peptic ulcer disease or small bowel tumor. Lesions causing occult blood are usually located proximal to the midcolon, such as from carcinoma of the cecum or Crohn's disease.

The amount and character of the stools may also vary with the location of the problem. Large, bulky stools are a result of a disorder such as Crohn's disease or malabsorption in the small intestine or right colon. Greasy, light colored, bulky, foul-smelling stools may be a result of steatorrhea from pancreatic insufficiency or

Table 6-10. Pathophysiology of diarrheas

Type of diarrhea	Mechanism	Characteristics of diarrhea and composition of diarrheal fluid	Examples
Osmotic	Unabsorbable (i.e., oligosac-charide) or poorly asorb-able (i.e., Mg^{++}; $SO_4^=$) solute in the alimentary tract	24-hr stool volume usually < 1 L Stool volume decreases with fasting 2x [Na] + [K] stool < stool osmolality (gap > 40) Stool pH decreased < 7	Lactose intolerance; cathartic abuse; excessive antacid use; postgastrectomy or partial gastrectomy; diabetes melli-tus
Secretory	Increased secretory activity of the alimentary tract, with or without inhibition of ab-sorption of intestinal con-tents; may also result from inhibition of electrolyte and water absorption	24-hr stool volume usually > 1 L Stool volume does not de-crease with fasting 2x [Na] + [K] stool approxi-mates stool osmolality (gap ≤ 40 mOsm/Kg) Stool pH ~ 7	Cholera; infection with toxin-producing *E. coli;* non beta islet cell tumors of the pan-creas; Zollinger-Ellison syn-drome; villous adenoma; medullary carcinoma of the thyroid
Mixed	Increased rate of transit as in hypermotility states; os-motic effect of ingested solutes may result from rapid intestinal transit and decreased net absorption	Variable	Hyperthyroidism; carcinoid syndrome; cholinergic drugs

From Greenberger, N.J., and Winship, D.H.: Gastrointestinal disorders: a pathophysiologic approach, ed. 2, Chicago, 1981, Year Book Medical Publishers, Inc.

celiac disease. Frothy, liquid stools may be a re-sult of a disorder in the small intestine such as lactase or sucrase deficiency or monosaccharide malabsorption. Watery stools from a disorder in the colon, small intestine, or stomach may be caused by villous adenoma, protein-losing en-teropathy, Zollinger-Ellison syndrome, lax-atives, gastrocolic fistulas, or diabetic neurop-athy.

INTERVENTIONS

The alimentary canal functions to provide the body with adequate water, electrolytes, and nutrients. To accomplish this task, food and fluids must be moved through the system while digestive enzymes are secreted at various points to break down ingested particles into usable form that can be absorbed. Undigested materials are passed in the feces. Digestive disorders, as well as other systemic defects, can necessitate another method of alimentation to provide ade-quate nutrition. In the pages that follow, the nutritional needs of the acutely ill will be identi-fied and alternate methods of nourishment re-viewed. Temporary or permanent diversion of the fecal pathway will also be discussed as will additional therapeutic interventions used to treat acutely ill patients with GI disorders.

Nutritional requirements

The body is an energy machine that main-tains a stable weight if the energy taken in is equal to the energy used. Weight loss and mal-nutrition develop if nutritional needs, including those for energy, are not met. Degree of hyper-metabolism and current nutritional status de-termine the rate at which malnutrition develops. Factors that determine the amount of energy re-

Table 6-11. Estimation of standard metabolic rates

	kcal/m²/hr		kJ/m²/hr	
Age in years	Men	Women	Men	Women
1	53.0	53.0	222	222
2	52.4	52.4	219	219
3	51.3	51.2	215	214
4	50.3	49.8	211	208
5	49.3	48.4	206	203
6	48.3	47.0	202	197
7	47.3	45.4	198	190
8	46.3	43.8	194	183
9	45.2	42.8	189	179
10	44.0	42.5	184	178
11	43.0	42.0	180	176
12	42.5	41.3	178	173
13	42.3	40.3	177	169
14	42.1	39.2	176	164
15	41.8	37.9	175	159
16	41.4	36.9	173	154
17	40.8	36.3	171	152
18	40.0	35.9	167	150
19	39.2	35.5	164	149
20	38.6	35.3	162	148
25	37.5	35.2	157	147
30	36.8	35.1	154	147
35	36.5	35.0	153	146
40	36.3	34.9	152	146
45	36.2	34.5	152	144
50	35.8	33.9	150	142
55	35.4	33.3	148	139
60	34.9	32.7	146	137
65	34.4	32.2	144	135
70	33.8	31.7	141	133
75 and over	33.2	31.3	139	131

Fleisch, A.: Le metabolisme basal standard et sa determination au moyen du "Metabocalculator," *Helv. Med. Acta*, 18:23, 1951.

quired are nutritional state, extent of catabolism associated with the specific disease process, and the duration of the disease and/or hypercatabolic state. Postoperative patients with sepsis, multiple trauma, or burns, for example, lose calories and protein at a greater rate than do active postoperative patients. All stress, including the aforementioned, aggravates any existing protein deficiencies, increases the requirements and decreases the efficiency of usage of nutrients, and requires that protein-wasting be limited as much as possible.

In light of all of this, nutritional intervention assumes great importance. This, however, presents a dilemma, for while meeting nutritional requirements is of the utmost importance for a successful recovery and while all kinds of guidelines and suggestions are available, the level of our knowledge in this area is very preliminary. Much more research is needed regarding nutritional requirements of the critically ill, as well as regarding nutritional requirements when they are being provided by methods other than oral consumption of food, before definitive information can be determined. The following information reflects the state of the art (or science) of determining energy requirements. These methods are for the most part suggestions about determining requirements for energy, protein, fat, vitamins, and trace minerals.

Energy requirements (calories)

It is uncertain why energy requirements increase so much in the critically ill, but we know that they do.

Wilmore suggests the following method for estimating energy requirements of the critically ill.

1. Estimate the basal metabolic rate of the patient based on height, weight, age, and sex (Table 6-11, Fig. 6-32). This predicted value is an estimate of basal energy requirements when the individual is free of disease. Locate this value on the left-hand scale (Fig. 6-33).
2. Determine the impact of the disease state on basal metabolism by locating the disease on the right-hand scale (Fig. 6-34).
3. By connecting the two points with a straight-edge, the estimated metabolic rate is determined from the middle bar. Recommended caloric intake consists of estimated metabolic rate + 25%, and can be read from the left side of the middle bar.[73]

Basal Metabolic Rate (Basal Energy Expenditure) can also be calculated using the Harris Benedict Formula (Table 6-12).

For men: BEE = 66 + (13.7 × W) + (5 × H) − (6.8 × A)

For women: BEE = 655 + (9.6 × W) + (1.7 × H) − (4.7 × A)

When W = Actual weight in kg, H = Height in centimeters, and A = Age in years

Caloric intake can then be expressed as a multiple of BEE.

Caloric intake as % BEE =

$$\frac{\text{Caloric intake}}{\text{Basal energy expenditure}} \times 100$$

Caloric intake is then evaluated by comparison to the values in Fig. 6-34.[5]

Wilmore identifies the following steps for determining requirements for caloric intake of hospitalized patients:

Steps for determining caloric intake in patients:

1. Determine the total caloric requirements of the individual based on height and weight or weight alone.
2. To achieve positive caloric balance and initiate weight gain, predict actual daily caloric requirements. Alternately, measure the oxygen consumption of the patient and determine the actual metabolic requirements.
3. For weight maintenance, provide the energy requirements as estimated or measured (+ 25% to cover requirements of daily activities above basal).
4. To achieve weight gain, increase the caloric intake to "safe" levels over and above the estimated or measured metabolic requirements. In most patients, a weight gain of 2 lb/week (positive energy

Fig. 6-32. Surface area from height and weight.

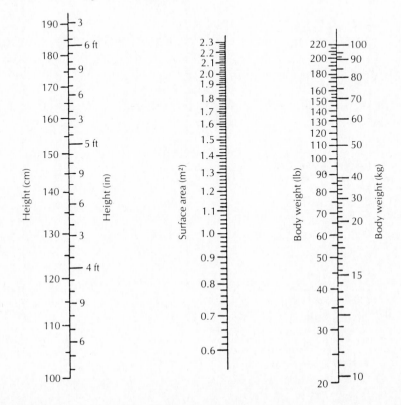

Fig. 6-33. Daily metabolic requirements.

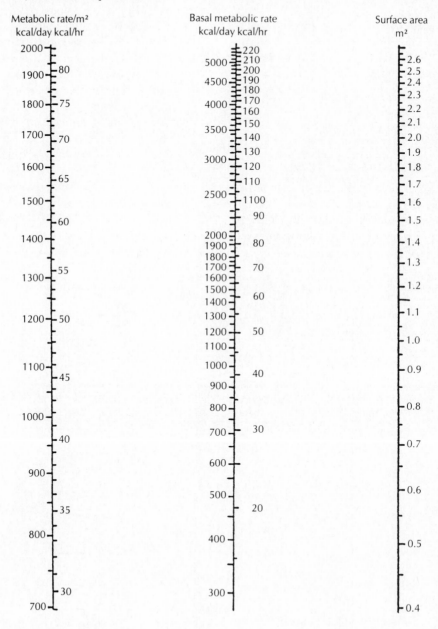

Table 6-12. Nutritional therapy requirements based on BEE nutritional therapy

Type of therapy	Energy requirements (calories required per 24 hr)	Prescriptions for anabolism*	
		Protein (g/day)	Calories (kcal/day)
Parenteral anabolic	1.75 × BEE		
Oral anabolic	1.50 × BEE		
Oral maintenance	1.20 × BEE		
Oral protein-sparing		1.5 × weight†	
Total parenteral nutrition		(1.2 to 1.5) × weight	40 × weight
Oral hyperalimentation		(1.2 to 1.5) × weight	35 × weight

Adapted from Blackburn, G.L., et al.: Nutritional and metabolic assessment of the hospitalized patient, JPEN 1:15, 1977.
*Levels of protein intake are to be adjusted according to blood urea nitrogen values and nitrogen balance.
†Weight = actual weight in kg.

Fig. 6-34. An estimate of energy requirements for critically ill patients.

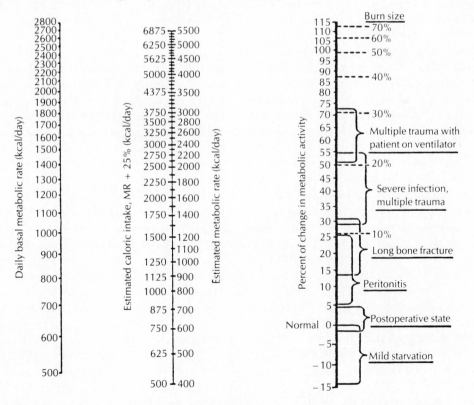

balance of 7000 kcal/week) is a reasonable goal. Nutritional rehabilitation requires time to restore body mass, and 3-6 weeks of intensive nutritional therapy are often required to replete the depleted patient. Nutritional prophylaxis should be utilized whenever possible, for it is much more efficient to prevent disruption of body mass than be forced to actively replete the wasted catabolic individual.[73]

According to Meng,[53] the recommended daily dietary allowances of calories for moderate physical activity for a man are 2810 calories and for a woman 2050 calories. When parenteral nutrition is used for the person in a reasonably good nutritive state, about 30 to 35 calories/kilogram of body weight daily are needed, while even more calories are needed to achieve weight gain in those people who have lost weight.

Long and Blakemore[48] state that the normal healthy man, resting in bed, requires 23 kcal/kg of body weight/day (or 1600 calories/day for a 70 kg man), whereas the same normal healthy man involved in light physical activity requires 30 kcal/kg of body weight/day or 2100 calories. Ordinary surgery does not alter the requirements for energy much during a convalescence lasting only 3 to 4 days because the insult is minimal. However, if the person is septic, the resting energy expenditure is increased up to 25% on the average, and as much as 50% (35 kcal/kg of body weight/day). Burns of 60% of the body surface can double requirements for long periods.

The point is made by many authorities that adequate calories are needed in order for protein or nitrogen to be used for protein synthesis. In addition, it is detrimental when administering TPN to exceed the optimal rate of glucose administration because it can result in fatty liver and an increased metabolic rate due to the energy needed for fat synthesis. No matter how much glucose is given there will still be utilization of fat as an oxidative substrate so that calories should be administered as both fat and carbohydrate.[7]

More specific methods for calculating the energy expenditure of the critically ill can be accomplished using indirect calorimetry. This technique measures the respiratory quotient (RQ), comparing the amount of carbon dioxide produced to the amount of oxygen consumed:

$$RQ = \frac{CO_2 \text{ produced}}{O_2 \text{ consumed}}$$

The RQ reflects the amount of carbohydrates, proteins, and fats being used for energy production. The RQ for the listed substrates is as follows:

Substrate	RQ
Carbohydrates	1.0
Proteins	0.8
Fats	0.7

An RQ greater than 1.0 indicates an increase in fatty acid synthesis, with a concurrent decrease in fat utilization for energy. Carbon dioxide is an end product in fat synthesis, and ventilatory complications and acid-base imbalance may result from the accumulated CO_2.

Indirect calorimetry may be employed to provide a guide for nutritional support. Although expensive and not universally used, it is a means by which the effectiveness of treatment can be documented, and it also provides a mechanism to compare predicted and measured kilocalorie requirements in an effort to prevent overfeeding or underfeeding.

Protein requirements (nitrogen)

Essential amino acids are the building blocks for protein. They are not synthesized in the liver and must be obtained from exogenous sources. The rate of essential to nonessential amino acids varies with age and nutritional state. During regrowth or after trauma children and adults require 40% of the nitrogen supply as essential amino acids, whereas normal adults require 20% of the nitrogen supply as essential amino acids.[73]

Wilmore determines dietary protein requirements in two ways: (1) by measuring all loss of nitrogen on a protein-free diet or (2) by determining the minimal quantity of nitrogen necessary to achieve nitrogen equilibrium.[73] The results of the second method are compared to a table with norms for adults, children, and traumatized individuals. The ratio of nitrogen to total energy intake is normally (for maintenance) 1:350, but it changes to 1:150 (range 1:100 to 1:200) in the critically ill person and in the person for whom restoration is the goal because protein economy is decreased.

According to Meng[53] the recommended daily dietary allowance of protein for an adult is 65 grams/day or 0.9 grams/kilogram of body weight. The nature of change with age is uncertain. When administering TPN, 8 to 16 grams/day of protein are required with essential amino acids all being given in adequate amounts and proportions and nonessential amino acids being given in combination to be effective. The optimal amino acid profiles to sustain visceral protein synthesis and the amount of nonprotein calories required are unknown.

Long and Blakemore[48] list the following nitrogen losses for the various insults: the elective postsurgical patient may lose 8 to 10 grams of nitrogen per day; the severely septic patient may lose 15 to 20 grams of nitrogen per day; the patient suffering skeletal trauma or severe burns may lose 20 to 30 grams of nitrogen per day; and the person receiving steroids may lose up to 40 grams of nitrogen per day.

Fat requirements

Fat provides a concentrated energy source of 9 calories/gram. Essential fatty acids are needed and can be provided by the administration of fat emulsion 2 to 3 times/week. Fat emulsions are isotonic and may be infused peripherally.

Vitamin requirements

Knowledge about vitamin requirements in the critically ill patient is meager. Fat-soluble vitamins (A, D, E, K) are stored in limited quantities while the water-soluble vitamins (B complex and C) are not stored in appreciable quantities. Major injuries or stress may increase the requirements for vitamin C, niacin, thiamine,

and riboflavin.[73] Table 6-13 gives vitamin requirements for normal and critically ill people.[73]

Electrolytes, minerals, and trace element requirements

Electrolyte requirements vary widely depending upon the volume and type of fluid loss; preexisting deficits; cardiovascular, renal, and endocrine status; and the types and amounts of nutrients given.

Minerals are essential to the nutritional and physiologic support of the critically ill. Levels can be monitored frequently by checking serum levels or assays of other biological fluids or tissues. Repleted patients or normal patients undergoing prolonged nutritional supplementation require minerals and trace elements, although definite requirements are undetermined.

Alternate modes of alimentation

For the patient who cannot or will not eat or cannot consume the quantities necessary to meet metabolic needs, alternate means of feeding have become available and are being used increasingly in recent years. After the patient's nutritional requirements have been determined, a decision can be made about the best method of feeding him while considering the options available. In general, people can receive nutrition enterally by oral food or tube feeding (nasogastric tube, esophagostomy, gastrostomy, or jejunostomy); by a peripheral intravenous route with an isotonic glucose and amino acid solution and/or fat emulsion; or by a central intravenous route administering hypertonic solutions of glucose and amino acids.

Once the need for nutritional support has determined the type of supplementation required, the decision about what method or combination of methods for feeding should be used is guided by mechanical considerations, economical considerations, and patient symptomatology and condition. Another factor to be considered is the goal of feeding—whether for maintenance or repletion. Frequently, enteral hyperalimentation alone or in combination with

Table 6-13. Vitamin requirements in normal and critically ill individuals

Vitamin	Biochemical action	Signs of deficiency or toxicity	Clinical history, predisposing deficiency	Requirement*		
				Normal†	Moderate injury‡	Severe injury‡
A (Retinol)	Maintains epithelial integrity and retinal pigments	Night blindness, xerosis; toxicity usually associated with food faddism, manifested by malaise, dermatitis, peripheral edema and yellow tint to skin	Protein deficiency, fat malabsorption	5 000 IU	5 000 IU	5 000 IU
D	Metabolism of calcium and phosphorus	Rickets, hypocalcemia; toxicity manifested by elevation of serum calcium and phosphorus, soft tissue calcification and renal calculi	Malnutrition, fat malabsorption	400 IU	400 IU	400 IU
E (Tocopherol)	Antioxidant preventing oxidation of polyunsaturated fatty acids	Hemolytic anemia in children, impaired red cell survival in adults	Fat malabsorption	15 IU	—	—
K (Phylloquinone)	Catalyzes prothrombin synthesis in the liver	Decreased prothrombin time	Prolonged antibiotic therapy, bile fistula, obstructive jaundice	0.4 mg	2 mg	20 mg
C (Ascorbic acid)	Maintains intracellular matrixes of cartilage and bone, important in collagen synthesis	Poor wound healing, hemorrhage, infection	Malnutrition	45 mg	75 mg	300 mg
Thiamine (B_1)	Decarboxylation of alpha keto acids—requirement proportional to carbohydrate in diet	Beriberi, decreased appetite, cardiomyopathy, neurological symptoms	Alcoholism, sepsis, trauma	1.5 mg	2 mg	10 mg

	Function	Deficiency Symptoms	Deficiency Conditions			
Riboflavin (B$_2$)	Contributes flavoproteins involved in oxidative process	Cheilosis, bleeding gums, seborrheic dermatitis, magenta-colored tongue	Kwashiorkor, severe malnutrition	1.8 mg	2 mg	10 mg
Niacin	Coenzyme in carbohydrate metabolism	Pellagra, dermatitis, dementia, toxicity manifested by flushing and burning sensations	High-corn diets, diets low or lacking in tryptophan	20 mg	20 mg	100 mg
Pyroxidine (B$_6$)	Participates in a variety of enzyme systems associated with amino acid metabolism	Mental depression, dermatitis, increased excretion of tryptophan metabolites	Malnutrition, pyroxidase antagonists (isoniazid used in treatment of tuberculosis)	2 mg	2 mg	40 mg
Pantothenic acid	Converted to coenzyme A which participates in biological acetylation reactions	Decreased antibody production in man, fatigue, nausea	Severe malnutrition	5-10 mg	18 mg	40 mg
Folic acid	DNA synthesis, transfer of one-carbon units	Megaloblastic anemia	Malnutrition, malabsorption, folic acid antagonist	0.4 mg	1.5 mg	2.5 mg
Vitamin B$_{12}$	Maintains normal folic acid metabolism, myelin synthesis, reducing agent, participates in metabolism of fat, carbohydrate, and protein	Pernicious anemia, neurological symptoms	Malnutrition, malabsorption, ileal resection, HCl and intrinsic factor also necessary for absorption	3 μg	2 μg	4 μg

*Deficiency states may require additional vitamin intake to achieve acceptable tissue concentrations.

†Normal requirements based on the 1974 Recommended Daily Dietary Allowances of Food for Men 23-50 Years of Age, Nutrition Board, National Academy of Sciences, National Research Council.

‡From *Therapeutic Nutrition with Special Reference to Military Situations.* National Academy of Sciences, National Research Council, January, 1951.

peripheral parenteral fluid is sufficient. The general rule to be followed is that if the gut works, it should be used in order to supply energy and essential nutrients.

Enteral alimentation

Enteral alimentation by tube involves the administration of liquid formulas or combinations through a tube inserted into the stomach or jejunum, such as a nasogastric tube, esophagostomy, gastrostomy, or jejunostomy; this is done when the person is unable to consume food orally. The goal is to provide essential nutrients, fluids, and adequate protein and calories for the individual.

Indications. Enteral tube alimentation may be called for in various circumstances such as the following: facial injuries; fractures of the jaw; stricture of the esophagus; weakness of the mastication muscles from various neurological disorders; tracheostomy; oral lesions; radical surgery of the upper alimentary tract, neck, upper respiratory system, or oropharynx; paralysis; unconsciousness; mental disturbance; or refusal of the patient to eat.

Contraindications. The enteral route should not be used in the face of severe gastrointestinal disturbances such as obstruction, intractible vomiting, and upper gastrointestinal bleeding. Diarrhea and ascites are not necessarily reasons to exclude the enteral route, although they may require modification of the method of administration or contents of the feeding as well as administration of other agents (for example, antidiarrheal agents). The patient whose level of consciousness is depressed so that he would be unable to handle vomiting without aspiration or with marked impairment of swallowing and gag reflexes is a poor candidate for enteral alimentation with either gastric or jejunal feeding.

Administration. Recent years have brought welcome advances to enteral alimentation by the development of nasogastric tubes of smaller size and new materials, as well as new and more diverse solutions. The new feeding tubes are of smaller diameters and much softer materials,

such as silicone rubber or polyurethane. Suitable feeding tubes currently available include the Keofeed tube, the Dobbhoff enteral feeding tube, and the Med Pro. The Keofeed stomach tube is made of silicone rubber, weighted at the distal end with a short column of mercury, and comes in sizes of 6 to 18 French (7 to 9 French are most commonly used). Most formulas require only gravity to drip through the Keofeed tube. The Dobbhoff tube, capable of passage into the distal duodenum or proximal jejunum, is made of polyurethane and has a mercury weight. The Med Pro is the smallest, made of silicone rubber and enclosed in a stiff outer tube of polyvinyl chloride. After passage of the tube, the outer portion is withdrawn and used as part of the administration set. A pump is usually required to infuse formulas through this tube.

Enteral therapy administration sets are commercially available or can be improvised from enema bags, resterilized IV bottles, or sterile plastic irrigation containers.

Many commercially prepared dietary products are currently available for tube feedings: nutritionally balanced blenderized formulas, milk-based formulas, lactose free formulas, protein hydrolysates or amino acid mixtures, and those containing medium chain triglycerides (MCT). Nutritionally complete liquid diets in the purified form have frequently been labeled *chemically defined* formulas or *elemental* diets, but because they are not elemental and vary widely in composition, it is generally felt that the term *defined formula* is better. The nutritionally balanced, blenderized formulas are cheap and readily available but not used much anymore because they require a large bore tube, which is uncomfortable and even dangerous to the patient, and they provide an excellent medium for bacterial growth.

Feeding mixtures suitable for enteral alimentation are *complete* or *modular*. The complete feedings are monomeric or polymeric. Polymeric products contain protein, fat, and carbohydrate in high molecular weight form. They have a lower osmolality, require normal lipolytic and proteolytic digestive functions, are less expensive, and contain about 1 kcal/ml. Monomeric products contain amino acids as the protein source, oligosaccharides or monosaccharides as the carbohydrate source, and contain little or no triglyceride or starch. They are hyperosmolar, low residue, do not require proteolytic or lipolytic digestive activity, and furnish about 1 kcal/ml. Monomerics are moderately expensive. High density feeding modules are the third type of preparation for enteral alimentation. They are prepared by mixing products available commercially to supply carbohydrate, protein, or fat in a calorie-concentrated (2 kcal/ml) source, or to add to other food or preparations. Monomeric products include Vivonex, Vivonex HN, and Flexical. Polymeric preparations include Citrotein, Precision LR and HN, Isocal, Ensure, Ensure Plus, and Precision Moderate N. Modular products include brands of carbohydrate (Controlyte, Hycal, and Polycose), fat (medium chain triglyceride oil), and protein (Casec and EMF).

Factors related to clinical status that should be considered in selecting the enteral feeding mixture are gastrointestinal tract function, metabolic rate, ability to eat, and the nature of gastrointestinal tract dysfunction. In addition to these factors, the desired constituents, which vary with different preparations, should be considered. Commercial products have certain advantages over hospital- or home-prepared products. These include the following: (1) decreased possibility of gross bacterial contamination, (2) certainty about diet standardization and known nutrient compositions, (3) inclusion of essential nutrients, (4) controlled osmolality, and (5) individualization of concentration in light of digestive or absorptive insufficiency. Disadvantages of commercial products are cost and limited adaptability to individual needs.

Various suggestions are made regarding the actual administration of enteral alimentation by tube. The patient's ability to tolerate and absorb the enteral fluid is determined by the osmolality of the solution and rate of flow. Usually a pump is used to guarantee a constant rate/volume of infusion. Continuous infusion is thought to be more desirable than bolus infusion as it decreases the likelihood of gastric retention or dumping. Initiating the infusion can be accomplished with a decreased rate or with a combination of decreased rate and dilute solution. If the latter approach is used, the volume is increased until the maximum desired volume is obtained and then the concentration is increased. With this approach full volume and concentration are usually achieved within 72 hours. If only the volume is limited, but full concentration is given, the volume is begun at about 50 to 75 cc/hr and is advanced gradually until the full volume is administered.

Potential problems during administration include: (1) mild abdominal distress (nausea, cramping), (2) diarrhea, (3) "tube-feeding syndrome," (4) aspiration, (5) fluid and electrolyte abnormalities, and (6) hypoglycemia. Mild distress of nausea and cramping can be controlled by changing the rate and/or concentration of administration. Nausea may also indicate delayed gastric emptying. The feeding should be stopped and gastric residual measured. Any·volume greater than 150 ml is considered evidence of delayed gastric emptying. Because of the electrolyte content of gastric fluid, any amount less than 150 ml that has been withdrawn should be reinstilled. Delayed gastric emptying also increases the risk of vomiting and aspiration. Diarrhea can occur as a result of bacterial contamination, increased lactose, too rapid introduction, improper insertion of the feeding tube, administration of cold feedings, high fat content, or high osmolarity. High osmolarity draws fluid into the GI tract from the blood in an effort to dilute the solution, which then stimulates peristalsis and diarrhea. The therapy for diarrhea and cramping when it results from the patient's inability to assimilate the large load of nutrients includes reducing the flow, diluting the solution, considering a different type of solution, or adding an antidiarrheal medication. "Tube-feeding syndrome" includes hypernatremia, hyperchloremia, azotemia, and dehydration. Signs and symptoms of this syndrome are thirst, weight loss, decreased hematocrit, and increased serum osmolarity. Treatment involves decreasing the protein load and giving water to remove the solute load and decrease hypernatremia. Aspiration can be prevented by elevating the head of the bed and checking residuals. Blood and urinary glucose levels should be monitored for hyperglycemia or glucosuria. The rate should be decreased and insulin possibly given. Glucosuria can result in osmotic diuresis and dehydration. Intake and output should be monitored to detect fluid abnormalities. Essential fatty acid deficiency is common and can be avoided by administering linoleic acid supplement orally or fat emulsion IV.

When enteral tube alimentation is given intermittently, the following considerations should be remembered: (1) elevate the head of the bed at least 30 degrees prior to and one half hour following each feeding, (2) check the tube's position before each feeding, (3) check the gastric residual before each feeding, and (4) give the feeding by gravity with a syringe or bag with the solution at room temperature. When administered continuously, these items should be considered: (1) elevate the head of the bed at least 30 degrees at all times; (2) stop feeding if the head must be lowered; (3) check the tube's position at least every 8 hours; (4) check the gastric residual every 2 to 4 hours; and (5) give the feeding at a consistent infusion rate, checking the rate frequently. Hang no more than a 4 to 8 hour supply at any one time. If the tube lumen is clogged by solution, it should be flushed with water and the tube replaced if necessary.

Parenteral alimentation

Parenteral alimentation is accomplished through a peripheral or central vein. Frequently the term *hyperalimentation* has been used, but because it may give the impression that the nutrition it provides is in excess of that indicated for achievement (either maintenance or reattainment) of normal body weight and nutrition, the preferred terms are *total parenteral nutrition* or *total parenteral alimentation*. The purpose of this procedure is to maintain an adequate nutritional state for patients who cannot utilize food through the gastrointestinal tract. In the broadest sense, it involves any route for feeding other than the gastrointestinal tract.

Peripheral intravenous alimentation. Peripheral intravenous alimentation is at best a short-term measure for the person who is nutritionally depleted. It is almost impossible to improve nutritional status in the deficient person through a peripheral route.

Maintaining an optimal nutritional state is also difficult except when fat emulsion is added. Then it may be possible to give sufficient kilocalories in an isotonic solution in order to spare protein and achieve adequate nourishment for patients in resting starvation and who are without contraindications to increased lipid intake. Amino acids are given, but the limitations on the glucose concentration in terms of fluid volume make it impossible to provide sufficient kilocalories to permit effective amino acid utilization for protein synthesis. The body can usually only handle about 3 L of fluid/day. When 3 L of the standard intravenous solution of 5% glucose is given, only 600 calories are provided. If 3 L of 10% glucose solution is given, that only provides 1200 calories. Limitations on peripheral intravenous alimentation include tonicity of the nutrients infused into the peripheral vein, volume of solution tolerated, and cost.

Total parenteral nutrition (TPN). TPN is the use of an indwelling central venous catheter for infusion of protein as amino acids (nitrogen), hypertonic glucose, and additives (vitamins, minerals, trace elements). High blood flow in the area allows rapid dilution so that the hypertonic solutions are tolerated without the problems that would occur in the peripheral veins. The TPN line is usually inserted into the right subclavian vein and threaded until the tip is in the superior vena cava. Alternately, the left subclavian or one of the jugular veins is used. TPN is given to provide needed calories; restore nitrogen balance; and replace essential vitamins, minerals, electrolytes, and trace elements. De-

Table 6-14. Suggested protein, calorie, and fluid regimens for TPN administration

Patient group	Protein intake (gm/kg/day)	Caloric intake (gm/day)		Fluid volume (ml)
		Glucose	Fat	
Intensive care unit	1.5-2.0	400	50-100	2000
Postoperative	1.0-1.5	500		2-3000
Renal failure				
Without dialysis	0.7-1.0	350	50	1000
With dialysis	1.5-2.0	400	50-100	2000
Liver failure	0.5-1.0	400	50-100	2-25,000

Courtesy Blackburn, G.L.: 67th Annual Clinical Congress of the American College of Surgeons, San Francisco, Oct. 13-16, 1981.

signing the appropriate TPN regimen requires estimation of patient's needs for the above in light of the patient's medical condition. Suggested regimens to meet requirements are delineated by Blackburn in Table 6-14.

Indications. TPN is indicated when oral tube feedings are impossible or when oral and tube feedings are inadequate to provide for the nutritional needs of the patient. Examples of conditions that might warrant TPN are: obstructive lesions of the gastrointestinal tract for which surgery cannot be immediately performed; following massive bowel resections prior to initiation of tube or oral feedings; GI fistulas; hypermetabolic states, such as extensive burns, major trauma, and serious infections; acute stages of inflammatory bowel disease; congenital anomalies of the newborn before correction; prolonged coma, if hope for recovery is retained and danger of aspiration is a major concern; acute renal failure with ileus or enteritis; and hepatic failure.

Dangers or complications. Infection is the most commonly cited complication of TPN. Its incidence correlates with the length of time the catheter is in place and is decreased by aseptic technique and proper maintenance. Infection can occur in the form of catheter site infection, bacteremia, endocarditis, systemic fungemia, and metastatic abscesses. Other potential complications include: perforation of the heart and major vessels (usually at the time of catheter insertion); extravasation of blood or solution; obstruction of the major vessels; pneumothorax or hemothorax; air embolism; hyperglycemia; hypoglycemia; elevated BUN from excessive administration of nitrogen or dehydration; disorders of electrolytes, essential fatty acids, vitamins, or minerals (excesses or deficits); and cardiac arrhythmias (usually from a displaced catheter).

Insertion of the catheter. The patient and family should be included when possible in a discussion of the purpose of the catheter, as well as what is involved in its insertion, and possible risks and benefits.

The patient is placed in Trendelenberg's position with a towel rolled behind the cervical thoracic vertebrae. Such positioning makes localization of the subclavian easier, increases venous pressure, dilates blood vessels, and helps prevent air emboli. The patient's chest and neck will be covered with a surgical drape, and the people involved in the insertion wear a gown and mask. Such positioning is, in general, not comfortable and should be done as late as possible. It is particularly uncomfortable for people with degenerative arthritis of the cervical spine or cardiopulmonary problems.

The skin is shaved and prepped with betadine and alcohol. Drapes are in place and at the time of insertion the patient's head should be facing the side opposite the insertion site. A local anesthetic is administered—1% lidocaine without adrenalin. A large bore needle on a syringe is inserted into the subclavian, during which time it is important that the patient not move in order to avoid pneumothorax or venous or arterial laceration. The catheter is threaded through the needle, during which time the patient who can cooperate should perform a valsalva maneuver to help prevent air emboli. After the catheter is threaded, the needle is removed and the catheter is stabilized in place by suturing. Ointment, usually iodophor, is applied at the insertion site, and a sterile occlusive dressing is applied.

An x-ray of the chest should be obtained to determine catheter placement. An isotonic solution should be infused slowly until it is confirmed that the catheter tip is located correctly.

Common complications of catheterization include pneumothorax, carotid or subclavian artery laceration, mediastinal hematoma, or phrenic or brachial plexus nerve damage. Other complications, though less common, include air embolism, bleeding, cardiac irritability, tamponade, and vascular damage.

Air embolism should be suspected if the following symptoms are evident: cyanosis, hypotension, tacchycardia, loss of consciousness. A whooshing sound may be heard during catheter insertion. If this problem is suspected, the patient should be placed on his left side, in Trendelenberg's position. This helps confine the air in the right atrium. Oxygen is administered and any life supports necessary are instituted.

Catheter maintenance. Care of the catheter is primarily focused at preventing bacterial and fungal infection as a result of contamination. It is generally felt that this is best accomplished by having a limited number of people, usually nurses on the hyperalimentation team, care for the TPN catheter by regular aseptic maintenance of the catheter site. It should be noted that while slight variations exist in these procedures in terms of cleansing agents, ointments, and intervals, they are essentially similar across institutions. In addition, there is little conclusive evidence that one way is better than another. Controlled studies are sorely needed in this area.

In most institutions the tubing is changed at least daily, and the dressing at the insertion site changed every 48-72 hours. The person chang-

ing the dressing wears a face mask and the patient either wears a face mask or has his head turned to the other side.

Sterile gloves are worn after the old dressing is removed. The catheter insertion site is cleansed with acetone to remove old adhesive and defat the skin. The area is then cleansed with iodine for two minutes, after which the iodine should be allowed to dry to allow time for antibacterial and antifungal action. Iodophor can be substituted for iodine in the allergic patient but should be washed off with alcohol in order to prevent burns. Iodophor ointment and sterile gauze should be placed over the insertion site. Benzoin can be applied to encourage adherence of the final air occlusive dressing. Recently, the use of transparent dressing in place of the occlusive type has been reported. Other sprays such as those used with ostomies are available to encourage adherence. Finally, an air occlusive dressing is applied.

All tubing junctions should be secured and the filter secured to prevent tension on the catheter. The following information should be noted in the chart: skin condition, catheter position, needle guard placement, sutures, and time and date of dressing change. It is helpful if these observations and dressing changes are performed by the same people so that differences are readily noted.

Three-way stopcocks should never be used with central TPN lines. These lines should be maintained as a closed system.

Monitoring the patient. The infusion should begin slowly (50 to 80 cc/hr) and gradually increased. Infusions should ultimately be given at a constant flow rate, being checked every 30 minutes. An IVAC pump and time tapes are helpful in controlling this.

Other aspects of monitoring the patient receiving TPN are also important. While the determination of appropriate observations has not been established by controlled studies, the following suggestions for acutely ill inpatients are currently common across institutions. Urine samples are checked every 4 to 6 hours for glucose. Daily blood glucose levels are monitored until stable. After they are stable, they should be checked two to three times per week. Assessment of electrolyte status should be carried out daily. Nitrogen balance studies are often performed two times per week but are not universally felt to be essential.

Care of soft tissue wounds

Wound healing is often compromised in the acutely ill patient with multisystem problems. Healing starts right after injury and continues for long periods. For the sake of discussion wound healing is divided into stages, but in reality it is a continuum. The healing process has the same components for all wounds but does vary in terms of duration and effectiveness with location, severity, extent of injury, and regenerative capacity of the cells involved. Healing involves the regeneration of tissue. If this does not occur, scar tissue is formed.

Types of wounds

Wounds can be described as surgical or traumatic, closed or open. *Closed wounds* heal by primary intention, with no tissue loss and little scarring. In healing by primary intention, shreds of fibrin connect the approximated edges of the wound, epithelialization and collagen formation occurs, and a small amount of granulation tissue fills the area. Little suppuration or infection occurs. *Open wounds* involve tissue loss and heal by secondary intention. Secondary intention, or *healing by granulation,* occurs as a result of wound edges that cannot be approximated because of extensive tissue damage and loss. Granulation tissue forms to fill the void between wound edges and to allow epithelial cells to migrate across the wound surfaces. This type of healing takes longer and results in greater scarring.

Closed traumatic wounds involve tissue damage without a break in the skin, such as a hematoma. Closed surgical wounds are those created by a surgical incision that has been sutured. They may or may not be covered with a dressing postoperatively. Serous drainage may be present for about 48 hours. Open traumatic wounds are a break in the skin, such as burns, traumatic injuries, varicose ulcers, and pressure lesions. An open surgical wound is an incision not closed primarily by sutures, occurring after contaminated or dirty procedures. Open surgical wounds might also result from infected or re-opened closed wounds that are then allowed to heal by granulation. Excessive amounts of drainage may require drains and/or extensive dressings.

Another way of classifying surgical wounds is in the terms: clean, clean-contaminated, or contaminated-infected. Table 6-15 describes each category, giving examples and risk of infection rates.

Healing process

The healing process of incised wounds varies from that of open wounds. The healing process of incised wounds involves three phases that may overlap: defensive, reconstructive, and maturative.

The defensive phase begins at the time the wound occurs and lasts about 4 to 6 days. It includes hemostasis, inflammation, and cell migration in order to control bleeding, seal the wound, protect the tissues from bacterial contamination, remove debris resulting from cell injury, and provide a support structure for later collagen depository.

The reconstructive phase starts around day 3 or 4 and continues for about 2 weeks. During this period, proliferation of epithelial cells and fibroblasts occurs in order to protect the wound from contamination, phagocytize necrotic tissue, and seal the wound edges.

The maturation phase may continue for up to 2 years. The scar undergoes a slow progressive change in size and shape for months. Fibroblasts decrease, collagen synthesis stabilizes, and the fibers organize to result in increased tensile strength. Visceral wounds usually regain strength more quickly than skin wounds.

Healing of wounds with tissue loss by secon-

Table 6-15. Surgical wounds: clean or contaminated

Category	Description	Examples	Risk of infection
Clean	Procedures in which the surgeon enters a sterile body cavity and exits through the same cavity, makes no contact with areas having bacterial populations (such as the gastrointestinal and upper respiratory tracts), encounters no inflammation or pus, and experiences no break in sterile technique	Open heart surgery, herniorrhaphy, mastectomy	1-2%
Clean-contaminated	Surgery, during which no major break in sterile technique occurs, performed on organs or areas with a bacterial population but no inflammation or pus, or on sterile organs or cavities connected with areas containing bacteria. This includes procedures in which the surgeon enters a sterile body cavity and exits through another cavity with a bacterial population	Appendectomy, gastric and small bowel resections, abdominal hysterectomy, cesarean section (sterile uterus connects to bacterially contaminated vagina), open fractures less than eight to 10 hours old	Approximately 5%
Contaminated-infected	Surgery performed on areas where there's acute inflammation and/or pus and on wounds containing foreign matter; procedures during which drainage spills from one organ or body cavity to another, or a significant break in sterile technique occurs	Appendectomy, with perforation; colon, rectal, and vaginal surgery; bowel resection with peritonitis or perforation; lacerations and open fractures more than eight to 10 hours old; oral surgery, incision and drainage of abscesses, boils, and infected pilonidal cysts	30% or greater

Meshelany, C.M.: RN 42(5):25, 1979.

dary intention differs from healing by primary intention in terms of duration of repair time, extent of scarring, and susceptibility to infection. These wounds have a greater tendency to develop chronic inflammation, extensive granulation tissue, and contraction. Healing by secondary intention occurs as granulation tissue forms and matures, providing a base over which marginal epithelial cells migrate and proliferate. When such an area is unable to be used by such epithelialization, the open area becomes covered with dried plasma protein and dead cells to form eschar.

Factors affecting wound healing

Wound healing is affected by host resistance factors, local environmental factors, and the presence or absence of bacteria.

Factors related to host resistance include: the person's overall health, weight, age, length of the surgical procedure, length of hospitalization prior to surgery, smoking, diabetes mellitus, medications, liver function, and nutrition. The obese person has more avascular fatty tissue that will impair healing, as well as being more prone to problems of immobility and pulmonary function. The elderly are more likely to have problems resulting from increased nutritional and pulmonary deficiencies and impaired immune function. The longer a person is hospitalized prior to surgery, the greater is his opportunity of colonization with nosocomial organisms.

Medications with the potential to affect wound healing include steroids, aspirin, cancer chemotherapy, oral anticoagulant therapy, and antibiotics. Chemotherapeutic agents can retard cell proliferation and thus wound healing. Aspirin causes decreased platelet aggregation and therefore prolongs bleeding time. It should be withheld for approximately 1 week prior to surgery. Oral anticoagulant therapy should usually be discontinued several days prior to surgery. Antibiotics are given prophylactically for certain surgical sites in order to prevent infection; they are indicated for surgery involving invasion of any area with extensive microflora (vaginal hysterectomy, colonic surgery, head and neck procedures). Narrow spectrum antibiotics should be given short-term to avoid overgrowth of nosocomial pathogens.

The liver performs several functions that are necessary for normal wound healing to occur, such as synthesis of clotting factors, production of albumin, and metabolism of drugs.

Nutrition influences wound healing in numerous ways. Protein depletion results in decreased antibodies, complement, and cells of the reticuloendothelial system. This renders the person more susceptible to sepsis, and healing is delayed. Adequate vitamin C is necessary for collagen formation. Adequate calories are needed for proper protein utilization. Adequate fluids, electrolytes, minerals, and vitamins are also essential for wound healing to occur. Table 6-16 is a summary of information about nutrients related to wound healing.

Factors related to the local environment of the wound that affect healing include: blood supply; temperature and humidity; presence or absence of necrotic debris; edema; dead space; hemorrhage; degree of tension; location of the incision; type of surgery; use of foreign materials, hemostasis, or drains; and skin preparation (a broad spectrum antibiotic soap should be used).

The presence or absence of bacteria can affect wound healing. Certain flora are normally present in various parts of the body. Additional sources of bacteria may be exogenous and endogenous. Exogenous sources include the local air and environment or a break in sterile technique during surgery or dressing changes. Urine, feces, and secretions are endogenous sources.

Dressings

Purposes of dressings. Dressings are used to create an optimal environment for wound healing. Different dressings may be needed as the wound changes over time. Dressings can serve many purposes, as enumerated below:

1. Protect the wound from contamination and trauma
2. Support and immobilize the wound
3. Absorb drainage and maintain a dry environment to decrease maceration
4. Debride the wound
5. Conceal disfigurements from patients until they are ready to deal with them
6. Provide pressure to minimize fluid accumulation in intercellular spaces (transudates, exudates)
7. Provide a physiologic environment
8. Serve as a passageway and as storage for drainage, secretion, pus, and necrotic debris

Dressings that support and immobilize the wound may help decrease pain, decrease interference with wound healing and scar formation, or prevent disruption of clots and newly formed capillaries.

Dressings used for debridement work by

Table 6-16. Nutrients affecting wound healing

Nutrient	Specific component	Contribution to wound healing
Proteins	Amino acids	Needed for neovascularization, lymphocyte formation, fibroblast proliferation, collagen synthesis, and wound remodelling
		Required for certain cell-mediated responses including phagocytosis and intracellular killing of bacteria
	Albumin	Prevents wound edema secondary to low serum oncotic pressure
Carbohydrates	Glucose	Needed for energy requirement of leukocytes and fibroblasts to function in inhibiting activities of wound infection
Fats	Essential unsaturated fatty acids	Serve as building blocks for prostaglandins that regulate cellular metabolism, inflammation, and circulation
	a. Linoleic	
	b. Linolenic	Are constituents of triglycerides and fatty acids contained in cellular and subcellular membranes
	c. Arachidonic	
Vitamins	Ascorbic acid	Hydroxylates proline and lysine in collagen synthesis
		Enhances capillary formation and decreases capillary fragility
		Is a necessary component of complement that functions in immune reactions and increases defenses to infection
	B complex	Serve as cofactors of enzyme systems
	Pyridoxine, pantothenic and folic acid	Required for antibody formation and white blood cell function
	A	Enhances epithelialization of cell membranes
		Enhances rate of collagen synthesis and cross-linking of newly formed collagen
		Antagonizes the inhibitory effects of glucocorticoids on cell membranes
	D	Necessary for absorption, transport, and metabolism of calcium
		Indirectly affects phosphorus metabolism
	E	No special role known: may be important if there is a fatty acid deficiency
	K	Needed for synthesis of prothrombin and clotting factors VII, IX, and X
		Required for synthesis of calcium-binding protein
Minerals	Zinc	Stabilizes cell membranes
		Needed for cell mitosis and cell proliferation in wound repair
	Iron	Needed for hydroxylation of proline and lysine in collagen synthesis
		Enhances bactericidal activity of leukocytes
		Secondarily, deficiency may cause decrease in oxygen transport to wound
	Copper	Is an integral part of the enzyme, lysyloxidase, that catalyzes formation of stable collagen crosslinks

Developed from Levenson, S., and Seifter, E.: Dysnutrition, wound healing, and resistance to infection, Clin. Plast. Surg. 4(3):375, July 1977.

combining capillary action and capturing necrotic debris within the mesh. The greater the gauge of the mesh, the greater the debridement.

Combining pressure dressings with elevation of the body part involved can help to decrease transudate accumulation.

Types of dressings. Wounds change throughout the healing process. As these changes occur, the type of dressing required needs to be constantly assessed and redetermined.

Dressings may be nonocclusive, occlusive, adhering, nonadhering, or medicated. Nonocclusive dressings let air circulate to the wound site in order to aid healing by keeping the wound dry. Such dressings are commonly used. Occlusive dressings keep air and moisture from the wound and are less commonly used. They are most often used to prevent fluid loss from burn sites and some skin grafts and plastic surgery wounds, as well as to treat dermatologic conditions. A nonocclusive dressing can be made occlusive by putting plastic wrap, a plastic bag, or waterproof fabric over the dressing or by covering it completely with nonporous tape. A nonadherent dressing will not stick to the wound surface or surrounding skin. They are usually made of absorbent rayon fabric impregnated with petroleum emulsion or wrapped in a thin layer of material such as telfa. Nonadherent dressings are used on open wounds and on primary wounds to prevent the dressing from adhering to the wound and destroying new tissue. Medicated dressings are prepared ahead with a medicated solution or normal saline. They may be used to debride wounds and treat open wounds, or to treat infections or dermatologic conditions. Wet-to-dry dressings are an example of medicated dressings. Wet-to-dry dressings are used on open wounds, promoting healing by secondary intention. They debride necrotic tissue and inhibit bacterial growth by a bactericidal solution. Their effectiveness is determined by proper application. If the dressing is properly moistened so that it has dried by the time it is removed, the layer of moistened gauze will trap necrotic material in its interstices as it dries.

When removed, it takes the debris along with the dressing. The solution used varies with the condition of the wound. Frequently, normal saline, acetic acid 0.25%, providone iodine (Betadine), or hydrogen peroxide 3% are used. Dakins' solution, a very dilute neutral solution of sodium hypochlorite, may also be used. Normal saline has no bactericidal action and thus is used only on clean wounds. Acetic acid is effective against a variety of gram positive and gram negative organisms, including pseudomonas, but not against staphylococcus and anaerobic bacteria. Betadine is particularly effective against staphylococcus and anaerobes. Hydrogen peroxide may be used on grossly contaminated wounds. Although it is beneficial because it speeds separation of necrotic tissue from the wound bed, hydrogen peroxide can be harmful because it lifts newly formed epithelium away from the dermis, thus harming granulation tissue.

Changing the dressing. The importance of maintaining aseptic technique during dressing changes cannot be overemphasized because of the danger of introducing exogenous organisms and causing infection. Epidemiologic principles regarding disposal of old dressings and supplies are equally important. Old dressings should be handled by isolation technique and always removed from the room. Strict handwashing with soap and water between patients is essential.

The old dressing should be removed slowly. The rate at which it is removed depends on whether the goal is to debride the wound or to protect granulation tissue. Granulation tissue can be protected by wetting the dressing and removing the dressing very slowly. Debridement can be accomplished by removing the dressing dry and more quickly, though still not too fast in order to avoid excessive bleeding.

The condition of the wound and dressing should be noted. Erythema, swelling, bleeding, smell, drainage, and necrotic tissue should be observed and described.

Packing may be used in an open wound. It may be moistened with normal saline, medication, Betadine, or hydrogen peroxide. Betadine may be used for its bactericidal qualities whenever this benefit outweights its action as an inhibitor of epidermal regeneration. Material used for packing should not contain cotton, which might be held in the wound.

The area around the wound should be cleaned in order to prevent local skin irritation and promote circulation. The wound is cleansed starting at the incision and working out, using a new gauze pad after each stroke. If the wound is deep and narrow, cotton-tipped swabs may be used.

Deep wounds may be irrigated with a bulb syringe. A sterile gauze pad is used to catch or direct the fluid. If there is a clean area and dirty area, the fluid should drain from a clean to a dirty area.

Drains may be inserted into the wound to prevent a nidus for bacterial growth. The drain should be cleansed as often as the dressing is changed. The stab wound should be cleansed from the center out, using a new swab for each new small area. The entire area is cleansed with gauze pads to remove any drainage that might damage healthy tissue. The safety pin is replaced if rusty or crusted. Cultures, when indicated, should be taken after cleansing of the drain in order to get fresh drainage. It is placed in a culture tube immediately and not allowed to dry. The culture tube should be refrigerated. A gauze pad should be placed under the pin to prevent rubbing and to draw drainage away from the skin surrounding the wound. If there is a large amount of drainage, a drainage collection bag such as for a stoma, can be used by slipping the drain through the opening and then fastening the bag to the skin. If no bag is used, enough gauze pads should be placed over the drain to absorb all fluids until the next dressing change.

Any incisions should have gauze pads placed over them, preferably in such a fashion as to prevent them from touching those over other incisions or drain sites. If needed, ABD pads, may then be placed over the gauze pads.

The completed dressing can be secured with tape or Montgomery straps. Straps are the best choice when the wound requires frequent dressing changes and needs more air circulating to the wound. The straps should be moved occasionally to prevent skin irritation. Tape is best used when dressing changes are not required too frequently. Paper or silk tape is best for long-term use or on people with fragile skin or allergies.

Dressings should be changed when saturated but preferably not more frequently than every four hours because of the increased risk of introducing other contaminants and disturbing regeneration of tissue.

Alternate modes of elimination

The construction of a stoma, or ostomy, is the creation of an artificial opening of the intestinal or urinary tract out onto the abdominal wall.* It can be created for cure or palliation of benign or malignant disease. It is important for the critical care nurse to be familiar with the more common types of ostomies—ileostomies, colostomies, and urinary diversions—because their care varies. While the ostomy may be done under emergency circumstances and the patient may be seriously debilitated, making it unrealistic to expect patient participation in providing care, it remains important to explain as much as is reasonable about the purpose and care of the ostomy to the patient as well as the family.

Types of ostomies

Ileostomies. Ileostomies are done most frequently for the treatment of inflammatory bowel disease. To create an ileostomy the surgeon brings a portion of the terminal ileum out onto the abdominal wall, everts a length of ileum, and sutures it to the skin to make a spoutlike stoma. It is important to have the stoma project an adequate amount (about 3.5 cm) in order to avoid skin trouble from contract of the stump drainage with the skin. Ileostomies are usually located on

---

*For more detailed information, the reader is referred to Broadwell and Jackson's *Principles of ostomy care* (St. Louis, 1982, The C.V. Mosby Co.)

the right side, usually permanent, and by nature of their location drain semiliquid materials.

The slightly acidic ileostomy drainage contains digestive enzymes and bile salts with great potential to damage the skin, so it is most important to carry out good skin and stoma care. Close surveillance of intake and output is important initially to guard against fluid and electrolyte imbalances. An ileostomy drains continuously so that a bag must be worn at all times. A disposable collection device is used initially because the stoma will shrink with time. It should be open-ended to allow easy emptying of the contents because of the frequency and consistency of the output.

The continent ileostomy was developed by Kock in 1968. An intraabdominal ileal pouch is created from the terminal ileum to serve as a reservoir for ileal contents. It is intubated with a catheter several times per day. Usually a pad is worn over the stoma. The creation of a continent ileostomy is contraindicated with short gut syndrome, Crohn's disease, obesity, and psychologic instability.

Colostomies. Colostomies may be temporary or permanent and are located most commonly in the ascending, transverse, or sigmoid colon. Temporary colostomies are performed as a measure to divert the colonic flow or to decompress the colon. In this case, the colostomy is usually formed by a loop stoma in the transverse colon. A permanent end colostomy is usually constructed when the rectum must be removed and is usually located in the left lower quadrant.

A temporary decompressing colostomy allows relief of obstruction and release of gas distending the colon. It is used to treat colonic dilation from mechanical obstruction such as from cancer, diverticular disease, and megacolon. Drainage during the first 24 hours may be copious. A decompressing colostomy may take the form of a loop colostomy or a "blowhole" colostomy.

To create a transverse loop colostomy, a loop of bowel is brought through the abdominal incision and a rod or bridge slipped under the loop to hold it out on the abdomen. This is usually done as an urgent or emergency procedure. It may be opened during the surgery but usually is opened a few days later by cautery, which is painless. The transverse loop colostomy requires an especially large appliance because of the stoma plus the rod. It is ideally constructed in the middle of the transverse colon.

Temporary diverting colostomies are performed to divert the fecal flow in cases of distal inflammation or perforation, or to protect a precarious anastomosis. These may end up becoming permanent, so location is an important consideration. A temporary diverting colostomy is constructed in similar fashion to a decompressing loop colostomy, with care being taken to allow a wide opening with protrustion of the exterior wall, separating the functional and nonfunctional parts.

A transverse double-barrel colostomy creates two distinct stomas, side by side. The active proximal stoma is to the patient's right side and the inactive distal stoma is to the patient's left side. One or two appliances may be worn, depending on the distance between the openings.

Sigmoid or descending colostomies may be permanent or temporary. Sigmoid colostomies, the more commonly performed, have more solid output. They are usually single-barrel-end-type and may have a flush or raised stoma. They may become regulated with or without irrigation. The first few days postoperatively the drainage is usually watery. Once it becomes thicker and formed, a closed-end bag may be used and changed only as needed.

Ileal loop. The ileal loop is a urinary diversion, also called an ileal conduit or ileal bladder. A stoma that is an inch or more in diameter is created and is usually permanent. The bladder may be removed (cystectomy). These stomas always have output, requiring a collection device. A tampon, dental wick, or rolled gauze may be held over the stoma to absorb urine, to keep the skin dry during the changing of the bag. Edema of the stoma is common for the first few days. In a week or so, a reusable appliance with a valve for emptying the drainage tube can be selected.

Stoma characteristics

The normal color for a stoma is dark pink to red. Blanching or lightening of the color may be indicative of interference with stomal circulation. Damage to the stoma's blood supply causes a red-to-purple color.

Bleeding in small quantities may be normal in the first few days due to surgical trauma, but in general, bleeding around the stoma or stem should be minimal. Appreciable bleeding from the peristomal area or from the opening of the stoma is abnormal.

Edema of the stoma should be assessed carefully and is of special concern if excessive. The condition of the skin around the stoma should be carefully observed and guarded.

The drainage and function of the stoma in terms of quality and amount should be watched carefully. Fluid status (intake and output) as well as electrolytes should be monitored and abnormalities corrected.

Care of the stoma

As one reviews the literature and talks to those experts involved in ostomy care, it becomes obvious that in most instances there is more than one acceptable way to manage care. There are many, many products and methods to use in this endeavor. In fact, the method or equipment that is appropriate for each individual may change over time as their stomas and personal abilities change. The following is a review, by no means all-inclusive, of some of the suggestions and options available in terms of protecting the skin, appliances, dilation, irrigation, and adhesives.

Protecting the skin is one of the prime concerns in ostomy care, no matter who the person is, where the ostomy is located, or what type of ostomy is present. There is no replacement for intact, healthy skin around the stoma. Once skin breakdown occurs, encouraging healing and preventing further breakdown is a real battle.

The abdominal skin of most people has not been exposed to the elements much and therefore is especially vulnerable to irritation from drainage, tape, appliances, and adhesives.

The appliance should be changed only as often as is necessary, as indicated by beginning leaking around the bag. The instant that leakage is noted, the bag and/or appliance should be changed. The bag should be removed carefully to avoid damaging the skin. Warm water or solvent can be used if needed to help loosen the bag from the skin. Solvent, if used, should be washed away. The area around the stoma should be cleaned with water or soap and water and patted dry.

A protective skin barrier, such as Stomahesive; karaya gum, powder, or paste; Colly-Seal; Relia-Seal; or Stomaguard (crixiline) may be applied. The bag should fit snugly, but not tightly, around the stoma in order to prevent drainage from coming in contact with the skin. When measuring the stoma, $^{1}/_{16}$ to $^{1}/_{8}$-inch clearance should be allowed. The size of the stoma will decrease as the amount of time after the surgery increases.

Mahoney gives the following general instructions for applying a postoperative appliance.

1. Empty contents and then gently remove old appliance. If it does not come off easily, loosen with drops of water or solvent if necessary. Wash solvent from skin.
2. Wash peristomal skin gently with mild soap and warm water.
3. Rinse and dry skin thoroughly.
4. Measure stoma with a measuring guide.
5. On the paper covering the adhesive backing, trace a circle $^{1}/_{16}$ to $^{1}/_{8}$ inch larger than the stoma.
6. Cut around the tracing. This should leave a hole, inside the adhesive, the right size to fit around the stoma. Remove paper backing.
7. Spray skin with Skin Prep or a similar product. Allow to dry and spray again.

8. Insert one hand into bag and position the hole over the stoma. For a few days after surgery, while the patient is confined to bed a large part of the time, put the bag on sideways to make it easier to drain and empty.

9. Press adhesive around stoma to form a seal. Be sure to press gently but firmly on area immediately adjacent to the stoma. Be careful to have NO wrinkles in adhesive. If you are dealing with a large piece of adhesive, fold back only the lower half of the paper covering. Put the lower half of adhesive on the skin carefully, then peel the rest of the paper off and apply the upper half of the adhesive.

10. Insert deodorant, either liquid or tablets.

11. Close bottom of pouch with elastics or a specially designed closure clip. Fold bottom up carefully, so you will have a clean part of the pouch to handle when emptying it.

12. Empty bag as needed. Wash it out at least once daily, preferably each time it is emptied.

13. Leave pouch on for 2 or 3 days, unless it leaks.

14. When it is removed (to be replaced), expose skin under the adhesive to the air for a few minutes.

Numerous measures to treat irritated skin have been suggested in the literature, although little or no formal investigational evaluation of their effectiveness exists. In order to protect the skin and prevent further damage, karaya powder or gel may be applied prior to the cement and/or bag. Various sizes of karaya rings may also be available and be preferred. Other products to protect the skin are available as discussed earlier. Skin prep may be applied to act as a protective skin barrier. Allowing the skin to be exposed to the air is a method that is thought to promote healing.

Adhesion can be ensured by using surgical cement or adhesive, double-faced adhesive, or a disk such as Colly-Seal. The method chosen should depend chiefly on whichever is least irritating and most effective for the individual. This may vary with individuals or with the same individual over time. If adhesives are difficult to remove from the skin with ease, a couple of methods can be tried. Warm water can be dripped between the skin and adhesive. Adhesive solvent can be dripped between the skin and faceplate or adhesive area. Solvent should never be used on irritated skin.

Numerous appliances are available in order to protect the skin, contain ostomy output, and control odor. Disposable or temporary appliances are available, as reusable or permanent appliances. Initially an open-ended drainable disposable appliance is used. As the output changes and depending on the type of ostomy, the type of appliance used may change.

The disposable bags have an open-ended drainage pouch in order to decrease the number of times the bag is removed from the skin. They are usually made of polyethylene material, have a square or oval adhesive backing, and an opening that may or may not be precut. A ring or belt may be needed to hold the bag in place. If there is a collar or flange, it may need to be reinforced in place with tape, usually done by a "picture-framing" method.

Reusable or permanent appliances come in two basic styles—one piece or two piece—and in a wide range of sizes and shapes. The two-piece models allow removal of the pouch for emptying and cleaning while the faceplate or mounting ring remains undisturbed. One-piece styles are easier and faster to apply and good for people with decreased manual dexterity. The pouches may be available in various colors of rubber or plastic, but are usually vinyl. The length of time they last varies with the type of material. These can be worn several days without washing. The end or tail can be closed or sealed in several ways—special clip, elastics, or an improvisational alligator clamp.

The disk or mounting ring for a two-piece

Table 6-17. Commonly used antacids

Trade name	Drug composition	Comments
Maalox	Magnesium and aluminum hydroxide	Preferred antacid Good buffering effect Good taste Nonconstipating Low sodium content Can cause hypermagnesemia in persons with renal failure
Maalox Plus	Magnesium and aluminum hydroxide Simethicone	Same as above Antiflatus
Mylanta	Magnesium and aluminum hydroxide Simethicone	Same as Maalox Plus
Amphogel	Aluminum hydroxide gel	Constipating Can interfere with absorption of anticholinergic drugs Contains sodium Decreases absorption of phosphate Good antacid effect Give with water so that medication reaches stomach Can be given by continuous drip (1 part amphogel to 2 or 3 parts water)
Gelusil	Magnesium trisilicate Magnesium and aluminum hydroxide	Slower buffering effect Gelatin effect in stomach to coat and protect the ulcer Nonconstipating
Riopan	Magaldrate (chemical combination of magnesium and aluminum hydroxide)	Rapid antacid action High acid-buffering effect No acid rebound Nonconstipating Low sodium content Can cause hypermagnesemia in persons with renal failure
Marblen	Magnesium and calcium carbonate Aluminum hydroxide Magnesium trisilicate	Neutralizes more acid than other antacids Nonconstipating Low sodium content
Alka-2	Calcium carbonate	Rapid neutralization of acid Constipating May cause hypercalcemia May cause acid rebound Not suitable for long-term therapy

From Phipps, W.J., Long, B.C., and Woods, N.F.: Medical surgical nursing, ed. 2, St. Louis, 1983, The C.V. Mosby Co.

appliance can be measured once any edema subsides. There are various types: (1) rigid or flexible, (2) precut or cut to exact specifications, (3) flat or convex. Other factors to consider in choosing an appliance are size, whether it is odorproof, cost, skin protection, and patient preference.

Pharmacologic interventions

Acutely ill patients subjected to major stress often develop stress ulcers. Their treatment consists of relief of symptoms, healing of the ulcer, and prevention of additional complications. Medical management uses antacids, anticholinergic drugs, and histamine antagonists as well as avoidance of irritating drugs or foods.

Antacids

Antacids are used to reduce gastric acidity by physical absorption or chemical neutralization. Although they do not facilitate healing, they do reduce pain. Table 6-17 outlines commonly used antacids. Nonsystemic antacids that are poorly absorbed from the stomach are most widely used because they do not alter the pH of the blood or impair normal acid base balance.

Anticholinergic drugs

Anticholinegic agents decrease gastric motility by blocking the action of acetylcholine. As a result, HCl release is decreased directly and indirectly, the latter by suppression of gastrin.

Histamine antagonists

Histamine antagonists inhibit the action of histamine at the histamine receptors of the parietal cells. As a result, gastric acid secretion is reduced. These drugs decrease pain and have been shown to promote healing.

Patients with digestive disorders must be followed during their convalescence to make sure adequate nutrition is maintained. Several members of the health team should work with these patients until they regain their strength completely and can resume full activity. Often education and supportive therapy are required.

BIBLIOGRAPHY

1. Arey, L.B.: Developmental anatomy, ed. 7, Philadelphia, 1974, W.B. Saunders Co.
2. The assessment of nutritional status. In Krause, M.V., and Mahan, L.K., editors: Food, nutrition, and diet therapy, ed. 7, Philadelphia, 1984, W.B. Saunders Company.
3. Bates, B.: A guide to physical examination, ed. 3, Philadelphia, 1983, J.B. Lippincott Co.
4. Bennion, M.: Clinical nutrition, New York, 1979, Harper & Row.
5. Besst, J.A., and Wallace, H.L.: Wound healing intraoperative factors, Nurs Clin North Am 14:701, Dec. 1979.
6. Blackburn, G.L.: Calorie-nitrogen relationship in total parenteral nutrition. In Proceedings of 67th Annual Clinical Congress of the American College of Surgeons—Pre- and Post-operative care: nutritional support in abnormal metabolic states, Oct. 11-16, 1981.
7. Blackburn, G.L., et al.: Nutritional and metabolic assessment of the hospitalized patient, JPEN 1:11, Jan.-Feb. 1977.
8. Blackburn, G.L., Maini, B.S., and Pierce, E.C.: Nutrition in the critically ill patient, Anesthesiology 47:181, Aug. 1977.
9. Block, G.J., Nolan, J.W., Dempsey, M.K.: Health assessment for professional nursing: a developmental approach, New York, 1981, Appleton-Century-Crofts.
10. Broadwell, D.C., and Jackson, B.S.: Principles of ostomy care, St. Louis, 1982, The C.V. Mosby Co.
11. Bruno, D.: The nature of wound healing—implications for nursing practice, Nurs Clin North Am 14:667, Dec. 1979.
12. Bryant, W.D.: Wound healing, CIBA Clinical Symposia 29:2, 1977.
13. Byrne, C.J., et al.: Laboratory tests, implications for nurses and allied health professionals, Menlo Park, CA, 1981, Addison-Wesley Publishing Co.
14. Capell, P.T., and Case, D.B.: Ambulatory care manual for nurse practitioners, Philadelphia, 1976, J.B. Lippincott Co.
15. Castle, M.: Wound care: clear-cut ways to speed healing, Nursing 1975 5:40, Aug. 1975.
16. Colley, R., and Wilson, J.: Meeting patients' nutritional needs with hyperalimentation, Nursing 79 9:76, May 1979.
17. Colley, R., and Wilson, J.: Meeting patients' nutritional needs with hyperalimentation, Nursing 79 9:57, June 1979.
18. Colley, R., and Wilson, J.: Meeting patients' nutritional needs with hyperalimentation, Nursing 79 9:50, July 1979.
19. Cooper, P.M., and Schumann, D.: Post-surgical nursing intervention as an adjunct to wound healing, Nurs Clin North Am 14:713, Dec. 1979.

20. Cope, Z.: The early diagnosis of the acute abdomen, ed. 5, London, 1979, Oxford University Press.

21. Costa, G., and Dnalson, S.: The nutritional effects of cancer and its therapy, Nutr Cancer 2:22, 1980.

22. Davenport, H.W.: Physiology of the digestive tract, ed. 4, Chicago, 1977, Year Book Medical Publishers, Inc.

23. DeWys, W.: Working conference on anorexia and cachexia of neoplastic disease, Cancer Res 30:2816, 1970.

24. DeWys, W.D.: Anorexia as a general effect of cancer, Cancer 43:2013, 1979.

25. Donoghue, M.M.: Anorexia in nursing care of the cancer patient with problems, Columbus, OH, 1981, Ross Laboratories.

26. Fischer, J.E.: Parenteral and enteral nutrition, DM 24:4, June 1978.

27. Fowkes, W.C., and Hunn, V.K.: Clinical assessment for the nurse practitioner, St. Louis, 1973, The C.V. Mosby Co.

28. Ganong, W.F.: Review of medical physiology, ed. 11, Los Altos, CA, 1983, Lange Medical Publications.

29. Geels, W., Bagley, K., and Vader, L.: The entercutaneous fistula: supplanting surgery with meticulous nursing care, Nursing 78 8:52, April 1978.

30. Given, B.A., and Simmons, S.J.: Gastro-enterology in clinical nursing, ed. 4, St. Louis, 1984, The C.V. Mosby Co.

31. Goldfinger, S., Phillips, S., and Rogers, A.: Diarrhea: a practical guide to diagnosis and management, New York, 1976, Projects in Health, Inc.

32. Greenberger, N.J., and Winship, D.H.: Gastrointestinal disorders: a pathophysiologic approach, ed. 2, Chicago, 1981, Year Book Medical Publishers, Inc.

33. Griggs, B.A.: A nursing guide for the adult T.P.N. patient, monograph printed for the 3rd Annual Clinical Congress of the American Society for Parenteral and Enteral Nutrition, Boston, Jan. 30-Feb. 3, 1979.

34. Griggs, B.A., and Hoppe, M.C.: Update: nasogastric tube feeding, Am J Nurs 79:481, March 1979.

35. Gross, L., and Bailey, Z.: Enterostomal therapy: developing institutional and community programs, Wakefield, MA, 1979, Nursing Resources, Inc.

36. Guyton, A.C.: Textbook of medical physiology, ed. 7, Philadelphia, 1986, W.B. Saunders Co.

37. Harvey, A.M., et al.: The principles and practice of medicine, ed. 21, New York, 184, Appleton-Century-Crofts.

38. Heymsfield, S.B., et al.: Enteral hyperalimentation: an alternative to central venous hyperalimentation, Ann Intern Med 90:63, Jan. 1979.

39. Ivey, M.F.: The status of parenteral nutrition, Nurs Clin North Am 14:285, June 1979.

40. Jacob, S.W., Francone, C.A., and Lossow, W.J.: Structure and function in man, ed. 4, Philadelphia, 1978, W.B. Saunders Co.

41. Johnson, L.R., editor-in-chief: Physiology of the gastrointestinal tract, vol. 2, New York, 1981, Raven Press.

42. Jones, D.A., Dunbar, C.F., and Jirovec, M.M.: Medical-surgical nursing: a conceptual approach, New York, 1978, McGraw-Hill Book Co.

43. Kaminski, M.V., et al.: Intravenous hyperalimentation in modern hospital practice, Tuckahoe, NY, 1977, USV Laboratories.

44. Kaminski, M.V., and Ruggiero, R.P.: Nutritional assessment: a guide to initiation and efficiency of enteral hyperalimentation, Int Surg 64:33, March 1979.

45. Kenner, C.V., Guzzetta, C.E., and Dassey, B.M.: Critical care nursing: body-mind-spirit, Boston, 1981, Little, Brown & Co., Inc.

46. Kraus, M.V., and Mahan, K.: Food, nutrition and diet therapy: a textbook of nutritional care, ed. 7, Philadelphia, 1984, W.B. Saunders Co.

47. Lamanske, J.: Helping the ileostomy patient to help himself, Nursing 81 7:34, Jan. 1977.

48. Langmon, J.: Medical embryology, ed. 4, Baltimore, 1981, Williams & Wilkins.

49. LeMaitre, G.D., and Finnegan, J.A.: The patient in surgery: a guide for nurses, ed. 4, Philadelphia, 1980, W.B. Saunders Co.

50. Long, C.L., and Blakemore, W.S.: Energy and protein requirements in the hospitalized patient, JPEN 3:69, March-April 1979.

51. Macleod, J., editor: Clinical examination, ed. 5, Edinburg, Scotland, 1979, Churchill Livingstone.

52. Mahoney, J.M.: Guide to ostomy nursing care, Boston, 1976, Little, Brown & Co., Inc.

53. Mahoney, J.M.: What you should know about ostomies, Nursing 78 8:74, May 1978.

54. Martin-Scott, I.: Skin care for ileostomists, The Practitioner 222:237, Feb. 1979.

55. Meng, H.C.: Parenteral nutrition: principles, nutrient requirements, and techniques, Geriatrics 30:97, 1975.

56. Meshelany, C.M.: Post-op wound dressings: your guide to impeccable technique, RN 42(5):25, 1979.

57. Noe, J.M., and Lamb, D.R.: The functions of a dressing: wound healing, a dynamic approach, Hospital Care 5:5, May 1974.

58. Nursing care of the cancer patient with nutritional problems, Report of the Ross Oncology Nursing Roundtable, Columbus, OH, 1981, Ross Laboratories.

59. Orr, M.E., Shinert, J., and Gross, J.: Acute pancreatic and hepatic dysfunction, Bethany, CT, 1981, Fleschner Publishing.

60. Ota, D.M., Imbembo, A.L., and Zuidema, G.D.: Total parenteral nutrition, Surgery 83:503, May 1978.

61. Phipps, W.J., Long, B.C., and Woods, N.F.: Medical surgical nursing, ed. 2, St. Louis, 1983, The C.V. Mosby Co.

62. Prior, J.A., Silberstein, J.S., and Stang, J.M.: Physical

diagnosis: the history and examination of the patient, ed. 6, St. Louis, 1981, The C.V. Mosby Co.

63. Robins, A.H.: GI series: physical examination of the abdomen, Richmond, VA., 1978, A.H. Robins Co.

64. Ropka, M.E.: Nutritional assessment of the person with cancer. In Nursing care of the cancer patient with nutritional problems, Columbus, OH, 1981, Ross Laboratories.

65. Ropka, M.E.: Nutrition. In Johnson, B.L., and Gross, J., editors: Handbook of oncology nursing, New York, 1985, John Wiley & Sons.

66. Salmond. S.W.: How to assess the nutritional status of acutely ill patients, J Nurs 80:922, May 1980.

67. Schilling, J.A.: Wound healing, Surg Clin North Am 56:859, Aug. 1976.

68. Schumann, D.: Preoperative measures to promote wound healing, Nursing 79 14:683, Dec. 1979.

69. Schumann, D.: How to help wound healing in your abdominal surgery patient, Nursing 79 10:34, April 1980.

70. Shils, M.E.: Enteral nutrition by tube, Cancer Res 37:2432, July 1977.

71. Shils, M.E., Bloch, A.S., and Chernoff, R.: Liquid formulas for oral and tube feeding, J Parenteral and Enteral Nutr 1:89, Feb. 1977.

72. Sleisinger, M.H., and Fordtran, J.S.: Gastrointestinal disease: pathophysiology, diagnosis management, ed. 3, Philadelphia, 1983, W.B. Saunders Co.

73. Spiro, H.M.: Clinical gastroenterology, ed. 2, New York, 1977, Macmillan Publishing Co.

74. Thorn, G.W., et al., editors: Harrison's principles of internal medicine, ed. 9, New York, 1979, McGraw-Hill Book Co.

75. Wallach, J.: Interpretation of diagnostic tests, ed. 3, Boston, 1978, Little, Brown & Co., Inc.

76. Widmann, F.K.: Clinical interpretation of laboratory tests, Philadelphia, 1979, F.A. Davis Co.

77. Wilmore, D.W.: The metabolic management of the critically ill, New York, 1977, Plenum Publishing Co.

78. Wilpizeski, M.D.: Helping the ostomate return to normal life, Nursing 81 11:62, March 1981.

79. Wound suction: better drainage with fewer problems, Nursing 75 5:52, Oct. 1975.

7 Coagulation

ROSEMARY HUME

Each year more disease processes are found to be associated with derangements in hemostasis and coagulation. Little information is available on the actual incidence of crises related to coagulation and hemostasis, because many of the cases are secondary phenomena resulting from primary disease states. Whatever the case may be, the challenge is great when the critical care practitioner works with a patient who is bleeding or thrombotic.

Thorough knowledge of the normal physiologic mechanisms and the pathophysiologic changes of hemostatic and coagulation abnormalities provides the basis for accurate and precise judgments when the patient's history is taken and a physical examination is done.

Laboratory monitoring by the practitioner is enhanced by thorough knowledge of the tests and their implications. Good management of specific regimens and interventions related to hemostasis and coagulation produces the best possible outcome for the patient.

During the past 10 years, research and development have added to the wealth of information about hemostasis and coagulation, especially in relation to critically ill patients. However, many unanswered questions remain to be studied. The critical care practitioner should be challenged to add to the understanding of this complicated yet rewarding field.

EMBRYOLOGY
Blood cells and vascular system

Primitive blood cells, called *blood islands,* are first seen in the 2-week-old embryo. These blood islands function during the next few weeks (the mesoblastic period) as the fetal erythropoietic system. Later the liver becomes the chief hemopoietic organ. Blood remains static and consists of erythroblasts suspended in plasma derived from extravascular spaces during the mesoblastic period. Circulation is established later in embryonic life after the vascular spaces are well defined.[13]

As the mesoblastic period proceeds, the blood islands begin to connect to the endothelial tubes that are forming the vascular system. Thus the primitive blood cells or blood islands become enclosed in endothelium-lined spaces at about 8 weeks of fetal life. The endothelium-lined vascular tubes are formed by the restructuring of peripheral mesenchymal cells into endothelial cells.

All of the arteries and veins begin as capillaries in the human embryo. The main vessels begin as clefts between germ layers lined by special mesenchymal cells, which become the first endothelial cells. Other vessels bud from the previous capillary-type vessels.

Once a vessel is established, it grows and thickens. The special mesenchymal cells around the endothelial cells become smooth muscle cells. Media form from multiplication of the smooth muscle cells and the addition of new muscle elements forms from mesenchyme.

The adventitia results from condensation of surrounding connective tissue and later differentiates into three separate layers. Eventually the external elastic lamina forms between the adventitia and the media.

By the third month of fetal life, mesoblastic hemopoiesis is replaced by blood formation chiefly in the liver; the spleen, thymus, and lymph nodes also contribute. In the adult, hemopoiesis is almost entirely a function of bone marrow; however, when abnormal requirements develop, blood cell formation occurs from the liver, spleen, and other organs. Thus the fetal type of hemopoiesis returns in postnatal life when the need arises.

Bone marrow hemopoiesis begins at about the fifth month of fetal life, when the blood vessels differentiate from the blood cells. During the last trimester, hemopoiesis increases in the bone marrow, and then the bone marrow remains the chief organ of blood cell derivation and maturation.

Platelet embryology

Megakaryocytes, cell precursors of platelets, are seldom found during the mesoblastic phase of blood cell formation. Megakaryocytes are seen later in fetal life, but it is not certain that these function normally in platelet production. The newborn exhibits defective platelet aggregation reaction and slightly abnormal release reaction.

PHYSIOLOGY
Hemostasis and coagulation

Hemostasis is the process whereby spontaneous or induced escape of blood is abated. Several complex mechanisms are involved in the maintenance of an intact vascular and hemostatic system.

Primary hemostasis involves platelet reactivity with subendothelial and endothelial tissues.

Secondary hemostasis results with the activation of the blood coagulation mechanisms, which produce a fibrin clot. Hemostasis is altered when components of the complex processes are absent, defective, or overproduced. When alterations are experienced, major or minor problems may result. Critically ill persons are especially vulnerable to altered hemostatic mechanisms.

Platelets

The hemopoietic stem cell is apparently the precursor of various types of blood cells. Some stem cells produce specific blood cell types. Glycoproteins induce and stimulate these stem cells to produce specific cell types. One glycoprotein is called *thrombopoietin* or *thrombopoietic stimulating factor (TSF)*. The production of platelets is induced by thrombopoietin.

Platelets are fragments of a specialized cell, the megakaryocyte, derived from bone marrow, pulmonary, or peripheral regions. Platelets are formed in the Golgi region of the cytoplasm of megakaryocytes. When the cytoplasm fragments, the platelets are released into the blood. The humoral factor, TSF, stimulates thrombocytosis. Platelets inactivate TSF. Thus the amount of platelets is controlled by circulating platelets.

About 20,000 to 40,000 new platelets per cubic millimeter (0.02 to 0.04 $\times$ 10^{12}) of blood are produced each day; the life span of platelets is 8 to 9 days. After release of platelets into the circulation, two thirds of them circulate while one third is in the spleen. The one third that sequesters in the spleen relates to the sluggish blood flow through the spleen. Platelet destruction normally occurs in the spleen, but if there has been a splenectomy, the liver becomes the organ of destruction.

The platelet is a contractile cell that, as stated earlier, is derived from megakaryocytes normally found in the bone marrow, lungs, and peripheral circulation. The normal range of platelets in the blood at any one time is between 200,000 and 450,000 per cubic millimeter. The normal neonate platelet count is similar to that of the adult.

Anatomically the platelet membrane connects with the inner parts of the cells by means of a complex canal-like network. The secreted substances flow through this canal-like structure during the release function. The membrane itself contains proteins. Many of the plasma clotting factors are able to adhere to the spongelike fluffy coat of mucopolysaccharide. Factors I, V, VIII, XI, XII, and XIII can all adhere to the platelet membrane.

Within the cytoplasm of the platelet, microtubules contract when stimulated, causing the disk to take on a spherical transformation. Granules within the cytoplasm contain many important products. The alpha granules contain platelet factor IV, beta thromboglobulin, smooth muscle stimulating factor (mitogenic factor), fibronectin, factor VIII—related antigen, fibrinogen, and platelet factor V. The "dense body" granules contain calcium, serotonin, ADP, and adenosine triphosphate (ATP). The third type of granule contains numerous acid hydrolases that are comparable to lysosomes in other cells. Glycogen, phagocytic material, and mitrochondria are found in platelet cytoplasm.

Venous system

Superficial veins and deep veins make up the peripheral venous system, which acts as a peripheral reservoir for blood. The deep vein reservoir is within muscles that serve as the chamber of the venous pump system. The superficial and deep veins are connected by communicating veins and the sphenofemoral and sphenopopliteal junctions. All of the vein systems contain valves.

Contraction of the calf muscles generates high pressures to help propel blood toward the heart, but this pressure can be transmitted backward into the venous reservoir when the valves function inadequately. About 10 mmHg is left over from arterial flow when the patient stands. This arterial inflow pressure, and the calf pressure, combine to transmit blood back to the heart.

The venous system and all of the problems

Table 7-1. Coagulation factors and commonly used synonyms

Factors	Synonyms
I	Fibrinogen
Platelet factor	
II	Prothrombin
IV	Calcium
V	Proaccelerin, plasma accelerator
VII	Proconvertin
VIII	Procoagulant VIII, von Willebrand VIII (plasma factor)
IX	Christmas factor
X	Stuart factor, Stuart-Prower factor
XI	Plasma thromboplastin antecedent
XII	Hageman factor
XIII	Fibrin stabilizing factor

related to it can be compared to disorders in failure of the left side of the heart. Mitral valve incompetence is similar to vein valvular problems in communicating veins. Aortic stenosis is similar to venous obstruction. Aortic insufficiency is similar to deep-vein valvular problems. When there is calf muscle paralysis, an analogy could be made to a myocardial infarction.

Whenever venous stasis changes in the wall of the vein and a state of hypercoagulability occurs or when an insult to the vein occurs from trauma or sepsis, primary and secondary hemostatic mechanisms result.

Liver

The liver plays a definite role in the hemostatic and coagulation mechanisms; therefore when liver function is altered, hemostasis may be altered.

The major site of coagulation factor synthesis is the hepatocyte of the liver. A feedback mechanism for factor production in the liver is not low concentrations of factors in the blood, but rather by-products formed when the factor is depleted during coagulation.

Except for a few, coagulation factors are synthesized in the liver (see Table 7-1). Apparently only the procoagulant portion of factor VIII is synthesized by the liver; the antigenic portion and the von Willebrand factor are synthesized by endothelial cells. Platelet factor XIII is apparently synthesized in the megakaryocyte. Four of the vitamin K–dependent factors are made in the liver. Factors II, VII, IX, and X are synthesized in the liver.

Vitamin K

Vitamin K is a fat-soluble vitamin that is obtained in a balanced diet. Vitamin K is also synthesized by certain intestinal tract bacteria in adults but not in newborns. Once ingested or manufactured internally, vitamin K depends on bile for absorption, because it is fat soluble. Prothrombin synthesis within the liver is catalyzed by vitamin K.

Vitamin K oxidizes to vitamin K_2 3-epoxide in the presence of carbon dioxide. Vitamin K_2 3-epoxide carboxylizes protein for calcium binding. When decreased vitamin K exists, the vitamin K–dependent coagulation factors cease to bind with calcium and are inactive in coagulation.

Prostaglandins

Although prostaglandins are made by all tissues, they were named because it was thought that they were made only by the prostate gland. In the coagulation process prostaglandin production is stimulated when the platelet adherence to collagen liberates the essential fatty acid arachidonic acid from a cellular site or from plasma. Arachidonic acid is a precursor of several physiologically active compounds that make up the prostaglandin family.

Enzymes transform arachidonic acid into a cyclic endoperoxide that is further transformed by other enzymes into thromboxane A_2 (Fig. 7-1). Thromboxane A_2 is a potent platelet-aggregating agent and a vasoconstrictor. The vasoconstrictor activity of thromboxane A_2 may account for the vasospasm necessary for normal hemostasis.[5]

While arachidonic acid metabolizes into thromboxane A_2, another metabolite, epoprostenol, is also produced through enzyme processes. Epoprostenol is a potent inhibitor of platelet aggregation, a vasodilator, and blocks binding of von Willebrand factor to platelets (Table 7-2).

When exogenous chemicals such as aspirin are given, the enzyme reactions that allow the arachidonic acid to metabolize to thromboxane A_2 are inhibited. The effect of aspirin as a platelet-inhibitory drug is very dose dependent, particularly since it appears that the enzyme is inhibited at low dose only. At higher doses epoprostenol may also be affected. Thus prostaglandin synthesis and inhibition within all tissues of the body are quite complicated, and endogenous and exogenous substances can affect prostaglandin activity.

Factors

Through international agreement, the coagulation factors are named by Roman numerals. When the factors are activated, the Roman

Table 7-2. Actions of prostaglandins

Thromboxane A_2	Epoprostenol
Vasoconstrictor	Vasodilator
Platelet-aggregating agent	Inhibitor of platelet aggregation
Binds with von Willebrand factor	Blocks von Willebrand factor

Fig. 7-1. Production of prostaglandins: epoprostenol and thromboxane A_2.

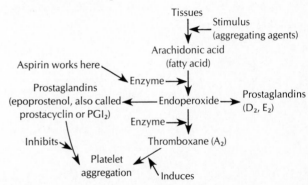

numeral is followed by the letter "a" in subscript.

Factor XII (Hageman factor)

Hageman factor is thought to be the first factor activated in the intrinsic pathway. The site of synthesis is unknown, but activated factor XII activates factor XI and activates prekallikein to kallikrein. Factor XII is probably activated by exposed collagen and other subendothelial connective tissue. Factor XII_a activates the kinin system and increases vascular permeability and leukocyte migration.

Kallikrein (Fletcher factor)

Kallikrein is a proteolytic enzyme that participates in the activation of plasma kininogens into bioactive kinins and plasminogen into plasmin and contributes as an activator in the complement system. The specific site of prekallikrein synthesis is not known. Fig. 7-2 shows the interrelationships among factors XI and XII, prekallikrein, kininogens, plasminogen, and complement.

Kinins

Kinins are small polypeptides that are split from alpha 2 globulins in plamsa or tissue fluids. Kallikrein, an enzyme, can activate the kininogen when certain physical or chemical effects occur in the blood. Kallikrein acts on alpha 2 globulin to release bradykinin. Bradykinin is a potent vasodilator and increases capillary permeability. Both kallikrein and bradykinin are destroyed by inhibitors present in body fluids.

Fig. 7-2. Interrelationships among factors XI, XII, kallikrein, kinins, and plasmin.

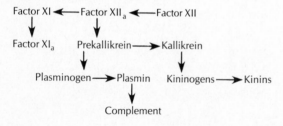

Factor XI

Factor XI is a glycoprotein that is activated by factor XII_a and possibly by several other substances, such as trypsin, prekallikrein, and kininogen. Probably factor XII_a in the presence of kininogen is the potent activator of factor XI to XI_a.

Factor IX (Christmas factor)

Factor IX is a glycoprotein activated by factor XI_a in the presence of calcium. Factor IX is apparently necessary for the formation of thromboplastin. Factor IX_a, in the presence of VIII_a, calcium, and phospholipids, activates factor X.

Factor X (Stuart-Prower)

Factor X takes part in the intermediate reactions of both the intrinsic and extrinsic systems. Factor X is a glycoprotein and is activated by either factor VII_a in the presence of tissue factor or by the combination of factors IX_a and VIII_a, calcium, and phospholipids. Factor X_a activates prothrombin (II) with the aid of factor V_a, calcium, and phospholipids (Fig. 7-3).

Factor V

Factor V is considered a cofactor (once called "accelerators"). It is involved in intermediate reactions, while it complexes with X_a and phospholipids to convert prothrombin to thrombin. In the literature factor V has been called "labile factor," " proaccelerin," or " plasma accelerator," but factor V is the accepted term. Factor V is synthesized in the liver. Some researchers feel that factor V is only a precursor of factor VI, but generally factor VI is no longer considered in a discussion of factors.

Factor VII

Factor VII is traditionally associated with the extrinsic system of coagulation and has appeared to be separate from the intrinsic system. However, observations show that factor VII can be activated by XII_a and kallikrein. Therefore these pathways are interrelated.

Factor VII is also activated by tissue thromboplastin, and activated factor VII plays a role in activating factor X.

Factor II (prothrombin)

No clot can form unless prothrombin is converted to thrombin. Prothrombin is synthesized in the liver with the aid of vitamin K. Factor X_a (a proteolytic enzyme), factor V (a cofactor), phospholipid, and calcium activate prothrombin. Calcium bridges form on the prothrombin binding sites. When this binding does not occur, as in vitamin K deficiency, an incomplete prothrombin molecule occurs.

Thrombin

Thrombin is the active agent that clots fibrinogen. It is inhibited by antithrombin III and heparin. The action is very powerful, but as thrombin is absorbed by the fibrin, an antithrombin reaction stops the action.

Fibrinogen

Fibrinogen is the glycoprotein clotted by thrombin. The molecule appears to be made of three globular portions. Complex molecular arrangements are involved in the fibrinogen-to-fibrin change. The clotting of fibrinogen by thrombin involves the splitting away of terminal fibrinopeptides A and B. The remaining portion of the fibrinogen molecule is considered a fibrin monomer. The fibrin monomer molecules attach to each other loosely at first and then more tightly with the aid of a fibrin stabilizing factor, which acts as an enzyme to bind the monomers. Most of the circulation fibrinogen is formed in the liver; liver disease decreases the concentration of fibrinogen in the blood. Fibrinogen is a large molecule that does not leak into interstitial fluids unless the capillary permeability is increased. Thus clotting is rare in interstitial fluids unless fibrinogen leaks out of the damaged capillaries. Fig. 7-3 illustrates the conversion of prothrombin to thrombin under the influence of prothrombin activator and calcium ions. The figure also shows how factor XIII affects fibrin.

Factor XIII

Factor XIII stabilizes the fibrin. A plasma glycoprotein, factor XIII is synthesized in the liver. Apparently factor XIII is also isolated from disrupted platelets. Thrombin converts factor XIII to the activated substance in the presence of calcium ions. Factor XIII_a acts as a transglutaminase. It stabilizes the fibrin clot by forming cross-linkages between glutamine and lipine residues of fibrin monomers. When factor XIII is deficient, wound healing may be impaired.

Factor VIII

A deficiency of factor VIII has long been associated with hemophilia; however, Factor

Fig. 7-3. Conversion of prothrombin, thrombin, and fibrinogen into fibrin threads. Factor XIII acts as a fibrin stabilizer.

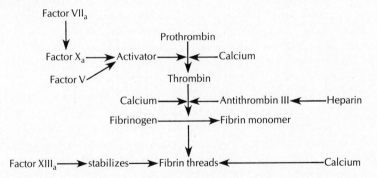

VIII has several other activities. It is necessary for proper platelet function and also contributes an immunologic reaction not involved in coagulation. Therefore factor VIII_F refers to the antihemophilic activity or the procoagulant activity. Factor VIII_{Ag} refers to the antigenic activity that can be quantified by various immunologic methods. Factor VIII_{vW} activity is lacking in severe classic von Willebrand's disease; the factor mediates the aggregation of platelets and adhesiveness of platelets to subendothelium. Factor VIII_{vW} is also increased in myocardial infarction and postoperative states.

Factor VIII is probably synthesized in the liver, but some evidence reveals that the spleen converts a precursor that is synthesized in the liver. The amount of factor VIII synthesized depends on the proportion of cells having an active X chromosome.

Factor IV (calcium)

Calcium acts as a cofactor in the activation of factors IX, X, and fibrin. Calcium also stabilizes factor V and is required for platelet aggregation. Generally the calcium ion concentration never gets low enough to prevent clotting. However, whole blood is prevented from clotting by the addition of citrate, which binds with the calcium to inactivate it.

Blood coagulation

Blood coagulation is described as a chain reaction involving factors, serine proteases, and cofactors. A discussion of some of the elements relating to blood coagulation follows.

Serine proteases. Enzymes involved in coagulation are serine proteases, like other enzymes in the body. The serine proteases of the system are factor XII (Hageman), prekallikrein, and factors XI, X, IX, and II (prothrombin).[1] Activation of the clotting serine proteases occurs when the first enzyme is activated. The activated serine protease is able to split the peptide bonds of the next enzyme in the cascade. Finally thrombin makes splits in the fibrinogen molecule, initiating the fibrin conversion. Other proteins that do

---

CLASSIFICATION OF BLOOD COAGULATION PROTEINS	
Serine proteases	**Cofactors**
XII	Kininogen
Prekallikrein	Factor VIII
XI	Factor V
IX	Tissue factor
X	
VII	
II	

---

not possess enzymatic activity but do help the proteolytic activity are kininogen, factor VIII, factor V, and tissue factor. These factors are called *cofactors*.

Cofactors. Cofactors are proteins that do not possess enzyme activity but that boost other clotting factors. Kininogen aids activated XII to activate factor XI. Factor VIII acts as a cofactor with activated IX to activate factor X. Factor V along with factor X convert prothrombin to thrombin. Tissue factor activates factor X with the help of factor VII (see Fig. 7-4).

Factor XIII is a fibrin-stabilizing factor, which is a transpeptidase. This enzyme can form new peptide bonds. Fibrinogen, which is converted into fibrin by thrombin, has no enzymatic activity.

Intrinsic and extrinsic pathways. When the coagulation cascade occurs within the vascular system, the components are from within the blood. Tissue factor from tissue trauma comes in contact with coagulation factors to begin the extrinsic cascade. Intrinsic, as well as extrinsic, coagulation must occur with ionized calcium. Coagulation actually occurs on the surface of the platelets, which release phospholipids that act as potent accelerators (Fig. 7-5).

Primary hemostasis. Primary hemostasis usually occurs when vascular injury disrupts the endothelial layer of the vessel and blood is exposed to subendothelial connective tissue. Platelets in the blood are attracted to the denuded

Fig. 7-4. Conversion of prothrombin to thrombin; subscript *a* represents activated state.

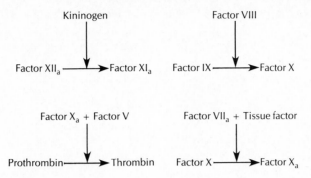

Fig. 7-5. Diagram of the coagulation cascade. Roman numerals indicate the factors. Roman numerals with the subscript letter *a* indicate the activated factors.

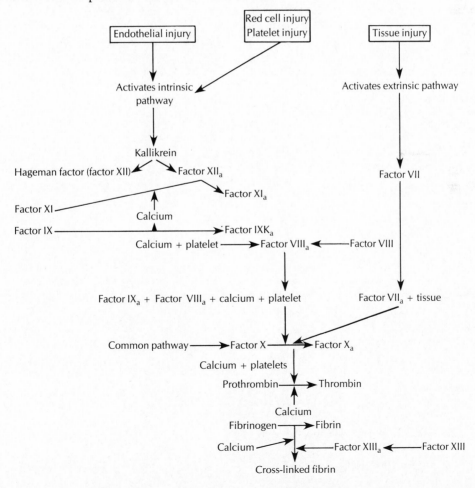

endothelial lining and begin to adhere to the collagen fibers. Platelets then undergo alterations, and a release reaction occurs. Nucleotide adenosine diphosphate (ADP) is released and causes the platelets to swell and adhere to each other. As the swelling and adhesion occurs, more ADP is released; the ADP acts as a chemical mediator and continues the process. Besides ADP, other chemicals are released from the platelet membrane. Phospholipases are activated that cause arachidonic acid to be released from platelet phospholipids. A second platelet enzyme, cyclooxygenase, transforms arachidonic acid into a cyclic endoperoxide.

A third platelet enzyme, thromboxane synthetase, acts on the cyclic endoperoxide to make thromboxane A_2 (Fig. 7-6). Thromboxane A_2 is a strong platelet-aggregating agent. It also probably helps to maintain a vasospasm by causing a vasoconstriction during primary hemostasis. A platelet plug is produced at the injury site with the aid of ADP, thromboxane A_2, and von Willebrand factor.

Normally the disk-shaped platelets circulate approximately 10 days. When platelets are activated by endothelial damage, they adhere to various elements of the vascular wall, principally collagen, basement membrane, and the microfibril. Thus a damaged vessel is the first process in the sequence of platelet adhesion. Shape change, release reaction, and platelet contraction are the other processes.

Shape change involves the transformation of the platelet from a disk to a sphere. The transformation probably involves actin filaments anchoring to the platelet membrane and exerting a force pulling the cell surface toward the center of the platelet. Calcium ions trigger the actin-myosin interaction within the platelet.

After shape change, platelets begin a secretory reaction and release the alpha granules, liposomes, and dense bodies. The release or se-

Fig. 7-6. Prostaglandin synthesis.

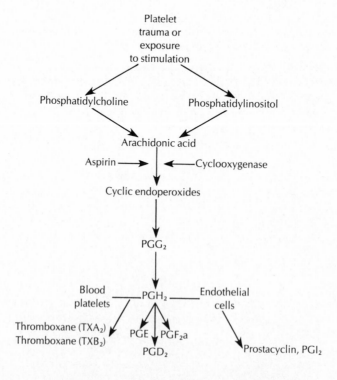

cretion from the alpha granules is called the *mitogenic factor*. This mitogenic factor is thought to be responsible for the movement of smooth muscle cells from the medial layers of arteries into the intimal layers, forming fibrous plaques characteristic of atherosclerosis.

Aggregation of platelets requires calcium. Probably external proteins or lipids cause alterations in the membrane of platelets to allow sticking of platelets to one another.

Three mechanisms probably involved in platelet aggregation and the release action are membrane adenylate cyclase activity changes, intraplatelet ionic calcium fluxes, and unstable endoperoxides and thromboxane A_2 synthesis. The interactions among these mechanisms are not completely understood.

Prostaglandins have been known to affect platelet aggregation and also to inhibit aggregation. Prostaglandins also play a part in the release of dense bodies, the irreversible phase of platelet aggregation. Although prostaglandins are not present in circulating platelets, whenever the platelet is injured or exposed to thrombin, collagen, epinephrine, or ADP, the prostaglandins are produced. Prostaglandins probably are produced when phospholipases C and A_2 catalyze the release of arachidonic acid from phosphatidylinositol and phosphatidylcholine. PGG_2 and PGH_2 are then formed from arachidonic acid by another catalyst, cyclooxygenase. Thromboxane A_2, the most potent activator, is formed in platelets with the aid of PGH_2. Epoprostenol, the most potent inhibitor of platelet activation, is formed in the endothelial cells. Epoprostenol can be called a circulating hormone. The lung releases it into the circulation. Thus a ratio between thromboxane A_2 and epoprostenol maintains control over thrombosis (Fig. 7-6).

Other platelet functions

Besides platelet function with primary and secondary hemostasis, there is some evidence that platelets are taken up by the endothelial cells and become part of the cytoplasm and contribute to the integrity of the vascular system. Plate-lets may also play a role in wound healing and inflammation through locomotor functions in response to chemotatic agents such as collagen and cyclic adenosine monophosphate. Phagocytic and pinocytic properties are also attributed to the platelet membrane.

Secondary hemostasis
Intrinsic pathways

Plasma protein enzyme systems rarely function by themselves. They are parts of a domino-like dropping action. Factor XII (Hageman) must attach to a negatively charged surface. In the body, the negatively charged surface is the subintimal vascular connective tissue or the platelet membrane surface. Hageman factor reacts with prekallikrein and kininogen, both proteins. Besides acting as clotting factors, prekallikrein and kininogen produce bradykinin and other kinins. The kinins dilate small blood vessels, increase permeability, and generally respond to injury. The presence of prekallikrein and kininogen in the clotting cascade became apparent when persons with deficiencies of those proteins developed prolonged clotting times.

After Hageman factor becomes activated, factor XI is activated, which further activates prekallikrein into kallikrein. Kallikrein, as stated earlier, releases bradykinin, and it may convert the fibrinolytic proenzyme plasminogen into the active plasmin. Kallikrein may also activate the extrinsic clotting system through factor VII activation.

The conversion of factor XI to XI_a and factor IX to IX_a are the next steps in the intrinsic pathway activation system. When activated Hageman factor splits factor XI, factor XI becomes activated. Factor XI_a then splits factor IX and activates it.

Factor X can be activated by IX_a of the intrinsic system or by factor VII of the extrinsic system. The intrinsic activation of factor X is complex. It involves factor IX_a, factor X, ionized calcium, and platelet phospholipid becoming a complex, while factor VIII acts as a cofactor (Fig. 7-5).

Extrinsic pathways

Factor X can also be activated in the extrinsic system by factor VII_a. Factor VII requires a cofactor (tissue factor) to become VII_a. Factor VII_a combines with factor X, phospholipid, and ionized calcium to activate factor X (Fig. 7-7).

Factor VII_a in combination with factor X can also activate factor IX. Factor X_a can also activate factor VII.

Common pathways

The conversion of prothrombin into thrombin takes place next with the aid of factor X in the presence of platelets or phospholipids, ionized calcium, and factor V (Fig. 7-8).

When thrombin is produced, a fragment of prothrombin remains and has been associated with preclinical or clinical thrombotic states, especially when elevated levels of the fragment are assayed.

The final phase of blood coagulation, the fibrinogen to fibrin formation, is aided by thrombin. Fibrinopeptides are released from the fibrinogen molecule by thrombin-forming fibrin monomers.

The fibrin monomers line up with each other, causing a network of gel fibrin to form. To stabilize the fibrin, factor XIII is needed. Factor XIII is activated by thrombin and ionized calcium. If factor XIII is not available, the cross-linked fibrin is much weaker and becomes much more susceptible to breakdown by plasmin. Plasmin can alter fibrinogen or fibrin by breaking them into smaller peptides and fragment X.

Platelet function in secondary hemostasis

Platelets actively participate in the coagulation cascade. Coagulation is a surface-dependent process that takes place on the platelet membrane. A membrane phospholipid, platelet factor 3, allows factor X_a, calcium, and factor V_a to form a complex that enzymatically converts prothrombin to thrombin.

Factor V_a is released from the alpha granule of the platelet and plays a role in providing a receptor site for factor X_a. This factor V_a is in addition to factor V circulating in the plasma.

With factor XI present, the exposure of platelets to ADP activates factor XII (Fig. 7-9).

An alternate pathway allows collagen-stimulated platelets to initiate coagulation that utilizes factor XI without factor XII. Platelets also provide phospholipids in the factor IX_a, calcium, and factor VIII interaction, ultimately converting factor X to factor X_a (Fig. 7-10).

Fibrinolysis – secondary hemostasis inhibitors

Coagulation and fibrinolysis are interrelated from the beginning of the clot-forming process. Plasminogen, probably produced by the liver, parallels the plasma level of fibrinogen. Plasminogen tends to adhere to fibrinogen so that it becomes incorporated into the clot with fibrinogen. Proteolytic enzymes (possibly kallikrein) activate plasminogen into plasmin. Plasmin, in turn, digests fibrin, clearing it into soluble fragments. The digestion takes place slowly through cleavage of arginyl-valine bonds. In addition to fibrinogen and fibrin, plasmin digests factors II, V, VIII, and XII. In the digestion process, frag-

---

Fig. 7-7. Activation of factor X in the extrinsic system.

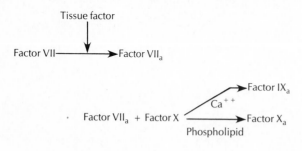

Fig. 7-8. Platelet contribution to conversion of prothrombin to thrombin.

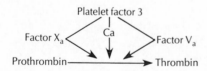

ment X plus small-molecular-weight peptides are produced. Fragment X splits into fragments Y, D, and other small peptides. Further, fragment Y splits to form other fragments, D and E. These fragments are commonly called *fibrin split products (FSP)* or *fibrin degradation products (FDP)*. These fragments then become anticoagulants in the circulation. The reticuloendothelial cells of the liver remove these fragments.

Inhibitors to fibrinolysis

Antiplasmin activity occurs from some of the substances that inhibit coagulation, including antithrombin III, alpha-antitrypsin, and protein C− inhibitor. Alpha$_2$ macroglobulin is by far the most significant inhibitor of plasmin. The mechanism of inactivation is a competition between thrombin and plasmin for the binding sites on the alpha$_2$-macroglobulin molecules.

Inhibitors of blood coagulation
Liver and lung

The normal liver is capable of clearing the body of activated coagulation factors. Fibrin and fibrinogen-fibrin complexes are probably removed by the reticuloendothelial cells of the liver, whereas activated factors are believed to be removed by hepatocytes. The pulmonary system may also remove tissue factor and fibrin.

Antithrombins

Several inhibiting proteases also exist in the plasma. The most important plasma inhibitor is antithrombin III. Antithrombin III inhibits thrombin, factors XII$_a$, I$_a$, IX$_a$, X$_a$, and probably VII$_a$. By itself, antithrombin III is an ineffective inhibitor but becomes effective with the addition of heparin. In fact, for exogenous heparin to work, antithrombin III must be present. With deficiencies of antithrombin III, persons become prone to thrombosis, and heparin therapy is ineffective.

Another serine protease, protein C, inhibits clotting by inactivation of factor V and VIII. Factors XI and XII are also inhibited by products in the serum and plasma.

Heparin

Endogenous heparin produced by basophilic mast cells of the precapillary connective tissue acts in conjunction with antithrombin to inhibit coagulation. Heparin combines with its cofactors to inhibit factors X$_a$, IX$_a$, XI$_a$, and XII$_a$.

When prothrombin is converted to thrombin, a fragment, F$_a$, is formed that inhibits the activation of prothrombin by factor X$_a$. Other feedback systems abound within the coagulation system. As new and more complex feedback mechanisms are found the total understanding may change. In fact, the distinction between intrinsic and extrinsic systems may be dissolved because of the complex intertwining of the systems.

In summary, primary hemostasis involves vascular contraction and platelet activation. Platelet activation is followed by aggregation, degranulation, and finally the release of endogenous ADP recruiting other platelets, causing irreversible platelet aggregation and formation of the platelet clot. Secondary hemostasis refers to the activation of the coagulation cascade by collagen or platelet phospholipid, ending in a fibrin clot. Along with coagulation, fibrinolysis is also activated.

Fig. 7-9. The role of platelets in the activation of factor XII.

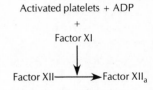

Fig. 7-10. Platelets combine with calcium, factor IX$_a$, and factor VIII$_a$ to activate factor X.

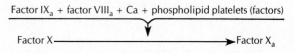

ASSESSMENT
History

It is often necessary to combine clinical assessment with laboratory data when evaluating hemostatic abnormalities. For example, factor XII (Hageman factor) deficiency may not present with significant bleeding, but the laboratory tests will show striking abnormalities. On the other hand, thrombopathy may initially be seen with significant bleeding, but the disease may be extremely difficult to demonstrate with laboratory tests. Therefore historical inquiry remains of prime importance in evaluating a bleeding or thrombosis problem.

The history helps to decide whether a patient has a significant bleeding problem. The type, onset, severity, site, and duration of bleeding or pain are important criteria to begin the questioning for historical data.

Bleeding and bruising related to minor trauma

If bruising or bleeding has occurred, especially if the bruise is 3 cm or larger, the episodes are probably associated with vascular abnormalities, but they can occur with coagulation and platelet disorders also. A significant history of bleeding following a dental extraction should be explored. Bleeding associated with platelet diseases causing a problem following a dental extraction is usually immediate and transient.

Exact amounts of bleeding and the number and type of extractions will help to define the cause. If the patient has had no bleeding episodes with teeth extractions, valuable information has been gathered. However, if the bleeding after an extraction was delayed and prolonged, a coagulation disorder may be the cause.

A family history of bleeding is especially important, because deficiencies of factors VIII, IX, and X are often linked, especially in males, to congenital abnormalities.[8] There may be cases in which there is a severe bleeding history, but the patient's primary screening tests yield normal results.

Since patients do not always respond to the question, "Are you a bleeder?" with detailed information, specific questions are mandatory about past bleeding in response to trauma. Mucous membrane bleeding, such as epistaxis, is a common symptom that both children and adults might discuss. Questioning about length and severity of bleeding becomes quite important, since epistaxis may or may not be of significance.

Several systemic diseases may be accompanied by abnormalities of the blood vessels, platelets, and coagulation factors. In liver disease, malignancies, systemic lupus erythematosus, and uremia, bleeding may be the symptom initially seen.

Another important facet of the history, when bleeding is the symptom for which the patient is initially seen is the medication history. Aspirin taken during the previous week could interfere with platelet function and contribute to the bleeding disorder. Other drugs discussed in a later section of this unit can also contribute to platelet dysfunction. Questions should be asked about any over-the-counter preparations being used by the patient. The patient's use of coumadin or heparin must also be determined. Patients who ingest bone marrow suppressant drugs or drugs that interfere with platelet function may have bleeding as a symptom at initial examination.

Sudden hemorrhage related to bleeding disorders

Sudden hemorrhage is less commonly associated with bleeding disorders than oozing of long duration. When there is a history of excessive bleeding with surgical procedures, a congenital coagulation disorder is suggested. Sudden hemorrhage is also associated with surgical procedures and is caused by a mechanical problem rather than a bleeding disorder.

Pain associated with bleeding and thrombosis

The history taker has a challenge when trying to gather information that will help to relate pain to possible bleeding or thrombosis. The nature of the pain, its severity, chronicity, and cause are important to know. Diagnostic clues can be obtained by further questioning the patient about the attributes of the pain. Pain associated with body movement is often associated with inflamed tissues or joints. Inflamed tissues or joints may be associated with bleeding disorders or coagulation problems, such as seen in hemarthrosis.

The quality of the pain must be determined. Deep, boring, pounding, sore, heavy, constricting, gnawing qualities may be associated with deep pain, as is seen with internal hemorrhage. Shooting pain usually results from the irritation of a nerve trunk, whereas a throbbing pain is often associated with inflamed tissues surrounding a pulsating artery.

Pain in the calves (claudication) is associated with walking, not with rest. The individual usually has a fixed distance of walking that produces the pain. As there is progressive narrowing of the artery or anemia occurs, pain occurs earlier. Angina pain occurs in a similar fashion, with narrowing of the arteries of the heart resulting from deposits, thrombosis, or spasm. Pain in the chest may also be caused by pulmonary emboli. Therefore specific questions regarding the pain as well as the history of pain in individuals is valuable information for diagnosis of bleeding or coagulation problems.

In conclusion, the history of hemorrhage or pain is very valuable to the diagnosis and treatment of any bleeding anomaly. The following areas should always be discussed during history taking:

1. Is there any history of spontaneous or posttraumatic (surgery or trauma) in the patient or his or her family?
2. What medications has the patient been taking (including over-the-counter drugs)? Be sure to ask about coumadin and aspirin.
3. Is there evidence on physical exam or history of liver disease or hepatic decompensation with or without splenomegaly?

4. What is the transfusion record of the patient? Banked blood quickly becomes deficient in factors I, II, V, VIII, and platelets.
5. Where is the bleeding? Localized bleeding after surgery probably reflects a technical complication. Generalized bleeding or oozing may mean coagulation abnormalities.
6. Is there evidence of thrombosis and bleeding? Neurologic impairment, renal failure, or circulatory problems may be the cause.

Physical examination
Skin assessment

When the practitioner examines a patient with a disorder in hemostasis or coagulation, three main approaches should be considered. Examination that evaluates (1) the blood vessels, (2) the platelets, and (3) the coagulation process will help to identify key information for diagnosis.[12] Most physical findings of bleeding are manifested in the skin.

Skin assessment includes inspection and palpation. Proper lighting while assessing the skin is mandatory. Describing and documenting skin lesions by their location, distribution, size, contour, and consistency are suggested.

Signs and symptoms

Vascular abnormalities. Vascular lesions result from changes in the superficial vasculature of the skin or bleeding lesions that result from hemorrhage into the skin.

Manifestations of blood vessel and platelet disorders result in petechiae, ecchymoses, epistaxis, and gastrointestinal, genitourinary, and vaginal bleeding. Minimal oozing following surgery or trauma may also be seen.

Petechiae. Petechiae are small capillary hemorrhages usually resulting from disorders in blood vessels or platelets. They are tiny red or red-brown capillary hemorrhages located within the skin papillae. Petechiae are most conspicuous in dependent areas of the body where there is increased venous pressure. Dependent parts of the body or areas constricted by a girdle or tight stockings are examples of areas of petechiae eruptions. When petechiae are seen on the thorax and abdomen and these areas have not been constricted by garments, an infectious disease is usually involved. Petechiae are common in the newborn as a result of trauma of delivery and are completely unrelated to bleeding disorders. Petechiae in the skin do not blanch under pressure.

Telangiectasia. Telangiectasia is a condition charactrized by dilation of the capillary vessels and minute arteries, forming a variety of angioma. The small red to violet lesions consist of thin, dilated, tortuous vessels that blanch on pressure and tend to bleed spontaneously or as a result of trivial trauma. They are usually found on the lips, tongue, and tips of fingers and toes, but may be found in visceral vessels.

Spider telangiectasia is charactrized by circular or stellate, bright red, faintly pulsatile lesions that branch from the arterial system into the subcutaneous and dermal layers of the skin. These are often seen in liver disorders and are considered vascular or bleeding lesions.

Ecchymoses. Ecchymoses are extensions of lesions usually indicating that extravasated blood has transversed fascial planes. An ecchymosis involves a larger hemorrhagic area than do petechiae. When these intradermal hemorrhages occur in larger groups, the condition is called *purpura.*

Purpura. Purpuric lesions are often pruritic. Fever and malaise are often present, and effusions into the joints or viscera produce symptoms such as joint pain (Schönlein's purpura) or, bouts of abdominal pain (Henock's purpura). Purpura is usually associated with one of the common manifestations of allergy such as erythema or urticaria.

Purpuric lesions do not cause elevation of the skin or mucosa. When defects in platelets or coagulation factors cause purpura, it is usually seen in the lower extremities. Purpura may result

from vessel damage or rupture or from a platelet deficiency.

The clinical picture of platelet abnormality is different from bleeding as a result of coagulation factor disorders. Petechiae in the skin and mucous membranes and possibly throughout the internal organs is typical with platelet dysfunction. The bleeding associated with platelet abnormalities stops rapidly with local pressure and fails to recur when pressure is withdrawn. When a coagulation factor deficiency occurs, hemorrhage results in subcutaneous or intramuscular areas; it responds to pressure and will recur when pressure is released. Hemarthrosis is an example of a coagulation factor bleeding disorder.

Hemarthrosis. Hemarthrosis is bleeding into a joint cavity. It can affect ankles, elbows, wrists, fingers, hips, shoulders, and knees. Hemarthrosis accounts for almost all the morbidity associated with hemophilia. Each patient usually experiences bleeding into specific joints. Presumably the blood causes a foreign body reaction in the joint, which becomes chronic and continually exudes fluid into the joint. The inflammation recurs with each minor trauma to the joint. In fact, bleeding may appear to result spontaneously because minimal trauma can cause bleeding.

Bony joint changes result from repeated hemarthrosis; these result in decreased function of the joint. The decreased function often results in flexion contractures and an inability to fully extend the joints. When the joint has decreased function, minor trauma tends to increase and therefore hemorrhage increases. Furthermore, as hemarthrosis occurs in one joint, other joints become vulnerable to mechanical stress and potential joint bleeding.

Hemarthrosis does not usually develop in a child until 3 or 4 years of age. Hemarthrosis is rare in disorders of blood vessels or platelets or in acquired coagulation disorders. It is usually diagnostic of severe hereditary coagulation disorders.

Internal hemorrhage. Faintness, tachycardia, hypotension, confusion, disorientation, and air hunger may be subtle signs of internal hemorrhage. Tarry stools, bright red stools, or smoky-colored urine may evidence bleeding in the gastrointestinal or genitourinary tract. Melena is the passage of dark, pitchy stools stained with blood pigments. Melena may also be seen in the newborn.

Visceral hemorrhage. Visceral hemorrhages take place in open spaces rather than closed spaces, as in hemarthrosis. Early symptoms are therefore infrequent. Deep subcutaneous and abdominal visceral bleeding is more common in hereditary deficiencies of coagulation factors.

Hematoma. A hematoma is an area in which underlying hemorrhage causes elevation of the skin or mucosa from extravasated blood. The skin surface usually becomes colored. In a child, hematoma may only be seen when the child is active.

Umbilical cord or scalp bleeding. Umbilical cord or scalp bleeding is common in hemorrhagic disease of the newborn. Generally this bleeding occurs as a result of coagulation factor disorders. After platelet and coagulation factors are consumed, initial signs and symptoms of any of the hemorrhagic problems of platelet or coagulation factors are seen. Disseminated intravascular coagulation and acrocyanosis are examples of problems with platelet and coagulation factor consumption.

With the consumption of platelets and coagulation factors a hemorrhagic state ensues. The fibrin that has been generated breaks down into fibrin split products (FSP) or fibrin degradation products (FDP), which inhibit the action of thrombin-activating fibrinogen to fibrin, thus intensifying bleeding.

Acrocyanosis. Acrocyanosis is a condition marked by symmetrical cyanosis of the extremities, with persistent, uneven, mottled blue or red discoloration of the skin of the digits, wrists, and ankles, with profuse sweating and coldness of the digits. Acrocyanosis is often associated with disseminated intravascular coagulation; it results from bleeding out of the small capillaries of the extremities.

Other skin changes

Jaundice. When increased bilirubin accumulates in the skin or sclera, a yellowish discoloration occurs. Jaundice is associated with liver disease. Liver disease is associated with coagulation disorders.

Pallor. Pallor is the whitish tint or absence of a reddish coloration of the skin in a light-skinned person. In a brown-skinned person, pallor results in yellowish-brown skin; in black skin, pallor appears as ashen gray. Pallor is caused by a marked decrease in the hemoglobin level of the blood.

Assessment of blood loss

Fluid and electrolyte status is altered when a patient loses blood. Direct and indirect methods of assessing blood loss are attempted by the practitioner so that accurate documentation can be made.

Direct methods

Gravimetric method. Blood-soaked linen or dressings can be weighed on a scale that is accurate to 0.1 g. The dry weight is subtracted from the weight of the item with blood. One gram of blood equals 1 ml.[3] If evaporation occurs during the time the blood-soaked item is exposed to air, an inaccurate weight may be derived.

Suction. Suction devices such as Hemovac or wall suction are used to draw blood into a container for measurement. When the container is large and the amount of blood suctioned is small, inaccuracies are possible.

Indirect methods

Patient weight. If the patient can be weighed before and after a blood loss, such as surgery, an estimate can be made of the loss; however, the number of grams of loss does not equal the number of milliliters of loss. Insensible water loss, removal of tissue during surgery, drains or catheters inserted, and IV fluids infused all increase or decrease body weight.

Blood pressure. Often a decrease in arterial blood pressure is considered an indicator of blood loss. However, homeostatic mechanisms such as vasoconstriction, increased heart rate, shifts of extravascular fluids into the intravascular space, and retention of sodium and water may prevent a drop in pressure even when considerable blood has been lost. Three pints of blood may be lost before a significant drop in pressure occurs. In general, 500 ml can be lost without effect on the blood pressure. When bleeding occurs slowly, the blood pressure is of little value as an indicator of blood loss.

Heart rate. The heart rate is useful when large amounts of blood are lost rapidly; however, when there is slow, oozing bleeding over an extended period, the heart rate may not increase.

Hemoglobin and hematocrit. With chronic blood loss, the body may not be able to absorb necessary quantities of iron from the intestines to form hemoglobin as it is lost. After a rapid blood loss, however, the composition of the blood may stay the same. When the body replaces the plasma in 1 to 3 days, the concentration of blood cells is reduced, resulting in low hematocrit and hemoglobin levels. Other indirect methods of measuring blood loss are the urinary output, central venous pressure, and pulmonary capillary wedge pressure. Observation of the patient may reveal pallored skin that is diaphoretic or bruised. Anxiety, pain, or edema may be other signs of insidious bleeding episodes.

Spleen assessment

The normal adult spleen lies immediately under the vault of the left side of the diaphragm with its convex surface separated from the thoracic cage by the costophrenic sinus of the pleura, which contains the lung only during deep inspiration. When the spleen is normal, it is not accessible to abdominal palpation.

When it is enlarged, the spleen is displaced downward from behind the thoracic cage and along its oblique axis toward the right iliac fossa. To palpate the spleen, the examiner stands on the left side of the patient, facing the feet. The patient could either place his left fist under the left eleventh rib, or a rolled towel could be placed so that the patient's thorax is forced upward. The examiner positions both hands around the left costal margin with the fingers curled up under the ribs, while the patient takes a deep inspiration. The spleen's lower margin should be felt by the fingertips.

Laboratory evaluation

Within the past 10 to 12 years, new laboratory advances have allowed clinicians to diagnose and treat thrombotic and hemorrhagic abnormalities of the hemostatic mechanism with more accuracy and skill. Techniques such as affinity chromatography and amino acid sequencing are available to analyze the various coagulation proteins.

Laboratory evaluation in disorders of hemostasis is directed toward determining whether a vascular, platelet, or coagulation abnormality is the cause of the bleeding (Table 7-3). Four primary tests provide this information. The tests measuring bleeding time and platelet count assess the vascular and platelet phases of hemostasis, whereas the partial thromboplastin time (PTT) and prothrombin tests evaluate the coagulation phase.

Once the clinical history and physical examination are concluded, laboratory testing should begin to identify and evaluate any hemostatic changes. A group of tests is used, because no single test can evaluate the whole system.

The usual tests begin with evaluations of prothrombin (PT), activated partial thromboplastin time (APTT), bleeding time, and platelet count. Thrombin time and peripheral smear tests are also frequently given. With these tests one can identify a specific part of the coagulation system as the source of the abnormality. Although the coagulation process is very complex and very difficult to separate into distinct sec-

Table 7-3. Laboratory tests and systems tested

System tested	Test
Platelets and capillaries	Template bleeding time
Platelets	Platelet count
Intrinsic	Activated partial thromboplastin time
	Factor assays
	Plasma clotting time
Extrinsic	Prothrombin time
	Factor assays
	Stypven time (except factor VII)
Fibrinolytic	Fibrin split/degradation products
	Euglobulin lysis time
	Fibrin monomer tests
Fibrinogen	Thrombin time
	Reptilase time

tions, the tests described here will be separated into sections according to the traditional intrinsic, extrinsic, and fibrinolytic systems. Platelet testing will also be reviewed.

Platelet tests

Platelet adhesion to red blood cells and to glass tubes that have been coated with collagen or other proteins is a test that can be performed to study adhesion. Measurements of adhesion-aggregation identify the normality of the primary phase of hemostasis. The platelet retention test screens for platelet function and is especially helpful in patients with von Willebrand's disease who have received transfusions or oral contraceptives. Apparently, with pregnancy, transfusions, or the use of oral contraceptives, the levels of factors VIII:C, VIII R:AG and VIII R:WF may be normal in von Willebrand's disease but should show abnormal results. Platelet retention tests would, however, show abnormal results.

Intrinsic system of coagulation tests

The intrinsic system includes factors XII, XI, IX, X, VIII, V, II, I (fibrinogen), prekallikrein (Fletcher), and kininogen (Fitzgerald). Factors VII and XIII are not measured by the following tests.

Partial thromboplastin time (PTT). The PTT is the most sensitive test of coagulation. It is most useful as a screening test to detect a deficiency of factors VIII, IX, X, XI, or XII. Test results are also abnormal in the presence of an anticoagulant such as heparin. Therefore a PTT evaluates the intrinsic pathway of coagulation.

A partial thromboplastin is the lipid portion of tissue extracts and reacts like platelet factor 3. It is sensitive to factors VIII, IX, X, XI, and XII, although the PTT is also prolonged in severe deficiency of factor V and hypofibrinogenemia.

Plasma clotting time. The plasma clotting time test relies on a normal platelet count and normal platelet function for accurate results. Calcium chloride is added to platelet-rich plasma, and clotting time is measured. A platelet abnormality will result in an abnormal plasma clotting time even though normal clotting proteins exist.

Whole blood clotting (Lee and White). Whole blood is added to three test tubes at 37° C (98.6° F) and then tilted at various time intervals until the blood clots. The procedure is time consuming and is insensitive to all but the very severe factor deficiencies. Some clinicians still use this test to monitor heparin therapy, but the heparin dose must be quite high.

Activated clotting time (ACT). An activator such as silica is added to whole blood, which causes better activation of factor XII. Abnormal results do reflect severe as well as mild factor deficiencies. Thus the ACT test is more effective than the Lee and White test.

Extrinsic system of coagulation tests

Factors VII, X, V, II, and fibrinogen (I) are evaluated in the extrinsic system tests. Factor VII is unique to the extrinsic system, whereas the others are in both systems.

Prothrombin time (PT). The prothrombin time test measures the rate of the extrinsic and common pathways. It measures factors VII, X, V, prothrombin, and fibrinogen. An abnormal PT suggests the use of oral anticoagulants or an acquired coagulation disorder. Hereditary deficiencies rarely affect the extrinsic system. Vitamin K deficiency can also affect the extrinsic factors and result in an abnormal PT.

Each laboratory uses its own thromboplastins, normal range, and therapeutic range for oral anticoagulants. Prolonged PT can result from deficiencies of factors VII, X, V, II, or I, vitamin K deficiency, and anticoagulants.

Fibrinogen tests

Thrombin test is an assay to determine fibrinogen level. The test shows abnormal levels when fibrinogen is decreased or when anticoagulants are present. If there is an abnormal structure of fibrinogen, the test will also be abnormal.

Fibrin degradation products

Some fibrin degradation products are present in normal serum, but their concentration is too low to be detected by usual methods. A positive result is associated with extensive clot formation and activation of the fibrinolytic system. Often a positive result relates to disseminated intravascular coagulation. Deep venous thrombosis and pulmonary embolism may also increase levels and yield a positive test result.

Fibrin monomers tests

These tests aid in diagnosis of primary fibrinolysis and disseminated intravascular coagulation (DIC). Protamine sulfate splits the soluble fibrin complexes of fibrin monomers attached to fibrin split products.

Other hemostatic abnormalities tests

Individual factor assays can be tested when abnormal PT and APTT are found. Factor deficiency is suspected when PT and APTT are abnormal.

Stypven time. The Stypven time test distinguishes between factor VII and factor X deficienices when a PT is abnormal. It may also be abnormal with factor I, II, or V deficiencies.

Reptilase time. The reptilase time test is used because it is not affected by the presence of heparin, whereas the thrombin time is sensitive to heparin. When the reptilase time is abnormal, the fibrinogen level is decreased, or the increased FDPs or soluble fibrin monomer complexes are present.

Euglobin lysis time. The euglobin lysis time test detects increased fibrinolytic activity. The increased plasminogen activators in fibrinolytic states cause increased plasmin. The euglobin in plasma contains plasmin, fibrinogen, plasminogen, and plasminogen activators. In increased fibrinolytic states a shortened lysis time is seen.

Disseminated intravascular coagulation tests

There are many procedures used in research laboratories that identify the many biochemical events of DIC. In the clinical laboratory the following tests are performed. Prothrombin time and the activated thromboplastin time are prolonged in DIC. The fibrinogen and platelets are decreased. For confirmation, the fibrinogen-fibrin split products should be highly elevated in the serum. Early indication of DIC may be studied by measuring the antithrombin III and cold-insoluble globulin (CIG) levels. Both would be decreased in DIC. Cold-insoluble globulin is associated with soluble fibrin complexes. CIG supposedly facilitates the removal of circulating particles through the reticuloendothelial system, especially in conditions such as trauma, burns, and malignancies. In DIC the depletion of CIG would result because of the increased particulate matter needing removal.

Diagnostic methods for thrombosis

Noninvasive methods. Thrombi generally occur in the capacitance veins of the soleus muscle and are difficult to identify without the aid of invasive techniques such as labeled fibrinogen evaluation. Once the thrombi extend outside the soleus, noninvasive tests are useful. If a noninvasive test is unquestionably positive, the probability is greater than 90% that venous thrombosis is present and thus anticoagulant therapy can be pursued. On the other hand, when test results are negative, other tests will be needed to confirm.

Doppler ultrasound. The Doppler ultrasound test probably provides the best noninvasive technique. This method depends highly on the skills of the observer. The observer needs to know the anatomy of veins and to recognize that normal venous flow is phasic with respiration. All major veins should be examined and compared in both limbs. When there is a continuous flow below an occlusion that is not influenced by respiration, obstruction is recognized.

Vascular test

TOURNIQUET TEST FOR CAPILLARY FRAGILITY (RUMPEL-LEEDE TEST). Stasis of blood in the skin causes some petechial hemorrhages to occur in normal individuals; however, when the capillaries are fragile, the petechial hemorrhages are more severe.

Capillary fragility is common in two types of disorders: (1) vascular disorders such as scurvy and senile purpura, and (2) platelet disorders such as thrombocytopenic purpura and thrombocytasthenia.

A pressure cuff such as a sphygmomanometer is inflated to halfway between the systolic and diastolic levels and maintained for 5 minutes, then released. Observation of the extremity is made 2 minutes after the release of the cuff. Petechiae are counted and recorded from a 2.5 cm diameter (quarter-sized) area of the forearm or a 4-cm area of the antecubital fossa. Normally the petechiae should not exceed ten in women and children or five in men.

Phleborheography. The phleborheographic technique for diagnosis of deep venous thrombosis of the lower extremities tests limb volume changes in response to increased volume load and respiration. Cuffs that sense volume change are placed on the thigh, calf, and foot. The thigh and calf cuffs measure the changes secondary to respiration. The results are measured by the respiratory wave activity and volume changes recorded from the cuff sites.

Impedance and strain gauge plethysmography assess emptying of the limb. A thigh cuff is inflated to 50 mmHg, then suddenly deflated releasing venous outflow, which is measured on the gauge. Studies using these noninvasive techniques have shown these methods are insensitive to thrombus only below the knee. Therefore more clinicians recommend the use of contrast phlebography to diagnose thrombophlebitis.

Invasive methods

Fibrinogen leg scanning. Fibrinogen leg scanning is a sensitive test for detecting calf vein thrombosis. Radioactive fibrinogen is injected and readings are taken over both legs. Venous thrombosis is suspected if an uptake increase of more than 20% occurs from one point to another.

ALTERATIONS

The pathophysiology related to the alterations in hemostasis and coagulation are varied. Blood vessel trauma or disruption and platelet abnormalities result in an abnormal primary phase of hemostasis. Coagulation factor abnormalities result in the secondary phase disruption. Vitamin K, drugs and disease processes may play a role in the clinical presentation that is seen in patients with disorders of hemostasis and coagulation.

Bleeding, arthritic pains, abdominal pain, hematuria, gastrointestinal hemorrhage, fever, and malaise related to purpura

Heredity, allergy, exposure to drugs and poisons, poor nutrition, infection, and hypertension may cause small blood vessels to rupture with undue pressure. Acute or chronic inflammation of blood vessels supplying the skin, joints, gastrointestinal tract, and kidneys cause the symptoms.

Conditions that can result in secondary purpura include (1) serious tissue trauma arising from a blow or a burn, (2) arterial hypertension resulting in increased capillary pressure, (3) bloodstream infections that damage vascular epithelium, (4) vitamin C deficiency, which causes increased capillary fragility, and (5) uremia and cachexia, which result in vessel weakness.

When autoantibodies develop against platelets, megakaryocyte development is interrupted and platelet production is reduced or sensitized causing the spleen to destroy the platelets. Thus spontaneous bleeding may occur in the skin, mucous membranes, and internal cavities as a result of platelet purpura.

Drugs such as quinidine, quinine, the sulfonamides, phenylbutazone, and chorothiazide may also cause platelet destruction and purpura.

Moderate degree of mucous membrane bleeding, bleeding from superficial lacerations, easy bruising, or excessive bleeding after dental extraction related to platelet abnormalities

In some persons, factor VIII–related antigen is lacking, decreased, or qualitatively abnormal, resulting in inherited von Willebrand's disease. Other platelet disorders result from an abnormality of the membrane glycoproteins.

The use of aspirin induces a disorder that is similar to congenital abnormalities. There is an absence of the secondary aggregation in response to ADP and epinephrine. There is also a lack of response for collagen when aspirin is ingested.

Platelet defects also result from such conditions as uremia, cirrhosis, scurvy, leukemias, plasma cell myeloma, and macroglobulinemia. In some of these conditions the abnormal protein apparently coats the fluffy mucopolysaccharide surface of the platelet and prevents platelet response to stimulation. Plasmaphoresis is used to control this condition.

Deep dissecting hematomas, superficial ecchymoses, hemarthrosis, and delayed bleeding postoperatively related to congenital bleeding disorders

Modes of inheritance for specific inherited coagulation abnormalities are autosomal dominant, self-linked recessive, and autosomal recessive (see Table 7-4). Occasionally there are cases in which combined deficiencies are seen.

Table 7-4. Modes of inheritance for specific coagulation abnormalities

Deficiency	Mode of inheritance
Factor VIII	Set-linked recessive
Factor IX	Set-linked recessive
Factor II	Autosomal recessive
Factor V	Autosomal recessive
Factor VII	Autosomal recessive
Factor X	Autosomal recessive
Factor XI	Autosomal recessive
Factor XII	Autosomal recessive
Factor XIII	Autosomal recessive
von Willebrand syndrome	
Dysfibrinogenemias	Autosomal dominant
Passovoy factor deficiency	

As discussed earlier, the primary phase of hemostasis includes the constriction of the damaged vessel and the adhesion of the platelets to each other and to the exposed vessel wall. The secondary phase involves the actual coagulation as the fibrin and platelets become a clot. Defects related to congenital factor abnormalities are secondary phase defects. There are three possible pathophysiologic reasons for hereditary coagulation defects: (1) deficient biosynthesis of the factor occurs, (2) functionally inactive factors are produced, or (3) functionally abnormal factors are produced—or a combination of all three defects. In each of these cases, the secondary phase of hemostasis and coagulation will be affected. The family history, the laboratory tests, and the bleeding abnormality contribute to the diagnosis of congenital bleeding disorders.

Decreased wound healing related to factor XIII deficiency or decreased fibrinogen

Fibroblasts migrate along fibrin strands forming the fibrous scar of any wound. When deficiencies of factor XIII or fibrinogen occur, the fibrin network is loose and seems to have insufficient support for fibroblast migration. Wounds do not heal properly as a result.

PATHOPHYSIOLOGY OF INHERITED COAGULATION DEFECTS

Deficient biosynthesis	Functionally inactive factors	Functionally abnormal factors
Hemophilia A	Hemophilia A	Hemophilia B
Hemophilia B	Hemophilia B	von Willebrand
von Willebrand	von Willebrand	Dysfibrinogenemia
Afibrinogenemia	Dysfibrinogenemia	Hypoprothrombinemia
Hypoprothrombinemia	Hypoprothrombenemia	Factor VII
Factor V	Factor V	Factor X
Factor VII	Factor VII	
Factor X	Factor X	
Factor XI	Factor XII	
Factor XII	Factor XIII	
Fletcher (prekallikrein)	Fletcher (prekallikrein)	
Fitzgerald (kininogen)		

Melena, cephalohematomas, umbilical bleeding, and postcircumcision bleeding related to vitamin K deficiency

Hemorrhage in the neonate related to vitamin K–dependent coagulation factor deficiency results from a deficiency of these factors at birth. The levels usually fall during the first 2 to 5 days and rise between the seventh and fourteenth days. Normal levels are reached at 3 months of age.

Prematurity, inadequate intake, delayed colonization of the gastrointestinal tract by bacteria, maternal deficiency of vitamin K, and other obstetric and prenatal complications may contribute to the deficiency at birth.

Bleeding related to vitamin K deficiency

There are five possible reasons for the development of a vitamin K deficiency. They are (1) decreased nutritional intake, (2) defective bowel synthesis, (3) poor absorption from the bowel, (4) a diseased liver, and (5) the presence of anti–vitamin K compounds.

Nutritional deficiency of vitamin K is rare in the adult but may be frequent in the infant whose formula is deficient or in the infant who is breastfed without supplements. Synthesis problems can result from long-standing gastrointestinal disorders. Antibiotic therapy can reduce intestinal bacterial flora and produce a vitamin K deficiency. In the infant the bowel may not yet have sufficient bacterial flora or bile salts for absorption. Normal liver function is necessary for the synthesis of prothrombin and other vitamin K–dependent factors.

When there is a vitamin K deficiency, the liver continues to synthesize and release similar but inactive vitamin K–dependent factors. These inactive factors may exhibit clot inhibitory actions and become antagonists to vitamin K when it is available.

Spontaneous bleeding, ecchymoses, gastrointestinal hemorrhage, hematuria, and retroperitoneal hemorrhage related to heparin therapy

Duration of heparin therapy is frequently cited as a predisposing factor in hemorrhage. It is rare for hemorrhage to occur in the first 48 hours after instituting heparin therapy. The risk increases by about 1% per day. Elderly females are reported to have a higher incidence of bleeding with heparin therapy; however, studies show a tendency for both elderly men and women to have increased bleeding.

When such symptoms occur as an otherwise unexplained drop in hematocrit levels, lower back or abdominal pain, or even vague symptoms such as increasing anxiety, restlessness, or tachycardia, heparin-induced hemorrhage must be considered.

Hemorrhage related to antibiotic administration

Antibiotics may contribute to bleeding in three ways: (1) by causing hypoprothrombinemia; (2) by interfering with platelet aggregation, and (3) by reducing the number of platelets (thrombocytopenia), which is rare. It is believed that the most frequent antibiotic-associated bleeding event is hypothrombinemia.

Antibiotic-associated bleeding may result especially from drugs possessing significant activity against gram-negative organisms or anaerobes. The drug action is thought to alter the number or type of intestinal bacterial flora, with consequent reduction in synthesis in vitamin K. Inhibition of platelet function from antibiotic usage is usually dosage related. No evidence of inhibition of platelet prostaglandin synthesis has been seen with antibiotics. Possibly the suppression of platelet aggregation is caused by a nonspecific binding of the drug to the platelet membrane, resulting in blockage of aggregation agonist sites.[10]

Alterations in platelet function related to drugs other than antibiotics

Besides antibiotics, a few drugs have been studied for their effects on hemostasis or coagulation. The following drugs are some of those that have been studied.[9]

Heparin

As mentioned in another section, heparin affects anticoagulation by interacting with antithrombin III to potentiate its effect on thrombin

and factors X_a, IX_a, and XI_a. The inhibitory effect causes thrombin and other factors to decrease clotting formation. However, heparin also affects platelet function. Apparently heparin inhibits the interaction of platelets with collagen, preventing the platelets from aggregating onto the exposed collagen.

Dipyridamole and pyrimido-pyramidine compounds

These drugs inhibit platelet aggregation and the platelet release reaction. They probably inhibit platelet phosphodiesterase, which increases cyclic AMP levels inside platelets. Dipyridamole also inhibits platelet adhesion to collagen and subendothelial structures. When given at 400 mg in four divided doses, dipyridamole also prolongs platelet survival in some persons.

Hydroxychloroquine

Though given as antimalarial agents, hydroxychloroquine compounds have some antiinflammatory properties. They inhibit aggregation induced by ADP or collagen. The release reaction is also affected. In some cases hydroxychloroquine has been known to prevent venous thrombi.

Nonsteriodal antiinflammatory drugs

Drugs such as aspirin, indomethacin, phenylbutazone, and sulfinpyrazone inhibit aggregation induced by collagen, ADP, or epinephrine. It is suggested that these compounds influence platelets in two ways. First, they inhibit the cyclooxygenase, which blocks the conversion of arachidonate to PGG_2 and PGH_2, which produce thromboxane A_2. Second, these drugs affect platelet shape change, aggregation, and the release reaction.

Clofibrate and halofenate

Clofibrate and halofenate, which lower serum lipids, also inhibit collagen-induced and ADP-induced aggregation. Platelet survival is also prolonged.

Table 7-5. Red and white thrombi by vessel and cause of symptom

Thrombus	Vessel	Cause of symptoms
Red	Vein	Bulk and location
White	Artery	Critical location rather than size

Propranolol

Propranolol apparently inhibits ADP-induced aggregation, but it is unclear just how this takes place. Propranolol also inhibits platelet adherence to collagen.

Hydrocortisone and methylprednisolone

Inhibition of platelet aggregation and release induced by ADP, epinephrine, collagen, thrombin, and endotoxin are seen with these drugs.

Muscular aches, leg cramps, and mild ankle edema related to retrograde flow of blood down saphenous vein

When patients have venous insufficiency, there is usually an increase in the number of capillaries in the skin. In addition, fibrin is deposited around the capillaries in patients with poor calf muscle function. When there is an increased number of capillaries in the skin of the lower leg, an increased capillary permeability allows a leakage of fibrinogen into the pericapillary spaces. It has been reported that even though there is the fibrinogen leakage and fibrin deposit, fibrinolytic activity is significantly reduced.

Thus venous hypertension occurs, causing dilation and elongation of venules, resulting in increased size of capillary pores. The enlarged capillary pores allow fibrinogen to leak into the interstitial spaces. Extrinsic clotting factors convert the fibrinogen into fibrin. The fibrin then deposits around the capillaries. Fibrinolytic activity is decreased in interstitial fluid, so the fibrin deposit causes a barrier to the transport of

oxygen from the capillaries to the cells. Ulceration of the skin probably results from the death of cells, caused by the diffusion barrier. Edema, bursting pain during exercise, and thickening of the skin and subcutaneous tissues (lipodermatosclerosis) may also occur.

Pain associated with thrombus or emboli

Normal endothelium of blood vessels has a surface which does not react to circulating blood constituents. The passive nature of the luminal surface composition and the active synthesis of the potent antiplatelet agent epoprostenol are two factors that maintain a nonthrombogenic surface of endothelium.

Recent studies implicate platelets in the beginning and progression of atherosclerotic lesions, as well as the thromboembolic complications associated with atherosclerotic disease, resulting in stroke and myocardial infarction. Therefore when nonendothelial vascular surfaces are exposed to flowing blood, platelet and coagulation reactions result in thrombus formation. Within an arterial vessel that has been damaged, the formation of a thrombus includes large amounts of platelets ("white thrombus"), whereas thrombi formed in venous circulation include both platelets and red cells entrapped in a fibrin mesh ("red thrombus"); see Table 7-5. High pressure arterial blood flow may cause embolic fragments that cause vascular occlusion, ischemia, or infarction downstream. Pain may be the result of the initial thrombus formation or any emboli phenomenon. Therefore the pathologic events that occur begin with vascular injury and endothelial denudation. Platelets react to the exposed subendothelial surfaces. This resulting thrombus is a distortion of the normal process of primary hemostasis.

In red thrombus (in a vein) there may be no evidence of vascular injury to the vessel or the valve cusps in which they originate. Biochemical injury may exist. Possibly turbulent flow of platelet enriched blood selectively deposits platelets in eddies, and the coagulation process ensues. The thrombus grows and extends in the vessel lumen in areas of static blood.

The symptoms that are produced by a red thrombus are a result of its bulk and location. The white thrombus produces symptoms because of its critical location rather than its size.

In the forming of an arterial thrombus there is an intrinsic arterial wall abnormality that facilitates platelet adherence. In comparison to a primary hemostatic plug seen in extravascular vessel injury, a white thrombus (in an artery) forms on the luminal surface of the injured vessel extending along the vessel. As the thrombus becomes concentric, red cells and fibrin are deposited. Only when the total lumen becomes occluded does the coagulation mechanism become dominant.

Gastrointestinal hemorrhage, esophageal varices, and peptic ulcer related to liver disease

The liver has both clearance and biosynthetic functions. When liver disease occurs, coagulation defects occur. Generally vitamin K–dependent factors are deficient in hepatic disease. Administration of vitamin K is without benefit in persons with hepatic disease, in comparison to those persons with biliary tract obstruction. Factor V and fibrinogen will also decrease in advanced disease.

Since plasminogen activators are normally removed by the liver, fibrinolytic activity increases in cirrihosis. Fibrin split products are also increased that affect platelet function. Portal hypertension may also cause hypersplenism and platelet sequestration, resulting in decreased platelet function and count.

Thrombosis and bleeding related to risk factors of certain disease states

Cancer patients are frequently thrombocytopenic as a result of chemotherapy. Combinations of chemotherapy, thrombocytopenia, and DIC are also seen in cancer patients.

When the kidneys are impaired, a functional defect occurs in platelets. Antibiotics given to patients who have renal impairment or cancer or who are of advanced age will also increase the risk of bleeding events.

The risk of coronary disease is reportedly lower in premenopausal women than in men. Some researchers have attributed this reduced risk to the prostacyclin emanating from the uterus in premenopausal women. Apparently premenopausal women have increased circulating levels of prostacyclin compared to men of comparable ages.

Thrombosis and bleeding related to renal diseases

Mucosal bleeding, epistaxis, gingival bleeding, hematuria, and gastrointestinal bleeding occur in renal impairment, possibly as a result of platelet abnormalities. Factor changes also occur in renal disease. Elevation of factor VIII, fibrinogen, and inhibitors of plasminogen activations occur. Antithrombin III may be decreased, especially in patients with nephrotic syndrome. With the increase in levels of inhibitors of fibrinolytic activity, this fibrinolysis is decreased. Factor XIII activity may also decrease in renal insufficiency.

Since the kidney is the site of production of erythropoietin, some patients who suffer from renal failure may have decreased secretion of erythropoietic substances. Decreased erythropoietin production leads to decreased red cell production and possible anemia and lowered hematocrit levels. When the decreased hematocrit level results in symptoms of shortness of breath, dizziness, fatigue, angina, or increased pulse rate, blood component therapy may be recommended. The blood component therapy may be indicated because of the decreased red cell production rather than decreased numbers of platelets.

Bleeding tendency related to frequent blood transfusion

Platelets degenerate in stored blood, so a deficiency of platelets occurs in patients who require massive amounts of blood. Platelet transfusions and fresh whole blood may be used to add to the body's increased production of platelets in these situations.

Hemostasis and coagulation changes related to lung metabolism

In the last 10 years several metabolic processes have been attributed to the lung. These processes, such as clearance of serotonin and norepinephrine, inactivation of bradykinin, activation of angiotensin II, and the synthesis of prostaglandins may have a direct impact on systemic organ function. Under certain circumstances the lungs produce prostaglandins that could lead to severe hemodynamic instability and death.[6]

Pressure breathing with hyperinflation is an example of a potent pulmonary metabolic stimulus. Often this breathing maneuver has been shown to increase fibrinolytic activity. Positive end-expiratory pressure (PEEP) will further enhance the fibrinolytic state by increasing the pulmonary secretion of plasminogen activator. PEEP will also cause a lowering of cardiac output, which affects lung metabolism. Circulating substances are released during PEEP that produce a negative inotropic effect. Therefore respiratory failure or adjustment of lung metabolism may cause defects in lung metabolism as well as derangements in gas exchange.

Vascular complications and thrombosis related to diabetes mellitus

The precise relationship between abnormalities of hemostasis and coagulation and diabetes is unclear, but research has revealed some possible mechanisms. There is evidence that disordered platelet function exists, possibly in platelet biochemistry and platelet vessel wall interaction, in many diabetic patients.[11]

The balance between the epoprostenol and thromboxane (TXA_2) supposedly protect the body against vascular damage. Epoprostenol is the most potent endogenous inhibitor of platelet aggregation, whereas thromboxane promotes aggregation and degranulation of platelets. It is hypothesized that the balance between these two pathways is disturbed in diseases such as diabetes. In some studies the levels of epoprostenol have been elevated in diabetic patients with retinopathy.

Some evidence also suggests that glucose stimulation of insulin release may trigger a classic negative feedback loop that inhibits beta cell production. Prostaglandins are the proposed feedback loop that inhibits the beta cell production.

In addition to disturbances of platelet and prostaglandin behavior in diabetic patients, there is evidence that other hemostatic abnormalities are common in diabetic patients. These abnormalities include coagulation activation, impaired fibrinolysis, and altered blood viscosity. All of these changes could theoretically predispose an individual to a thrombotic state, as is seen in diabetic patients.

Alterations of hemostasis related to cardiopulmonary bypass surgery

Patients who have preoperative coagulation irregularities tend to have bleeding during or after surgery. Therefore the history and laboratory evaluation are quite important before surgery. The personal and family histories are valuable; a detailed drug history is also significant. The common drugs that inhibit platelet function are aspirin, antihistamines, phenylbutazone, aspirin-containing compounds, and papaverine-containing vasodilating drugs.

Pathophysiologically, the most frequent problems that occur with cardiopulmonary bypass surgery are (1) platelet problems, (2) heparin alterations, (3) DIC, and (4) primary fibrinolysis.

Platelet problems in cardiopulmonary bypass surgery

Platelet function may be altered with cardiopulmonary bypass through an activation process that releases and somewhat depletes the alpha-granule contents, while the dense granule constituents are not released. This activation results in occasional impairment of platelet function. In some patients the platelet function returns to normal within 1 hour postoperatively.

Possibly the platelet damage is a result of a shearing force or a contact with foreign material that causes the activation. The platelet membrane may become coated with nonspecific proteins or protein breakdown substances, causing a change in the platelet membrane function. In any case, platelets are usually affected during bypass surgery. Often platelet concentrates are recommended as a postoperative treatment for patients.

Decreased platelets may result from hemodilution, loss of platelets in the pump, formation of platelet thrombi in the vascular spaces, or consumption resulting from DIC.

Heparin

Heparin is used as an anticoagulant during open heart surgery. Occasionally neutralization of heparin with protamine sulfate does not result in reversal of the heparin action. Heparin rebound may be seen when the protamine sulfate metabolizes faster than heparin. The protamine-heparin bond is loose and thus is a possible reason for heparin rebound. Also, heparin in body tissues may have a delayed entry into the circulation postsurgically.

Protamine sulfate itself can act as an anticoagulant. The thrombin clotting time should correct after protamine has been given in a heparinized patient. If the test fails to correct, protamine may be the anticoagulant.

Disseminated intravascular coagulation and fibrinolysis

With the advent of more sophisticated techniques and procedures, DIC is not a common complication. Usually specific factors are decreased during surgery; replacement includes those that are needed.

Fibrinolytic activity decreases during most major surgeries but increases in cardiopulmonary bypass surgery. Thus some clinicians have

elected to use antifibrinolytic agents (like epsilon-aminocaproic acid). Postoperative hemorrhage may or may not be affected by the use of antifibrinolytic agents. Although the mechanism for increased fibrinolysis is unclear, some suggest that the stimulus may be in the oxygenation system, which activates the plasminogen-plasmin system.

Disseminated intravascular coagulation, fibrinolysis, and generalized bleeding tendency related to primary disease states

A sequence of events occurs in some primary disease states that triggers the coagulation mechanisms causing generalized bleeding, DIC, and fibrinolysis. Initially fibrin is deposited in the microcirculation, and clotting factors and platelets are consumed faster than the liver and bone marrow can synthesize new components. Therefore fibrinogen, factors II, V, VIII, XIII, and circulating platelets are decreased. The following pathophysiologic mechanisms have been proposed as possible trigger mechanisms or substances.

1. *Diffuse vessel wall injury* may result in profuse coagulation as subendothelial connective tissue is exposed. However, an exact mechanism is not known as yet.

2. *Activation of platelets* probably is not a major factor in the beginning of the intravascular coagulation, but activation and aggregation of platelets are a part of the process.

3. *Extrinsic pathway activation* by tissue thromboplastin during tissue trauma is thought to be associated with the generalized coagulation. However, there is no way to measure tissue thromboplastin in the blood.

4. *Activation of the intrinsic pathway* through factor XII activation is not conclusively essential to activate DIC. Some substances can activate factor XI without factor XII. One theory is that as Hageman factor (XII) is activated, the kallekrein-kinin system, the fibrinolytic enzyme system, and the complement system are also activated. Possibly the generation of bradykinin

during this process causes the circulatory collapse associated with DIC, but bradykinin is usually broken down quickly.

5. *Activation of leukocytes* may be a primary contributory event when endotoxin activates the procoagulant activity of leukocytes. Monocytes and promyelocytes of promyelocytic leukemia may also be activated to cause coagulant effects. However, no strong evidence is available to prove relationships to DIC.

6. *Activation of the complement system* probably occurs with some DIC development; however the complement system is not vital to the development of DIC.

7. *Activation of the coagulation system* by proteases that bypass normal activation is seen with snake venoms and trypsin released in acute hemorrhagic pancreatitis. Other proteases may activate procoagulants, which in turn may activate DIC.

Biochemically the plasma changes that occur during DIC are two: blood coagulation system activation and fibrinolytic enzyme system activation.

Activation of the blood coagulation system

Consumption. In certain primary disease states associated with DIC, the clotting factors fibrinogen and factors V, VIII, and XIII diminish or disappear altogether along with platelets as they are activated by thrombin in the microcirculation.

Soluble fibrin complexes. Microcirculatory thrombosis may be perpetuated in certain disease states, resulting in DIC. Soluble fibrin complexes may be precursors to intravascular deposits. First, the fibrinogen-fibrin reaction results in the thrombin-cleaving peptides to the N-terminal portions of fibrinogen. The residual portion of the molecule is called the fibrin monomer. Second, the fibrin monomer combines with other fibrin monomers or unused fibrinogen to form soluble fibrin complexes. These soluble fibrin complexes are something between fibrinogen and fibrin. Third, these soluble fibrin complexes aggregate and cause large amounts of coagulation in small vessels.

Enzyme systems and inhibitors

Levels of prekallikrein, plasminogen, kallikrein inhibitors, and plasmin inhibitors decrease as acute DIC develops. Activation of the kallekrein-kinin system and the fibrinolytic enzyme system occurs when the intrinsic coagulation system is activated. Also, in DIC the major physiologic clotting inhibitor, antithrombin III, binds in complexes, resulting in decreased levels of this clotting inhibitor.

Activation of the fibrinolytic enzyme system

When a trigger causes an increase of plasminogen activators, the cascade of events contributing to the bleeding tendency of DIC results. Vascular endothelium injury or fibrin formation in a vessel stimulates secretion of plasminogen activators.

As stated earlier, when the Hageman factor is activated, the fibrinolytic enzyme system is activated probably through prekallikrein. Thus, the Hageman factor starts the clotting mechanism and the breakdown mechanism leading to the dual states in DIC.

Plasminogen activators can be found in the blood and within the fibrin network. Thus lysis of a clot can come from within the clot itself or from the circulation. Bleeding that results in DIC can be related to the breakdown from within hemostatic plugs when plasmin is activated. Fibrinogen–fibrin split products result from the breakdown, even though there are plasmin inhibitors such as alpha$_2$-macroglobulin, alpha$_2$-plasmin, alpha$_2$-antitrypsin, and complement circulating in the blood.

Fibrinogen–fibrin split products

With enhanced plasmin activity, many fibrinogen fragments are released into the circulation. Fragments D, E, X, and Y are identifiable parts of fibrinogen. Fragment X probably acts as an anticoagulant by interfering with the fibrinogen-fibrin polymerization. The fibrinogen or thrombin fragments that are released by the enhanced plasmin activity are measured by laboratory means. The detection of fibrin split–degradation products in the blood, along with decreased platelets and increased clotting times, herald a possible DIC state.

INTERVENTIONS
Bleeding related to alterations in vascular, platelet or coagulation systems

Often medical treatment related to hemorrhagic conditions requires specific treatments, as will be outlined later. Nursing actions are vital and include both medical and general observations. The following points should be stressed when caring for patients who are bleeding.

1. Observe the patient continuously so that signs of bleeding, such as petechiae and ecchymosis, will be found. Petechiae and ecchymosis may be found on the skin or within the mouth. Bright red or tarry stools and hematuria signal bleeding. The severity and duration of nosebleeds should be reported. Signs of internal hemorrhage may be subtle. Faintness, tachycardia, hypotension, confusion, disorientation, and air hunger may herald internal hemorrhage.

2. Teach the patient to report symptoms early. Instructing the patient and a significant other helps prevent more serious complications.

3. Prevent excessive bleeding from an intramuscular injection by using a small needle followed by pressure to the site of injection several minutes after the administration. Close observation of the injection site should continue several hours after the injection.

4. Turn the patient gently and frequently. Weak or older adults should be assisted to the bathroom, especially at night, to prevent bumps or falls that could cause bleeding.

5. Encourage electric razors to avoid cuts. Soft toothbrushes soaked in warm water help prevent gum bleeding yet clean teeth.

6. Encourage the use of identification tags that communicate the bleeding disorder, the physician's name, and the patient's blood type.

7. Teach the patient the effects and dangers of medications that they take or might take.

8. Observe the laboratory data for any correlation between signs of bleeding and potential critical situations.

9. Ask questions that gather historical information about reasons for bleeding or pain signs or symptoms.

Bleeding, arthritic pains, abdominal pain, hematuria, gastrointestinal hemorrhage, fever, and malaise related to purpura

Treatment for purpura centers on treatment of the underlying cause and the bleeding. If toxic drugs are the cause, they must be discontinued.

Corticosteroids are given to reduce the bleeding tendency and to elevate the platelet count. Platelet transfusions are given when the platelet count falls below 20,000 to 30,000 per cubic millimeter.

If the hypothesis of autoimmunity is correct, the removal of the spleen probably halts the destruction of sensitized platelets. In children the splenectomy is not recommended until after the child is at least six years of age.

Melena, cephalohematoma, umbilical cord bleeding, and postcircumcision bleeding related to vitamin K deficiency

Administration of vitamin K to the newborn dramatically curtails the bleeding associated with vitamin K deficiency. The prothrombin time shortens within 6 hours and normal factor measurements are obtained in 24 hours.

The possible side effects of vitamin K overdose are hemolysis, hyperbilirubinemia, and kernicterus in the neonate.

Interventions for bleeding related to platelet and plasma coagulation factor deficiencies
Fresh frozen plasma

Whenever plasma coagulation factor deficiency exists, fresh frozen plasma (FFP) may be infused after the donor's plasma and the recipient's red cells are found compatible to ABO type. In patients with coagulation deficiencies, a needle smaller than 19 gauge should be used to decrease the chances of bleeding at the site of administration.

The rate of administration does not have to be rapid unless the patient is quite hypovolemic. Usually the administration is over 1 to 4 hours. Amounts of 5 to 20 ml/kg of body weight are administered. A standard unit is generally 225 ml.

Documentation should include the time the normal saline infusion was started, what gauge and type of needle was used, the venipuncture site, and the status of the infusion. The charting should also include the time the infusion was started, the number of the unit infused, and any other pertinent observations. Vital signs before and after the transfusion and the length of infusion should be included as well as any reactions, complications, lab tests, and the full signature and title of the nurse. Plasma and the normal saline should be included on the intake sheet.

Fresh frozen plasma contains rich amounts of factors V, VIII, and XI. In patients with undefined hereditary deficiencies of clotting factors, FFP may be used to control bleeding until diagnosis is made. Often platelet concentrates are given concurrently.

Platelets

The therapeutic importance in platelet disorders is to determine whether there is increased platelet destruction or decreased platelet production. Determination of platelet integrity is usually done with a bone marrow aspiration for evaluation of megakaryocytes. Increased megakaryocytes in the presence of a low platelet count indicates either immune destruction or hypersplenism.

Platelets are used to increase platelet counts and to prevent further bleeding from thrombocytopenia. One unit of platelets is given for every 10 kg of body weight. Normal saline is usually used as a starter solution, but the plate-

lets can be given without one. Platelets are usable up to 72 hours following the collection. Platelets should be ABO-Rh compatible, but transfusions are given that are not compatible.

A requisition for each unit or pool of platelets is usually required. The unit should be checked for aggregation in the bag. Gentle kneading until the aggregates disperse is acceptable. If the practitioner is unable to resuspend the platelets, the unit should be returned to the blood bank.

Proper identification according to hospital policy is mandatory. Platelets should be administered as soon as possible, but not over 4 hours after entering the platelet container. Platelets are usually given as rapidly as possible. If reactions are seen, chills, fever, and allergic reactions are the most common.

Some hazards may be associated with platelet transfusions. Alloimmunization, sensitization to red cell antigens, risk of hepatitis, volume overload, and allergic reactions to plasma proteins may occur.

When antibodies to antigens on the platelets (alloimmunization) occurs, the antibodies affect the human leukocyte antigens (HLA), which are the surface of the platelets. If a patient becomes sensitized, matching for antigens must be done. Antiplatelet antibodies may also result when drugs such as guanidine, quinine, or thiazide derivatives are taken.

Usually a blood sample is drawn 1 hour after platelet infusion and testing is done at 24 hours, to distinguish antiplatelet antibodies. The difference in destruction resulting from antiplatelet antibodies and increased platelet consumption resulting from coagulopathy is detected at the 1-hour testing. Antiplatelet antibodies will reduce the platelets in 1 hour; coagulopathy usually results in normal platelets at 1 hour but decreased platelets after 24 hours.

Other variables that affect platelet consumption are hepatosplenomegaly, pyrexia, infection, bleeding, and disseminated intravascular coagulation. The major factor, however, is the possible presence of platelet antibodies. Occasionally the donor with the correct HLA type may be subjected to a plateletpheresis to obtain single-donor platelets. Because the patient may depend on a family member for donor platelets, strain may develop among members of families.

Cryoprecipitate

Cryoprecipitate is used in the treatment of bleeding in factor VIII deficiency or hemophilia A, or to treat an antihemophilic factor (AHF) deficiency. Each unit of cryoprecipitate contains approximately 100 units of AHF activity.

Unless large volumes of plasma are given, determination of ABO and Rh compatibility is not necessary. However, reactions can occur, including urticaria or hives. Benadryl can be given if a reaction occurs.

For administration a large-gauge needle is not necessary, since there are no red cells to damage. A smaller needle is less damaging to the vein and soft tissue. Normal saline should be used to flush the cryoprecipitate from the bag. Factor VIII has an affinity for plastic but does wash with normal saline.

The number of bags and amount of solution should be included in the intake and output records. Vital signs and clinical status should also be included.

Antihemophilic factor (AHF) and plasma thromboplastin component (PTC)

Plasma thromboplastin component is used to treat factor IX deficiency (hemophilia B). Antihemophilic factor is used to treat factor VIII deficiency. These factors are often stocked in the pharmacy, but may also come from the Blood Bank. Both factors are in solid form and must be diluted for administration. Both factors are heat labile and must be refrigerated. PTC can become activated in the solid form at warm temperatures, possibly causing enzymes to activate intravascular thrombosis on administration.

When mixing the factors for administration, gentle shaking for up to 10 minutes may be needed to produce a clear solution. Vigorous shaking may make foam. A 25-gauge butterfly needle may be used for pediatric as well as adult patients. Administration of the solution over a 5-minute interval is accepted.

Reactions are rare. Charting should include the usual vital signs, time and length of administration, any untoward effects, and the manufacturer and lot numbers of vials. Hepatitis is a greater danger with these products, because they are multiple-donor products.

Proper disposal of needles, syringes, and vials is important. Hand washing before and after a procedure is vitally necessary. Hand-to-mouth contact may cause hepatitis if hands are contaminated. The nurse must record the lot number of the vials and the manufacturer's name when a needle stick incident is reported.

Prothrombin complex

When congenital factor V deficiency occurs or when acquired factor II, VII, IX, or X deficiencies occur, prothrombin complex is given to provide for coagulation. There is a high risk of hepatitis with this administration, because prothrombin complex is derived from a large pool of donors.

Prothrombin complex contains a concentrated stable powder that is especially capable of factor IX activity. The amount needed depends on the patient's condition. Therefore assays are needed before and during treatment with prothrombin complex.

Fibrinogen

Fibrinogen concentrates or cryoprecipitate are good sources of fibrinogen. The half-life of fibrinogen is approximately 90 hours, so the replacement need not be as frequent. Hepatitis is a risk with fibrinogen concentrates but much less so with the use of cryoprecipitate. Some patients develop antibodies against fibrinogen.

Hemarthrosis related to coagulation factor deficiency

Hemarthrosis is usually treated with antihemophilic factor (AHF) or fresh whole blood.

Rest for the joint is necessary and is sometimes accomplished with a protective cast. Ice is also used around the joint. Analgesics and corticosteroids may be given to reduce pain and edema. Aspiration of blood from the joint may be required. After edema and bleeding stops, the patient is encouraged to move the joint.

Spontaneous bleeding, ecchymosis, gastrointestinal bleeding, hematuria, and retroperitoneal hemorrhage resulting from vitamin K deficiency

Vitamin K catalyzes the production of clotting factors in the liver. Aquamephyton may be given intravenously, but dosage should not exceed 1 mg/minute. The possibility of shock or cardiac arrest exists with rapid infusion.

Bleeding related to vitamin K and antibiotics

When persons are treated with antibiotics possessing significant activity against gram-negative organisms or anaerobes, it is thought that there is an alteration in the number or type of intestinal bacterial flora, with consequent reduction in synthesis of vitamin K. Prophylactic administration of vitamin K may be indicated in some patients receiving antibiotic therapy.

Thromboembolic complications related to venous stasis or arterial changes

Advancing age, starting at age 45, presents a risk of thromboembolic complications so high that prophylaxis can be recommended for all patients undergoing surgery. Those who have had previous thromboembolism, varicosities, or malignancies have additional risk factors that may indicate the use of antithrombotics in younger patients.

Dextran is a plasma expander with antithrombotic properties. Dextran causes hemodilution and decreases blood viscosity while increasing the blood flow rate, particularly in veins. Albumin also causes hemodilution and reduces blood viscosity but does not produce antithrombotic effects. The following explanation has been reported to explain why dextran does have antithrombotic activities.

Dextran decreases the adenosine diphosphate–induced platelet adhesiveness and aggregation about 4 hours after the end of infusion. Apparently the dextran effect on the platelets is not direct.

The lysability of fibrin, formed from fibrinogen, is changed when dextran is given. Thrombi themselves are changed in structure and lysability, paralleling the decrease in platelet adhesiveness. Dextran changes factor VIII. Factor VIII is important for both platelet and coagulation function. While dextran affects factor VIII, platelet function becomes impaired and the structure of thrombi formed is changed. Thrombi usually have a "white" platelet-rich head and a "red," erythrocyte-rich tail. With dextran the "white" head disappears and the platelet aggregates disseminate throughout the thrombus. Since the head of a thrombus is usually the most resistant to plasmin-induced lysis, dextran allows for fibrinolysis to occur more readily.

Thus dextran is able to decrease the incidence of major thrombi, thrombi in the postoperative course, and pulmonary emboli. However, dextran will not prevent formation of thrombi.

There are side effects and contraindications for dextran. Renal damage occurs if dextran is given in excessive amounts to a dehydrated person. Pulmonary edema and overexpansion of the blood volume may be seen in patients with cardiac insufficiency. The risk seems to be greater with 10% dextran 40. The risk is also greater when dextran is given daily for several days. Increased bleeding may be caused when doses exceed 1.5 g/kg of body weight per day for dextran 70, or 2 g for dextran 40. The most dangerous side effect is anaphylactoid reactions. A reaction usually occurs immediately following the start of the infusion. Blood pressure drops and cardiac arrest may occur. Elderly patients seem to be more prone to this reaction. The anaphylactic reaction probably occurs because antibodies against dextran have been formed from previous dextran stimuli, resulting from bacterial action in dental cavities. Hapten dextran supposedly can be used to prevent anaphylactoid reactions.

Dextran should be avoided in patients with bleeding disorders, uremia, or impaired platelet function.

Deep vein thrombosis related to vein or artery changes

Anticoagulants serve as a secondary preventive measure only when used for proximal deep vein thrombosis of the lower extremity, including the popliteal, femoral, and iliac veins, or for pulmonary emboli. Anticoagulants slow thrombus formation by inhibiting extension of the venous thrombus. Anticoagulants do not affect original thrombi or emboli. Oral anticoagulants oppose the effects of vitamin K, an essential fat-soluble vitamin. Apparently a carboxyl group at the gamma end of the glutamic acid is required for coagulation factors that use vitamin K for synthesis. Factors VII, X, IX, and prothrombin (II) require vitamin K to be able to bind to calcium. Vitamin K converts into vitamin K epoxide in the course of synthesis of these factors. Oral anticoagulants apparently interfere with vitamin K regeneration from an inactive form.

It is not necessary to provide a loading dose when giving anticoagulants. In fact, a loading dose may cause an early deficiency of factor VII and a possible major bleeding complication. Typically the dose is begun with 10 mg of warfarin per day. This dose is continued for 2 or 3 days and then gradually reduced to about 5 mg/day, depending on laboratory results of prothrombin time.

It is important to continue heparin therapy along with the oral anticoagulant for at least a week because the protime reflects primarily the effect of the clotting factor that is most depressed, factor VII. However, the combined levels of the four vitamin K–dependent clotting factors are reflected in the prothrombin time only after about a week.

Clinical circumstances and other drugs may affect anticoagulant therapy. Sensitivity to warfarin (Coumadin) derivatives is increased with advanced age. Starvation (vitamin K is gained from dietary sources) and broad-spectrum antibiotics reduce synthesis of vitamin K by intestinal flora. A possible cause of postoperative bleeding is the combination of limited oral intake after operation, the use of broad-spectrum antibiotics, and failure to administer supplementary vitamin K. Postoperatively, the anesthesia may cause the liver to reduce the contents of vitamin K in the body. Thus anticoagulants may need to be reduced postoperatively.

Increase in dose may be required when barbiturates are consumed with anticoagulants. Barbiturates induce production of hepatic microsomal enzymes that metabolize vitamin K antagonists. Sudden discontinuance of barbiturates could cause bleeding episodes.

Anticoagulants cross the placenta and are excreted in the breast milk. Vitamin K antagonists are associated with fetal abnormalities. Anticoagulants may interfere with carboxylation of proteins involved in information and calcification of bone.

Thrombosis formation related to venous stasis or arterial changes

Heparin is produced by the body in most cells. However, there is no evidence that endogenous heparin can be extracted from normal human blood. The heparins in current use are extracted from hog intestinal mucosa or from partly purified beef lung.

The most common methods of administration are intravenous and subcutaneous. When used to treat patients with active thrombosis, heparin should be administered in doses sufficiently large to prolong an appropriate coagulation test. In most cases it is desirable to achieve an anticoagulant effect rapidly and then sustain it. An intravenous bolus injection of heparin followed by a continuous infusion, intermittent intravenous injection or subcutaneous injection. A dose of 5,000 to 10,000 units is injected intravenously, which produces levels higher than the therapeutic range. Following the initial injection, a dose of 20,000 to 40,000 units, depending on response, is given over 24 hours. When the patient is at risk of bleeding, lower doses are given. Subcutaneous injections may be used with venous thromboembolism. The heparin, usually 5,000 units, can be given two or three times daily in the fat of the subcutaneous tissues over the lower abdominal wall, using a small-gauge needle (25).

Heparin exerts its effect in the presence of plasma cofactor, an alpha-2 globulin known as *antithrombin III*. Antithrombin III is a natural inhibitor of a number of activated clotting factors—including factors XII, XI, IX, X, and thrombin—that have serine residue at their enzyme activity center. Antithrombin III, combined with heparin, inactivates coagulation enzymes in a progressive and irreversible manner.

The heparin action may not be the same for each coagulation enzyme. Thus the inactivation of X_a and thrombin may vary with the molecular weight of the heparin fraction. Heparin may also act directly in thrombin.

Low doses of heparin may be ineffective in preventing extension of established venous thrombi, but low doses are effective in preventing occurrence of venous thrombi in high-risk situations. This low-dose effectiveness in prevention is probably related to the fact that heparin is required to inhibit early stages of blood coagulation rather than to just inhibit thrombin formation. Heparin has also been shown to have effects on platelet function.

Heparin therapy is usually given over a period of 48 to 72 hours to overlap induction of oral anticoagulants. Monitoring of continuous infusions should be done with the activated partial thromboplastin time.

Checking the drip rate and time-taping the infusion of heparin should be done at least every hour. Attaching the heparin drip to a volume-controlled flow device is recommended. The staff must be alerted to report any bleeding around injection sites or for any blood in the stool or urine. Wound sites would also be moni-tored in trauma or surgical patients. The most common sites for bleeding are the mucous membranes, wounds, or cuts in the skin. Protamine sulfate must be available as an antidote for heparin.

Medication nurses should be alerted so that intramuscular injections or arterial punctures are used only when absolutely necessary. Intramuscular injections may lead to a hematoma in the muscle. The vastus lateralis muscle of the thigh should be used if intramuscular injections are needed. Injections into the gluteal muscle can produce retroperitoneal bleeding, which may insidiously accumulate. Possibly the first sign of retroperitoneal bleeding would be shock.

Some side effects of heparin may include hypersensitivity reactions and thrombocytopenia. Osteoporosis and suppression of kidney function have also been reported.

Spontaneous bleeding, ecchymosis, gastrointestinal bleeding, hematuria, and retroperitoneal hemorrhage resulting from heparin therapy

Protamine is the specific antidote to full-dose intravenous heparin. One milligram of protamine sulfate neutralizes 80 to 120 units of heparin. Plasma or plasma fractions are of no specific benefit in reversing heparin effect. The effects of protamine are very fast and last for approximately 2 hours. It is recommended that no more than 5 mg be infused per minute to prevent hypotension, bradycardia, dyspnea, and possible anticoagulant effects. Continuous laboratory studies should accompany the administration of protamine for excessive heparin therapy.

Thrombosis related to atherosclerosis

Researchers have found that aspirin has a protective effect against acute myocardial infarction in men with unstable angina, and they suggest that aspirin also has a preventive effect on mortality.[7]

Platelet aggregation apparently occurs in atherosclerosis. Aspirin inhibits cyclooxygenase and the secondary phase of platelet aggregation.

Acute deep vein thrombosis and pulmonary emboli related to venous or arterial changes

Thrombolytic therapy

With anticoagulation, thrombolytic therapy is utilized to manage proximal acute deep vein thrombosis, as well as the severe forms of pulmonary embolism. Because anticoagulants provide only secondary prophylaxis, thrombolytic therapy should be added to prevent persistent pulmonary hypertension, chronic venous hypertension, and recurrent episodes of thrombophlebitis and pulmonary emboli. With the removal of the offending thrombus or embolus, the circulation and anatomy can be restored to a more normal state. Surgical removal of thrombi or emboli is indicated in some cases. However, enzymatic lysis can be very successful for some patients, particularly when the lesion is less than 72 hours old.

Urokinase, streptokinase, and streptokinase-plasmin mixture are available thrombolytic agents that produce enzymatic lysis of thrombi and emboli. With the lysis of these thrombi and emboli, prevention of potential growth of new venous channels is accomplished. When large venous thrombi do not resolve quickly, new venous channels without valves proliferate or remaining valves become dysfunctional. Thus pain, swelling, and venous hypertension may become chronic. These chronic conditions might result in venous claudication and venous ulcers. Within the lung, pulmonary hypertension may result from an episode of pulmonary emboli. Fibrous webs and residual pathologic conditions are evident in autopsies of patients who had had large pulmonary emboli treated only with heparin. Permanent hemodynamic disturbances and defects in the pulmonary capillary blood volume have also been reported.

Therefore persons treated with anticoagulants only when extensive proximal deep venous thrombus or pulmonary embolism occurs benefit only from secondary prophylaxis. Thrombolytic agents thus offer some relief for appropriately selected cases.

Leg pain related to deep vein thrombosis and immobilization

Static methods

Static method such as elevation of legs to a 30-degree angle is a frequently used intervention but has not been studied in depth by itself. Early ambulation and physiotherapy are usually used in combination with elevation when prevention of thrombi is a goal.

Elastic compression with controlled, graded compression reduces (but does not abolish) the incidence of thrombosis in the lower leg.

Active methods

To promote venous blood flow, three methods are suggested. Manipulating the foot backward and forward, as if on a pedal, has been shown to increase venous blood flow in the femoral vein, as measured by an electromagnetic flow probe, and to reduce the incidence of isotopically detectable thrombi in the calf.

Electrical stimulation of calf muscles

Electrical stimulation of calf muscles has been studied; it has shown increased arterial inflow to muscles as well as the volume of venous blood flow and venous flow velocity. A study in 1968 revealed that electrical stimulation produced a reduction in the number of isotopically detectable calf vein thrombi.[2] Electrical stimulation seems to be effective for all types of patients, including those with malignant disease. Apparently elastic compression is not as effective in patients with malignant disease. A slight complication with electrical stimulation is an occasional blister at an electrode site.

Pneumatic compression

Pneumatic compression is a third active method of venous thrombosis prevention. Inflatable boots, driven by small pumps, deliver intermittent compression, which increases the volume and velocity of femoral vein blood flow. The ideal degree of compression is 40 mmHg reached in 5 seconds, followed by 1 minute of relaxation.

While all of these mechanical methods reduce the incidence of vein thrombosis, it is important to remember that none of these are as effective as the use of subcutaneous heparin therapy.

Alterations of hemostasis related to cardiopulmonary bypass surgery

When the appearance of oozing from intravenous sites accompanied by hematuria or petechiae occurs, a hemostatic abnormality should be suspected. If the chest tube bleeding increases, the problem is more likely a surgical technique problem.

Screening tests should be done by the laboratory to help identify the specific problem. Some clinicians routinely give platelet concentrates while awaiting final laboratory results. Protamine sulfate is calculated according to the amount of heparin.

Antifibrinolytic agents may be considered if the patient fails to respond to platelets or if fibrinolysis is suspected.

Bleeding tendency, intravascular coagulation, and fibrinolysis related to certain primary disease states

The interventions used in this situation have been controversial for some time. Therapy should always be directed toward treating the underlying disease state. Other controversial treatments will be discussed separately.

Epsilon aminocaproic acid (Amicar). Though this drug initially was encouraging to clinicians, it is seldom used. Epsilon aminocaproic acid competes with essential amino acids for transmembrane transport, reducing hepatocyte protein synthesis. Serious complications have been reported, and few clinicians use the drug for treatment of DIC.

Heparin given in doses of 150 to 600 units/kg of body weight over a 24-hour period has long been used in conjunction with replacement therapy. However, a high rate of failure has occurred with heparin. A possible reason for failure is the reduction of the heparin cofactor, antithrombin III. Antithrombin III becomes depleted in DIC and enhances coagulation. Furthermore, heparin's anticoagulant activity depends on antithrombin III. A heparin–antithrombin III therapy is presently used.

Some clinicians have suggested the use of CIG as a treatment of DIC. CIG, a protein that supports the reticuloendothelial system in removing particulate matter, becomes very depleted in DIC. When CIG levels are normal, removal of platelet aggregates and soluble fibrin complexes is improved, and the circulatory thrombosis of DIC should decrease.

Above all, the most important intervention for DIC is to treat the primary disease state, whether that disease is sepsis or shock or any of the many other disease states that would lead to DIC.

BIBLIOGRAPHY

1. Bang, N.U.: The biochemistry of blood coagulation. In Bang, N.U., et al.: Thrombosis and atherosclerosis, Chicago, 1982, Year Book Medical Publishers, Inc.
2. Browse, N.L., and Negus, D.: Prevention of postoperative leg vein thrombosis by electrical muscle stimulation, Br. Med. J. 3:615, 1970.
3. Clough, D.H., and Higgins, P.G.: Accurate assessment of blood loss, Crit. Care Update 10(1):19, 1983.
4. Goldfarb, W., and Yates, A. (editors): Critical care medicine, I. Pittsburgh, 1978, Broudy Corp.
5. Deykin, D.: Thrombosis and antithrombotic therapy. In Harrison's principles of internal medicine, ed. 9, New York, 1982, McGraw-Hill Book Co.
6. Hechtman, H.B., and Shepro, D.: Lung metabolism and systemic organ function, Circ. Shock 9(4):457, 1982.
7. Lewis, D., et al.: Protective effects of aspirin against acute myocardial infarction and death in men and unstable angina, N. Engl. J. Med. 309(7):396, 1983.
8. Miale, J.B.: Laboratory medicine hematology, ed. 6, St. Louis, 1982, The C.V. Mosby Co.
9. Owen, C.A., et al.: The diagnosis of bleeding disorders, ed. 2, Boston, 1974, Little Brown & Co., Inc.
10. Packham, M.A., and Mustard, J.F.: The journal of the American Society of Hematology, Blood 50(4):555, 1977.
11. Panwalker, A.P., and Rosenfeld, J.: Hemorrhage, diarrhea and superinfection associated with the use of moxalactam, J. Infect. Dis. 147(1):171, 1983.
12. Preston, F.E.: Disorders of haemostasis in diabetes mellitus, Ric. Clin. Lab. 12(3):425, 1982.
13. Sanders, J.H., and Gardner, L.B.: Handbook of medical emergencies, ed. 2, 1978, Garden City, N.J., Medical Examination Publishing Co., Inc.

8 Thermoregulation

LINDA ABELS

The human body is subjected to numerous stresses in everday life. Some of these stresses, in excess, are capable of destroying life. However, complexly interrelated mechanisms exist in the body that strive to establish, or reestablish, and maintain a homeostatic state. The temperature-regulating mechanism is an example of one such mechanism. The human body is limited in its ability to withstand extremes in temperature change. Metabolic activities are inhibited with very low temperatures (those below 35° C, or 95° F). Some cellular proteins are inactivated with very high temperatures (greater than 45° to 50° C, or 113° to 122° F), which destroy tissue faster than it can be repaired. This chapter will review the role of temperature regulation and control in critically ill people.

EMBRYOLOGY

The thermoregulatory system can be traced embryologically to the ectoderm in the developing embryo. The ectoderm, which is the outermost germ layer in the embryo, gives rise to the nervous system tissues, which are integrally involved in regulating body temperature. These tissues develop approximately 17 days after fertilization. The ectoderm first differentiates into a neural groove and neural ectoderm and subsequently separates from the remaining ectoderm to form a neural tube with two parallel neural crests. This process is referred to as *neurulation*.

The neural crests develop into cells that later become neurons, or Schwann cells, which ultimately give rise to autonomic postganglionic neurons, the adrenal medulla, and afferent neurons of the cranial and spinal ganglia, as well as preganglionic neurons and motor neurons of the cranial and spinal nerves.

The cephalic end of the neural tube develops into the brain, becoming the prosencephalon (forebrain), the mesencephalon (midbrain), and the rhombencephalon (hindbrain). It is the prosencephalon that finally differentiates into the diencephalon, which among other structures contains the hypothalamus, the area so vitally involved in temperature regulation.

PHYSIOLOGY
Temperature gradients

Three thermal zones exist in the body. The innermost zone, or *core zone,* consists of all structures that lie within the body cavities and is the crux of the entire thermal system. The core temperature, often referred to as the set point, is 37° C ± 0.5° (98.6° F ± 1.0°) and, under normal conditions, fluctuates very little.[9] There is a difference of approximately 0.5° to 1.0° C (1.0° to 2.0° F) between temperatures in the core zone and those in the middle, or *intermediate zone,* which consists of the skeletal muscles.[5] Ordinarily the skeletal muscles play only a small role in heat production. However, when the core temperature is in danger of dropping, the skeletal muscles become actively involved in the production of heat. The outermost *superficial zone,* composed of the skin and subcutaneous tissues, is approximately 2° to 3° C (4° to 6° F) lower than the core temperature, or about 34° to 35° C (93.2° to 95° F).[8] The superficial zone serves as a buffer layer to protect the core from ambient temperature changes. Its temperature varies with blood flow, the environmental temperature, the humidity, and air velocity. Temperature fluctuation over a fairly wide range occurs in response to environmental factors and to the rate of heat production and/or heat loss by the body.

Control mechanisms

Thermostatic regulation is accomplished through both physical and chemical mechanisms and involves positive and negative feedback systems. The nervous system serves as a communication center by means of a series of relay stations and a central component. Messages are interpreted and integrated, and the appropriate response—to increase heat loss, conserve heat, or increase heat production—is activated. The circulatory system sets in motion the machinery for carrying out the desired activity either through vasodilation, vasoconstriction, or stimulation of the endocrine system. Chemical mechanisms are controlled chiefly by the endocrine system. Secretions of the thyroid-stimulating hormone (TSH) and the adrenocorticotropic hormone (ACTH) from the anterior pituitary gland influence the thyroid gland and the adrenal cortex, respectively, regulating the metabolic rate and gluconeogenesis. The adrenal medulla is also involved, secreting adrenaline and norepinephrine in response to sympathetic stimulation. The specific functions of these physical and chemical mechanisms are discussed in the pages that follow.

To understand exactly how these mechanisms operate in the regulation of body temperature, it is necessary to review the principles involved in the production and loss of heat.

Heat balance

Body temperature is determined by the balance between the amount of heat gained by the body and the amount of heat lost to the environment. If heat gain is exactly equal to heat loss, the body temperature remains the same. When heat gain exceeds heat loss, the body temperature rises. exceeds heat loss, the body temperature rises. When heat loss is greater than heat production, the body temperature falls. The delicate balance between the rates of heat production and heat loss is maintained by the autonomic nervous system; this system varies the blood supply (and ultimately the amount of heat loss) at the body surface and controls either the autonomic or somatic motor outflow tracts, which produce sweating or shivering, respectively.

Heat can be taken up from the environment under certain conditions, or it can be produced in the body. Heat is generated by all of the body tissues. It is produced in the mitochondrion,* often referred to as the "powerhouse" of the cell. The actual amount of heat produced by different tissues varies. At rest, the major amounts of heat are produced by those body tissues that have rapid chemical reactions such as the tissues of the heart, liver, brain, and endocrine glands. This accounts for the proportionally higher temperature in these areas. Heat is also produced by the skeletal muscle although the amount is less than that produced in the core. Therefore the temperature of skeletal muscle is somewhat less than the temperature of the core. This can be misleading because references often report that skeletal muscle accounts for almost 40% of the body's heat production.[5] Remembering the ratio of muscle mass to core, however, is useful in explaining this discrepancy.

Mitochondria (singular, *mitochondrion*) are cell organelles (little organs) found scattered throughout the cytoplasm; they produce the chemical energy used by most cells.

Because the entire mass of the body is composed of muscle, the overall contribution of the skeletal muscle in heat production is great.

Newborns have a large amount of brown adipose tissue that is high in mitochondria and is extremely active in thermogenesis in the presence of cold. This mechanism is responsible for a significant amount of heat generation.[38]

Heat, or chemical energy, is released through a series of chemical reactions. Ingested food (carbohydrates, fats, and protein) is converted through a series of catabolic processes into usable organic molecules. Chemical bonds in these organic molecules contain potential energy and are easily broken, resulting in the subsequent release of energy. Released energy is used at the cellular level to convert adenosine diphosphate (ADP) to adenosine triphosphate (ATP), which is a high-energy compound. ATP is the immediate source of energy for the cells and, when energy is released, is converted back to ADP.

Carbohydrates and fats are the favored fuels for energy formation because carbohydrate and fat molecules contain carbon-hydrogen bonds that are unstable and energy rich. Carbohydrates have less energy than fats because the latter contain more of these energy-rich carbon-hydrogen bonds. Protein fuels are used only when carbohydrate and fat fuels are inadequate. Approximately 45% of energy is derived from carbohydrates, 40% from fats, and 15% from proteins.[8] These percentages are misleading unless the amount of energy released by 1 gram of each of the respective fuels is considered. For example, the amount of energy released by 1 gram of fat (9.3 calories*) is almost twice the amount released by 1 gram of carbohydrate (4.1 calories) or 1 gram of protein (4.1 calories).

Energy transformation is accomplished in several steps that require a small energy input for the transformation to proceed. The two-stage process begins with a simple glucose molecule and necessitates the investment of two molecules of ATP. The first stage is an anaerobic process referred to as *glycolysis* (or the Embden-Meyerhof pathway), which takes place in the cytoplasm. In glycolysis, glucose is oxidized to pyruvic acid, which is a keto acid. The steps and enzymes involved in glycolysis are illustrated in Fig. 8-1. The major reactions that take place can be summarized in a relatively simple way. The glucose molecule is fairly stable and requires some energy to be activated. This activation energy is provided by an ATP molecule, which donates the terminal phosphate group to glucose in a process called *phosphorylation*. The ATP becomes ADP and the original glucose molecule becomes glucose-6-phosphate. The glucose-6-phosphate is converted to fructose-6-phosphate, which reacts with another ATP molecule. This reaction results in the formation of a diphosphorylated six-carbon compound that splits to form two three-carbon compounds known as glyceraldehyde-3-phosphate and dihydroxyacetone-3-phosphate. These two compounds are interconvertible and subsequently form phosphoglyceraldehyde. Ultimately, in ensuing reactions, the compounds are oxidized when a total of four hydrogen atoms are removed (two from each compound) and phosphorylated when a molecule of inorganic phosphate is added to each compound. The hydrogen atoms are picked up by two nicotinamide adenine dinucleotide (NAD)* molecules; these molecules form two NADH molecules and are transported via one of two shuttles to the electron transport chain in the mitochondria, where they are used in the formation of ATP. The two high-energy phosphate groups are used to convert the ADP molecules to ATP. In the remaining steps, the phosphate bonds of the three-carbon compounds that are left are converted into high-

---

*Calories are used to express the amount of heat released. A *calorie* is defined as the amount of heat needed to raise the temperature of 1 gram of water 1° C. Thermodynamics uses the term *large calorie (Calorie)*, or *kilocalorie*, which is the amount of heat needed to raise 1 kg of water 1° C.

---

*NAD (nicotinamide adenine dinucleotide) is a coenzyme, that is, a small organic molecule necessary for many enzymatic actions to proceed.

Fig. 8-1. Glycolysis (Embden-Meyerhof pathway). Glucose is oxidized to pyruvate or lactate in a series of enzymatically catalyzed reactions. ATP is invested and converted to ADP, releasing high-energy phosphate bonds when energy is required for a reaction sequence. NAD is a coenzyme that serves as a hydrogen carrier. It is reduced to NADH + H$^+$ during glycolysis. NADH and hydrogen are transferred from the cytosol to the respiratory chain in the inner mitochondrial membrane. As they pass along the electron transport system, more energy will be produced. A net gain of two ATP molecules occurs for each molecule of glucose that passes through the glycolytic pathway.

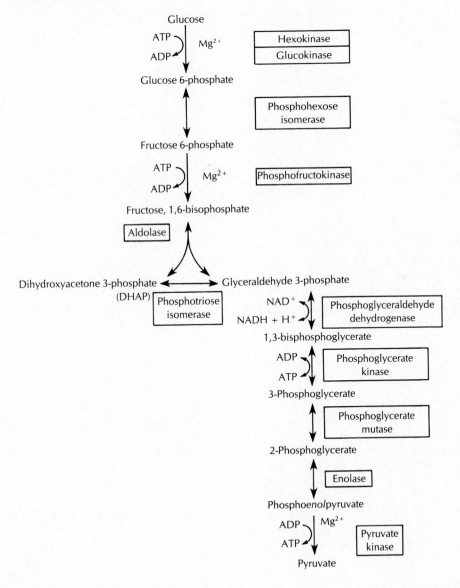

Fig. 8-2. Tricarboxylic acid cycle (TCA cycle). Also referred to as the citric acid cycle or Krebs cycle, this series of reactions in the mitochondria is the final common pathway for the oxidation of carbohydrates, proteins, and fats. Acetyl-CoA is oxidized to oxaloacetate. During the TCA cycle, reducing equivalents are formed and transferred to the respiratory chain, where large amounts of high-energy phosphate bonds are generated in a process known as oxidative phosphorylation. A net gain of two ATP molecules occurs in one complete revolution. (GTP can be formed from GDP, producing another high-energy compound.) Enzymes that catalyze specific reactions are boxed.

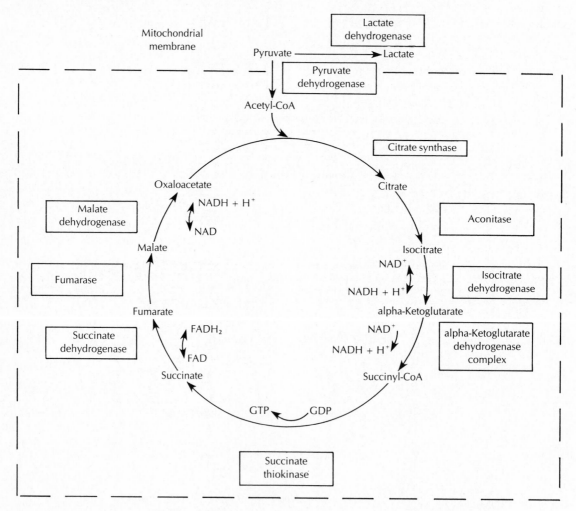

energy bonds that are subsequently transferred to two more ADP molecules for conversion to ATP. Thus a total of four ATP molecules are produced, but because two must be invested to begin the process, the net gain is two molecules. The waste product is lactic acid, which is oxidized during the aerobic process.

The second stage of the energy transformation process is an aerobic process described in Fig. 8-2. Initially, the two pyruvic acid molecules produced in glycolysis must be prepared to enter what is called the Krebs cycle, or the tricarboxylic acid cycle. These molecules must be oxidized (one hydrogen atom is removed) because the Krebs cycle only accepts two carbon compounds. At the same time the molecules are oxidized, carbon dioxide is released, leaving a two-

carbon compound. This two-carbon compound is subsequently connected with coenzyme A and is called acetyl-CoA. (A coenzyme is necessary for enzymatic action to proceed.)

Acetyl-CoA enters the Krebs cycle and is oxidized via a series of reactions to regenerate oxaloacetate, the compound with which it originally combined to form citrate. During the course of the Krebs cycle, three molecules of NADH, one molecule of $FADH_2$,* two molecules of carbon dioxide, and one molecule of ATP are formed. Because two molecules of acetyl-CoA are formed for every one glucose molecule, each glucose molecule involves two turns

---

*FAD (flavin adenine dinucleotide) is another coenzyme. It is found in oxidized form (FAD) and in a reduced state ($FADH_2$).

Table 8-1. Energetics in the catabolism of glucose

Pathway	Reaction	Method of ATP production	Number of ATP molecules formed/ molecule of glucose
Glycolysis	Glyceraldehyde-3-P ↔ 1,3-bisphos-phoglycerate	Respiratory chain oxidation of 2 NADH	6*
	1,3-bisphosphoglycerate ↔ 3-phosphoglycerate	Oxidation at substrate level	2
	Phospho*enol*pyruvate ↔ Pyruvate	Oxidation at substrate level	2
		TOTAL	10
			− 2
		NET TOTAL	8
	Pyruvate → Acetyl-CoA	Respiratory chain oxidation of two NADH	6
Krebs (TCA) cycle	Isocitrate ↔ alpha-Ketoglutarate	Respiratory chain oxidation of two NADH	6
	alpha-Ketoglutarate → Succinyl-CoA	Respiratory chain oxidation of two NADH	6
	Succinyl-CoA ↔ Succinate	Oxidation at substrate level	2
	Succinate ↔ Fumarate	Respiratory chain oxidation of two $FADH_2$	4
	Malate ↔ Oxaloacetate	Respiratory chain oxidation of two NADH	6
		NET TOTAL	30
TOTAL (per molecule of glucose under aerobic conditions)			38

Modified from Martin, D.W., Mages, P.A., and Radwell, V.W.: Harper's review of biochemistry, ed. 19, Los Altos, 1983, Lange Medical Publications.
*Only 4 ATP molecules will be formed from NADH if the glycerophosphate shuttle is used.

of the Krebs cycle. Therefore the net result is six NADH molecules, two $FADH_2$ molecules, four CO_2 molecules, and two ATP molecules for each glucose molecule. Because each NADH yields three ATP and each $FADH_2$ yields two ATP, 24 ATP molecules are ultimately formed from products of the Krebs cycle.

Energy transformation also is accomplished by an electron transport system, which transfers high-energy hydrogens with their electrons from the NAD molecule to successive acceptors. At the end of the chain, hydrogen atoms that have become ions form water, whereas the high-energy electrons are donated to oxygen. In the electron transport system, ADP again becomes ATP via oxidative phosphorylation.[9]

In summary, 38 ATP molecules are formed for every one glucose molecule invested. NADH formed during glycolysis is usually transported via the malate shuttle. If the glycerophosphate shuttle is used, two less molecules of ATP are formed, reducing the total net production to 36

Fig. 8-3. Entry of carbon skeletons of amino acids into the energy pathways. Amino acids must undergo deamination (removal of an amino group) or transamination (transfer of an amino group) before entering one of the energy pathways.

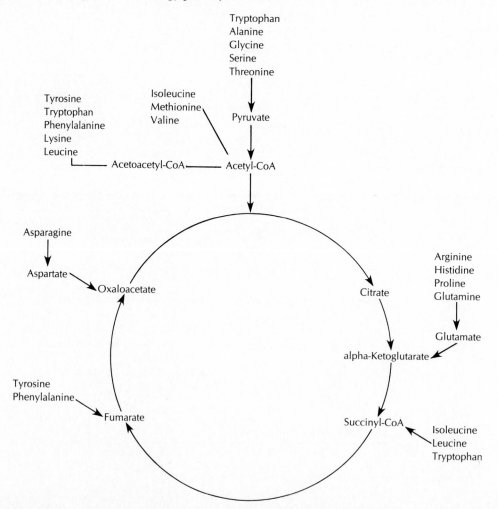

instead of 38. Table 8-1 summarizes the energetics of these pathways.

Fat (lipids) also enter the glycolytic cycle. Lipids are converted to glycerol and fatty acids; each is subsequently oxidized in the cytoplasm of the cell. Glycerol is converted via oxidative phosphorylation to phosphoglyceraldehyde and enters the glycolytic pathway, proceeding similarly to glucose. Fatty acids are activated by linking the terminal end with coenzyme A. This long-chain compound undergoes beta-oxidation, resulting in the formation of acetyl-CoA, which enters the Krebs cycle. A large amount of energy can be obtained via this pathway because many molecules of acetyl-CoA are formed from each long-chain fatty acid.

Proteins that have been converted to amino acids are occasionally used as energy fuel. Amino acids must be deaminated (that is, the amino group removed) or transaminated to enter energy pathways. The end products are keto acids; they enter glycolysis or the Krebs cycle (Fig. 8-3). Fig. 8-4 summarizes the energy pathways of carbohydrates, fats, and proteins.

Fig. 8-4. Energy pathways of carbohydrates, fats, and proteins. Carbohydrates undergo hydrolysis to form glucose, which enters the glycolytic pathway. Fats are hydrolyzed to fatty acids that can undergo beta oxidation to form acetyl-CoA, which can then enter the tricarboxylic acid cycle. Proteins are hydrolyzed to amino acids that are subsequently deaminated or transaminated to form substances that can enter the TCA cycle either directly or indirectly.

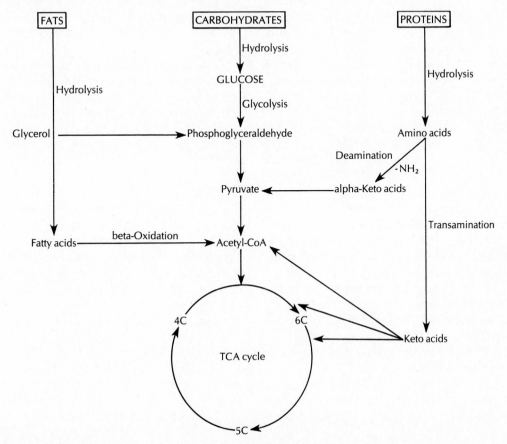

The chemical reactions involved in energy transformation are relatively inefficient.[8] No energy is lost because, according to the first law of thermodynamics, energy cannot be gained or lost when it is converted from one form to another. However, approximately 75% to 90% of the energy liberated in catabolic activities becomes heat before it can be used by the cells. The remaining 10% to 25% is used for cellular activities.[47]

The rate at which heat in the body is produced, or *metabolic rate,* is determined principally by the amount of muscular activity, the external temperature, and food digestion. If all of these variables are removed, the metabolic rate can be correlated with the amount of energy exchanged during minimal functional activity.

Changes in muscular activity can exert a dramatic effect on the metabolic rate. For example, strenuous exercise can, when associated with maximal muscular contraction increase heat production to about 50 times the normal amount for short intervals of a few seconds. Normal or substained exercise can increase the rate of heat production approximately 20 times the normal amount for a period of several minutes.[48,52]

Environmental temperatures influence the rate of heat production in an indirect manner. A decrease in the environmental temperature causes an individual to feel cold. If the temperature is low enough, the person begins to shiver in an effort to produce more heat and subsequently increases her metabolic rate. A significant lowering of the body temperature can also slow the metabolic rate if no compensatory mechanisms, such as shivering, are activated. An elevated environmental temperature that can cause an elevation in the person's temperature can also increase the metabolic rate. Studies have shown that there is approximately a 10% to 13% increase in the metabolic rate for every 1-degree rise in body temperature.[36,52]

Digestion of foodstuffs obviously affects the rate of heat production. The rate of absorption of carbohydrates, lipids, and proteins will determine just how quickly energy will be transformed. Of the various end products of carbohydrate metabolism, the primary monosaccharides—glucose, fructose, and galactose—exhibit rates of absorption that differ from one another. The difference in the rate of uptake can be attributed to differing affinities for the carrier mechanism. Lipid absorption is related to the specific substrate because lipase, the enzyme that controls lipolysis, demonstrates substrate specificity, whereas the rate of amino acid absorption is controlled by amino acids' structural configuration.[8]

Other factors can also influence the rate of heat production. The amount of circulating thyroxine directly influences the metabolic rate because this hormone is responsible for controlling the rate of all chemical reactions in body cells. Maximal quantities of circulating thyroxine can increase the metabolic rate up to 100% above normal, whereas a loss of this hormone can decrease the basal metabolism down to 50% below normal.[22]

The adrenal medullary secretions of epinephrine and norepinephrine exert a direct effect on the muscle and liver cells, thus increasing the rate of glycogenolysis. Norepinephrine also increases the rate of brown fat metabolism, thereby increasing the infant's metabolism up to 100%.[11,22]

Energy use

The energy derived from the catabolism of food is used by the body tissue for metabolic activities. The actual rate of movement dictates the amount of energy needed. Energy requirements are smallest during the resting state and greatest during strenuous exercise or extreme emotion. Moderate work, that is, the work of the average, everyday job, utilizes about three times the amount of energy used by the resting metabolism, or approximately 4 kcal/min. Hard work utilizes almost 9 kcal/min, whereas during maximal work—that is, work that can only be maintained for a short period of time—the demand for oxygen needed for chemical reactions far exceeds the supply.[9] This shortage leads to anaerobic metabolism.

Energy is supplied to the tissues from the central organs. The amount of energy used by the tissue is not always equal to the amount of energy produced by the body. There must be a way to account for any discrepancies between energy production and utilization because, according to the first law of thermodynamics, energy cannot disappear. These energy differences can be explained by food storage depots. A carbohydrate such as glucose is polymerized to glycogen in a process referred to as glycogenesis

(Fig. 8-5). Although glycogen formation occurs in practically all body tissue, glycogen is stored chiefly in the liver and muscle.[47] Liver glycogen aids in the maintenance of blood glucose, particularly between meals. Muscle glycogen serves as a source of hexose units for glycolysis within the muscle itself. The rate of glycogen synthesis is regulated by 3':5'-cycle adenylic acid (cyclic AMP, or c AMP), an intracellular intermediate compound through which many hormones appear to act. C AMP is formed from ATP by an enzyme, adenylate cyclase, which is found on the inner surface of cell membranes. Adenylate cy-

---

Fig. 8-5. Pathway of glycogen synthesis and glycogenolysis in the liver. Enzymes that catalyze reactions are boxed. Cyclic AMP inhibits glycogen synthase, "turning off" glycogenesis. It activates phosphorylase, promoting glycogenolysis.

Adapted from Martin, D.W., et al.: Harper's review of biochemistry, ed. 19, Los Altos, CA, 1983, Lange Medical Publications.

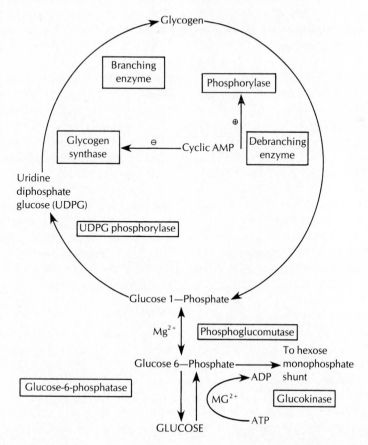

clase is activated by epinephrine, norepinephrine (via beta-adrenergic receptors on the cell membrane), and glucagon (through an independent receptor). C AMP inactivates the enzyme glycogen synthase, thus inhibiting the formation of glycogen. Thyroid hormones increase the synthesis of adenylate cyclase and ultimate of c AMP by potentiating the effects of epinephrine. Glucose in excess of that which is converted to glycogen is converted into fat from acetyl-CoA (fatty acid synthesis). Fats (lipids) are stored as triglycerides in adipose tissue in the liver and are found in small amounts in the muscles. Proteins are stored in a variety of tissues, including muscle, liver, and lymph, because there is no special storage organ for protein. Proteins in excess of what can be stored are also converted into fat and stored in adipose tissue. All of this potential energy can be stored indefinitely until the moment it is needed.

When food intake is adequate to meet metabolic needs, food stores are conserved, but in times of need, storage depots must be used to prevent tissue damage. When food intake is inadequate, these stores are mobilized. Glycogen stores are used to reform glucose in a process known as glycogenolysis (Fig. 8-5). During glycogenolysis, each glucose molecule is split away by a catalyzed process. The catalyst in this reaction, phosphorylase, is activated by the hormones glucagon and epinephrine via cyclic AMP. Glucagon is secreted by the alpha cells of the pancreas when the blood glucose level falls below normal. Epinephrine is released by the adrenal medulla in response to sympathetic stimulation and increases the availability of glucose for rapid metabolism. Once glucose is released, it enters glycolysis.

Moderate amounts of glucose can also be formed from amino acids and from the glycerol portion of fats. The process in which this happens is called *gluconeogenesis* (Fig. 8-6). Gluconeogenesis is stimulated by a reduction in available carbohydrates and a decrease in the blood glucose. Under these conditions, protein and lipid stores are mobilized, permitting the conversion of deaminated amino acids and glycerol into glucose.

Gluconeogenesis is also under hormonal control. The anterior pituitary gland, in response to a reduction of available carbohydrates, releases quantities of corticotropin, a hormone that stimulates the adrenal cortex to release glucocorticoid hormones in large quantities. One of these glucocorticoids, cortisol, mobilizes proteins from all cells of the body. Many of these proteins are deaminated by the liver and serve as substrates for conversion into glucose. Thyroxine also influences gluconeogenesis. It is thought to mobilize both proteins and fats from storage depots. The proteins are subsequently deaminated and, with the glycerol portion of fats, are all converted into glucose.

Fats that have been stored as triglycerides in the body must be transported to other tissues when necessary to provide energy. These triglycerides are hydrolyzed to fatty acids and glycerol, which can once again enter the glycolytic pathway, or Krebs cycle. The procedure is apparently initiated in the presence of decreased glucose availability. The reduction in glucose decreases the amount of alpha-glycerol/phosphate, a substance necessary for the synthesis of new triglycerides, and increases the amount of the enzyme lipase, a substance that promotes rapid hydrolysis of triglycerides.[47]

Protein stores must be deaminated before entering the energy pathways. Once deaminated, they enter via gluconeogenesis or ketogenesis. Of the 20 available amino acids, five are converted directly to fats, whereas 14 must first be converted to carbohydrates and then to fats to enter the appropriate pathways.[47]

Heat loss

In a steady state, the heat lost from the body is balanced by the heat produced by the body. Therefore the energy produced by the catabolism of carbohydrates, fats, and proteins is either stored or converted into heat or external work. The heat is subsequently lost to the environment via three mechanisms: (1) radiation,

Fig. 8-6. Major pathways of gluconeogenesis in the liver. Entry points of glucogenic amino acids after transamination are indicated in boldface print. Key gluconeogenic enzymes are italicized. The bold arrows indicate the main pathway of gluconeogenesis. The ATP required is supplied by the oxidation of acetyl-CoA from long-chain fatty acids or lactate via pyruvate.

Adapted from Martin, D.W., et al.: Harper's review of biochemistry, ed. 19, Los Altos, CA, 1983, Lange Medical Publications.

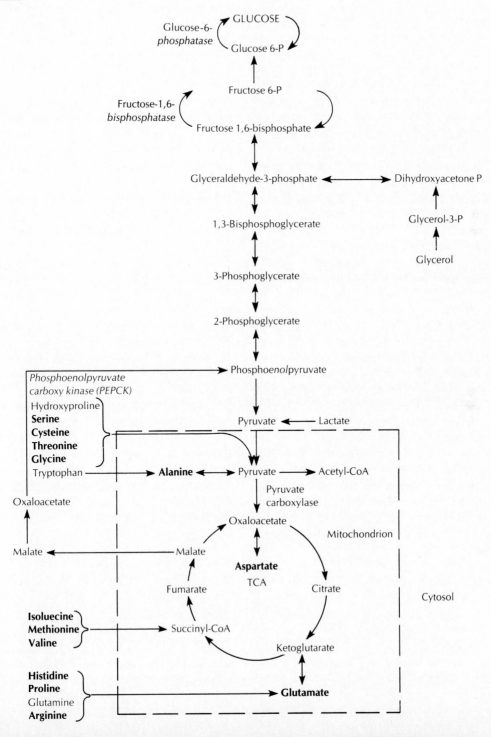

(2) conduction and/or evaporation, and (3) convection.

Heat loss resulting from radiation accounts for approximately 60% of the heat lost to the environment.[28] Heat loss of this type can be explained by the principle that objects located near each other will radiate toward one another. The exchange of heat depends on the temperature and the nature of the radiating surfaces. A black body will absorb all types of radiation and reflect nothing. The perfect reflector, in contrast, will absorb nothing. An object that reflects some light at all wavelengths is said to be a *gray body*. Human skin can be compared to a gray body because its reflecting power varies with wavelength. In the infrared region of the light spectrum (1000 to 1,000,000 nm),* reflectivity is the same for both skin colors. Therefore all skin is black in the dark. In the visible spectrum, however, there is a difference in reflectance. Darker skin absorbs more heat than white skin. The net transfer of heat by radiation is the difference between the radiation emitted by the surface and the radiation it receives. Heat will radiate from a warmer object to a cooler object.

Heat loss by conduction occurs only through direct contact with an object. Heat is transferred from a warmer object to a cooler object. No other material is exchanged in the process. The rate at which heat is transferred is directly proportional to the thermal conductivity† of the object, its area, and the change in temperature and is inversely proportional to the object's density. Heat loss via conduction can be reduced with the use of insulation. The degree of reduction depends on the amount and effectiveness of the insulation. Superficial conduction losses vary inversely with the type and thickness of external clothing worn. Conduction losses from internal organs to the skin are inversely related to the degree of fat or adipose tissue in the body.

The convection of heat depends on the presence of a liquid or gaseous medium between hot and cold objects and on the exchange of warm and cold molecules between warm and cold surfaces. Convection may be natural, or it may be forced, such as that which occurs with a fan. Initially, heat must be conducted through the air layers next to the skin from molecule to molecule. As the distance from the skin increases, heat is transferred by convections of air, either naturally or in a forced manner. The rate of heat loss by convection depends on the thermal gradient (which is the difference between the temperatures of the skin and the air) and the velocity of the air.

Evaporative heat loss occurs when water from the lungs or perspiration from the surface of the skin is converted to water vapor. Vaporization accounts for the loss of approximately 0.6 kcal of heat/gram of water. The evaporative heat loss varies with the environmental temperature. The body continuously loses some heat from the skin and respiratory tract by evaporation. At environmental temperatures below 30° C (86° F), the evaporative heat loss is fairly constant at a rate of 12 to 15 grams/square meter/hour.[28] About one half of the heat is lost from the respiratory tract as moisture in breathing. The other half is lost slowly through the sweat glands as insensible* perspiration with apparent dry skin or by active sweating.[65] With a surrounding temperature of 30° C (86° F), the evaporative heat loss amounts to 25% of the total heat loss, which at this temperature equals basal heat production. Above 30° C (86° F), the evaporative heat loss exhibits a linear relationship with the increase in temperature, and the loss occurs primarily as perspiration. When the temperature of the environment is hotter than that of the skin, the heat loss by evaporation must also take care of metabolic heat and heat absorbed by radiation

---

*One nm (nanometer) is equal to 1×10^{-9} meters.
†Thermal conductivity is a constant. It is determined by the area, density, temperature gradient, and amount of heat flowing through an object. The conductivity of body tissue is relatively close to that of water because body tissue is approximately 95% water.

---

*Insensible heat loss cannot be felt or seen but consists of water lost as a result of its diffusion through the epidermis. This fluid is not formed by the sweat glands; it is formed over the entire body surface independent of the environment. It amounts to a heat loss of approximately 600 kcal in 24 hours.

and convection. As these temperatures equalize, all metabolic heat must be lost by evaporation because there can be no loss by radiation and convection.

Temperature control

Body temperature is regulated primarily by the hypothalamus (Fig. 8-7), although several other systems are also involved.[10,11,13,64,65] The hypothalamus has two distinct regions that regulate temperature. Cells in the supraoptic area in the anterior hypothalamus are *thermolytic,* controlling heat loss, whereas nuclei in the tuberal area of the posterior hypothalamus are *thermogenic,* controlling heat conservation.

Hypothalamic temperature-regulating centers are influenced reflexly by the skin and by the temperature of blood flowing through them. Once the sensory receptors have been stimulated, a message is transmitted to the hypothalamus, where it is integrated and processed. After the message is processed, the appropriate response is initiated, and an effector organ is stimulated.[9,10]

Cutaneous, subcutaneous, and deep connective tissue thermoreceptors, located in the dermal layer of the skin, are sensitive to either hot or cold.[11,22,28] Cold receptors are generally more numerous than warm receptors.[10] Both cold and warm receptors are more common on the face and hands than anywhere else on the body. Sensitivity is greatest where receptors are most dense.[31] Once stimulated, these receptors relay information via sensory fibers in the lateral spinothalamic tract to synaptic relays in the reticular system of the medulla oblongata and finally to the posterolateral ventromedial nuclei of the thalamus. The information is projected to the cerebral cortex, where processing takes place.[22] Warm receptors increase their rate of firing with an increase in temperature greater than 0.1° C in the range of 30° to 43° C (86° to 109.4° F) and cease firing in cold; cold receptors increase their rate of firing with cold temperatures, responding to decreases of greater than 0.1° C in a range from 35° to 15° C (95° to 59° F). The sensation of

cold persists even after the stimulus has been removed because these receptors will continue to discharge as long as the temperature is below a certain level. These receptors stop firing in the presence of heat. Additional thermoreceptors can be found in the tongue, respiratory tract, viscera, and spinal cord.[28] They also respond to localized temperature changes, adjusting their rate of discharge accordingly. Thermoreceptors are distributed in a punctate manner and actually respond to the presence or loss of heat because the temperature is only a measurement of the amount of heat. Thermoreceptors respond to stimuli at the depth at which they are located; thus they respond to external and internal stimuli.

Deep body receptors found in the spinal cord, veins, and viscera also respond to local

Fig. 8-7. Hypothalamic centers involved in temperature regulation.

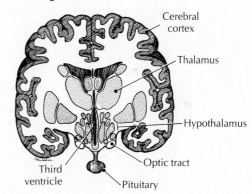

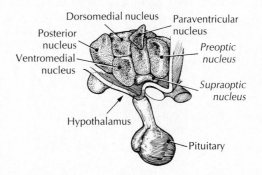

temperature changes.[22,28] They are connected with the anterior and posterior portions of the hypothalamus via the central thermoreceptors in the hypothalamus and respond to local changes in the temperature of the circulating blood.[29] Because the temperature of circulating blood varies closely with the overall core body temperature, the hypothalamus is able to monitor and respond to minimal temperature fluctuations.

Recent studies indicate a possible relationship between the relative ratio of sodium to calcium ions within and around the posterior hypothalamus and temperature regulation. Excessive sodium results in an elevation in the body temperature, whereas excess calcium has the opposite effect. The exact mechanism for these occurrences is still being investigated.[6]

Stimulation of thermolytic nuclei in the supraoptic area initiates activities that increase heat loss.[10,11] Thermolytic responses include cutaneous vasodilation and sweating. Vasomotor stimulation changes the distribution of circulation, shunting large amounts of blood to the periphery. As the blood vessels of the skin dilate, the temperature of the skin increases, and heat is lost rapidly by radiation. Sweating is initiated as a cooling mechanism to increase heat loss by evaporation; it is most effective in hot, dry climates because the rate of evaporation depends on the difference between the vapor tension of water on the surface of the skin and that in the air. Sweating enforces the vasodilative process by chilling the skin as water is evaporated. Sweat release from the exocrine glands is controlled by the sympathetic postganglionic cholinergic diversion of the autonomic nervous system and occurs simultaneously in most areas on the surface of the body. This sweat release is a form of forced convection because body heat is first conducted to the glandular fluids and then transported to the body surface via the pumping action of contractile elements in the glands' ducts.

The sweating mechanism in adults occurs at lower environmental temperatures than it does in full-term newborns. Adults sweat at temperatures above 32° to 34° C (89.6° to 93.2° F), whereas full-term infants sweat at temperatures above 35° to 37° C (95° to 98.6° F). Premature infants do not have well-developed sweat mechanisms and use an increase in respiratory rate as a method of losing heat.[37]

A significant loss of body water can occur with sweating. Two mechanisms (the thirst center and osmoreceptors) are activated by the hypothalamus in response to significant water loss and body dehydration. The thirst center in the hypothalamus, responding to a dry mouth and to dehydration, activates the thalamus and the cortex to initiate a sensation of thirst and a desire for water. In addition, osmoreceptors in the supraoptic area respond to an increase in the serum osmolality associated with dehydration; these osmoreceptors then increase the production and release of ADH. Once released, ADH results in water reabsorption in the kidneys (see Unit 5 for a more detailed explanation). Thus the hypothalamus, while promoting heat loss by radiation and evaporation, can also compensate for additional problems that may develop.

Heat promotion, production, and conservation are aided by vasoconstriction, increased metabolism, increased shivering, and increased thyroid hormone production and occur with stimulation of the tuberal area in the posterior hypothalamus (Fig. 8-8).

Activation of the tuberal area, or sympathetic stimulation, results in an increase in the release of the catecholamines epinephrine and norepinephrine.[10,11] Epinephrine is secreted from the adrenal medulla secondary to autonomic sympathetic stimulation. Norepinephrine is produced at the postganglionic terminals in response to sympathetic innervation. Both epinephrine and norepinephrine influence circulatory and metabolic mechanisms to alter the body temperature. The release of catecholamines results in vasoconstriction of cutaneous vessels. This vasoconstriction decreases the flow of warm blood from the internal structures to the

Fig. 8-8. Summary of thermoregulatory mechanisms involved in heat production.

Modified from Reuler, J.B.: Hypothermia: pathophysiology, clinical settings and management, Annals of Internal Medicine **89:**519, 1978.

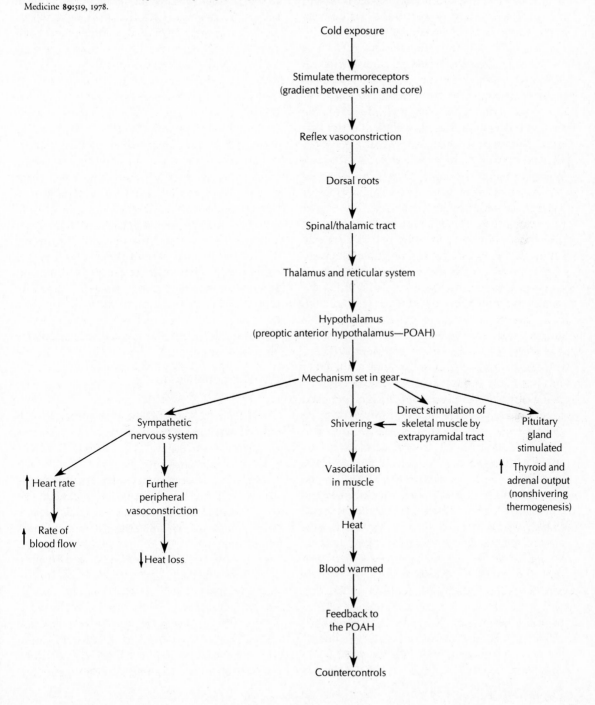

skin, ultimately decreasing the transfer of heat. Skin temperature falls, heat is conserved, and the internal core temperature rises. Catecholamine release also increases the metabolic rate because catecholamines have a stimulant effect on the catabolism of carbohydrates and fats.

Prolonged exposure to cold, such as happens at the beginning of winter, causes a hormone in the hypothalamus to be secreted into the anterior pituitary gland. The thyroid-stimulating hormone TSH is released, stimulating the thyroid gland to produce increased quantities of the thyroid hormones. Thyroxine affects the metabolic rate by influencing the rate at which cellular oxidation takes place. Thyroxine also exerts a synergistic effect with epinephrine.[22]

Stimulation of the thermogenic center can also initiate shivering as a compensatory mechanism for heat production when cutaneous vasoconstriction proves to be inadequate. Newborns and premature infants, however, do not demonstrate shivering thermogenesis in response to cold. Rather, they become restless and irritable and increase their metabolic heat production and ultimately their oxygen consumption.[11]

The actual mechanism by which shivering produces heat is thought to be involuntary.[34] It is believed that cold exposure increases muscle tone indirectly as a result of stimulation of the thermogenic center; this stimulation subsequently extends down the brainstem into the spinal cord to the anterior motor neurons. These impulses increase skeletal muscle tone. As the muscle is stretched and muscle tone is increased, the stretch reflex is elicited and oscillates, causing the muscle to contract. This contraction stretches an antagonistic muscle, which also develops a stretch reflex. The process continues with the second muscle stretching and the first muscle again creating a continuous shaking movement. Heat is produced by the muscles as muscle tone increases.[28] Shivering can produce moderately large amounts of heat but is not effective in maintaining body heat for a prolonged time period.

ASSESSMENT
History

A complete history should be obtained from the patient with an alteration in body temperature. Particular attention should be given both to details of the onset of the present illness, with a chronologic description of developing symptoms, and to the past history for indications of multisystem involvement. Information about precedent acute infections or infectious diseases should be documented. Patients should be asked about preexisting diarrhea and boils. Special consideration should be paid to epidemiologic factors and potential exposures that might help establish a diagnosis, such as place of residence, contact with animals or birds, or contact with people with suspected infections. Questions about the possibility of recent trauma, both surgical and accidental, should be noted because the former may predispose the patient to infection and the latter to central nervous system malfunction. Inquiry should also be made about drug intake because some drugs may cause a problem (drug hypersensitivity reactions), whereas other drugs may mask one.

Physical examination
General inspection

The physical examination can provide valuable information in establishing the cause of the temperature alteration.[32] Therefore it should be performed systematically.

Initially, objective data such as the patient's weight and vital signs should be obtained. The weight should be compared to a baseline "normal" weight; unexplained weight losses should be documented. Vital signs should also be recorded. The body temperature should be measured, recognizing that diurnal variations do exist and may be as great as 0.5° to 1.0° C (1.0° to 2.0° F), ranging from 36.5° to 37.5° C (97.6° to 99.6° F). In addition, different recordings can be made depending on whether the method for obtaining the temperature is oral, rectal, or axillary. Rectal temperatures are most reliable and average 0.5°

to 1.0° higher than oral temperatures. They may, however, be contraindicated in the presence of certain cardiovascular disorders. Axillary temperatures are least reliable, averaging 1° below oral temperatures. The pulse rate should also be evaluated because a rapid rate and rhythm often accompany febrile illnesses. Respiratory rates should be observed unobtrusively. A tachypnea may be seen as a compensatory maneuver to increase heat loss in hyperpyretic states. Blood pressure should be measured but does not usually directly reflect temperature changes.

A general "head-to-toe" survey, which should follow the initial obtaining of objective data, is helpful in evaluating the patient's general health because it may reveal compensatory chilling and shivering or sweating. Inspection of the skin for flushing or localized redness (erythema) may reveal vasodilatory changes that occur with increased heat production. Skin rashes, lesions, or eruptions may be significant, indicating infection, ulceration, or cellulitis. Petechial hemorrhages may develop in the ocular fundi, conjunctivae, nail beds, and skin secondary to increased capillary permeability.

Lymphatics

Careful examination of the lymph nodes should be made, with special attention paid to the supraclavicular, axillary, and epitrochlear areas. Supraclavicular nodes are part of the deep cervical chain and drain lymph from the head, arms, chest wall, and breast area. Enlargement of these nodes on the right side occurs with granuloma or neoplasm from the lung or esophagus, whereas on the left side enlargement is associated with neoplasms in the abdominal cavity. Axillary nodes may be enlarged with neoplasms or infections within the regional drainage. Enlarged epitrochlear nodes in close proximity to the medial humeral epicondyle, between the biceps and triceps brachii, are found with local infections within the regional drainage and with inoculation of generalized infections within the drainage area.

Heart

Hyperpyretic states can lead to alterations in the heart sounds themselves. For example, abrupt ventricular contractions may produce a more intense first heart sound. In addition, the presence of abnormal findings may provide invaluable diagnostic clues. The finding of a previously nonexistent heart murmer is significant and could indicate subacute bacterial endocarditis. Inflammation of the pericardial sac may result in the development of a pericardial friction rub, which is a to-and-fro grating sound caused by the rubbing together of the parietal and visceral surfaces of the inflamed pericardium.

Abdomen

Abdominal palpation is essential and may reveal a direct area of tenderness caused by localized inflammation that involves the abdominal wall, the peritoneum, a viscus, or even a distended solid organ. Checking for Blumberg's sign (rebound tenderness) can be used to confirm the presence of peritoneal inflammation. Light palpation may also detect subcutaneous crepitus, a tactile sensation caused by gas bubbles that are produced by anaerobic microorganisms growing in the subcutaneous tissue or underlying muscles. Reflex muscle spasms caused by peritoneal irritation may result in involuntary rigidity of the muscle, leading to its resistance to palpation. This resistance is characterized by a firm, boardlike abdomen and is an attribute of peritonitis.

Deep abdominal palpation is helpful in evaluating the liver and spleen and may be necessary to identify areas of deep tenderness or masses not previously suspected. A smooth and tender liver is suggestive of acute hepatitis, amebic hepatitis, amebic abscess of the liver, or multiple hepatic abscesses. The spleen is not tender except when the peritoneum is inflamed from infection or infarction; rather the spleen, in acute infections, is moderately enlarged and soft. Splenomegaly occurs in bacterial, viral, and protozoal infections. Slight enlargement of the spleen is present in subacute bacterial endocarditis and other acute and subacute infections. Moderate enlargement is found in hepatitis abscesses and the leukemias, whereas great enlargement occurs in, among other disorders, chronic myelocytic leukemia.

One finger is used to evaluate the kidney and paranephric region. The finger is pressed into the soft tissues enclosed by the costovertebral angle, which lies between the spine and the twelfth rib in a radial direction. Costovertebral angle, or CVA, tenderness indicates inflammation in this area.

Percussion of certain areas of the abdomen may yield diagnostic information. In addition to being useful in delineating organ borders and sizes, percussion is also helpful in locating areas of tenderness. Percussion tenderness occurs in acute hepatitis and cholecystitis.

Pelvis

Digital examinations of the rectum and vagina are necessary to gain information about the lower part of the peritoneal cavity and about adjacent structures, including the male and female genitourinary tracts. In the male a tender prostate, as well as a pelvic abscess, can be identified, the latter being manifest as a tender round mass felt through the anterior rectal wall superior to the prostate gland. In the female tenderness of the normally impalpable rectouterine pouch is evidence of an abscess. Pain in the lateral fornices and adnexa indicates salpingitis; when limited to the right side, it must be distinguished from the pain of acute appendicitis. A painful mass in one or both lateral fornices suggests pyosalpinx with peritonitis.

Data base lab

Both invasive and noninvasive tests can be used in evaluating a patient with temperature alterations. The baseline studies that are done depend on the patient's presenting symptoms. For example, chest roentgenograms and sputum examinations are indicated in the presence of respiratory symptoms, whereas urine studies are used with urinary tract symptoms. Cerebrospinal fluid evaluations, blood cultures, skull and sinus roentgenograms, and lactate dehydrogenase (LDH) measurements should be obtained with central nervous system pathology. In the presence of fever or hypothermia without associated symptoms, the following studies are usually performed.

Complete blood count (CBC)

In obtaining the complete blood count, or CBC, special attention is given to the white blood cell count (WBC). An elevation in the number of leukocytes, called *leukocytosis,* is generally found in bacterial infections, whereas a reduction in the number of leukocytes, *leukopenia,* is usually characteristic of viral infections. Microscopic examination of the leukocytes is performed with the white cell count differential. All of the white blood cells—neutrophils, eosinophils, basophils, lymphocytes, and monocytes—are counted, and the relative percentage out of a total of 100 is determined. The aberrations reported in the following discussion are reviewed in connection to their relevance to thermoregulatory pathology.

Neutrophilia, which is an increase in the number of circulating neutrophils, occurs with infections caused by most Gram-positive bacteria and by many Gram-negative organisms, as well as by some viruses. An elevation in the number of neutrophils often includes immature forms, referred to as a *shift to the left*. A state of *neutropenia,* which is a reduction in the amount of neutrophils, is associated with most viral diseases, including influenza and hepatitis. Neutropenia usually accompanies splenic enlargement and may be caused by a massive infection by any organism. In general, the more debilitated the patient, the less severe the infection needs to be to precipitate neutropenia.

Eosinophilia refers to an increase of circulating eosinophils and occurs with parasitic infestation. It has also been reported with some poststreptococcal conditions. *Eosinopenia* is seldom noteworthy.

An increase in basophils is easily recognized, whereas a decline is scarcely noticeable. *Basophilic leukocytosis* occurs in chronic myelocytic leukemia and colitis. A decrease in the basophil count can be found in any stress reaction associated with increased corticosteroid production.

Lymphocytosis can be described in two ways. *Relative lymphocytosis* occurs when the number of circulating lymphocytes is unchanged but the WBC is low because of neutropenia. *Absolute lymphocytosis* refers to an increase in the number of circulating lymphocytes. The former accompanies most conditions associated with neutropenia, whereas the latter is related to many viral infections. A mild lymphocytosis occurs subsequent to many viral infections and sometimes after a bacterial infection during the convalescent period. Marked lymphocytosis is characteristic of chronic lymphocytic leukemia, whereas a somewhat less marked lymphocytosis occurs in most lymphomas. Low lymphocyte counts are found following small doses of radiation or adrenal corticosteroids. Atypical lymphocytes are noted in viral and allergic conditions. These cells tend to be larger than normal and have a vacuolated cytoplasm and a coarse chromatin network in the nucleus. Lymphocytosis with a moderate leukocytosis may be normal in infants and young children from the ages of 4 months to 4 years.

Monocytosis occurs in some protozoal or rickettsial infections. The number of mature and early monocytes is increased markedly in monocytic leukemia.

Cultures and microscopic examination

The ultimate diagnosis of any infectious disease depends on the isolation, cultivation, and identification of the offending organism. Different culture media can promote or discourage bacterial growth. A good culture medium must meet several criteria, as follows: it must contain the essential nutrients in the appropriate concentration. It must have an adequate amount of salt and water and must be of proper consistency. It must be sterile and free of any substances that could inhibit the growth of the organism being cultured and must be of a pH that would promote the metabolic activities of the offending organism. Once cultured, attention must also be given to temperature requirements and environmental conditions for incubation because some organisms require aerobic conditions, others require anaerobic conditions,* and still others need CO_2-enriched environments. The medium that is selected depends on the organism(s) most likely to be found in the specimen and, to some extent, on the source of the specimen.

Rich culture media that contain blood are often used because they provide relatively nonselective conditions under which a variety of pathogens will flourish. Nutrient broth can also be used. In many cases, however, selective and differential media are required to isolate a specific organism. *Selective media* permit the growth of single organisms or a group of closely related organisms while virtually inhibiting the growth of all other organisms. These types of media are useful in showing the presence of the organism of interest. *Differential media* allows several or many organisms to proliferate. These types of media contain dyes or other ingredients on which different organisms act in a variety of ways to produce variations in color.

Once the organism has been isolated, it can be obtained in pure culture and characterized taxonomically by means of morphological, physiologic, and other more specialized tests. One such specialized test that is used frequently is the test of antibiotic sensitivity of a culture. This test provides information about the sensitivity of a particular organism or organisms to antibiotics and is of value in identifying antibiotic resistance, which develops because of genetic mutations. Ultimately the test may be used to identify the appropriate antibiotic for therapy.

Microscopic procedures can also be enlisted to aid in the identification of the pathogen. Spe-

---

*Anaerobic infections have increased in frequency over the past few years, resulting in part from improved collection techniques. The most frequently isolated organisms are of the species *Bacteroides* and *Fusobacterium*.

cific techniques may be required to facilitate reaching a diagnosis.

Staining procedures can be used to identify the presence of some pathogenic organisms. Although direct examination of a specimen is possible, many organisms are small and too difficult to examine without being stained.

The Gram stain uses a purple-blue complex, which enters the organism when the slide of the smeared specimen is flooded with crystal violet and iodine. Once the dye complex has entered the cell, it can either remain, imparting a purple-blue color, or it can be washed away with a decolorizer. Just what occurs depends on the characteristics of the cell wall. The cell walls of Gram-positive bacteria have a low lipid content and are impermeable, thus preventing the escape of the intracellular dye complex when the decolorizer is applied. Gram-negative bacteria have a high lipid content, much of which is removed by the decolorizer. Consequently, the intracellular dye complex can be washed away. A contrasting counterstain (carbol-fuchsin or safranin) can be applied to color the Gram-negative organisms. Both organisms can be studied microscopically in an effort to establish or confirm a diagnosis based on morphological characteristics, including shape, relative size, and growth configuration. Some Gram-positive organisms with absent or damged cell walls will appear to be Gram-negative.

The acid-fast stain, which also relies on cell wall properties, can be used to identify acid-fast bacteria. In this procedure, carbol-fuchsin is introduced into the cell with heat and acid. Once stained, acid-fast organisms resist decolorizing with an acid decolorizer because of a waxy material in their cell walls. Mycobacteria and bacteria of the genus Nocardia are sought using this technique.

Culture sources

Blood. Blood is cultured on broth media because bacteremias are seldom mixed, making mixed flora discrimination unnecessary. Gener-ally, three to five cultures should be obtained over a 24- to 48-hour period although, if antibiotic therapy has been initiated, the number of cultures obtained should be doubled. This is necessary to ensure adequate sampling and to preclude the institution of treatment for a contaminant. Meticulous technique is essential. The site must be cleansed appropriately (with detergents and alcohol sponges) and treated with tincture of iodine unless severe iodine sensitivity exists. Blood should be obtained from different sites via direct venipuncture or, if necessary, arterial puncture. The use of indwelling arterial or venous catheters to obtain samples is contraindicated because of the likelihood of contamination. Growth of the same organism from several different cultures taken at different times is usually clinically significant. Growth of *Staphylococcus* epidermis or diptheroids, although usually considered contaminant, could indicate a bloodstream invasion in patients with endocarditis or prosthetic heart valves. In debilitated or immunosuppressed patients, all organisms should be considered significant.

Cerebrospinal fluid (CSF). Analysis of the cerebrospinal fluid (CSF) consists of chemical tests and a microscopic examination that includes a cell count, Gram stain, and culture, the last used to confirm a presumptive diagnosis made on the basis of a cell count and Gram stain alone. Chemical tests are useful in determining the amounts of protein, glucose, chlorides, calcium, and enzymes that are present in the spinal fluid. Only small amounts of protein are normally found because protein molecules do not cross the blood-brain barrier. Elevations in the protein concentration may occur with increased permeability of the blood-brain barrier caused by inflammation, when there is blood in the spinal fluid, or in the presence of degenerative disease of the central nervous system. This last condition is usually indicated when relatively few cells are present. The concentration of calcium in the spinal fluid is directly proportional to the amount of protein because calcium is bound to protein. The CSF glucose concentration is normally 50% to 80% of the blood glucose level. A reduction in the spinal fluid glucose level accompanies inflammation and infection, degenerative diseases, and most tumors. The most significant reduction occurs in the presence of infectious disorders because all types of organisms consume glucose. Although spinal fluid chloride determinations are less important now than they used to be, their alterations are frequently of value in diagnosing tuberculosis meningitis when the neurologic findings are nonspecific. In this situation, CSF chloride and glucose levels are depressed, and there is a mild elevation of proteins and mononuclear cells. CSF chloride determinations are invalidated if the patient is receiving an intravenous infusion of electrolyte solutions. Enzyme determination in the CSF is not routinely determined. Mild to moderate enzyme changes often accompany various neurologic disorders. The enzyme most affected is the glutamic-oxaloacetic transaminase (GOT), which rises in inflammatory, hemorrhagic, and degenerative diseases of the central nervous system.

Because cerebrospinal fluid normally contains only a few cells, a cell count is performed to identify the presence of any abnormalities. Up to 20 small lymphocytes/mm^3 may be normal, although this number varies and is age dependent. The presence of granulocytes, large mononuclear cells, or red cells is always considered abnormal. Red cells may result from a hemorrhagic process or from trauma during the puncture.

Macroscopic examination of the CSF can differentiate grossly purulent from clear fluid, but even seemingly clear fluid can harbor microorganisms. Spinal fluid specimens are routinely cultured on several media to identify the etiologic organism. Spinal fluid should be cultured as soon as possible after the specimen is obtained and should not be refrigerated because some organisms are sensitive to the cold temperatures. Different environments are required for incubation because some organisms are anaerobes,

some are aerobes, and some require CO_2 enrichment.

Sputum. Bronchial and pulmonary secretions or exudates are often studied by examining the sputum. Unfortunately, admixture of secretions with saliva and nasopharyngeal material is common, making sputum examination misleading at best. Sputum specimens can be collected from coughing, transtracheal aspiration, or directly via bronchoscopy. Because most children and some adults swallow their sputum, some samples may be obtained by aspirating stomach contents. If this is necessary, the stomach should be aspirated early in the morning before any food or water is ingested.

Sputum collection should be preceded by specific instructions to the patient; good oral hygiene must be carried out before obtaining the sample to minimize contamination by mouth flora. Because true sputum originates below the larynx, the specimen should be expelled after deep coughing. If necessary, nebulized aerosols can be used. A 20% solution of saline in distilled water should be heated for this purpose. The heated vapor condenses on the surface of the tracheobronchial mucosa, thereby stimulating the production of secretions. An early-morning specimen is best because it represents an overnight accumulation. In addition, more sputum is usually raised in the morning, and this sputum produces the most organisms. Generally, specimens should be collected daily for at least 3 separate days.

Transtracheal aspiration may be helpful in obtaining a sputum specimen. Although this procedure may be unduly traumatic for an unintubated patient, it is the technique of choice for patients with artificial airways. The equipment should be sterile to minimize contamination. A sputum trap can be used to collect the sample. Again, specimens should be collected daily for at least 3 days.

Bronchial secretions collected via bronchoscopy should be followed by specimen collection for at least 3 days.

Sputum specimens are routinely treated with a preparation of sodium hydroxide (or its substitute) to liquefy mucus and exudate and to achieve maximal destruction of other microorganisms. The specimen is subsequently examined microscopically, using both Gram-staining and acid-fast staining techniques. The sample is also cultured, using both blood agar and selective and differential media. Fungal infections can also be identified with the appropriate culture medium.

Urine. The urinary tract does not normally harbor bacterial organisms. Bacteria found at the urethral meatus do not usually ascend into the urinary tract. However, urinary tract infections are very common and derive from many sources. Many of the offending organisms are inhabitants of the intestinal tract. Others can be traced to instrumentation.

A urinalysis with a culture and colony count is most often obtained after preliminary findings from a routine urinalysis suggest the presence of infection. Good technique in collecting the specimen is essential to minimize the growth of contaminants from periurethral tissues. A sample from catheterized patients should be obtained, without interrupting the closed system, by sterile aspiration of the catheter with a needle and syringe. Specific instructions should be given to the uncatheterized patient to collect a clean specimen that is voided midstream. Although satisfactory specimens can be collected in this manner, catheterization may be unavoidable. Suprapubic aspiration may be necessary in infants and young children. Cystoscopy is rarely required in the critical care setting. It is preferable to collect urine that has been in the bladder for at least 2 hours to evaluate the degree of bacteriuria. Dilute urine will have a lower population of bacteria than will urine that has remained in the bladder for several hours. Urine for culture can be refrigerated for several hours without altering the validity of the results.

Because the mere presence of bacteria in the urine is not sufficient evidence to establish a diagnosis, quantitation becomes a very important part of the procedure. Quantitation is accomplished by plating approximately 0.1 ml of urine. After 24 hours, a colony count can be made. A colony count of less than 10,000 viable bacterial units/ml is insignificant. Counts greater than 100,000 colonies/ml indicate the presence of infection, whereas counts between 10,000 and 100,000 are questionable and must be repeated with a fresh specimen. Such counts obtained repeatedly usually reflect persistent, chronic, or suppressed infection; if found only once, they usually indicate contamination. Negative cultures in the presence of clinical signs of urinary tract infection may occur with anaerobic infections or some obstruction. It should be noted that specimens obtained from the ureters or the renal pelvis may culture fewer colonies because bacteria multiply while urine is being held in the bladder. When a significant number of colonies are cultured, a sensitivity is performed to determine the appropriate antibiotic therapy.

Throat smears. Cultures of the throat are most reliable if inoculated promptly after collection. The throat swab must be taken from each tonsillar area before a swab is taken from the posterior pharynx.

Microscopic examination of throat smears is of no value in streptococcal infections because normal throat flora are predominantly streptococcal. Throat smears can, however, be helpful in fusospirochetal disease and diptheria.

Wound specimens. In closed wounds or undrained abscesses, the pus often contains only one group of organisms, most commonly staphylococci, streptococci, anaerobes, or coliforms. This is also true of bone and joint infections. However, a multitude of organisms can be found in open, draining wounds, often making a definitive diagnosis difficult. When deep suppurative wounds drain onto exterior surfaces through a sinus or fistula, care must be taken to avoid mistaking the flora of the surface drainage for those of the deep lesion. The sterile swab used to obtain the specimen should be inserted deeply into the draining wound. Specimens are taken from the edge of a cellulitis in an effort to identify the etiologic organism. Both microscopic examination and cultures are used to identify the pathogen. Yeast or fungus can be seen microscopically in smears and scrapings from a suspicious lesion and can be grown in cultures. Viral antigens can sometimes be identified from surface lesions by the fluorescent antibody method. This method uses fluorescent dyes that bind to globulin molecules, making identification under the fluorescent microscope possible.

Microscopic studies of smears and cultures of specimens from wounds, bone and joint infections, and abscesses often assist in the identification of the offending organism or organisms and help in the choice of the appropriate antimicrobial drug.

Gastrointestinal specimens. Specimens from the gastrointestinal tract are relatively easy to obtain. Stool specimens and bile obtained from duodenal drainage can be examined microscopically and cultured. Although stained smears may reveal a prevalence of abnormal organisms, they cannot be used to differentiate enteric bacterial pathogens from normal flora. Repeated examinations with fresh specimens are needed to identify intestinal ova and parasites.

Routine selective and differential cultures are used for the separation of nonlactose-fermenting organisms from coliform bacteria. Blood is drawn concurrently for serologic diagnosis. Viral organisms are isolated from fecal specimens and accompanied by serum specimens, using very specialized techniques beyond the scope of this text.

Skin tests

The intracutaneous introduction of an antigenic stimulus from an infectious agent can elicit a hypersensitive skin reaction, manifested as induration with or without erythema. A positive skin reaction indicates that the patient, at some time in the past, has been exposed to the agent. Only when conversion from a negative to a positive test occurs during or just preceding the current illness can the infection be considered current. Skin reactivity diminishes significantly during very advanced stages of many infectious diseases; this is called *anergy*. Skin reactivity is also reduced if the patient is being treated with corticosteroids or other immunosuppressive drugs. Anergy may also be encountered in malnutrition or in the presence of certain other diseases (measles, chicken pox, sarcoidosis, Hodgkin's disease, uremia, and other advanced neoplasms).

Skin testing does not use pure antigens but rather introduces a mixture of potentially reactive substances. Consequently, both immediate and delayed reactions can occur; the latter become most significant in establishing the diagnosis of an infection.

The interpretation of a skin test takes place 48 hours after the intracutaneous injection of the antigenic material. Readings may also be taken at 24 and 72 hours, but those taken at 48 hours are usually most significant. Induration size is the factor to be considered in making a reading. Erythema alone is insignificant. Erroneous interpretations can be made if some of the test volume is injected subcutaneously or leaks onto the skin surface. The injection should raise a well-circumscribed bleb for the most accurate result. Tests should be repeated when several strengths of the antigenic preparation are available and the initial test was negative. In such instances, the smallest concentration of the test preparation should be applied first and then followed with increasingly higher concentrations if preceding tests remain negative. Antigenic preparations most frequently used include tests for histoplasmosis and tuberculosis.

Serologic tests

Some infectious diseases are accompanied by serologic responses that demonstrate a significant increase in antibody levels specifically directed toward a given microorganism.[4,39] Because the serologic demonstration of an antibody can reflect exposure in the recent past, as well as the present, a rise in the antibody level in the second of two specimens, obtained 10 to 20 days apart, is necessary to establish a diagnosis of a current infection. Both specimens must be examined at the same time for meaningful results. Specimens must be obtained via venipuncture or (in rare instances) arterial puncture, using strict asepsis. Antibody titers are most often obtained in mycoplasmal pneumonia, histoplasmosis, infectious mononucleosis, parasitic disorders, staphylococcal infections, and streptococcal infections. Viral infections can be identified in a similar manner, but it is important to realize that some viruses persist in their hosts for long periods of time.

Roentgenographic studies

Roentgenographic studies enjoy limited use in the diagnosis of an infectious disease.[21,24] Their value lies in the identification of malignancy-induced fevers.

The chest roentgenogram is useful but of questionable value in the early detection of a chest infection because some patients with acute disease have a normal chest film. In addition, because the severity of many conditions necessitates the use of portable equipment, the clarity of the film is often compromised. Careful review of the normal chest roentgenogram may facilitate or augment the diagnosis. Some of the abnormal signs that may be visible include the silhouette sign, the air bronchogram sign, and Kerley-B lines. They are often found with areas of consolidation manifested by areas of whiteness resulting from increased density.

The silhouette sign occurs when there is a loss of contrast between two adjacent structures and indicates that the densities of the structures have become the same. The silhouette sign is helpful in the localization of processes that increase the water content of the lungs, such as happens with pneumonia and in the presence of pulmonary infiltrates. When conditions such as these occur, the areas involved are not clearly defined. For example, anterior upper or middle lobe disease is manifested by loss of the cardiac silhouette. A shadow that overlaps a border but fails to obliterate the silhouette suggests that the problem involves the posterior lower lobes, the

posterior mediastinum, or the posterior pleural cavity.

Conditions that make the lung tissue more water dense create the air bronchogram sign. The air bronchogram sign occurs when the lungs are filled with secretions. Because air density is darker than water density, the bronchi are easily visualized unless they are also filled with secretions or are destroyed. The appearance of the air bronchogram sign verifies the presence of an intrapulmonary disorder. An air bronchogram sign cannot be seen in areas that do not have bronchi.

Kerley-B lines are believed to represent fluid in or thickening of the interlobular septa and appear as short, linear shadows perpendicular to the pleural surface.

Ultrasound tomography

Ultrasonography or computerized tomography can be used in febrile patients to demonstrate the presence or absence of an abscess.[62] When an abscess is identified, these studies provide valuable information about the relationship between the abscess and the surrounding viscera. The studies are indicated when symptoms or physical findings are localized to a particular area. In the absence of localizing symptomatology, radionuclide scanning using gallium-67 is the procedure of choice. The injected radionuclide binds to iron-binding proteins, which are in turn bound to local inflammatory cells. Gallium-67 may accumulate in the normal liver and in the skeleton, but the density of this substance at the site of infections of the liver or bone is much greater than in uninvolved areas. When there is a question, the gallium-67 scan can be correlated with another radionuclide scan of the liver or bone to facilitate a diagnosis.

ALTERATIONS

Under normal conditions, the set point and the actual body temperature are essentially the same, approximately 37° C (98.6° F).[35,64] This is referred to as *normothermia*. To maintain this constant level, the temperature-regulating center responds to ambient or internal temperature increases or decreases, processes the information, and makes the appropriate response. Thermoregulatory mechanisms are not always successful. Alterations in body temperature are classified as hyperthermia, fever, and hypothermia.

Malignant hyperthermia

Malignant hyperthermia is a rare,[40] sudden dysfunction of muscle metabolism precipitated by general anesthesia or muscle relaxants.[5-7,16,25] It is characterized by a rapid increase in muscle metabolism that is thought to be caused by an elevation in the myoplasmic calcium concentration.[16] Glycogenolysis ensues, with the production of lactic acid, carbon dioxide, and heat. Some of the lactate that is absorbed by the liver is metabolized to glucose, but the majority is converted to carbon dioxide, water, and heat. Oxidative phosphorylation is uncoupled by the increase in calcium that proves toxic to the mitochondria.[25] As a result, ATP production decreases, whereas lactic acid, carbon dioxide, and heat increase. The body cannot handle the great amount of heat produced, and hyperthermia and heat stroke ensue. Heat dissipation is also prevented by a peripheral vasoconstriction that is thought to occur.[25,54]

An underlying inborn error of muscle metabolism has been found in patients who experience malignant hyperthermia. This dysfunction is thought to be transmitted as an autosomal dominant trait.[25]

The drugs thought to precipitate this catastrophic event include most general anesthetics, succinylcholine, gallamine, cardiac glycosides, calcium salts, and caffeine.[15,25]

Fever (hyperpyrexia)

Fever develops when an individual attempts to regulate his body temperature at a higher level.[2,33,46] With fever, a person's heat production is accelerated, while at the same time heat loss is diminished. The set point is elevated and activates thermoregulatory mechanisms that evoke a thermogenic response (such as peripheral vasoconstriction or shivering).[3,6] This is called the *chill phase* and is characterized by rapid heat production. During this phase, there is an approximate 10% increase in heat production for every 1-degree rise in body temperature. Heat production decreases once the new set point is reached. At this equilibration point, heat production once again equals heat loss. This phase is referred to as the *plateau phase* and can continue for a few hours or a few weeks, depending on the cause of the fever. The *defervescence phase* begins when the set point is lowered to its previously normal position.[28,46,62] Heat loss ensues so that this new set point can be reached. Thermolytic mechanisms such as vasodilation and sweating are activated. When the new set point is attained, heat production and heat loss become equal once again, and the body temperature stabilizes. The return of the preexisting set point may occur with correction of the underlying problem or as a result of the institution of adjunct pharmacologic therapy.

Fevers can result from bacterial or viral infections or from any other antigen-antibody reaction that causes moderate to severe inflammation.[43] Although the exact mechanism by which the set point is elevated remains unclear, it is believed that a variety of substances serve as activators for a sequence of events that lead to a fever.[6,46,62] In the process of phagocytizing these activators, which are also referred to as exogenous pyrogens, the host's leukocytes produce and release small-molecular-weight proteins identified as "leukocytic" or "endogenous" pyrogens. These endogenous pyrogens initiate several biochemical reactions in the brain of the host that elevate the set point.[3,6,62,64]

One of the most common substances known to initiate the febrile pathway is a component of the cell wall of Gram-negative bacteria known as an *endotoxin*.[6,63] Endotoxins, in addition to causing fever, have other effects on their host, including a reduction in the number of circulating white blood cells (leukopenia) followed by the production of new white blood cells (leukocytosis), protection against the effects of irradiation, mobilization of interferon, enhancement of nonspecific immunologic resistance, a reduction in serum iron levels, and a lowering of the blood pressure. Endotoxins contain several components, with a lipopolysaccharide portion considered to be the most instrumental in the initiation of the physiologic events attributable to endotoxins. More specifically, the lipopolysaccharides are comprised of three regions: two polysaccharides and a lipid called lipid A. Studies reveal that lipid A is responsible for many of the effects of endotoxins.

Phagocytosis of the lipid A component of the cell wall, whether the bacteria are dead or alive, results in the release of endogenous pyrogens. These endogenous pyrogens produce a fever within 1 hour after inoculation. The magnitude and duration of the fever are diminished with repeated inoculation of the endotoxin.[63]

Gram-positive bacteria are also srongly pyrogenic, although they are not believed to contain endotoxins. As with endotoxin-induced fevers, Gram-positive fevers are believed to be triggered by the production of endogenous pyrogens. The onset of fever occurs within several hours after inoculation. Studies have shown that repeated inoculation with Gram-positive organisms does not diminish the febrile response, as is characteristic with Gram-negative bacteria.[63]

Viruses are also thought to induce fevers via the production of endogenous pyrogens that are indistinguishable from bacterially induced endogenous pyrogens. The latency period with viruses is several hours. Virally induced fevers are associated with a decrease in the circulating lymphocytes, as opposed to the decreasing granulocytes associated with bacterially induced fevers. Tolerance to viruses occurs rapidly.[63]

Hypersensitivity-induced fevers operate via the production of endogenous pyrogens through one of two routes, both of which involve antigen-antibody reactions.[63] An antigen is defined as any substance that elicits the production of antibodies. Antibodies are specialized proteins that are synthesized in response to the contact of specialized white cells, or lympho-

cytes, with these antigens. Some of the thymus-independent lymphocytes, or B-cell* lymphocytes, secrete antibodies known as gamma globulins, or immunoglobulins, that form the basis for humoral immunity. Another group of lymphocytes, the thymus-dependent lymphocytes (or T-cell lymphocytes), are responsible for cell-mediated immunity and have antibody-like cells on their surface. Following an initial contact, an organism produces antibodies of sensitized lymphocytes specific for that antigen. The individual is then said to be sensitized. In humoral immunity, a second exposure to these antigens results in rapid antibody production. In cell-mediated immunity, lymphocytes are already sensitized. In either situation, the following events can occur: a series of reactions triggered when specific antibodies come in contact with specific antigens can result in an enhancement of the inflammatory response leading to phagocytosis of the antigens, direct killing of microorganisms without prior phagocytosis, or neutralization of bacterial toxins and viruses.

The hypensensitivity-induced fever may be the result of the reaction of antigens with circulating antibodies in the previously sensitized organism or may be caused by all mediated processes, the latter being called *delayed hypersensitivity*. The exact mechanism by which both of these hypersensitivity-induced fevers produce endogenous pyrogens is unclear, although in delayed hypersensitivity it has been suggested that a nonpyrogenic intermediate called *lymphokine* is produced when specific antigens come in contact with certain cell-bound antibodies. This lymphokine induces endogenous pyrogen production from special types of effector cells, resulting in a fever.

Fever may also be a symptom of many types of malignancies. Although the specific activator for a tumor-induced fever is still unknown, endogenous pyrogen has been demonstrated.[6] Sev-

---

*B-cell lymphocytes were first detected in the bursa of Fabricius in chickens. Although there is no similar structure in humans, it is believed that lymphoid tissue in the tonsils, Peyer's patches of the intestine, and the appendix are equivalent sites.

eral hypotheses have been suggested to explain these fevers; some of them may be attributed to secondary bacterial or viral infections. However, because some others occur without identifiable infectious agents, other explanations are needed. It has been postulated that some of these tumor-induced fevers are the result of a toxin produced by the tumor, of tissue necrosis with the release of some pyrogenic materials, or of an undiagnosed infection.[6]

As is evident, all activators of fevers appear to trigger the formation of endogenous pyrogens.[43] Activation of leukocytes initiates the production of an endogenous pyrogen precursor, which is subsequently converted to the active form of endogenous pyrogen that is secreted by the leukocytes.

Endogenous pyrogens act directly on sites within the brain, entering directly from the bloodstream. The areas most sensitive to endogenous pyrogens seem to be the preoptic area and the anterior hypothalamus. Although it is somewhat less sensitive to endogenous pyrogen, the brainstem is also affected. The posterior hypothalamus appears to be insensitive. The exact mechanism by which endogenous pyrogens alter the set point remains a matter of speculation. Fig. 8-9 describes the process by which this is thought to occur.

Recently a group of fatty acids called prostaglandins have been implicated in febrogenesis.[6,42] Prostaglandins are present in brain tissue and other tissues and are released in response to many different kinds of insults to the body. Some studies have proposed that prostaglandins serve as intermediaries between endogenous proteins and the raised set point. Others have suggested that a breakdown product of the pre-

---

Fig. 8-9. Proposed mechanism for the increase of thermoregulatory set point and elevation of body temperature. The intermediates between endogenous pyrogen and the thermoregulatory set point are the subject of investigation. Intermediaries being studied include the extracellular ratios of Na^+ to Ca^{2+} as well as hormones and neurotransmitters such as cyclic AMP, norepinephrine, and dopamine.

Adapted from Kluger, M.J.: Is fever a nonspecific host defense response? In Powand, M.C., and Canonico, P.G.: Infection: the physiologic and metabolic response of the host, New York, 1981, Holland Biomedical Press.

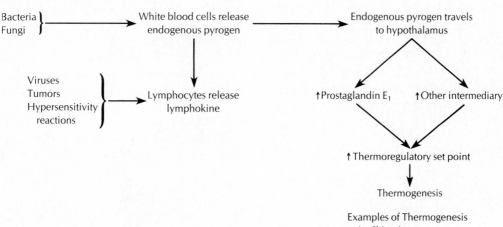

FEVER ACTIVATORS OR INDUCERS

cursor of prostaglandins, arachidonic acid, leads to the production of two pyrogenic substances, endoperoxide or thromboxanes, and that either may be responsible for the development of a fever.[42] A generally accepted point is that prostaglandins mediate pyrogen-induced fevers but that their role in naturally occurring fevers is questionable.[6] Clearly, more work must be done before the exact role of prostaglandins in febrogenesis can be determined.

Various cations such as sodium and calcium also affect body temperature. Initial studies suggested that these ions might play a part in the adjustment of the set point by stimulating warm-sensitive neurons.[6] Although this has yet to be proven, it is generally accepted that the ratio of these two ions, not the absolute values of each, can alter the temperature.[6,42] When sodium to calcium ratios are increased, shivering and peripheral vasoconstriction occur and the temperature increases. The ratio changes necessary to produce these alterations are well above normal physiologic levels. This may be because the warm-sensitive neurons described above are not located near the ventricles of the brain, and changing the CSF levels of sodium and calcium might only slightly raise the cation levels near the neurons.

Hypothermia

Hypothermia is defined as a lowering of the body temperature to below 35° C (95° F).[49] It can be induced by surface cooling or bloodstream cooling or can be attributed to anesthesia, especially in conjunction with the use of barbiturates. Surface cooling occurs when the environmental temperature is drastically lowered or the body is unprotected and subjected to prolonged exposure.* Bloodstream cooling requires intravascular techniques and cools the core first, thereby reducing the gradients; it is used principally in major surgeries, such as open-heart procedures. Barbiturate anesthesia depresses heat production.

Regardless of cause, hypothermia occurs only when heat loss exceeds heat production. Heat loss can occur as heat is transferred from the body to a colder medium or when heat production is reduced.

When a person is subjected to prolonged exposure, the superficial skin temperature drops as heat is transferred. Superficial skin sensors alert the anterior hypothalamus, which activates thermogenic mechanisms. Skin vessels constrict secondary to sympathetic stimulation. This decreases blood flow to the periphery, thereby reducing heat loss. At the same time, vessels in the intermediate zone dilate to increase the flow of blood and oxygen to the muscles. Shivering begins as the body attempts to compensate for the heat loss by producing more heat. During this time, an increase in the heart rate is also noted; this is necessary to ensure an adequate blood flow. The thyroid gland and the adrenals are also activated to increase metabolic activity and the rate of glycogenolysis. After a short period of time, peripheral vasoconstriction is replaced by peripheral vasodilation, and the cold skin is flooded with warmed blood. The heat of this blood is lost to the cold skin, resulting in the return of cold blood to the core. The process continues, with heat being given up by the core to the cold blood. Cold exhaustion ensues as the core temperature falls.

Although the principles of heat exchange remain similar, bloodstream cooling is actually the reverse of surface cooling. The blood is cooled externally and returned to the core via intravascular cannulation. Gradients are set up, but in this case they proceed from the superficial zone inward. A steady state cannot be reached with this method unless it is combined with surface cooling techniques.

Accidental hypothermia in anesthesia is most often found in infants, apparently because of suppression of central mechanisms or the in-

---

*The amount of time that it takes for someone to become hypothermic depends on the surface area exposed and the degree of adipose tissue.

complete development of the thermoregulatory mechanisms. The most common example of the latter is the immaturity of the skeletal muscle and the consequent inability to produce enough heat when the body temperature falls.

The frequency of accidental hypothermia is difficult to predict. Certain individuals, however, are more prone to experience it. The elderly person in a poor state of health is certainly a likely candidate to develop hypothermia on exposure. The acutely intoxicated alcoholic exhibits an even greater risk because alcohol intoxication is associated with several factors that accelerate the reduction in body temperature. These factors include (1) peripheral vasodilation, causing an increased rate of heat loss; (2) depression of the heat production center; and (3) an alteration of the temperature coefficient of the blood, leading to more rapid cooling. Finally, the neonate, with an immature thermoregulation center, is at risk.

The physiologic effects of hypothermia, either accidental or induced, are widespread. Almost every system of the body is affected. In general, the greatest reduction in metabolic activities occurs between 37° and 30° C (98.6° and 86° F). Between 20° and 30° C (68° and 86° F), organ function decreases exponentially, whereas below 20° C (68° F), the decline levels out.

Circulation

The heat continues to be oxygenated throughout hypothermia, although myocardial oxygen uptake is reduced progressively as the temperature falls. This discrepancy is manifest in changes in the heart rate and in slower resting metabolism, which continue until the heart ceases beating at a body temperature of around 5° to 10° C (41° to 50° F).

Dysrhythmias are most common.[27] In the absence of underlying cardiovascular pathology, however, rhythm disorders are usually not manifest until the core temperature is 32° C (89.6° F) or below. Atrial fibrillation is usually the first dysrhythmia to develop and is most apt to appear at temperatures below 28° C (82.4° F).[51]

First-degree AV block often develops at around 25° C (77° F), especially in persons with preexisting pathology.[27] Ventricular ectopy is also fairly common; it can be seen at any time but is most frequent around 25° C (77° F) or below.[51] As the temperature continues to drop, ventricular fibrillation* and ventricular asystole usually develop. The former is most common around 28° C (82.4° F), whereas the latter occurs at 10° C (50° F) and below.

Changes in the electrocardiogram are also visible during hypothermia.[27,61] The PR interval increases progressively with the decreasing temperature. The QRS interval initially increases in amplitude around 30° C (86° F), declines at 25° C (77° F), and widens, becoming almost two times greater than normal at 29° C (84.2° F).[61] Below 26° C (78.8° F), the QT interval lengthens and the ST segment begins to elevate. T-wave changes are visible around 25° to 26° C (77° to 78.8° F).[37]

Both blood flow and cardiac efficiency are altered in the presence of hypothermia. Blood flow is generally decreased, with coronary flow being reduced less than elsewhere. The direct effect of cold causes the coronary arteries to dilate, thereby maintaining adequate circulation. Myocardial contractility is enhanced with temperatures of around 32° C (89.6° F) because of cold-precipitated bradycardia. However, even with increased contractile effort, stroke volume and cardiac output fall progressively.

Peripheral circulatory changes occur below 34° C (93.2° F). Initially, there is a rise in the arterial blood pressure to between 32° and 34° C (89.6° and 93.2° F). This response can be directly traced to the cold. As temperatures decrease, peripheral resistance increases, with changes most apparent in the pulmonary system. This is caused by the reduced blood flow, cold vasoconstriction, and increased viscosity of the blood. At about 28° C (82.4° F) the blood pressure returns

---

*The disturbance could be attributed to anoxia or reduced coronary perfusion but is most likely caused by the direct effects of cold or, in the case of elective hypothermia, by drugs, anesthesia, or manipulative surgery.

toward normal, and below 25° C (77° F) it begins to fall. The pulse pressure remains unchanged until the temperature decreases to below 28° C (82.4° F).

Changes in the peripheral venous system are less pronounced. The venous pressure is increased at first but ultimately returns to normal. It reaches a maximum peak at about 30° C (86° F). This elevation is caused by the direct effect of cold because blood flow is significantly reduced.

Cardiovascular reflexes are impaired below 28° C (82.4° F). Both carotid and aortic baroreceptors are depressed at around 28° C (82.4° F) and are absent at 20° C (68° F). This is because of diminished transmission at the ganglion. Vasomotor and venomotor reflexes are altered at 25° C (77° F) and totally abolished below 20° C (68° F). The latter can be traced to reduced catecholamine production or a restrictive effect.

Irregularities are also manifest in the blood during hypothermia.[16] These changes occur below 26° C (78.8° F) but are apparently reversible. Hematologic alterations include an increase in blood viscosity, an elevation in the hematocrit, leukopenia, and thrombocytopenia.[14] In addition to the direct effect of cold, sequestration (of the liver and spleen) and fluid shifts in and out of the cells have been implicated as probable causes of these aberrations. The function of the cardiovascular system generally returns to normal with rewarming.

Respiration

Changes in ventilation and perfusion are not consistent during hypothermia.[49] Initially, ventilation is depressed progressively, with falling temperatures. The respiratory rate is decreased to around 28° to 30° C (82.4° to 86° F). This can be attributed to decreasing metabolic requirements, the direct effect of cold on the central and peripheral reflexes, and structural effects. With continued falling temperatures, respiratory arrests usually occur between 16° and 20° C (60.8° and 68° F). However, other changes are noted if moderate temperatures are maintained. With prolongation of moderate hypothermia, ventila-

tory rates increase, returning to normal. The threshold to stimuli is restored, thereby reactivating central and peripheral reflex mechanisms.

Pulmonary blood flow is reduced during hypothermia in accordance with total flow. However, because resistance is increased in the smaller pulmonary vessels to a greater extent, the actual volume of blood in the lungs is increased. This can be explained in terms of depressed vasomotor tone, and it can be a serious problem if the pulmonary bed becomes more and more distended because perfusion would be so adversely affected by congestion.

Arterial blood gas and acid-base alterations are manifest below 28° C (82.4° F).[49] An acidosis invariably develops as ventilation decreases and may, according to studies, persist even after rewarming. Its persistence can be attributed to inadequate tissue perfusion, leading to hypoxia and lactic acid accumulation. Respiratory acidosis is coupled with a nonrespiratory (metabolic) acidosis, with prolonged hypothermia and temperatures below 25° C (77° F).

The oxygen dissociation curve shifts to the left as hypothermia becomes progressively deeper. As a result, oxygen is not released by the hemoglobin to the tissues. Under ordinary conditions this would lead to hypoxia, but with reduced metabolic needs it is not a problem.

Central nervous system

The effects of hypothermia on the central nervous system depend on the degree of cooling. The sensorium is depressed below 33° C (91.4° F) with further reduction at 30° C (86° F) and marked changes noted at 25° C (77° F). Reflexes (both sensory and motor), on the other hand, are increased at 34° C (93.2° F) and depressed below 30° C (86° F). Chemoreceptor activity changes between 21° and 25° C (69.8° and 77° F). Hypoxic reflexes are altered below 21° C (69.8° F), whereas hypercarbic reflex mechanisms are present until 25° C (77° F). Neuromuscular activity is normal until 25° C (77° F). All central nervous systems alterations return to normal with rewarming.[20]

Kidneys

The kidneys exhibit a highly developed system of autoregulation, designed to maintain homeostasis even in the face of adversity; their response to hypothermia is quite remarkable. When body temperature is reduced, blood flow to the kidney is only somewhat diminished, being exceeded primarily by coronary flow. The glomerular filtration rate is decreased, but the filtration fraction remains constant unless plasma flow is greatly altered. This serves to keep the electrolytic composition of the blood within normal limits. When there is a significant reduction in plasma flow (30° to 32° C, or 86° to 89.6° F), however, renal function does become depressed. The damage that occurs, however, is not always totally irreversible. Rewarming results in the return of approximately 75% of normal function. Complete recovery may take up to 24 hours, if it occurs at all.

Urine output can increase during hypothermia because of the presence of an isosmotic diuresis. Sodium and chloride are excreted because of tubular depression, resulting in reduced water reabsorption, or a "cold diuresis." Potassium excretion is also reduced. Therefore there is an increase in intracellular potassium and a decrease in the serum potassium. These changes may be the cause of some of the ventricular ectopy noted earlier.

The depressed tubules are unable to handle glucose very efficiently. Glycosuria increases as the temperature decreases. With a reduction in the glomerular filtration rate and decreased utilization, hyperglycemia can be a problem. However, because reabsorption is more often depressed to a greater degree, glucose may be lost at an alarming rate, and replacement may even be necessary.

Alimentation

Gastrointestinal function is depressed progressively as the temperature falls. Blood flow in the stomach is decreased but not significantly so until 10° C (50° F). Peristalsis is reduced at 34° C (93.2° F) and can result in a paralytic ileus. Blood flow to the liver also decreases with hypothermia in a characteristic linear fashion, but the rate of decline is still less than for other organs. The most significant effect is a reduction in the detoxifying and conjugating activities of the liver. As a result, the half-life of drugs normally broken down in the liver is increased. Pancreatic secretions are reduced early when body temperature falls and are totally absent at 28° C (82.4° F). Synthesis continues, however, so that on rewarming, pancreatic activity flourishes.

Endocrine system

Because cold is in itself a stress stimulus, the body's immediate reaction to cold surface temperatures is to increase the production of catecholamines, glucocorticoids, and thyroxine, releasing these hormones into the bloodstream in large quantities. If these thermoregulatory efforts fail, the core temperature subsequently falls as thermoregulation is depressed. A depressed thermoregulatory set point serves to ameliorate the stress response and gives rise to a different endocrine response, the same response that occurs initially with bloodstream cooling. With anesthesia, the response depends on the specific anesthetic agent.

Hormonal secretion usually decreases and in some cases may be markedly suppressed or, at very low temperatures, may even be inactivated. Adrenal, cortical, and medullary activities are affected. For example, the adrenal-cortical response is absent in the presence of hypothermia and barbiturate anesthesia, unaltered with ether, and progressively depressed with other agents. In general, both cortical and medullary activity is repressed at approximately 30° C to 32° C (86° to 89.6° F) and inactivated at 20° C (68° F). Thyroxine production and release are also decreased. In the pancreas, endogenous insulin production is reduced. At the same time, the action of exogenous insulin is significantly retarded.[15] In addition, in the pituitary gland ACTH, TSH, and ADH are all reduced.

The systemic effects of altered or absent hormonal production and release are varied. As an example, during hypothermia the metabolic role of norepinephrine becomes more important than that of epinephrine. At 30° C (86° F), the pressor effect of norepinephrine is diminished, whereas at 20° C (68° F), it disappears. Therefore the hypothermic heart becomes unusually sensitive to epinephrine. Its positive inotropic effect is enhanced, easily inducing ventricular fibrillation. Reduced TSH and thyroxine are not as significant because energy requirements are also decreased with hypothermia, but the hypothermic effect on endogenous and exogenous insulin activity may lead to hyperglycemia.[15] ADH reduction leads to a hypothermic diuresis, the effects of which have already been described in Unit 5.

During rewarming, endocrine function usually returns to normal. In some instances there may be an exaggerated response to exogenous agents, but this reaction is most often transient.

In summary, there are many complications from accidental or induced hypothermia. Superficial tissue damage can occur secondary to prolonged exposure. Fat necrosis can develop, resulting from the hypothermia itself. Inadequate perfusion can lead to hypoxia, which may result in brain damage. Cardiac dysrhythmias have been reported and can be attributed to the direct effect of cold and hypoxia.

INTERVENTIONS

Thermoregulatory alterations may be treated symptomatically or by correcting the underlying cause. In many situations, palliative therapy is begun before a definitive diagnosis can be established. Treatment of hyperthermic and febrile states in critically ill people must be more vigorous and more sustained than in less severely ill patients. However, care must be taken to avoid inadvertently lowering the body temperature below normal. The euthermic state is preferred except in some instances in which therapeutic hypothermia is desired to prevent brain damage during hypoperfusion or brain edema.[59]

Palliative therapy

Palliative therapy for fever frequently consists of external cooling, in addition to the use of antipyretic drugs.[19] In patients with impaired heat loss (hyperthermia), external cooling is mandatory.

External cooling

External cooling alone is usually of little value in the management of fever because the body will continue to try to maintain a temperature that is congruent with the elevated set point. In situations in which antipyretic drugs are contraindicated, however, external cooling is the treatment of choice.[45]

Tepid and cool water baths and cooling mattresses or blankets can be used to promote external cooling. Ice baths are rarely indicated in the treatment of fever but constitute the intervention of choice for malignant hyperthermia and heat stroke. Alcohol sponging is not advisable, especially for infants and young children, who often dislike the odor and the sensation of cold that alcohol imparts to the skin.[58] In addition, there are documented reports of coma in children following sponging with isopropyl alcohol, probably secondary to fumes absorbed via the lungs.[58]

Both tepid and cool water baths reduce body temperature by conduction. Tepid baths maintain a constant water temperature of 32.2° C (90° F), whereas cool water baths begin at 32.2° C (90° F) and are gradually lowered to 18.3° C (65° F) during the course of therapy by adding ice chips. The use of ice tends to induce shivering and peripheral vasoconstriction, which lead to increased heat production and offset some of the benefits of the procedure.

Soaked washcloths should be applied first to the face and then to alternating portions of the body surface, from the shoulders to the knees. Sponging is more effective than submergence because evaporation from exposed areas hastens cooling.[58] If a tub is used, it should only be filled with a few inches of water. Vigorous rubbing is containdicated because it will encourage vaso-dilation.

Cool applications must be continued for at least 30 minutes to prevent the production of heat in response to short periods of cooling. A fan can be employed to increase surface cooling by evaporation. Body temperature should be checked every 10 to 15 minutes to evaluate the effectiveness of treatment.

The cooling mattress or cooling blanket provides a convenient and efficient means for lowering body temperature.[46] It is, however, less efficient than the ice bath or packing in ice, contraindicating it as the initial therapy for malignant hyperthermia or heat stroke. It is used in the treatment of the patient with sustained hyperpyrexia or with hyperthermia secondary to neurologic impairment. When implemented, it permits accurate titration of the body temperature.

The cooling apparatus consists of a fluid-filled mattress and a control unit. The fluid in the control unit is cooled to the desired temperature and circulated through the coils in the mattress. The patient is placed in a supine position on the mattress and may either be naked or covered with a thin gown. Only a sheet should be used to protect the mattress. A thin layer of an oil lubricant must be applied to patients' skin to prevent thermal burns if they are to be positioned in direct contact with the mattress. The mattress should never be folded because this causes rewarming. The mattress should be removed once the desired temperature is attained to avoid overcooling.

The time required to attain the desired temperature varies according to the technique used and the age and size of the patient. Infants and children are cooled more rapidly than adults are. Cooling should proceed so that the temperature drop is no greater than approximately 1° C (2° F) every 15 minutes to avoid ventricular ectopy. During cooling, shivering must be controlled to prevent increased heat production. Drugs used most commonly to control shivering contain a mixture of meperidine (Demerol), prometh-azine (Phenergan), and chlorpromazine (Thorazine), given intravenously at 15- to 20-minute intervals.

Cold enemas also have sometimes been used to induce cooling in the past. Today, however, their indications are few and far between.[47] Cooling enemas are inappropriate for patients' hyperpyretic states but are of value on the rare occasion in malignant hypertension and heat stroke, when traditional modes of therapy fail. Electrolyte imbalance can occur if large volumes of enema fluid are used.

Refrigerated saline administered intravenously can also be used to lower body temperature. However, because cold saline is not readily available, an alternative is to place the intravenous tubing between the patient and the bottle in an ice-water solution. Cooled parenteral fluid should not be infused through a central line because of the effect of direct cooling on myocardial function. Caution is important because this therapy can cause cardiac dysrhythmias.

Some researchers have suggested the use of cooled peritoneal lavage or peritoneal dialysis in lowering body temperature, based on animal and human studies, respectively.[12] Another researcher has reported the use of sodium nitro-prusside to produce peripheral dilation, thereby exposing a greater portion of the patient's blood volume to either a cooling mattress or an ice bath.[41] In addition, others have described the institution of extracorporeal circulation (cardiopulmonary bypass) to reduce fever.[23,56,57] Currently, these approaches are rather untraditional and are used only when conventional therapy is ineffective.

Antipyretics

Antipyretics are pharmacologic agents that restore the normal hypothalamic set point when body temperature is elevated.[63] Restoration of the normal set point initiates a series of activities that will promote heat loss so that the temperature and set point will be congruent with each other. Mechanistically, these drugs appear to inhibit prostaglandin synthesis by blocking the enzyme prostaglandin synthetase* in the preoptic anterior hypothalamus.[17,44,46] Prostaglandins, as discussed previously, are thought to play a part in set point elevation in response to endogenous pyrogen. Because prostaglandins have no role in the regulation of normal body temperature, these antiprostaglandin drugs will have no effect in the absence of fever. They will not reduce body temperature below normal. A secondary mechanism, vasodilation, may also occur with antipyretic administration.

Controlled investigations have revealed no differences in antipyretic efficiency between acetylsalicylic acid (aspirin) and acetaminophen, the two most commonly used antipyretics. The effects of each are basically identical when compared milligram for milligram. An appreciable antipyretic effect is seen within 30 to 60 minutes after the administration of a therapeutic dose. A nadir effect is reached within 3 hours, with some antipyresis still found at 6 hours.

The antipyretic effect of these drugs is proportional to the dosage or blood level but only within a therapeutic range. Excessive administration in the case of acetylsalicylic acid has been associated with hyperpyrexia.[18] There is some evidence that the effects of these two drugs may be additive. When acetylsalicylic acid and acetaminophen are administered together, there appears to be a greater reduction in temperature and an increased duration of antipyresis.

Antipyretic therapy is prescribed in pediatrics on the basis of age, although a weight-based dosage schedule is also published. Acetylsalicylic acid and acetaminophen should be used with caution in neonates and young infants because the half-life of each drug is prolonged during that time.

Both of the described antipyretic agents are almost completely absorbed from the gastrointestinal tract. They are metabolized in the liver to some degree. Acetaminophen is almost completely metabolized by hepatic tissue, whereas acetylsalicylic acid, in contrast, is broken down in the liver (rate limited) and excreted by the kidneys in amounts dependent on the pH. High urine flow and alkaline urine result in an increased salicylate elimination. Therefore patients with an alkaline pH may require more salicylates to achieve a therapeutic level.

The toxic effects of salicylates and acetaminophen differ. A complex acid-base disturbance is notorious with aspirin toxicity.[18,60] It appears as a mixed respiratory alkalosis and nonrespiratory (metabolic) acidosis. The respiratory alkalosis occurs because of a direct effect of salicylates on the central nervous system and as a secondary response to the metabolic acidosis. The primary respiratory alkalosis can be traced to the hyperventilatory effect of salicylates on the respiratory center. The secondary effect occurs as compensatory response. Respiratory alkalosis is more transient in infants under the age of 1 year.

Metabolic acidosis is produced by increased peripheral concentrations of lactic and pyruvic acid, which accumulate because the salicylates inhibit the Krebs cycle enzymes alpha-ketoglutaric dehydrogenase and succinic acid dehydrogenase. Acidosis also results from an increased lipid metabolism, which elevates the amount of ketone bodies. In addition, there is an inhibition of aminotransferases leading to aminoacidemia and aminoaciduria. All of these factors together produce a profound nonrespiratory acidosis.

Other metabolic changes also take place. Toxic levels of aspirin uncouple oxidative phosphorylation,[18,60] thereby increasing oxygen consumption and tissue glycolysis. This occurs in the muscle and in the brain and may lead to increased heat production and depleted glucose, the latter occurring in spite of normal serum glucose levels.

Dehydration can also be seen. Both sweating and insensible water loss occur with fevers. Hyperventilation leads to increased water loss from

---

*Salicylates also inhibit prostaglandin synthetase elsewhere in the body; therefore they are of value as generalized anti-inflammatory agents.

the respiratory tract, whereas aciduria and acidemia promote renal fluid loss. This fluid loss cannot always be replaced because many patients with salicylate intoxication are lethargic or even comatose. Many also vomit. Electrolyte imbalance is common, manifested as hyponatremia, hypernatremia, and/or hypokalemia.

Central nervous system dysfunction is also characteristic of salicylate intoxication. It is manifest as tinnitus, disorientation, hallucinations, irritability, lethargy, seizures, and coma and can be traced to the following respiratory and metabolic derangements: (1) direct effect of salicylates on brain cells; (2) acid-base imbalance; (3) electrolyte derangement; (4) systemic hypoglycemia; (5) depletion of brain glucose; and (6) cerebral arterial vasoconstriction secondary to decreased carbon dioxide.

Toxic signs are also manifest in the gastrointestinal tract.[60] Hemorrhagic gastritis can occur if aspirin penetrates the lipoproteins of the cells lining the stomach. This takes place because the cellular biochemistry is altered, permitting diffusion of hydrochloric acid into the gastric lining. The hydrochloric acid causes inflammation, erosion, and finally bleeding. Some studies have also exhibited damaged jejunal mucosa with salicylate intoxication.

Interference with prothrombin formation and platelet aggregation has been found during salicylate therapy.[18,60] The problem with prothrombin formation was associated with chronic high-dose therapy, whereas the thrombocytic disorder was reported with a regular dosage of only 5 grains of salicylate. Platelet dysfunction was traced to an inhibition of prostaglandin synthesis that resulted in the prevention of adenosine diphosphate (ADP) release. An increase in fibrolytic activity has also been documented.

Pulmonary edema may be seen in salicylate poisoning.[45] It occurs without generalized fluid retention and is thought to be noncardiac in origin, being caused by an increase in pulmonary capillary permeability. Aspirin intoxication has also precipitated asthmatic attacks. Broncho-

spasm is believed to be induced by the biochemical inhibition of the synthesis of prostaglandins in the E series.

Aspirin can depress renal function, especially in patients with kidney disease. A decrease in urine volume and an increase in tubular reabsorption of free water has been seen.[18] Also noted was a decrease in creatinine clearance and an elevation in the blood urea nitrogen.[60]

Although hepatic damage with aspirin is rare and apparently limited to patients with connective tissue disorders, a number of studies have attempted to link salicylates with Reye's syndrome. The American Academy of Pediatrics issued a statement in 1982 that suggested aspirin not be given to children with viral infections.

A depressed immunologic response has been documented with aspirin therapy.[60] At the time of this writing, the immunosuppressant effects of salicylates are still being investigated.

Acetaminophen and salicylate intoxication differ greatly, even in terms of dose relationships. Many of the side effects of aspirin therapy are visible with normal doses; however, acetaminophen toxicity is primarily limited to overdosage.

The primary effect of acetaminophen overdose is hepatic damage.[50,55] Hepatotoxicity is manifest in three stages, beginning with nausea, vomiting, pallor, and diaphoresis. During the second stage, no clinical symptoms are visible. Jaundice, coagulopathies, encephalopathy, and hepatic enzymatic elevation are characteristic of the final stage, which may culminate in death. Identification of acetaminophen toxicity is made difficult by the fact that serum concentrations decrease rapidly. Hepatic injury is caused by a toxic metabolite that binds to liver cells, leading to centrilobular necrosis. Children appear to be less susceptible to hepatic damage than do adolescents and adults.

Reports of acute tubular necrosis and myocardial damage have also been documented with acetaminophen overdose.[50,57] Associated ECG changes included ST segment abnormalities and flattening of the T wave. There has been a case of pancreatitis in an adult with acetaminophen poisoning, two reports of elevation in the serum amylase level, and a report of hypoglycemia. Postmortem examination has revealed pericarditis, myocardial necrosis, and subendocardial hemorrhage.

Hypothermic drugs

Hypothermic drugs such as phenobarbitol and alcohol are used on rare occasions to lower the body temperature. Their use is limited to malignant hyperthermia and severe heat stroke, as a possible ancillary measure.

Dantrolene sodium

Dantrolene sodium (Dantrium) is used in the prevention or treatment of malignant hyperthermia. It decreases mycoplasmic calcium concentrations and seems to terminate the basic disturbance. The safety of long-term use of this drug, which is associated with weight depression, hepatopathy, and nephropathy, has not been established.[67]

Corrective therapy

Corrective therapy is instituted to treat the underlying cause of fever and hyperthermia. This category of therapy includes a variety of regimens (such as antibiotics, antiviral agents, and antifungal drugs, the discussion of which is beyond the scope of this book.

Therapy for the hypothermic patient

The hypothermic patient presents a unique therapeutic challenge. Effective management of hypothermia requires both supportive measures and specific rewarming techniques. Rewarming interventions may be passive or active, the latter involving both external and internal procedures.

Supportive measures

Supportive therapy is essential to keep patients viable while they are being rewarmed. Electrocardiographic monitoring is implemented to aid in identification of dysrhythmias that may result directly from the decrease in body temperature (that is, atrial flutter or atrial fibrillation) or may be attributable to the hypoxia or metabolic acidosis that ensues (that is, ventricular ectopy). Vital signs must be carefully recorded, with documentation of core temperature made. A low-recording thermometer should be available to permit accurate measurments. Routine laboratory studies are needed for judicious management. Included in these tests are platelet counts and tests for a prothrombin time and fibrinogen levels (see Unit 7), as well as serum glucose, amylase, and renal function studies (see Units 5 and 6). Arterial blood gases that are obtained must be corrected to the body temperature for accurate interpretation because normal values are measured at 37° C (98.6° F). Oxygen support or mechanical ventilation are instituted as needed. Frequent tracheal aspiration may be necessary to remove secretions produced by the effect of cold on the tracheobronchial tree.

The replacement of fluids and electrolytes is necessary to correct the volume depletion frequently associated with profound hypothermia. Intravenous therapy is dictated by the presence of any preexisting diseases. An intravenous catheter should not be positioned in the heart because of myocardial irritability. A blood-warming coil maintained at 37° to 43° C (98.6° to 109.4° F) will enable the administration of warmed fluids.

Pharmacologic therapy is implemented with caution. Sodium bicarbonate may be used to correct nonrespiratory acidosis but should be instituted prudently to avoid overcorrection of the rapidly changing metabolic conditions. Insulin administration is infrequent because of the risk of postwarming hypoglycemia. Because drugs often have little effect at low temperatures, they are used on a limited basis. The hazards of overmedication are always present because of delayed metabolism.

ECG abnormalities are frequent. As mentioned, atrial flutter or atrial fibrillation can often be seen. Both abnormalities appear to convert as the patient is rewarmed. The presence of premature ventricular contractions has also been noted. Ventricular ectopy may be abolished with the correction of hypoxia or metabolic acidosis but may also require lidocaine. The hypothermic heart is unresponsive to atropine, pacing, and electrical countershock. CPR can be performed indefinitely until adequate rewarming occurs and other therapy can be instituted.

Rewarming techniques

Passive rewarming techniques are limited to situations that occur away from medical facilities. These techniques include removing the patient from the environmental exposure and applying some kind of insulating material (such as blankets). The goal of passive therapy is to maximize basal heat production.

Active rewarming methods constitute a controversial subject in the management of hypothermic patients. In the past there was a generalized acceptance of external rewarming techniques; however, great disagreement has developed about the appropriateness of most internal rewarming procedures.

Active external rewarming includes the use of electric warming blankets, heated objects, and immersion of the patient in a heated water bath. Currently there is some question about the advisability of surface rewarming because of the inherent physiologic changes that may aggravate the effect of hypothermia on the core. Some researchers have found that the "afterdrop" of core temperature following the removal of a chronic cold stressor may be exaggerated with surface rewarming. This is believed to be attributable to the peripheral vasodilation that occurs with external rewarming, which causes paradoxical central cooling by shunting stagnant cold blood to the core. The myocardium is chilled even more and consequently is more vulnerable to ventricular fibrillation. In addition, hypovolemic shock may be precipitated; this takes place in the vascularly depleted patient when the circulating blood volume is decreased secondary to peripheral vasodilation. Immersion is also being re-

evaluated because the water interferes with hemodynamic monitoring, and the movement may precipitate ventricular fibrillation. In addition, CPR would be hampered should it become necessary. Electric heating mattresses and blankets pose the threat of thermal burns in unprotected areas.

There is no unanimity in the choice of techniques employed in core rewarming. Current studies advocate the implementation of core rewarming for temperatures less than 32° C (89.6° F) to preclude the hazards of afterdrop, dysrhythmias, and rewarming shock. External rewarming is adequate when the previously described pathophysiologic changes have not had a chance to develop.

Some of the techniques for core rewarming include gastrointestinal irrigations, hemodialysis, peritoneal dialysis, extracorporeal blood warming, and inhalation warming.

Gastrointestinal irrigation is accomplished using either an intragastric balloon or high-colonic infusions. Although there is some risk of precipitating cardiac dysrhythmias associated with passage of the intragastric balloon (nasopharyngeal stimulation), both gastrointestinal irrigation procedures require little in the way of equipment and can rapidly be expedited.

Both hemodialysis and peritoneal dialysis have been safely employed in central rewarming. Hemodialysis provides a mechanism for drug clearance, as well as core rewarming. Peritoneal dialysis is fairly easy to carry out. A routine dialysis protocol is followed using a potassium-free dialysate, which is warmed by being run through a blood-warming coil immersed in warm water. The temperature of the dialysate should be approximately 43.3° C (110° F). This can be accomplished by maintaining the water bath at 54.4° C (130° F). Successful return to normothermia has been reported with six to eight rapidly performed exchanges (quick instillation and immediate removal).

Extracorporeal blood rewarming is carried out using an arteriovenous shunt inserted between the femoral artery and vein. Blood can be heated to 40° C (104° F) without hemolysis. The blood is interposed with a heat exchanger; this procedure has had some degree of success.

The most recent innovation in internal core rewarming advocates the inhalation of warmed oxygen. This method uses the large alveolar surface area and the properties of the trachea, which enable it to withstand temperatures of up to 57° C (134.6° F). Warmed, humidified oxygen can be administered via a face mask or endotracheal tube. The temperature of the inhalate must be monitored at the mouth and should be kept between 40.5° and 46.1° C (105° and 115° F).

In conclusion, better understanding of the pathophysiology of hypothermia have led to several treatment modalities. These modalities are still being evaluated to decide which of them are of most value and have the least associated risks.

REFERENCES

1. Arey, L.B.: Developmental anatomy, ed. 7, Philadelphia, 1974, W.B. Saunders Co.
2. Atkins, E.: Pathogenesis of fever, Physiological Review 40:580, 1960.
3. Atkins, E., and Bodel, P.: Fever, New England Journal of Medicine 286:27, 1972.
4. Baron, S., editor: Medical microbiology, Menlo Park, CA, 1982, Addison-Wesley.
5. Benzinger, T.H.: Heat regulation: homeostasis of central temperature, Physiological Review 49:671, 1969.
6. Bernheim, H.A., Block, L.H., et al: Fever: pathogenesis, pathophysiology and purpose, Annals of Internal Medicine 91:261, 1979.
7. Britt, B.A.: Etiology and pathophysiology of malignant hyperthermia, Federation Proceedings 38(1):44, 1979.
8. Brobeck, J.R.: Energy balance and food intake. In Mountcastle, V.B.: Medical physiology, ed. 14, St. Louis, 1980, The C.V. Mosby Co.
9. Brobeck, J.R., and DuBois, A.B.: Energy exchange. In Mountcastle, V.B.: Medical physiology, ed. 14, St. Louis, 1980, The C.V. Mosby Co.
10. Brooks, C.M., and Koizumi, K.: The hypothalamus and control of integrative processes. In Mountcastle, V.B.: Medical physiology, ed. 14, St. Louis, 1980, The C.V. Mosby Co.
11. Bruck, K.: Thermoregulation: control mechanisms and neural processes. In Sinclair, J.C.: Temperature regulation and energy metabolism in the newborn, New York, 1978, Grune and Stratton.
12. Bynum, G., Patton, J., et al.: Peritoneal lavage cooling in an anesthetized dog heatstroke model, Aviation, Space and Environmental Medicine 49(6):779, 1978.
13. Cabanac, M.: Temperature regulation, Annual Review of Physiology 37:415, 1975.
14. Chadd, M.A., and Gray, O.P.: Hypothermia and coagulation defects in the newborn, Archives of Disease in Childhood 47:819, 1972.
15. Curry, D.L., and Curry, K.P.: Hypothermia and insulin secretion, Endocrinology 87:750, 1970.
16. Denborousk, M.A.: Etiology and pathophysiology of malignant hyperthermia, International Anesthesiology Clinics 17(4):11, 1979.
17. Done, A.K.: Antipyretics, Pediatric Clinics of North America 19:167, 1972.
18. Done, A.K.: Aspirin overdosage: incidence, diagnosis, and management, Pediatrics 62(suppl.):890, 1978.
19. Done, A.K.: Treatment of fever in 1982: a review, American Journal of Medicine 74(6A):27, 1983.
20. Ehrmantraut, W.R., Ticktin, H.E., et al.: Cerebral hemodynamics and metabolism in accidental hypothermia, Archives of Internal Medicine 99:57, 1957.
21. Forrest, J.V., and Feigin, D.S.: Essentials of chest radiology, Philadelphia, 1982, W.B. Saunders Co.
22. Gale, C.C.: Neuroendocrine aspects of thermoregulation, Annual Review of Physiology 35:391, 1973.
23. Gjessing, J., Barsa, J., et al.: Possible means of rapid cooling in emergency treatment of malignant hyperthermia, British Journal of Anaesthesia 48:469, 1976.
24. Goodman, L.R., and Putman, C.E.: Intensive care radiology imaging of the critically ill, ed. 2, Philadelphia, 1983, W.B. Saunders Co.
25. Gordon, R.A.: International symposium on malignant hyperthermia, Springfield, IL, 1973, C.C. Thomas.
26. Gronert, G.A.: Malignant hyperthermia, Anesthesiology 53(5):395, 1980.
27. Gunton, R.W., Scott, J.W., et al.: Changes in cardiac rhythm and in the form of the electrocardiogram resulting from induced hypothermia in man, American Heart Journal 52:419, 1956.
28. Hardy, J.D.: Physiology of temperature regulation, Physiological Review 41:521, 1961.
29. Hardy, J.D.: Posterior hypothalamus and the regulation of body temperature, Federation Proceedings 32:1564, 1973.
30. Hardy, J.D.: Body temperature regulation. In Mountcastle, V.B.: Medical physiology, ed. 14, St. Louis, 1980, The C.V. Mosby Co.
31. Hardy, J.D., Gagge, A.P., et al.: Physiological and behavioral temperature regulation, Springfield, IL, 1970, C.C. Thomas.
32. Hart, F.D., editor: French's index of differential diagnosis, ed. 11, Chicago, 1979, Year Book Medical Publishers.

33. Hellon, R., and Townsend, Y.: Mechanisms of fever, Pharmacology and Therapeutics **19**(2):211, 1982.

34. Hemingway, A.: Shivering, Physiological Review **43**: 397, 1963.

35. Hensel, H.: Neural processes in thermoregulation, Physiological Review **53**:948, 1973.

36. Himms-Hagen, Jean: Cellular thermogenesis, Annual Review of Physiology **38**:315, 1976.

37. Houdas, Y., and Ring, E.F.J.: Human body temperature, its measurement and regulation, New York, 1982, Plenum Press.

38. Hull, D., and Smales, O.R.C.: Heat production in the newborn. In Sinclair, J.C., editor: Temperature regulation and energy metabolism in the newborn, New York, 1978, Grune and Stratton.

39. Jawetz, E., Melnick, J.L., et al.: Review of medical microbiology, ed. 14, Los Altos, CA, 1980, Lange Medical Publications.

40. Kalow, W., Britt, B.A., et al.: Epidemiology and inheritance of malignant hyperthermia, International Anesthesiology Clinics **17**(4):119, 1979.

41. Katlic, M.R., Ramos, L.G., et al.: Sodium nitroprusside in the treatment of extreme pyrexia, New England Journal of Medicine **299**:154, 1978.

42. Kauffman, R.E.: Fever. In Shirkey, H.C., editor: Pediatric therapy, ed. 6, St. Louis, 1980, The C.V. Mosby Co.

43. Kluger, M.J.: Temperature regulation, fever and disease, International Review of Physiology **20**:209, 1979.

44. Koch-Weser, J.: Acetaminophen, New England Journal of Medicine **295**:1297, 1976.

45. Lewis, F.J.: Treatment of fever with surface cooling, Surgical Clinics of North America **39**:177, 1959.

46. Lorin, M.I.: The febrile child: clinical management of fever and other types of pyrexia, New York, 1982, John Wiley & Sons.

47. Martin, D.W., et al.: Harper's review of biochemistry, ed. 19, Los Altos, CA, 1983, Lange Medical Publications.

48. Morehouse, L.E., and Miller, A.T.: Physiology of exercise, St. Louis, 1963, The C.V. Mosby Co.

49. Paton, B.C.: Accidental hypothermia, Pharmacology and Therapeutics **22**(3):331, 1983.

50. Piperno, E.: Pathophysiology of acetaminophen overdosage toxicity: implication for management, Pediatrics **62**(suppl.):880, 1978.

51. Reuler, J.B.: Hypothermia, pathophysiology, clinical settings, and management, Annals of Internal Medicine **89**(4):519, 1978.

52. Robertshaw, D., editor: Environmental physiology II, International Review of Physiology, vol. 15, Baltimore, 1977, University Park Press.

53. Robinson, S.: Physiology of muscular exercise. In Mountcastle, V.B.: Medical physiology, ed. 14, St. Louis, 1980, The C.V. Mosby Co.

54. Rodgers, I.R.: Malignant hyperthermia: a review of the literature, Mount Sinai Journal of Medicine **50**(1):95, 1983.

55. Rumack, B.H., and Matthew, H.: Acetaminophen poisoning and toxicity, Pediatrics **55**:871, 1975.

56. Ryan, J.F., Donlin, J.V., et al.: Cardiopulmonary bypass in the treatment of malignant hyperthermia, New England Journal of Medicine **290**:1121, 1974.

57. Smith, A.L.: The febrile infant, Pediatrics in Review **1**:35, 1979.

58. Steele, R.W., Tanka, P.T., et al.: Evaluation of sponging and of oral antipyretic therapy to reduce fever, Journal of Pediatrics **77**:824, 1970.

59. Stern, R.C.: Pathophysiologic basis for symptomatic treatment of fever, Pediatrics **59**:92, 1977.

60. Temple, A.R.: Pathophysiology of aspirin overdosage toxicity with implications for management, Pediatrics **62**(suppl.):873, 1978.

61. Trevino, A., Razi, B., et al.: The characteristic electrocardiogram of accidental hypothermia, Archives of Internal Medicine **127**:470, 1971.

62. Vickery, D.M., and Quinnell, R.K.: Fever of unknown origin, an algorithmic approach, Journal of the American Medical Association **238**:2183, 1974.

63. Villaverde, M.: Fever from symptom to treatment, New York, 1978, Van Nostrand Reinhold Co.

64. Werner, J.: The concept of regulation for human body temperature, Journal of Thermal Biology **5**:75, 1980.

65. Whittow, G.C.: Comparative physiology of thermoregulation, vol. II, New York, 1971, Academic Press.

66. Whittow, G.C.: Comparative physiology of thermoregulation, vol. III, New York, 1973, Academic Press.

67. Willner, J.: Malignant hyperthermia, Pediatric Annals **13**(2):128, 1984.

Appendix
Common Drug Interactions*

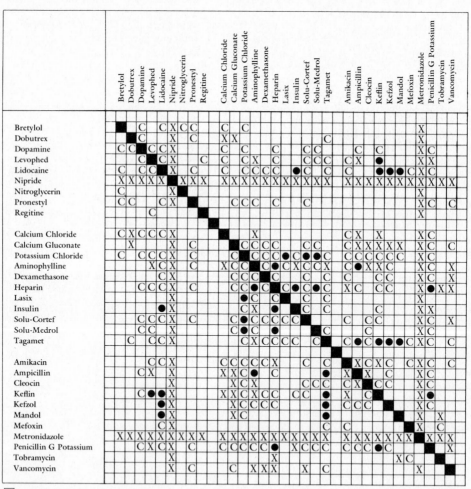

	Bretylol	Dobutrex	Dopamine	Levophed	Lidocaine	Nipride	Nitroglycerin	Pronestyl	Regitine	Calcium Chloride	Calcium Gluconate	Potassium Chloride	Aminophylline	Dexamethasone	Heparin	Lasix	Insulin	Solu-Cortef	Solu-Medrol	Tagamet	Amikacin	Ampicillin	Cleocin	Keflin	Kefzol	Mandol	Mefoxin	Metronidazole	Penicillin G Potassium	Tobramycin	Vancomycin
Bretylol	■	C		C	X	C	C			C		C																X			
Dobutrex	C	■	C		X		C			X	X									C								X			
Dopamine	C	C	■	C	C	X		C		C		C			C			C	C			C	C					X	C		
Levophed	C		C	■	X		C			C	C	C	C		C	X		C	C	C	X	X		●				X	X		
Lidocaine	C	C	C	X	■	C		C		C	C	C	C	C	●	C		C		C				●	●	●	C	X	C		
Nipride	X	X	X	X	X	■	X	X	X	X	X	X	X	X	X	X	X	X	X	X	X	X	X	X	X	X	X	X	X	X	X
Nitroglycerin	C	C		C		X	■																					X			
Pronestyl	C		C		C	X		■			C	C	C		C			C										X	C		C
Regitine			C			X			■																			X			
Calcium Chloride	C	X	C	C	C	X				■			X							C	X	X						X	C		
Calcium Gluconate		X		C	C	X		C			■	C	C	C	C			C	C		C	X	X	X	X	X		X	C		C
Potassium Chloride	C		C	C	C	X		C			C	■	C	C	C	●	●	●	C		C	C	C	C	C	C	C	X	C		
Aminophylline			X	C	X	X		C		X	C	C	■	C	●	C	X	C	C	X	C	●	X	X				X	C		X
Dexamethasone			C	X	C	X					C	C	C	■	C		C		C		C			C	C			X	C		X
Heparin			C	C	●	X		C			C	C	●	C	■	C	●	C	●	C	X	C		C	C			X	●	X	X
Lasix				X	C	X						●	C		C	■		C		C								X			
Insulin					●	X						●	X	C	●		■	C	C			C						X	X		
Solu-Cortef			C	C	C	X		C			C	●	C		C	C	C	■	C	C		C		C	C			X	C		X
Solu-Medrol			C	C		X					C	C	C	C	●		C	C	■			C			C			X	C		
Tagamet	C	C		C	C	X				C		C	X		C	C		C		■	C		C	●	C	●	●	●	C	X	C		C
Amikacin			C	X		X				C	C	C	C	X	X			C		C	■	X	C	X	C			C	X	C		C
Ampicillin		C	C	X		X				X	X	C	●		C		C			C	●	■	X		X			C			X	C
Cleocin				X		X					X	C	X							C	C	X	■	C	C				X	C		
Keflin		C	●	●	●	X					X	C	X	C	C			C		C	X		C	■					X		●
Kefzol			●		X	X					X	C		C	C			C	C		●	X	C		■	C	C	C			X	C
Mandol			●		X	X					X	C									●					■				X	X	
Mefoxin			C		X	X						C						C		C	C						■	C	X		
Metronidazole	X	X	X	X	X	X	X	X	X	X	X	X	X	X	X	X	X	X	X	X	X	X	X	X	X	X	X	■	X	X	X
Penicillin G Potassium		C	X	C	X	X		C		C	C	C	C	●		X	C	C	C		C	C	C	●	C			X	■		X
Tobramycin			X			X									X					C		X	C					X		■	
Vancomycin			X		C	X		C		C		X	X	X			X		C									X			■

C — Physically compatible.
X — Incompatible.
● — Conflicting reports of compatibility—call pharmacy for more information.
☐ — No information available—consider incompatible.

Courtesy St. Vincent Hospital and Health Care Center, Indianapolis, IN.

*Other reactions and interactions may occur that have not been noted. Pharmacologic textbooks should be consulted for further questions or more detailed information.

Index